Development
of the
Nervous System

Development of the Nervous System

DAN H. SANES

THOMAS A. REH

WILLIAM A. HARRIS

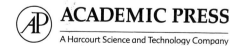

ACADEMIC PRESS
A Harcourt Science and Technology Company

San Diego   San Francisco   New York   Boston   London   Sydney   Tokyo

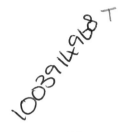

Cover photo: Courtesy of Dr. Chi-Bin Chien

This book is printed on acid-free paper.

Academic Press
A Harcourt Science and Technology Company
525 B Street, Suite 1900, San Diego, California 92101-4495, USA
http://www.academicpress.com

Academic Press
Harcourt Place, 32 Jamestown Road, London NW1 7BY, UK
http://www.hbuk.co.uk/ap/

Library of Congress Catalog Card Number: 00-101602

International Standard Book Number: 0-12-300330-X

PRINTED IN THE UNITED STATES OF AMERICA
03   04   05   CO   9   8   7   6   5   4   3   2

To our families

CONTENTS

CHAPTER 7 · · · · · · ·

Survival and Growth

CHAPTER 8 · · · · · · ·

Synapse Formation and Electric Function

CHAPTER 9
Refinement of Synaptic Connections

CHAPTER 10
Behavioral Development

Contents

PREFACE

The human brain is said to be the most complex object in our known universe, and the billions of cells and trillions of connections are truly wonders of enormous proportions. The study of the way that the cellular elements of the nervous system work to produce sensations, behaviors, and higher order mental processes has become a most productive area of science. However, neuroscientists have come to realize that they are studying a moving target: growth and change are integral to brain function and form the very basis by which we can learn anything about it. As the behavioral embryologist George Coghill pointed out, "Man is, indeed, a mechanism, but he is a mechanism which, within his limitations of life, sensitivity and growth, is creating and operating himself." To understand the brain, then, we need to understand how this mechanism arises and the ways in which it can change throughout a lifetime.

The construction of the brain is an integrated series of developmental steps, beginning with the decision of a few early embryonic cells to become neural progenitors. As connections form between nerve cells and their electrical properties emerge, the brain begins to process information and mediate behaviors. Some of the underlying circuitry is built into the nervous system during embryogenesis. However, interactions with the world continuously update and adapt the brain's functional architecture. The mechanisms by which these changes occur appear to be a continuation of the processes that sculpt the brain during development. Since the text covers each of these developmental steps, it is relatively broad in scope.

An understanding of the development of the nervous system has importance for biologists in a larger context. Studies of development have led to insights into the evolutionary relationships among organisms. The dogma of phylogeny and ontogeny of the last century has been superseded by a deeper understanding of the ways in which evolutionary change can be effected through changes in development. The brain is no exception to these rules. We should expect that insight into the evolution of that which makes us most human will be gained from an appreciation of how developmental processes are modified over time.

The goal of this text is to provide a contemporary overview of neural development for undergraduate students or those who have some background in the field of biology. This intent is not compatible with a comprehensive review of the literature. A recent MEDLINE search of publications in the field of neural development [(neural or neuron or nervous) and (development or embryology or maturation)] yielded 56,840 papers published between 1966 and 1999. We admit, up front, to having read only a fraction of these papers or of the thousands that were published before 1966. As a practical matter, we made use of authoritative books, contemporary review articles, hallway conversations, and e-mail consultations to select the experiments that are covered in our text. Even so, we expect that important contributions have been missed inadvertently. Therefore, advanced students will find themselves quickly turning to specialized texts and reviews. Another compromise that comes from writing an undergraduate biology book well after the onset of the revolution in molecular biology is that all subjects now have a rather broad cast of molecular characters. In addition, the most instructive experiments on a particular class of molecules have often been performed on nonneural tissue. Even if we chose to cover only the genes and proteins whose roles have been best characterized in the nervous system, most chapters would run the risk of sounding like a (long) list of acronyms. Therefore, we charted a compromise between the need to update students and our strong inclination to hold their attention. The book does not contain exhaustive lists of molecular families, and the most current review articles must serve as an appendix to our text.

Among the many scientists who helped us through discussions, unpublished findings, or editorial comment are (in alphabetical order) Chiye Aoki, Michael Bate, Olivia Bermingham-McDonogh, John Bixby, Sarah Bottjer, Martin Chalfie, Hollis Cline, Martha Constantine-Paton, Ralph Greenspan, Voker Hartenstein, Mary Beth Hatten, Christine Holt, Darcy Kelley, Chris Kintner, Sue McConnell, Ilona Miko, Ronald Oppenheim, Thomas Parks, David Raible, Henk Roelink, Edwin Rubel, John Rubenstein, David Ryugo, Nancy Sculerati, Carla Shatz, and Tim Tully.

Induction

Development and Evolution of Neurons

Even before metazoans arose on earth, single-celled eucaryotes and procaryotes had evolved mechanisms for responding to the environment. However, almost as early as multicellular animals evolved, neurons were part of their tissues. The forms of the metazoan nervous systems in the various phyla range in complexity from the nerve net of the jellyfish to the billions of specifically interconnected neuron assemblies of the human brain. Nevertheless, neurons and nervous systems of all multicellular animals share many common features. Voltage-gated ion channels are responsible for action potentials in the neurons of hydras, as they are in people. Synaptic transmission between neurons in nerve nets is basically the same as that in the cerebral cortex (Fig. 1.1). In this book, we describe the mechanisms responsible for the generation of these complex networks, highlighting examples from a variety of organisms when appropriate. In the past decade particularly, it has come to be realized that, despite the great diversity in the nervous systems of various organisms, the underlying principles of neural development have been maintained throughout evolution.

It is particularly appropriate to begin a book concerned with the development of the nervous system with an evolutionary perspective. The subjects of embryology and evolution have long shared an interrelated intellectual history. One of the major currents of late 19th century biology was that a description of the stages of development would provide the key to the path of evolution of life. *Ontogeny recapitulates phylogeny* was an important theory at the start of experimental embryology (Gould, 1970). Although careful study of embryos clearly showed that they did not resemble the adult forms of their ancestors, it was clear that new forms are built upon the structures of biological predecessors. One of the aims of this book is to show how an understanding of the development of the nervous system will give us insight into its evolution.

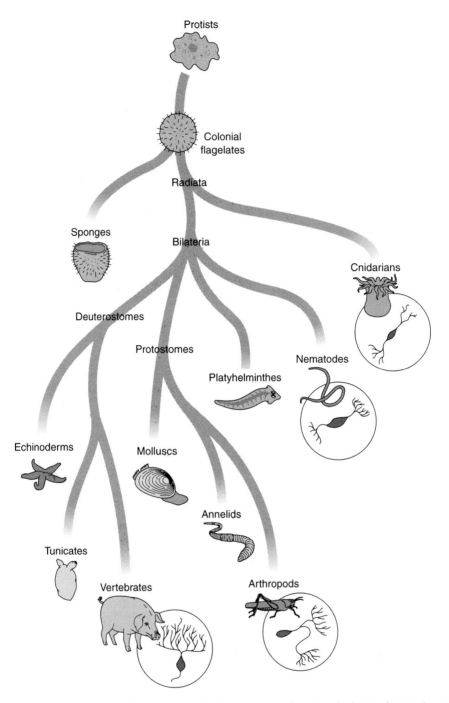

Figure 1.1   Neurons throughout the evolution of multicellular organisms have had many features in common. All animals other than colonial flagellates and sponges have recognizable neurons that are electrically excitable and have long processes. The Cnidarians have nerve networks with electrical synapses, but synaptic transmission between neurons is also very ancient.

It is also wise to remember, as pointed out by Dobzhansky (1951), that "nothing in biology makes sense except in the light of evolution."

Early Embryology of Metazoans

The development of multicellular organisms varies substantially across phyla; nevertheless, there are some common features. The cells of all metazoans are organized as layers. These layers give rise to the various organs and tissues, including the nervous system. These layers are generated from the egg cell through a series of cell divisions and their subsequent rearrangements (Fig. 1.2). The egg cells of animals are typically polarized, with an *animal pole* and a *vegetal pole*. This polarity is often visible in the egg cell since the vegetal pole contains the yolk, the stored nutrient material necessary for sustaining the embryo as it develops. Once fertilized by the sperm, the egg cell undergoes a series of rapid cell divisions, known as cleavages. There are many variations in cleavage patterns in embryos, but the end result is that a large collection of cells, the blastula, is generated over a relatively short period of time.

In many organisms the cells of the blastula are arranged as a hollow ball, with an inner cavity known as a blastocoel. Those cells at the vegetal pole will ultimately develop as the gut, while those at the animal pole will give rise to the epidermis and the nervous system. Cells in between the animal and vegetal poles will generate mesodermal derivatives, including muscles and internal skeletal elements. The rearrangement of this collection of cells into the primary (or germ) layers is called gastrulation. Gastrulation can occur via a variety of mechanisms, but all result in an inner, or endodermal, layer of cells; an outer layer of cells, the ectoderm; and a layer of cells between the two other layers, known as the mesoderm (Gilbert and Raunio, 1997). The middle layer can be derived from either the ectoderm (ectomesoderm) or the inner layer (endomesoderm).

During gastrulation, the cells of the mesoderm and endoderm move into the inside of the embryo, often at a single region known as the blastopore. Once the endoderm and mesoderm are inside the ball, they usually obliterate the blastocoel and form a new cavity, the archenteron, or primitive gut. Animals can be divided in two groups on the basis of whether the mouth forms near the point of this blastopore (in protostomes) or at a distant site (in deuterostomes). Once these three primary germ layers are established, the development of the nervous system begins. A more detailed description of the development of the other organ systems is beyond the scope of this text. Nevertheless, one should keep in mind that the development of the nervous system does not take place in a vacuum, but is an integral and highly integrated part of the development of the animal as a whole.

The next three sections deal with the embryology of several examples of metazoan development: nematode worms (*Caenorhabditis elegans*), insects (*Drosophila melanogaster*), and amphibians (*Xenopus laevis*). The development of these animals is described because it has been particularly well studied for historical and practical reasons. However, one should take these examples as representative, not as definitive. The development of the very simple nervous system of Cnidarians (hydra) is also instructive. The necessity of studying many diverse species has become critical to the understanding of the development of any one species.

Neural Tissue Is Derived from Ectoderm

The development of the nervous system begins with the segregation of neural and glial cells from other types of tissues. The many differences in gene expression between neurons and muscle tissue, for example, arise through the progressive narrowing of the potential fates available to blast cells during development. The divergence of neural lineages from other tissue lineages can occur in many different ways and at many different points in the development of an organism. However, the cellular and molecular mechanisms that are responsible for the

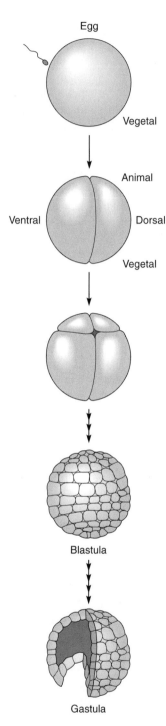

Figure 1.2 The early processes of animal development follow a conserved pattern. After fertilization, a series of cleavage divisions divide the egg into a multicellular blastula. The animal and vegetal poles represent an initial asymmetry in the oocyte, and the second axis, dorsal–ventral in this example, is established after fertilization. The process of gastrulation brings some of the cells from the surface of the embryo to the inside and generates the three-layer structure common to most multicellular animals.

divergence of the neural and glial lineages from other tissues are fundamentally conserved.

Hydra

The first generalization that can be made concerning neural segregation is that the nervous system is derived from the ectodermal germ layer in all triploblastic (three-germ layered) organisms. The organisms we discuss in this book are triploblastic; that is, they have three distinct primary layers. However, neurons are present in more primitive diploblastic (two layered) organisms like jellyfish and hydras. The jellyfish and hydras are among the organisms that belong to the Cnidarian phylum. These animals are among the most primitive multicellular animals, with no defined organs and only a tissue level of organization for the different cell types. The freshwater *Hydra* is one of the more well-studied examples of the phylum (Fig. 1.3A). Hydras have an outer layer, the epidermis, and an inner epithelium, the gastrodermis (Fig. 1.3B), and between these layers is an extracellular matrix similar in composition to the basement membranes of other animals. The gastric cavity has a single opening that serves as both a mouth and an anus, and the hydra uses the surrounding ring of tentacles to capture food. The nervous system of hydras and jellyfish is composed of bipolar neurons organized as a network. The neurons coordinate the activity of the animal via voltage-gated channels, action potentials, and chemical and electrical synaptic transmission. Thus, the basic features of the nervous system have been around for at least 600 million years and appear to have been present in animals ancestral to all metazoans except sponges.

Given the many similarities neurons have had since they arose in evolution, it is worthwhile to consider how they develop in these most primitive animals. Cnidarians can reproduce either asexually or sexually, and most biologists are familiar with the asexual budding of hydras (Fig. 1.3A). A bud forms as an evagination from a region of the body wall known as the

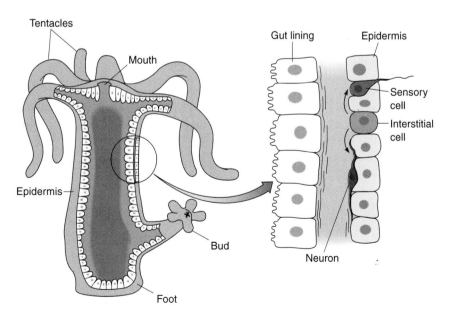

Figure 1.3 The nervous system shares a common cellular lineage with the ectoderm. In very simple animals, like the *Hydra,* the neurons are derived from a precursor in the epidermis, known as the interstitial cell, which can generate both neurons and other sensory cells.

bud zone. The bud elongates over the next 2 days and then separates from the parent organism. The neurons of these animals, like all the cells, arise from multipotent progenitor cells in the epidermal layer, known as the interstitial cells. The interstitial cells are a heterogeneous collection of true stem cells and progenitor cells differentiating along various cell-specific pathways. Are these interstitial cells similar to the precursors of the neurons in other phyla? Unfortunately, although the development of the nervous system has been described in some detail, little is known of the cellular and molecular mechanisms that give rise to neurons in these animals. Therefore, it is difficult to make direct comparisons between the Cnidarians and other metazoans. Recently, a gene related to the proneural genes (see below) of *Drosophila* and vertebrates has been discovered in *Hydra* (Grens *et al.,* 1995); however, much more study of the cnidarians is necessary to determine the degree to which the mechanisms for neurogenesis are common to all multicellular animals.

C. Elegans

The development of *C. elegans,* a nematode worm, also highlights the shared lineage of the epidermal and neural cell fates. These animals have been studied primarily because of their simple structure (containing only about 1000 cells), their rapid generation time (allowing genetic mutants to be made), and their transparency (enabling lineage relationships of the cells to be established). These nematodes have a rigid cuticle that is made of collagenous proteins secreted by the underlying cells of the hypodermis. The hypodermis is analogous to the epidermis of other animals, except that it is composed of a syncitium of nuclei rather than of individual cells. *C. elegans* have a simple nervous system, composed of only 302 neurons and 56 glial cells. These neurons are organized into nerve cords, instead of the nerve net of the jellyfish. The nerve cords are primarily in the dorsal and ventral sides of the animals, but there are some neurons that run along the lateral sides of the animal as well. The nematodes move by a series of lon-

gitudinal muscles and they have a simple digestive system. Fig. 1.4 shows a hermaphroditic female, but *C. elegans* also has rare males, which are somewhat smaller.

Developmental biologists have long been interested in nematodes. Theodore Boveri studied nematode embryology and first described the highly reproducible pattern of cell divisions in these animals in the late 1800s. Boveri's most famous student, Hans Spemann, whose work on amphibian neural induction is described below, worked on nematodes for his Ph.D. research. The modern interest in nematodes, however, was motivated by Sydney Brenner, a molecular biologist who was searching for an animal that would allow the techniques of molecular genetics to be applied to the development of metazoans (Brenner, 1974).

Due to the stereotypy in the pattern of cell divisions, the lineage relationships of all the cells of *C. elegans* have been determined (Sulston *et al.,* 1983). The first cleavage produces a large somatic cell, the AB blastomere, which will go on to give rise to most of the hypodermis and the nervous system, and the smaller germline P cell, which in addition to the gonads will also generate the gut and most of the muscles of the animal. Subsequent cleavages produce the germ cell precursor P4 and the precursor cells for the rest of the animal: the MS, E, C, and D blastomeres (Fig. 1.4). These cells all migrate into the interior of the embryo, while the AB derived cells spread out over the outside of the embryo completing gastrulation. The next phase of development is characterized by many cell divisions and is known as the proliferation phase. Then an indentation forms at the ventral side of the animal marking the beginning of the morphogenesis stage, and as this indentation progresses, the worm begins to take shape (Fig. 1.5). At this point, the worm has only 556 cells and will add the remaining cells (to the total of 959) over the four larval molts. The entire development of the animal takes about 2 days.

The neurons of *C. elegans* arise primarily from the AB blastomere, in lineages shared with the ectodermally derived hypodermis. An example of one of these lineages is shown in Fig.

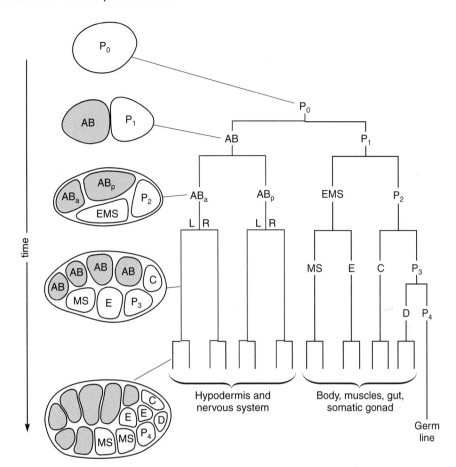

Figure 1.4 The nervous system shares a common cellular lineage with the ectoderm. The cell divisions that generate the *C. elegans* nematode worm are highly reproducible from animal to animal. The first division produces the AB blastomere and the P1 blastomere. The germline is segregated into the P4 blastomere within a few divisions after fertilization. The subsequent divisions of the AB blastomere go on to give rise to most of the neurons of the animal, as well as to the cells that produce the hypodermis of the animal.

1.5. The Abarpa blastomere can be readily identified in the 100-min embryo through its position and lineal history. This cell then goes on to give rise to 20 additional cells, including 9 neurons of the ring ganglion. The progeny of the Abarpa blastomere, like most of the progeny of the AB lineage, lie primarily on the surface of the embryo prior to 200 min of development; at this time, the cells on the ventral and lateral sides of the embryo move inside and become the nervous system, while the AB progeny that remain on the surface spread out to form the hypodermis. Most of the neurons arise in this way; of the

222 neurons in the newly hatched *C. elegans*, 214 arise from the AB lineage while 6 are derived from the MS blastomere and 2 from the C blastomere.

Drosophila

The development of *Drosophila* is characteristic of "long germ band" arthropods. Unlike the embryo of the nematode, where cleavage of the cells occurs at the same time as nuclear division, the initial rounds of nuclear division in the *Drosophila* embryo are not accompanied by

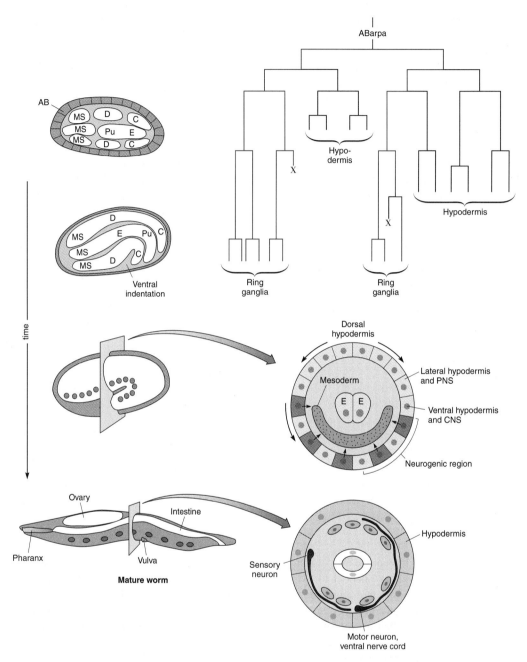

Figure 1.5 The next phase of development of *C. elegans* also highlights the shared lineages of hypodermis and neurons. During gastrulation, the MS, E, C, and D blastomeres all migrate into the interior of the embryo, while the progeny of the AB blastomeres spread out over the external surface. Once the embryo starts to take form, sections through the embryo show the relationships of the cells. The neurons are primarily derived from the ventrolateral surface, through the divisions of the AB progeny cells. As these cells are generated they migrate into the interior and form the nerve rings. A typical lineage is also shown. The Abarpa blastomeres, through five rounds of division, generate 9 neurons and 10 hypodermal cells.

corresponding cell divisions. Instead, the nuclei remain in a syncitium up until just prior to gastrulation, 3 h after fertilization. Prior to this time, the dividing nuclei lie in the interior of the egg, but they then move out toward the surface and a process known as cellularization occurs during which the nuclei are surrounded by plasma membranes. At this point the embryo is known as a cellular blastoderm.

The major part of the nervous system of *Drosophila* arises from cells in the ventrolateral part of the cellular blastoderm (Figs. 1.6A and 1.6B). Soon after cellularization, the ventral furrow, which marks the beginning of gastrulation, begins to form (Fig. 1.6). At the ventral furrow, cells of the future mesoderm fold into the interior of the embryo. The process of invagination occurs over several hours and the invaginating cells continue to divide and eventually give rise to the mesodermal tissues of the animal. As the mesodermal cells invaginate into the embryo, the neurogenic region moves from the ventrolateral position to the most ventral region of the animal (Fig. 1.6). The closing of the ventral furrow creates the ventral midline, a future site of neurogenesis. On either side of the ventral midline is the neurogenic ectoderm, tissue that gives rise to the ventral nerve cord, otherwise known as the central nervous system (Fig. 1.6). However, it is worth noting that a separate neurogenic region, known as the procephalic neurogenic region, gives rise to the cerebral ganglia or brain.

Drosophila neurogenesis begins in the neurogenic region when scattered cells within this region enlarge and begin to move from this layer into the inside of the embryo (Fig. 1.6). At the beginning of neurogenesis, the neurogenic region is a single cell layer; the first morphological sign of neurogenesis is that a number of cells within the epithelium begin to increase in size. These larger cells then undergo a shape change and squeeze out of the epithelium. This process is called delamination and is shown in more detail in Fig. 1.7. The cells that delaminate are called neuroblasts and are the progenitors that generate the nervous system. In the next phase of neurogenesis (Fig. 1.8), each neuroblast divides to generate many progeny, known as ganglion mother cells (GMCs). Each GMC then generates a pair of neurons or glia. The entire central nervous system of the larval *Drosophila* is generated in this way. However, the *Drosophila* nervous system is not completed in the larva, but rather additional neurogenesis occurs during metamorphosis. Sensory organs, like the eyes, are generated from imaginal discs, small cellular discs in the larva that undergo a tremendous amount of proliferation during metamorphosis to generate most of what we recognize as an adult fly. These structures are described more thoroughly in a later chapter.

Amphibian

The vertebrate embryo undergoes a similar process of development. After fertilization, a series of rapid cell divisions, known as cleavages, divide the fertilized egg into blastomeres. The embryo, now known as a blastula, then undergoes the process of gastrulation, in which the three primary or "germ" layers are formed. The point of initiation of gastrulation is identified on the embryo as a small invagination of the otherwise smooth surface of the blastula and this is called the blastopore (Fig. 1.9) and is in some ways analogous to the ventral furrow of the fly. In amphibians the first cells to invaginate occur at the dorsal side of the blastopore (Fig. 1.9), and, as described below, they have a special significance to the development of the nervous system. The mechanism of involution is complex, and it appears that a small group of "bottle" cells initiates the process by changing shape and creating a discontinuity in the surface.

The involuting cells lead a large number of cells that were originally on the surface of the embryo into the interior (Fig. 1.9). The part of the blastula that will ultimately reside in the interior of the embryo is called the involuting marginal zone (IMZ). Most of these cells will ultimately give rise to mesodermal derivatives, like muscle and bone. The first cells to involute crawl the furthest and ultimately give rise to the mesoderm of the anterior part of the animal (i.e.,

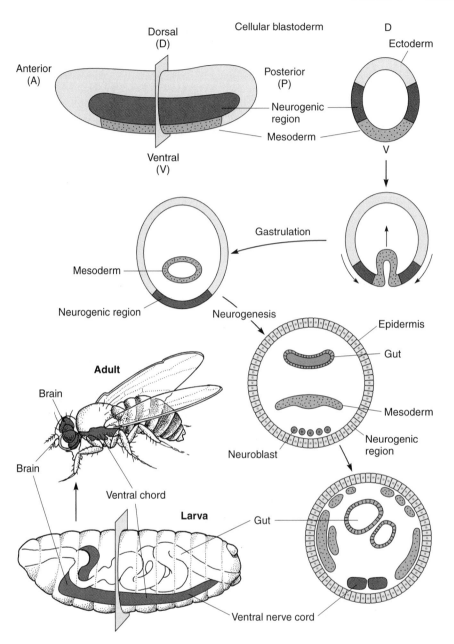

Figure 1.6 The nervous system of *Drosophila* is derived from the ventrolateral region of the ectoderm. The embryo is first (top) shown at the blastoderm stage, just prior to gastrulation. The region fated to give rise to the nervous system lies on the ventral–lateral surface of the embryo (red). The involution of the mesoderm at the ventral surface brings the neurogenic region closer to the midline. Scattered cells within this region of the ectoderm then enlarge, migrate into the interior of the embryo, and divide several more times to make neurons and glia. These neurons and glia then condense into the ganglia of the ventral nerve cord (or CNS) in the larva and the adult.

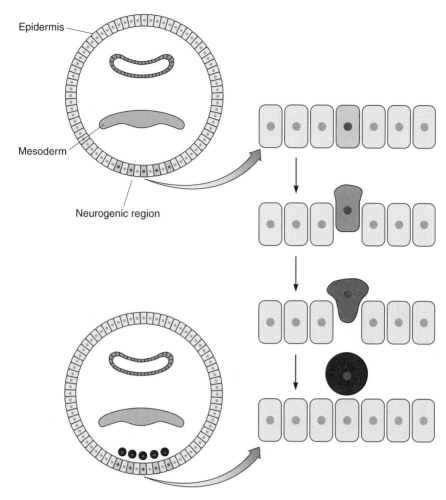

Figure 1.7 The neuroblasts of the *Drosophila* separate from the ectoderm by a process known as delamination (red). The neuroblasts enlarge relative to the surrounding cells and squeeze out of the epithelium. The process occurs in several waves; after the first set of neuroblasts has delaminated from the ectoderm, a second set of cells in the ectoderm begins to enlarge and also delaminates.

the head). The later involving IMZ cells ultimately produce the mesoderm of more posterior regions, including the tail of the tadpole.

At this point in development, the neural plate of the vertebrate embryo still largely resembles the rest of the surface ectoderm; however, shortly after its formation, the neural plate begins to fold onto itself to form a tube-like structure, the neural tube (Fig. 1.10). Much more will be said about the neural tube and its derivatives and shape changes. For now, suffice it to

say that this tube of cells gives rise to nearly all the neurons and glia of vertebrates. Another source of neurons and glia is the neural crest, a group of cells that arises at the junction between the tube and the ectoderm (Fig. 1.10). The neural crest is the source of most of those neurons and glia of the peripheral nervous system, whose cell bodies lie outside the brain and spinal cord. This tissue is unique to vertebrates and has the capacity to generate many diverse cell types; we say a great deal more about it in later chapters.

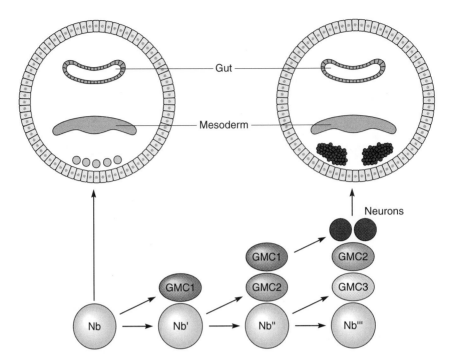

Figure 1.8 The delaminating neuroblasts then go on to generate several neurons through a stereotypic pattern of asymmetric cell divisions. The first cell division of the neuroblast produces a daughter cell known as the ganglion mother cell, or GMC. The first GMC divides to form neurons, while the neuroblast divides again to make another GMC. In this figure, the neuroblast is shown through its successive stages as Nb, Nb', Nb", and Nb"', while the GMCs are numbered successively as they arise.

Interactions with Neighboring Tissues Are Required for the Ectoderm to Make Neural Tissue in Many Animals

The three basic layers of the embryo, the endoderm, the mesoderm, and the ectoderm, arise through the complex movements of gastrulation. These movements also create new tissue relations. For example, after gastrulation in the frog, presumptive mesoderm underlies the dorsal ectoderm. A large number of experimental studies in the early part of this century revealed that these new tissue arrangements were of critical importance to the development of a normal animal. By culturing small pieces of embryos in isolation, it was possible to determine the time at which each part of the embryo acquired its character or fate (Fig, 1.11). When the dorsal ectoderm was cultured in isolation prior to gastrulation, the cells differentiated into epidermis, while when roughly the same piece of tissue was isolated from gastrulating embryos, the piece of ectoderm now differentiated into neural tissue, including recognizable parts of the brain and the spinal cord and even the eyes. These results led Hans Spemann, a leading embryologist of the time, to speculate that the ectoderm became fated to generate neural tissue as a result of the tissue rearrangements that occur at gastrulation (Hamburger, 1969). One possible source of this "induction" of the neural tissue was the involuting mesoderm, known at the time as the archenteron roof. As noted above, the involuting tissue is led by the dorsal lip of the blastopore. To test the idea that the involuting mesoderm induces the overlying ectoderm to become neural tissue,

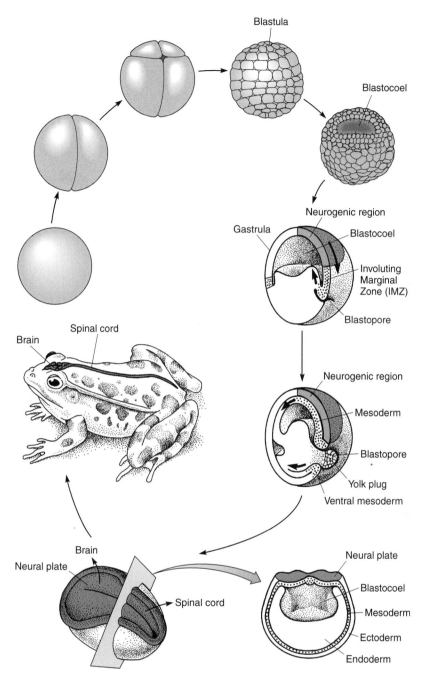

Figure 1.9 The development of the central nervous system, brain and spinal cord, in a vertebrate embryo is shown from the egg cell to the adult frog. After a series of cleavage divisions produce a blastula, a group of cells known as the involuting marginal zone, or IMZ, grows into the interior of the embryo at a point known as the blastopore. This process of gastrulation is shown in two cross sections. The involuting cells go on to form mesodermal tissues and induce the cells of the overlying ectoderm to develop into neural tissue, labeled as the neurogenic region (red). After the process of neural induction, the neurogenic region is known as the neural plate and is restricted to giving rise to neural tissue. A cross section of the embryo at the neural plate stage shows the relationships between the tissues at this stage of development. The neural plate goes on to generate the neurons and glia in the adult brain and spinal cord.

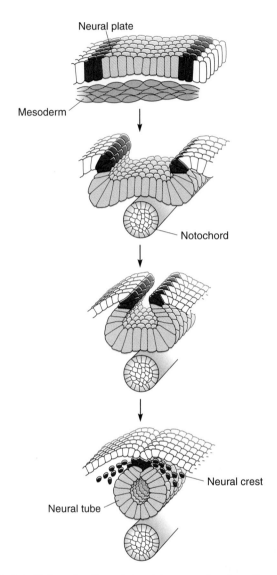

Neural plate

Mesoderm

Notochord

Neural crest

Neural tube

Figure 1.10   The neural plate (light red) rolls up into a tube separating from the rest of the ectoderm. The mesoderm cells condense to form a rod-shaped structure—the notochord—just underneath the neural plate. The neural plate begins to roll up and fuse at the dorsal margins. A group of cells known as the neural crest (dark red) arises at the point of fusion of the neural tube.

Spemann and Hilde Mangold carried out the following experiment (Fig. 1.12). The dorsal lip of the blastopore was dissected from one embryo and transplanted into the blastocoele of another, and the host embryo was allowed to develop further to the tadpole stage. Spemann and Mangold found that an entire second body axis, including a brain, a spinal cord, and eyes developed from the ventral side of the embryo where neural tissue does not normally arise. To determine whether the new neural tissue that developed in these twinned embryos came from the dorsal lip tissue, they transplanted the dorsal blastopore lip from a pigmented embryo into the blastocoel

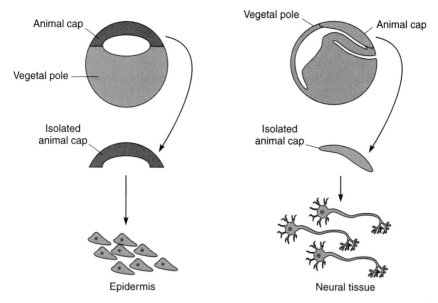

Figure 1.11   Isolation of fragments of embryos at different stages of development demonstrates when tissue becomes committed to the neural lineage. If the animal cap is isolated from the rest of the embryo, the cells develop as epidermis, or skin. If the same region of the embryo is isolated a few hours later, during gastrulation, it will develop into neural tissue (shown in the figure as red neurons). Experiments like these led to the idea that the neural lineage arises during gastrulation.

of a nonpigmented strain of frogs. They found that the new body axis was made of mostly non-pigmented cells, indicating that it came largely from the host blastula, not the transplanted dorsal lip. Thus, the grafted blastoporal cells have the capacity to induce neural tissues from a region of the ectoderm that would normally not give rise to the nervous system. In addition to the neural tissue in these embryos, they found that mesodermally derived structures also contributed to the twinned embryo. They concluded that the dorsal lip acts not only as a neural inducer but also as an "organizer" of the entire body axis. As a result of these experiments, this region of the embryo is known as the Spemann organizer.

In the years following these initial studies of Spemann and Mangold, several embryologists tried to further characterize the induction process, as well as to identify the inducing factor. One of the first realizations that came from these additional studies was that the organizer has subdivisions, each capable of inducing specific types of differentiation. Holtfreter subdivided the organizer region into pieces and, using the same transplantation strategy, he found that when more lateral aspects of the dorsal lip were used tails were induced, whereas when more medial regions of the organizer region were transplanted heads were induced (Fig. 1.13). In an attempt to more precisely define the heterogeneity of the region, Holtfreter also cultured small bits of the dorsal lip and found that that these develop into more or less well-defined structures, such as single eyes or ears! Holtfreter (1939) succinctly summarizes, "even at the gastrula stage the head organizer is not actually an equipotential entity, but is subdivided into specialized inductors although distinct boundaries between them do not seem to exist."

Neural induction does not appear to act solely through a vertical signal passed from the involuting mesoderm to the overlying ectoderm; there is also evidence that a neural inducing signal can be

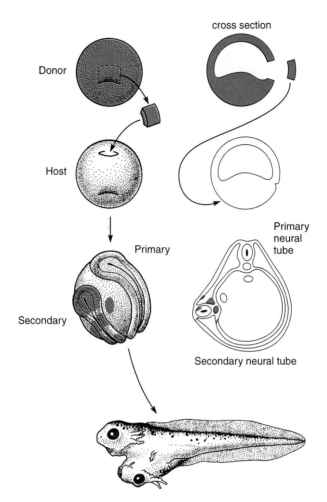

Figure 1.12   Spemann and Mangold transplanted the dorsal lip of the blastopore from a pigmented embryo (shown in red) to a nonpigmented host embryo. A second axis, including the neural tube, was induced by the transplanted tissue. The transplanted dorsal blastopore lip cells gave rise to some of the tissue in the secondary axis, but some of the host cells also contributed to the new body axis. They concluded that the dorsal lip cells could "organize" the host cells to form a new body axis, and they named this special region of the embryo the Spemann organizer.

passed through the plane of the ectoderm. When blastulas are placed in hypotonic solutions just prior to gastrulation, the IMZ cells fail to involute and instead evaginate to produce an "exogastrula." Under these conditions the process of signaling between the mesoderm and the ectoderm should be blocked, since the involuting mesoderm is no longer underneath the ectoderm. However, surprisingly, some neural induction does appear to take place. While this was difficult to determine in Holtfreter's time, the use of antibodies and probes for neural-specific proteins and gene expression clearly shows that organized neural tissue forms in such exogastrulae (Holtfreter, 1939; Ruiz i Altaba, 1992) (Figure 1.16). This so-called planar induction can also be demonstrated in a unique tissue combination invented by Ray Keller that bears his name, the Keller sandwich. In this preparation, the presumptive neural ectoderm and the dorsal lip are dissected

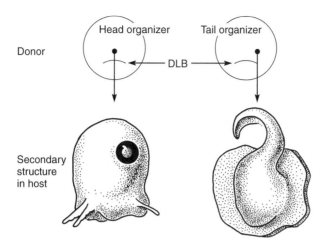

Figure 1.13 The tissue of the dorsal lip of the blastopore (DLB) contains multiple inducing activities. Holtfreter subdissected the organizer region of an amphibian embryo and transplanted the pieces to another embryo, as in the Spemann and Mangold experiment. When more medial parts of the organizer were transplanted, only heads developed from the secondary axis, whereas transplantation of more lateral pieces resulted in secondary axes made up primarily of tail tissue. (Adapted from Willier *et al.,* 1995)

from two embryos and sandwiched together. Remarkably, the convergence and extension movements of the neural ectoderm take place, and the tissue elongates (Keller *et al.,* 1992) (Fig. 1.14). However, the mesoderm does not move inside of the sandwich, but rather extends away from

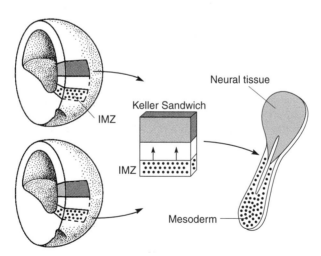

Figure 1.14 Planar neural induction can be contrasted from vertical neural induction by Keller sandwiches. The organizer region, including the IMZ cells, along with some of the surrounding ectodermal tissue can be cultured in isolation and will not involute. The tissue undergoes morphological changes similar to those that occur during gastrulation, except the tissue extends rather than involutes. Nevertheless, neural tissue (red) is induced in the attached ectoderm, indicating that the signals for neural induction can be passed through the small region that connects the mesodermal cells and the ectodermal cells.

the neurectoderm like an exogastrula. Only a thin bridge of tissue connects the mesoderm with the neural ectoderm, but, nevertheless, extensive and patterned neural development occurs in these cultures (Fig. 1.14).

The early efforts to further define the chemical nature of the neural inducer were unsuccessful. In the initial attempts at characterization, Bautzman, Holtfreter, Spemann, and Mangold showed that the organizer tissue retained its inductive activity even after the cells had been killed by heat, cold, or alcohol. Holtfreter subsequently reported that the neuralizing activity survived freezing, boiling, and acid treatment; however the activity was lost at temperatures of 150°C. Several embryologists then set out to isolate the active principle(s) in the dorsal lip of the blastopore using the following three approaches: (1) extracting the active factor from the dorsal blastopore cells, (2) trying out candidate molecules to look for similar inductive activities, and (3) testing other tissues for inductive activities.

The initial attempts at direct isolation of the inducing activity from the blastoporal lip cells were hindered by the small amounts of tissue that could be obtained and the limited types of chemical analysis that were available. From the initial report in 1932 to the late 1950s, over 100 studies tried to characterize the neuralizing activity. The search for the neural inducer was one of the major preoccupations of developmental biologists in this period. While one group reported that the active principle was lipid extractable, another would report that the residues were more active than the extracts. To obtain more tissue to work with, several investigators screened a variety of adult tissues for similar inducing activities. While some found a certain degree of specificity, liver and kidney being the most potent neural inducers, others found that "fragments from practically every organ or tissue from various amphibians, reptiles, birds, and mammals, including man, were inductive" (Holtfreter and Hamburger, 1955). Perhaps the most disconcerting to the investigators at the time was the results from the candidate molecule approach. Some of the factors found to have neuralizing activity made some sense: polycyclic hydrocarbon ster-

oids, for example; however, other putative inducers, such as methylene blue and thiocyanate most likely had their effects through some toxicity or contamination.

In the early 1980s a number of investigators began to apply molecular biological techniques to study embryonic inductions. The first of these studies attempted to test for factors that would trigger the process of mesoderm induction in the frog. As described above, the frog embryo is divided into an animal half and a vegetal half. The animal half will ultimately gives rise to neural tissue and ectodermal tissue, while the vegetal half gives rise primarily to endoderm; the mesoderm, which ultimately goes on to make muscle and bone and blood, arises in between these two tissues from the cells around the embryo's equator (see Fig. 1.15). It has been known for many years from the work of Peter Nieuwkoop that the formation of the mesodermal cells in the equatorial region requires some type of interaction between the animal and vegetal halves of the embryo. If this animal half or "cap" is isolated from the vegetal half of the embryo, no mesodermal cells develop. However, when Nieuwkoop (1973, 1985) recombined the animal cap with the vegetal half, mesodermal derivatives developed in the resulting embryos (Fig. 1.15). He postulated that a signal from the vegetal half of the embryo induced the formation of mesoderm at the junction with the animal half of the embryo. The identification of the molecular basis for this induction came from experiments in which isolated animal caps were exposed to a variety of factors and cell-conditioned media. Most factors failed to cause mesoderm formation in the animal caps; however, two factors, fibroblast growth factor (FGF) and transforming growth factor-β (TGF-β) had potent mesodermal inducing activities. These results have been followed up by a number of groups since that time, and the following picture of mesoderm induction has emerged. A TGF-β related molecule, either Veg1 or nodal-related 1 or 2, is released from the vegetal half of the embryo and together with eFGF, a member of the FGF family of proteins that is expressed in the early embryo, induces the equatorial region to develop

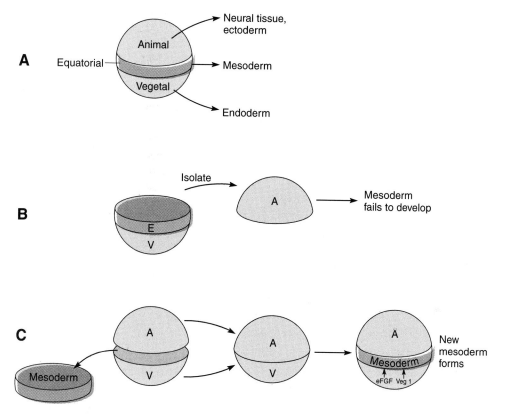

Figure 1.15 Interactions between the animal and vegetal cells of the amphibian embryo are necessary for induction of the mesoderm. (A) The regions of the amphibian embryo that give rise to these different tissue types are shown. The animal pole gives rise to epidermal cells and neural tissue; the vegetal pole gives rise to endodermal derivatives, like the gut, and the mesoderm arises from the equatorial zone. (B) If the animal cap and vegetal hemispheres are isolated from one another, mesoderm does not develop. (C) If the equatorial zone is removed from an embryo and the isolated animal and vegetal caps are recombined, a mesoderm forms at a new equatorial zone. Two of the molecules that may be essential for the induction of the new mesoderm are eFGF and Veg1.

mesodermal lineages (see Fig. 1.15). A second signaling system, involving a group of proteins known as Wnt proteins, induces the dorsal part of the equatorial zone to develop as the Spemann organizer. In this way the early embryo sets up the basic axes of the body.

At the same time these studies of mesodermal inducing factors were taking place, a number of investigators realized that the animal cap assay might also be a very good way to identify neural inducers. Not only do isolated animal caps fail to generate mesodermal cells, they also fail to develop into neuronal tissue. Several factors added to animal caps caused the cells to develop into neural cells as well as mesodermal tissue. However, since the organizer at the dorsal lip of the blastopore is made from mesoderm, it was not clear whether the neural tissue that developed in animal caps was directly induced by the exogenous factor or alternatively whether the factor first induced an organizer which subsequently induced neural tissue. (Fig. 1.16). Therefore, to refine the assay to look for direct neural induction, studies concentrated on identifying factors that would cause the increase in the expression of neural genes without the

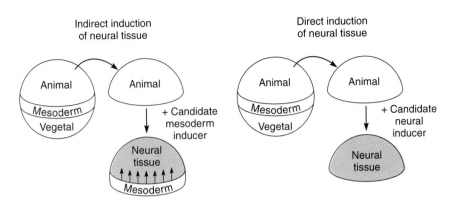

Figure 1.16   Indirect neural induction versus direct neural induction. The organizer transplant experiments show that the involuting mesoderm has the capacity to induce neural tissue in the cells of the ectoderm. When assaying for the factors released from mesoderm responsible for this activity it was important to distinguish between the direct and the indirect induction of neural tissue when animal caps were treated with a candidate factor. In the first example, mesoderm is induced by the factor and then neural tissue is induced by the mesoderm. Thus, both mesoderm and neural genes are turned on in the animal caps. However, in the case of a direct neural inducer, neural genes are turned on, but mesoderm-specific genes are not expressed.

concomitant induction of mesoderm-specific gene expression.

The animal cap assay was used for the isolation of the first candidate neural inducer. Richard Harland (Smith *et al.,* 1993; Lamb *et al.,* 1993) and his collegues used an ingenious expression cloning system to identify a neural inducing factor that they named noggin (Fig. 1.17). The cloning was done by taking advantage of the fact that X-irradiated frog embryos fail to develop a dorsal axis, including the nervous system, and instead develop only ventral structures. Nevertheless, the transplantation of a dorsal blastopore lip from a different embryo can restore a normal body axis to the UV-treated embryo, indicating that the UV embryo can still respond to the neural inducing factor(s). Further, injection of only the poly-A RNA from a hyperdorsalized embryo (Li-treated) can also restore a normal body axis. Harland's group took advantage of this fact and used pools of cDNA isolated from the organizer region to rescue the UV-treated embryos. By dividing the pools into smaller and smaller collections they isolated a cDNA that coded for a unique secreted protein, which they named noggin. When this protein was expressed and used to treat animal caps, they found that it was ca-

pable of inducing the specific induction of neural genes without the induction of mesodermal genes. *In situ* localization of noggin showed that it is expressed in gastrulating embryos, specifically expressed by the cells of the dorsal lip of the blastopore, precisely where the organizer activity is known to reside. Injection of noggin RNA into UV-treated embryos at the 4-cell stage can restore body axis and even hyperdorsalize the embryos to give bigger brains than normal.

At the same time that the noggin studies were being done, other labs were using additional approaches to identify the specific molecules that induce the nervous system. DeRobertis was interested in identifying genes that were expressed in the dorsal blastopore lip organizer region. A transcription factor, goosecoid, was one of the first such genes to be identified. Goosecoid was found to cause a secondary axis to form when the mRNA coding for the protein was injected into embryos. The axis duplication assay is essentially the molecular equivalent to the Spemann dorsal lip transplantation experiment. DeRobertis (Sasai *et al.,* 1994, 1995) reasoned that genes that were induced as a result of goosecoid expression might be important for inducing the axis. Therefore, they conducted a differential

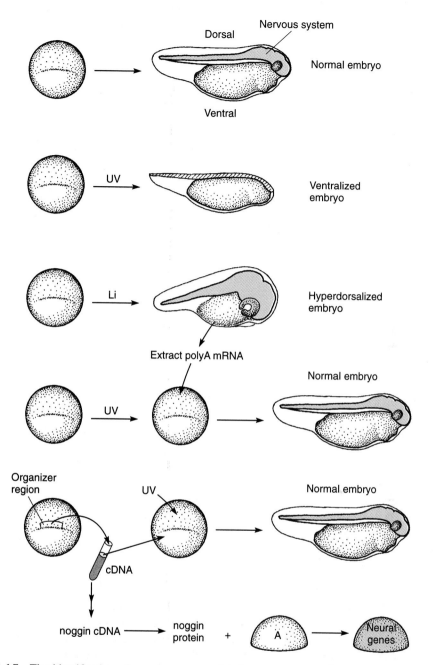

Figure 1.17 The identification of noggin as a neural inducer was accomplished through the use of an expression cloning strategy in *Xenopus* embryos. UV light treatment of the early embryo inhibits the development of dorsal structures by disrupting the cytoskeleton rearrangements that pattern the dorsal inducing molecules prior to gastrulation (ventralized). Lithium treatment of the early embryo has the opposite effect; the embryo develops more than normal dorsal tissue (i.e., hyperdorsalized). If messenger RNA is extracted from the hyperdorsalized embryos and injected into a UV-treated embryo, the messages encoded in the mRNA can "rescue" the UV-treated embryo and it develops relatively normally. Similarly, cDNA from the organizer region of a normal embryo can rescue a UV-treated embryo. The noggin gene was isolated as a cDNA from the organizer region that could rescue the UV-treated embryo when injected into the embryo, and, subsequently, recombinant protein was made from this cDNA and shown to induce neural tissue from isolated animal caps without any induction of mesodermal genes.

screen for genes expressed in the same region as goosecoid and they isolated a molecule they named chordin. Like noggin, this is a secreted protein that is expressed in the organizer during the period when neural induction is occurring. Overexpression of chordin in the ventral part of the embryo causes a secondary axis, similar to goosecoid. Thus, chordin appears to act similarly to noggin as a putative neural inducer.

A third candidate neural inducer was identified by Melton and Hemmati-Brivanlou as a previously identified reproductive hormone known as follistatin (Hemmati-Brivanlou and Melton, 1994). In the reproductive system, follistatin works as a regulatory factor by binding to and inhibiting activin, a TGF-β like protein that controls FSH secretion from the pituitary gland. During a screen for mesoderm inducing factors, Melton found that activin could act as a ventral mesoderm inducer. To study the mechanism of action of activin on mesoderm induction, he constructed a truncated activin receptor that when misexpressed in embryos would interfere with normal endogeneous activin signaling (Hemmati-Brivanlou and Melton, 1994) (Fig. 1.18). To the surprise of Melton and Hemmati-Brivanlou, interfering with activin signaling not only disrupted normal mesoderm development, it also induced the cells of the animal cap to develop as neurons without any additional neural inducing molecule. They proposed that activin—or something like it—normally inhibits neural tissue from differentiating in the ectoderm. They also suggested that perhaps neural induction was inhibiting this neural inhibitor; in other words, the Spemann organizer secretes a factor or factors that antagonize a neural inhibitor. These results led Melton to propose the idea that neural tissue is in some way the default state of the ectoderm and that it must be actively inhibited by activin-like activities.

The idea that the ectoderm is actively inhibited from becoming neural tissue has some additional support. In 1989, two groups (Godsave and Slack, 1989; Grunz and Tacke, 1989) reported that dissociation of the animal cap cells prior to neural induction caused most of the cells to differentiate as neurons (Fig. 1.19). Taking these lines of evidence together, it became clear that molecules that could inhibit activin signaling would make good neural inducers. Since follistatin was already known to inhibit activin signaling from the studies of these factors in the reproductive system, Melton tested whether follistatin could act as a neural inducer. Melton found that indeed follistatin could cause a secondary axis when misexpressed; moreover, recombinant follistatin could induce neural tissue from animal caps. Follistatin is also expressed in the organizer region of the embryo at the time of neural induction, like chordin and noggin.

Even more fascinating than the fact that three candidate neural inducing factors were identified in a relatively short period of time is the fact that these three factors may all act by a related mechanism and that this mechanism appears to be at least partially conserved between vertebrates and invertebrates (Fig. 1.20). The analysis of chordin's sequence revealed an interesting homology between chordin and a *Drosophila* protein called short gastrulation or sog. Sog is expressed in the ventral side of the fly embryo and mutations in this gene in *Drosophila* result in defective dorsal–ventral patterning of the embryo. In null mutants of sog, the epidermis expands and the neurogenic region is reduced. And like chordin, microinjection of sog into the nonneurogenic region of the embryo causes the formation of ectopic neural tissue. Thus, sog seems to be the functional homolog of chordin. At this point the advantages of fly genetics were important. From analysis of other *Drosophila* mutants it was possible to show that sog interacts with a gene called *decapentaplegic,* or dpp, a TGFβ-like like protein related to the vertebrate genes known as bone-morphogenic proteins, BMP-2 and BMP-4. Dpp and sog directly antagonize one another in *Drosophila.* Mutations in dpp have the opposite phenotype of sog mutations. In dpp mutants, the neurogenic region expands at the expense of the epidermis and ectopic expression of dpp causes a reduction in neural tissue. These *Drosophila* studies motivated studies of the distribution of the BMPs at early stages of *Xenopus* development, and a similar pattern has emerged. BMP-4 is expressed

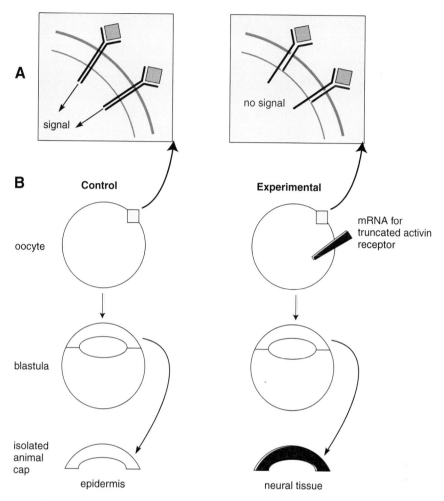

Figure 1.18   Expression of a truncated activin receptor blocks normal activin signaling through the receptor and induces neural tissue. (A) The normal activin receptor transmits a signal to the cell when activin binds the receptor and it forms a dimer. The truncated activin receptor still binds the activin (or related molecules) but now the normal receptor forms dimers with the truncated receptor. Lacking the intracellular domain to signal, the truncated receptor blocks normal signal transduction through this receptor. (B) Oocytes injected with the truncated activin receptor develop to the blastula stage, and when the animal caps are dissected from these embryos, they develop into neural tissue without the addition of a neural inducer. This result indicates that inhibiting this signaling pathway might be how neural inducers function.

throughout most of the gastrula, but at reduced levels in the organizer and neurogenic animal cap. As expected, recombinant BMP-4 can suppress neural induction by chordin, the vertebrate homolog of sog.

The studies of sog/chordin and dpp/BMP-4 lead to two conclusions. First, it appears that the dorsal–ventral axis of the developing embryo uses similar mechanisms in both the fly and the vertebrate; however, as discussed in the previous section, the neural tissue in the vertebrate is derived from the dorsal side of the animal, while the neurogenic region of the fly is on the ventral side (DeRobertis and Sasai, 1996; Holley *et al.,*

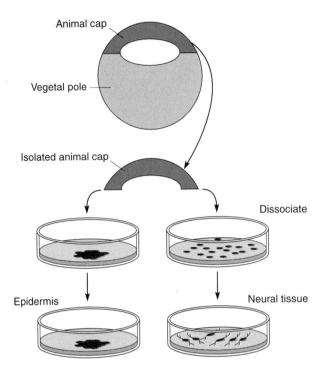

Figure 1.19   Dissociation of animal cap cells prior to gastrulation causes most of them to differentiate into neurons in culture. Animal caps can be dissociated into single cells by removing the Ca^{2+} ions from the medium. If these cells are then put onto a cell culture plate as isolated cells they develop into neurons, whereas cells cultured under similar conditions but left aggregated develop as epidermis. This result is consistent with the idea that the neural fate is actively suppressed by the cellular associations in the ectoderm.

1995). The idea that the vertebrate and arthropod body plans were inverted with respect to one another was first proposed by Geoffry Saint-Hillaire from comparative anatomical studies, and this appears to be confirmed by these recent molecular studies. Second, the antagonistic mechanism between sog and dpp in the fly also led to the hypothesis that the various neural inducers might work through a common mechanism, the antagonism of BMP-4 signaling. The following three key facts all indicate that this is indeed the case. First, BMP-4 inhibits neural differentiation of animal caps treated with chordin, noggin, or follistatin. Second, BMP-4 also inhibits neural differentiation of dissociated animal cap cells. Third, antisense BMP-4 RNA causes neural differentiation of animal caps without addition of any of the neural inducers. The dominant-negative activin receptor induction of neural tissue can also be understood in this context, since the activin receptor is related to the BMP-4 receptor and additional experiments have shown that the expression of the truncated receptor also blocks the endogenous BMP-4 signaling (Wilson and Hemmati-Brivanlou, 1995).

Do all three of these neural inducers act equivalently to inhibit BMP-4 signaling? Biochemical studies have demonstrated that chordin blocks BMP-4–receptor interactions by directly binding to BMP-4 with high affinity. Noggin also appears to bind BMP-4 with an even greater affinity while follistatin can bind the related molecules BMP-7 and activin. Therefore, it is likely that at least these three neural inducers act by blocking the endogenous epidermalizing BMP-4 and thereby allowing neural differentiation of the neurogenic ectoderm (Piccolo *et al.*, 1996) (Fig. 1.21). These factors are expressed in

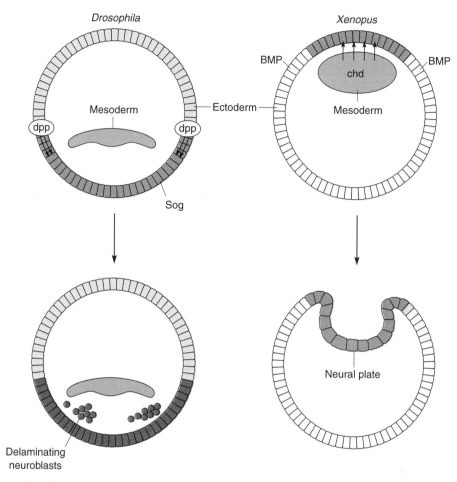

Figure 1.20 Vertebrate and invertebrates use similar molecules to pattern the dorsal–ventral axis. The *Drosophila* embryo in cross section resembles an inverted *Xenopus* embryo. As described in Fig. 1.6, the neurogenic region is in the ventral–lateral *Drosophila* embryo, whereas in the vertebrate embryo the neural plate arises from the dorsal side. In the *Drosophila* embryo, a TGF-β type molecule, dpp, supresses neural diifferentiation in the ectoderm, and in the vertebrate embryo, the related molecules, BMP-2 and BMP-4, suppress neural development. In *Drosophila,* sog (short gastrula) promotes neural development by inhibiting the dpp signaling in the ectoderm in this region. In *Xenopus* a related molecule, chordin (chd), is one of the neural inducers released from the involuting mesodermal cells. Chordin also inhibits BMP signaling, permitting neural development in these ectodermal cells.

a range of vertebrate organisms, including chick embryos and mammals; however, there is some evidence that they may have overlapping or re-dundant functions. The studies described in *Xenopus* embryos have provided evidence that these factors are capable of inducing neural tissue. There is less evidence that each one is normally required for the development of the nervous sys-tem. For example, deletion of both copies of the follistatin in mice does not cause a major disrup-tion of neural induction in this species. Simi-larly, while elimination of the noggin gene in mice causes some abnormalities in brain de-velopment, neural induction still takes place. Perhaps the best evidence that vertebrates re-quire an inhibitor of ventral fates for appropriate

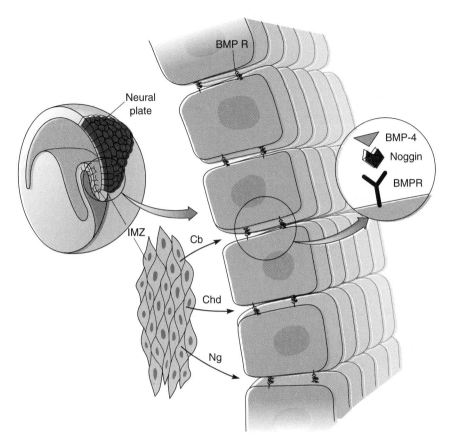

Figure 1.21   The current model of neural induction in amphibian embryos. As the involuting mesodermal cells of the IMZ grow past the overlying ectodermal cells, they release several molecules that interfere with the BMP signals between ectodermal cells. Ceberus (Cb), chordin (Chd), noggin (Ng), and follistatin all interfere with the activation of the BMP receptor (BMPR) by the BMPs in the ectoderm and thereby "induce" this region of the embryo to develop as neural tissue, ultimately generating the brain, the spinal cord, and most of the peripheral nervous system.

neural tube formation is the zebra fish chordin mutation, which results in animals with reduced neural tube and reductions in other dorsal tissues (Schulte-Merker *et al.,* 1997).

In addition to these three BMP antagonists, several additional neural inducers have emerged in the past few years, and these may act through other intracellular pathways to modify the signals from the BMP antagonists. Another secreted molecule, cerberus, is also expressed in the deepest part of the Spemann organizer and appears to act as both a BMP antagonist and a Wnt antagonist. eFGF, an activator of receptor tyrosine kinase signaling, is expressed in some

of the last cells to involute during gastrulation. As described in a previous section, several lines of embryological investigation dating back 50 years have suggested the existence of multiple inducers that selectively promoted different regions of the nervous system. Thus, it is likely that an understanding of the subtle differences in the activity of these inducers, coupled with the detailed molecular geography of the Spemann organizer, may ultimately explain some of the exquisite experimental embryology of Holtfreter's day (Fig. 1.21).

Thus, the model of neural induction that has emerged from these many lines of investigation is quite gratifying and at the same time somewhat surprising. Despite all of the experiments that were done to study the embryology of neural induction by a great many investigators, it has only been relatively recently that we have appreciated that neural tissue differentiation in the ectoderm is actively inhibited by BMPs and that neural induction is actually the reversal of this inhibition. In addition, what has also emerged from these studies is that the process of neural induction is coupled to the process of dorsal–ventral axis specification and that the "neural inducers" have more general effects on defining the dorsal axis of the embryo.

Interactions among the Ectodermal Cells Control Neuroblast Segregation

The generation of neurons from the neurogenic region of both vertebrates and invertebrates typically involves an intermediate step: a neural precursor cell is first produced and this cell goes on to produce many neurons. The neural precursor is capable of mitotic divisions, whereas the neuron itself is usually a terminally postmitotic cell. In the previous section, we saw how in both *Drosophila* and *Xenopus* the antagonism of the TGF-β-like factors BMP and dpp was critical in defining the neurogenic region of the embryo. This section describes some of the genes important in the next stage of the development of the nervous system, the formation of the neuroblasts in these neurogenic regions. Once again, the mechanisms are conserved in vertebrates and invertebrates, and so these mechanisms are very ancient ones. The production of these neural precursor cells is described first in *Drosophila,* where the mechanisms are most well understood. Some of the same mechanisms also appear to regulate this process in vertebrates, though much less is known about this class.

In *Drosophila,* as described in the previous section, the neural precursors or neuroblasts form by a process that starts with their delamination: certain cells within the neurogenic region enlarge and begin to move into the inside of the embryo. Next, each neuroblast divides to generate many progeny, known as ganglion mother cells. Each GMC then generates a pair of neurons or glia (Fig. 1.8). The neuroblasts form from the neurogenic ectoderm in a highly stereotyped array (Fig. 1.22), and each neuroblast can be assigned a unique identity based on its position in the array, the expression of a particular pattern of genes, and the particular set of neurons and glia that they generate (Doe, 1992). The first neuroblasts to form are arranged in four rows along the anterior–posterior axis and in three columns along the mediolateral axis. The types of neurons and glia generated by a particular neuroblast depends on its position in the the array, and so each neuroblast is said to have a unique identity. The next waves of neuroblasts to form are also organized in rows and columns. The genes involved in controlling the identity of several of the neuroblasts have been identified and are discussed in Chapter 4. However, at this point we describe the mechanisms that control the segregation of the neuroblasts from the ectoderm.

One class of molecules that is intimately involved in the segregation of the neuroblasts from the other epidermal cells is a member of a family of transcription factors, known as the basic-helix-loop-helix (or bHLH) factors. The bHLH family of transcription factors contains both activators and repressors of transcription. Many of the various tissues in the animal have cell-type-specific activators of this class. For example, muscle cells contain several different "myogenic" bHLH proteins, each of which serves somewhat overlapping functions to activate muscle-specific genes at various points in the development of muscle. A similar set of bHLH genes, the *achaete scute* gene complex, is required for the segregation of the neuroblasts in *Drosophila*.

The *achaete scute* genes were identified for their effects on the development of the bristles, or chaete, on the fly, each of which contain a neuron that signals to the fly brain when stimulated. These genes are organized in a complex of four (*achaete, scute, asense,* and *lethal of scute*) at a single locus in *Drosophila* (Alonso and

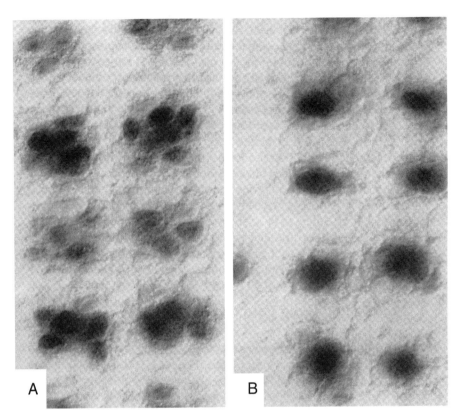

Figure 1.22 Neuroblast segregation in the *Drosophila* neurogenic region proceeds in a highly patterned array. Just prior to neuroblast delamination (A) a group of ectodermal cells expresses a proneural gene. One of the cells in this group maintains its expression of the proneural gene product, and that cell becomes the neuroblast (B). (From Doe, 1992, with permission.)

Cabrera, 1988). Deletion of this locus results in the absence of most of the neuroblasts in the fly, both in the central and peripheral nervous systems (Cabrera *et al.,* 1987), while animals with extra copies of these genes have ectopic neurons and sense organs (Campos-Ortega, 1998). Since these genes are required for the formation of neurons from the epidermal cells, they have been called the "proneural genes" (Fig. 1.23). An additional *achaete scute*-related gene, *atonal,* is a proneural gene for the internal chordotonal sensory organs and the eye (Jarman *et al.,* 1993).

How do the proneural genes function in neuroblast segregation? These genes, like other tissue-specific bHLH genes in other organs (Weintraub, 1993), activate transcription by binding to DNA at specific sites, known as E-boxes, with a palindromic consensus sequence of CANNTG. These cell-type-specific bHLH genes (otherwise known as class B) bind DNA as dimers; their dimer partners are similar but more ubiquitously expressed bHLH genes, known as class A. In *Drosophila,* the class A gene is called *daughterless* (Da), named for its role in the sex determination process (Caudy *et al.,* 1988). The dimerization occurs through one of the helices (Fig. 1.24), while the basic region is an extension of the other helix and interacts with the major groove of the DNA. The *achaete scute* transcription factors are thought to bind to E-boxes in the promoter regions of neuroblast-specific genes and activate their transcription to maintain that cell as a neuroblast. At this time

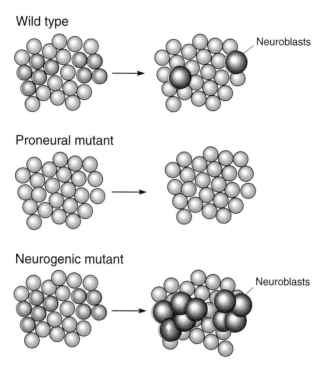

Wild type

Neuroblasts

Proneural mutant

Neurogenic mutant

Neuroblasts

Figure 1.23 Neurogenic genes and proneural genes were first identified in *Drosophila* due to their effects on neural development. In the wild type embryo, only one neuroblast delaminates from a given region of the ectoderm. However, in flys mutant for proneural genes, like *achaete scute,* no neuroblasts form. In contrast, in flys mutant for neurogenic genes, like *Notch* and *Delta,* many neuroblasts delaminate at the positions where only a single neuroblast is formed in the wild type animal. Thus, too many neurons form and these mutants are called "neurogenic."

only a few genes are known to be transcriptionally activated by the *achaete scute* genes (Singson *et al.,* 1994), and they all have a specific E-box in their upstream promoter region.

The process of neuroblast formation requires that a precise number of cells from the neurogenic region delaminate. Just prior to the delamination of the neuroblasts, *achaete* is expressed in a group of four to six epidermal cells (Skeath and Carroll, 1992). A combination of pair-rule genes and DV-patterning genes act on the promoter regions of the *achaete scute* genes to induce their expression in these regularly spaced clusters of cells along the neurogenic region (Skeath *et al.,* 1992). The four to six cells that express *achaete scute* are known as the proneural cluster (Fig. 1.22), and they all have the potential to form neuroblasts. Under normal cir-

cumstances, only a single cell from each cluster will delaminate as a neuroblast. The cell that delaminates to form the neuroblast continues to express the *achaete scute* proneural genes, while all of the other cells in the proneural cluster downregulate their expression of *achaete scute.*

In experiments designed to determine whether interactions among the cells were necessary for singling out one of the cells of the proneural cluster for delamination as the neuroblast, Taghert *et al.* (1984) used a laser microbeam to destroy the developing neuroblast at various times during its delamination (Fig. 1.25). They found that ablation of the delaminating neuroblast with a laser microbeam causes one of the other cells in the cluster to take its place and delaminate. These results led to the idea that the expression of *achaete scute* genes, and hence neuroblast

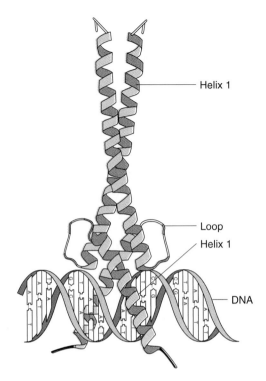

Helix 1

Loop
Helix 1

DNA

Figure 1.24 Several critical proteins that are necessary for the development of specific cell and tissue types are members of the bHLH transcription factor family of molecules. bHLH denotes the basic-helix-loop-helix structure of these molecules. The bHLH transcription factors dimerize via their first helix and interact with DNA via their second helix and their basic region.

potential, is regulated by a system of lateral inhibition. The cell that begins to delaminate maintains its *achaete scute* expression, and suppresses the proneural function in the other cells of the cluster. The other cells then remain as epidermal cells, while the *achaete scute*-expressing cell delaminates as the neuroblast.

The mechanisms by which the cell that ultimately develops as the neuroblast is singled out from the original cluster have been the subject of intensive investigation in recent years. Studies of this process have uncovered a unique signaling pathway that may underlie lateral inhibitory processes in many regions of the embryo. Molecules that figure prominently in this process are the *Notch* receptor and one of its ligands, Delta. *Notch* is a large transmembrane protein characterized by an extracellular portion with a large number of repetitive domains (36), known as

EGF-repeats because of their similarity to the cysteine-bonded tertiary structure of epidermal growth factor (EGF). However, despite this apparent structural similarity to an extended peptide mitogen, *Notch* has no apparent mitogenic activity, but rather act as a receptor for ligands with a somewhat similar structure, *Delta* and *Serrate* (Fehon *et al.,* 1990). These genes are expressed not only in the nervous system but also in many areas of the embryo where lateral inhibitory interactions are defining tissue boundaries. In fact, *Notch* and *Delta,* and the additional ligand *Serrate* were named for their effects on wing development, where lateral inhibition is also mediated by these genes and is necessary for the proper development of the wing morphology.

The *Notch/Delta* pathway is critical for singling out the neuroblast from the proneural clus-

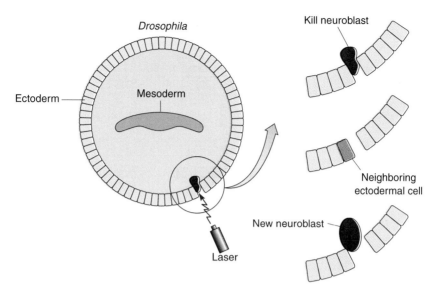

Figure 1.25 Ablation of the delaminating neuroblast with a laser microbeam directed at the ventral neurogenic region of the fly embryo causes a neighboring ectodermal cell to take its place. This experiment shows that the neuroblast inhibits neighboring cells from adopting the same fate via the mechanism of lateral inhibition.

ter and the fate of the cells in the neurogenic region depends on their level of *Notch* activity. Low *Notch* receptor activity in one of these cells causes them to become a neuroblast, while high activity results in the cell adopting an epidermal fate. In *Notch* null mutants, nearly all of the cells in the neurogenic region become neuroblasts. As a result the *Notch* null embryos have defects in the epidermis (Fig. 1.23). A similar phenotype occurs in Delta null mutants. Because of the phenotypes the mutant animals show, the *Notch* and *Delta* genes have been termed neurogenic, but activation of this system actually has the opposite effect and suppresses neuroblast formation.

One model for how the *Notch/Delta* signaling pathway mediates the lateral inhibitory interactions among the cells of the proneural cluster is shown in Fig. 1.26. Initially all of the *achaete scute*-expressing cells also express an equal amount of *Notch* and *Delta* (Hartley *et al.*, 1987; Hoppe and Greenspan, 1986). If by a stochastic process, the central cell in the proneural cluster expresses more *achaete scute* than the others, this cell will then concomitantly express a higher

level of *Delta* than the other cells of the cluster. When the *Delta* in the central cell activates *Notch* on the neighboring cells, it suppresses their *achaete scute* expression and further downregulates their *Delta* expression, preventing them from differentiation as a neuroblast. In this way only a single neuroblast develops from the proneural cluster at a particular location in the fly.

This model brings to mind several questions. First, how does *Notch* activation lead to the suppression of *achaete scute* in a neighboring cell? Second, what starts the central cell of the cluster down the path to increase its expression of *achaete scute*? In the past few years a considerable amount of effort has gone into working out the signal transduction cascade for the *Notch/Delta* signaling system and so a reasonable answer can now be given to the first question and this is described in detail below; however, the answer to the second question is still somewhat of a mystery.

The identification of the downstream signaling components of the *Notch* pathway took advantage of other *Drosophila* mutants as well

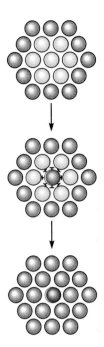

Figure 1.26 Just prior to the delamination of a neuroblast, a group of cells in the ectoderm express the proneural genes *achaete* and *scute* (light red); this group is the proneural cluster. Shortly after, one of the cells near the center (dark red) expresses a higher level of the proneural genes and through a process of lateral inhibition begins to block proneural gene expression in the cells around it. Finally, only this one cell is left expressing the proneural genes and it delaminates to form the neuroblast.

as of biochemical analysis of the homologous pathway in vertebrates. As described above, *Notch* is a transmembrane protein, with EGF repeats in the extracellular domain and a distinct intracellular domain, which contains a repeating motif known as cdc10/ankyrin repeats. The cdc10/ankyrin repeats in the intracellular domain of *Notch* are critical for signal transduction via this system. Mutations in *Notch* that delete the cdc10/ankyrin repeats in the intracellular domain block *Notch* signaling. Moreover, another neurogenic gene in *Drosophila, Supressor of hairless,* codes for a protein that binds to the cdc10/ankyrin repeats of *Notch* (Fortini and Artavanis-Tsakonas, 1994). A current hypothesis for how signal transduction works in this system is as follows (Fig. 1.27). When *Notch* is not bound to *Delta, supressor of hairless* (SuH) is tethered to the cytoplasm, bound to the cdc10/

ankyrin repeats of *Notch*. The activation of *Notch* by binding to *Delta* causes SuH to be released from *Notch*. SuH can then be translocated to the nucleus where it acts as a transcriptional activator at genes with a specific sequence in their promoters.

The genes activated by SuH should suppress neuroblast formation, since *Notch* activation in the epidermal cells prevents them from delamination. This expectation has been confirmed by the demonstration that SuH directly regulates the transcription of another class of bHLH proteins, the *enhancer of split* complex (E(spl)) of genes. The E(spl) proteins are similar to the proneural bHLH proteins of the *achaete scute* class, but instead of acting as transcriptional activators they are strong repressors of transcription. There are seven E(spl) genes in *Drosophila,* and their expression patterns overlap

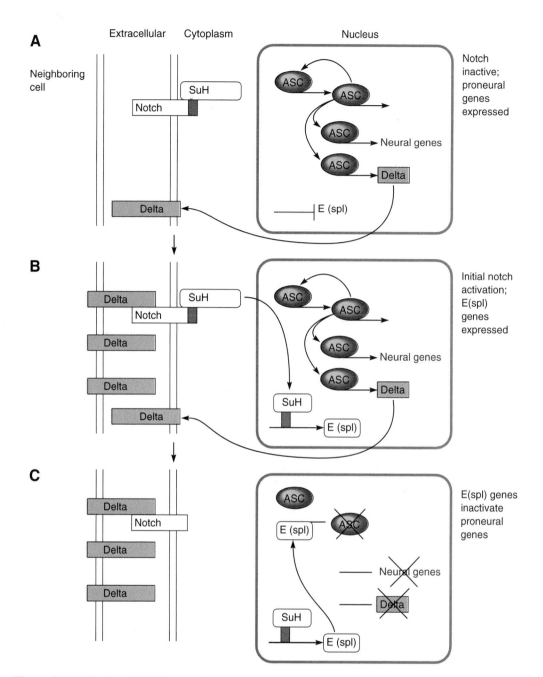

Figure 1.27 The lateral inhibitory mechanism involves the neurogenic genes *Notch* and *Delta*. In (A), a cell expresses *achaete scute* genes (ASC) and *Notch* is inactive. The ASC activates its own transcription to maintain its expression and also activates the expression of downstream neural-specific genes and the *Notch* ligand *Delta*. This cell would then become a neuroblast; however, if a neighboring cell expresses more *Delta* (B), this activates the *Notch* pathway in the first cell. The activated *Notch* leads to a release of *Suppressor of hairless* (SuH) which along with part of the intracellular domain of *Notch* diffuses to the nucleus and acts as a transcription factor on another gene's promoter, the *enhancer of split* complex (E(spl)) (C). The E(spl) proteins are repressors of ASC gene transcription and so they block further neural differentiation and reduce the levels of *Delta* expression. Thus, this cell is suppressed from the neural fate because of *Notch* activation by a neighboring cell that expressed more *Delta*.

considerably, so they are thought to be at least partly redundant. The proteins coded by these genes form heterodimers with the *achaete scute* proteins through their dimerization domains, but they can also form homodimers. The E(spl) proteins may directly interfere with *achaete scute*-mediated transcription, and in addition these proteins bind to nearby sites on the promoter and recruit additional repressor proteins, such as groucho. As might be expected by their function as transcriptional repressors, the E(spl) genes are expressed in the cells surrounding the delaminating neuroblast, and they act to prevent cells from adopting the neural fate.

E(spl) proteins can be added to the mechanism of *Notch/Delta* lateral inhibition in the following way (Fig. 1.27) (Bailey and Posakony, 1995). As described above, *Notch* activation by *Delta* causes the SuH translocation to the nucleus. Specific sequences in the promoters of E(spl) genes bind the SuH protein resulting in the expression of E(spl) in these cells. The E(spl) proteins bind to the E-boxes in the *achaete scute* promoter and repress transcription. Therefore, the amount of *achaete scute* protein in the cells with active *Notch* declines and the cell loses its potential to delaminate as a neuroblast. In addition, since *Delta* expression is activated by *achaete scute* genes, the reduction in the expression of *achaete scute* in the cells with activated *Notch* also results in a reduction of *Delta* expression in the same cells. Thus, the *Notch/Delta* pathway provides a negative feedback pathway for neuroblast formation and a molecular mechanism for lateral inhibitory interactions among cells.

Virtually all of the molecules described in the segregation of neuroblasts in the *Drosophila* have vertebrate homologs that are required for similar roles in the vertebrate. The *Notch/Delta* signaling pathway is one of the fundamental mechanisms by which neighboring cells become different in metazoans. Throughout development, there are numerous examples of cells with a common lineage differentiating into different cell types. It is likely that *Notch/Delta* signaling functions in most, if not all, of these cases.

Notch/Delta/Achaete Scute Genes in Vertebrates

Vertebrate homologs to the *achaete scute* genes have been identified in several species. Mammalian, chicken, *Xenopus,* and fish all have a similar gene, named *Mash1, Cash1, Xash1,* or *Zash1.* These genes are expressed in the developing nervous system in distinct subsets of neural progenitor cells. These genes have the same bHLH structure as the *Drosophila achaete scute* genes and can act as transcriptional activators when heterodimerized with the vertebrate daughterless homologs E12 and E47. These correlative data have all supported a role for *achaete scute*-like genes in the vertebrate that may be analogous to that in the *Drosophila.* In addition, similar genes have been identified in *C.elegans* and even Cnidarians, and so this seems to be a very ancient system for the segregation of neuroblasts from the epidermis.

Do the ash genes control the segregation of the neurectoderm from the epidermis in vertebrates? There is some evidence that these genes are critical to the process of neural plate formation in *Xenopus.* To test this possibility, Turner and Weintraub (1993) overexpressed *Xash1* in one half of the *Xenopus* embryo by injection of RNA coding for *Xash1* into one cell at the 2-cell stage. They found that the resulting embryos had a much larger neural plate on the injected side. The larger neural plate arose in these animals at the expense of the epidermis, just as an overexpression of *achaete scute* gene in *Drosophila* causes ectopic neuroblasts. Similar experiments with other vertebrate proneural bHLH genes have produced even more dramatic results. Figure 1.28 shows the results of overexpression of a bHLH gene called NeuroD, in which ectodermal cells are converted to neurons all over the lateral skin of the embryo. More recent experiments in mice by David Anderson and François Guillimont, and their colleagues, have shown that deletion of the genes for two other proneural bHLH genes, neurogenin1 and neurogenin2, block the development of the crainial ganglia neurons. Therefore, in verte-

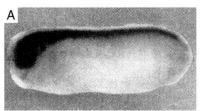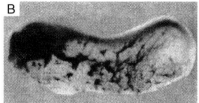

Figure 1.28 Experimental overexpression of NeuroD, a vertebrate proneural bHLH gene, in a frog embryo causes neurons to form throughout the lateral epidermis. Neurons are stained in both control (A) and experimental (B) with the neural specific protein N-CAM. (Reprinted with permission from Lee *et al.,* Conversion of Xenopus ectoderm into neurons by NeuroD, a basic helix–loop–helix protein. *Science* **268:** 836–844. Copyright 1995 American Association for the Advancement of Science.)

brates, proneural bHLH transcription factors appear to have a very similar role in the formation of neurons as their counterparts in *Drosophila.* (Fode *et al.,* 1998, Mae *et al.,* 1998)

What about the system of lateral inhibition, *Notch* and *Delta*? Here the vertebrate nervous system appears to be somewhat different from that of the fly. Instead of a single *Notch* receptor, vertebrates have at least four *Notch* genes, three of which are expressed in parts of the developing nervous system. In addition, vertebrates also have several ligands for *Notch* receptors, including two *Delta* genes and two *Serrate*-like genes, also known as jagged in mammals. *Notch1* may play a role in the cell fate decisions delimiting the lateral extent of the neural plate. Injections of mRNA for an activated form of *Notch* into the *Xenopus* embryo at the 2-cell stage, similar to that described for *Xash1,* causes the nervous system to expand on the injected side. Thus, it appears that *Notch* is important for the lateral interactions that define the boundary of the neural plate, but the result is contrary to that which would be expected. Active *Notch* in the fly

prevents neuroblast segregation, while in the *Xenopus* it expands the neural plate at the expense of ectoderm. Although these results seem contradictory, as is described later, *Notch/Delta*-mediated interactions are important in the differentiation of neurons from the neuroblast/progenitor cells as well as in the initial segregation process from the epidermis, and part of the explanation of the *Xenopus* results may lie in this later function of *Notch.*

Overall the data from the various experimental systems has revealed a common set of molecular mechanisms for the early development of the nervous system. Multiple interacting and partly overlapping mechanisms have been discovered, and while some species appear to have a greater reliance on particular molecular pathways than others, a rather gratifying picture is emerging of both neural induction and the initial stages of neural differentiation. The next challenge will be to analyze the interactions among these various molecular pathways for a full understanding of how the diversity of nervous systems arises.

Polarity and Regionalization

·   ·   ·   ·   ·

Regional Identity of the Nervous System

Like the rest of the body in most metazoans, the nervous system is regionally specialized. The head looks different from the tail, and the brain looks different from the spinal cord. There are a number of basic body plans for animals with neurons, and in this section we consider how the regional specialization of the nervous systems arises during the development of some these animals. At least some of the mechanisms that pattern the nervous system of an animal are the same as those that pattern the rest of an animal's body. Likewise, many different types of tissues play key roles in regulating the development of the nervous system.

In the vertebrate embryo, most of the neural tube gives rise to the spinal cord, while the rostral end enlarges to form the three primary brain vesicles: the prosencephalon (or forebrain), the mesencephalon (or midbrain), and the rhombencephalon (or hindbrain) (Fig. 2.1). The prosencephalon gives rise to the large paired cerebral hemispheres, the mesencephalon gives rise to the midbrain, and the rhombencephalon gives rise to the more caudal regions of the brain stem. The three primary brain vesicles become further subdivided into five vesicles. The prosencephalon gives rise to both the telencephalon and the diencephalon. In addition to generating the thalamus and the hypothalamus in the mature brain, an important feature of the diencephalon is the paired evaginations of the optic vesicles. These develop into the retina and pigmented epithelial layers of the eyes. The mesencephalon remains as a single vesicle and does not expand to the same extent as the other regions of the brain. The rhombencephalon divides into the metencephalon and the myelencephalon. These two vesicles will form the cerebellum and the medulla, respectively.

The most caudal brain region is the rhombencephalon, the region that will go on to develop into the hindbrain. At a particular time in the development of this part of the brain, the rhombencephalon becomes divided into segments known as rhombomeres (see below). The rhombomeres are defined as regularly spaced

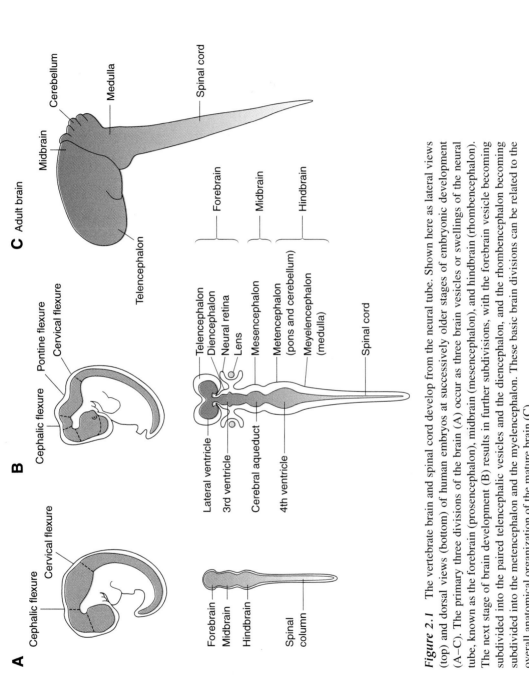

Figure 2.1 The vertebrate brain and spinal cord develop from the neural tube. Shown here as lateral views (top) and dorsal views (bottom) of human embryos at successively older stages of embryonic development (A–C). The primary three divisions of the brain (A) occur as three brain vesicles or swellings of the neural tube, known as the forebrain (prosencephalon), midbrain (mesencephalon), and hindbrain (rhombencephalon). The next stage of brain development (B) results in further subdivisions, with the forebrain vesicle becoming subdivided into the paired telencephalic vesicles and the diencephalon, and the rhombencephalon becoming subdivided into the metencephalon and the myelencephalon. These basic brain divisions can be related to the overall anatomical organization of the mature brain (C).

repeating units of hindbrain cells and are separated by distinct boundaries. Since this is one of the clearest areas of segmentation in the vertebrate brain, the study of the genes that control segmentation in rhombomeres has received a lot of attention and is discussed in detail in the next section as a model of how the anterior–posterior patterning of the nervous system takes place in vertebrates.

The insect nervous system is made up of a series of connected ganglia known as the ventral nerve cord. In many insects, the ganglia fuse at the midline. The segmental ganglia of the ventral nerve cord are not all identical, but rather vary from anterior to posterior in the number and types of neurons they contain. The insect brain is composed of three regions known as the pro-

tocerebrum, the deutocerebrum, and the tritocerebrum (Fig. 2.2). The compound eyes connect through the optic lobes to the rest of the brain. Thus, like in the vertebrate, there are quite distinct regional differences along the anterior–posterior axis of the insect nervous system, and so there must be mechanisms that make one part of the nervous system different from another part.

The Anterior–Posterior Axis and Hox Genes

In both vertebrates and invertebrates, the mechanisms that control the regional development of the nervous system are dependent on the

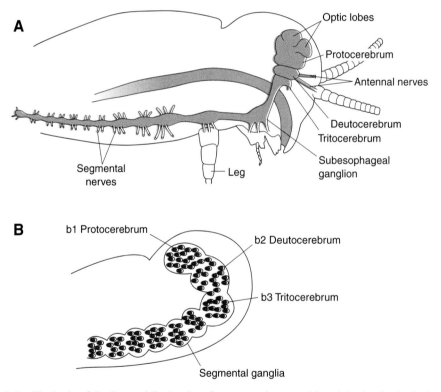

Figure 2.2 The brain of the *Drosophila* develops from extensive neuroblast delamination in the head. The adult is shown in (A) and the embryo is shown in (B). Three basic divisions of the brain are known as the protocerebrum, the deutocerebrum, and the tritocerebrum. These divisions are similar to the segmental ganglia, in that they are derived independently from delaminating neuroblasts in their respective head segments. However, they later fuse together and along with the optic lobes form a complex network.

mechanisms that initially set up the anterior–posterior axis of the embryo. Much more is known about these mechanisms in the *Drosophila* embryo, and so is described first; however, it appears that many of the same genes are involved in the specification of the anterior–posterior axis in the vertebrate.

The anterior–posterior axis of the fly is primarily set up by the distribution of two molecules: a transcription factor known as bicoid and a RNA-binding protein called Nanos, localized primarily to the posterior pole of the embryo (Driever and Nusslein-Volhard, 1988). The mRNAs for these genes are localized in their distribution in the egg prior to fertilization by the nurse cells in the mother. Shortly after fertilization, these mRNAs are translated, resulting in opposing protein gradients of the two gene products (Fig. 2.3).

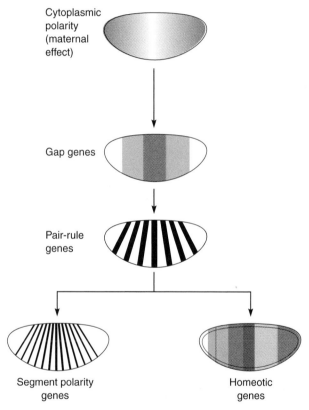

Cytoplasmic polarity (maternal effect)

Gap genes

Pair-rule genes

Segment polarity genes

Homeotic genes

Figure 2.3 The unique positional identity of the segments in *Drosophila* is derived by a program of molecular steps, each of which progressively subdivides the embryo into smaller and smaller domains of expression. The oocyte has two opposing gradients of mRNA for the maternal effect genes: bicoid and hunchback are localized to the anterior half, while *caudal* and *Nanos* messages are localized to the posterior regions. The maternal effect gene products regulate the expression of the gap genes, the next set of key transcriptional regulators, which are more spatially restricted in their expression. *Orthodenticle* (otd), for example, is a gap gene that is only expressed at the very high concentrations of bicoid present in the prospective head of the embryo. Specific combinations of the gap gene products in turn activate the transcription of the pair-rule genes, each of which is only expressed in a region of the embryo about two segments wide. The periodic pattern of the pair-rule gene expression is directly controlled by the gap genes, and along with a second set of periodically expressed genes, the segment polarity genes determine the specific expression pattern of the homeotic genes. In this way, each segment develops a unique identity.

The levels of these two proteins determine whether a second set of genes, the gap genes, are expressed in a particular region of the embryo. The gap genes, in turn, control the striped pattern of a third set of genes, the pair-rule genes. Finally, the pattern of expression of the pair-rule genes controls the segment-specific expression of the fourth set of genes, the segment polarity genes. This developmental hierarchy progressively divides the embryo into smaller and smaller domains with unique identities (Small and Levine, 1991; Driever and Nusslein-Volhard, 1988). This chain of transcriptional activations generates a stereotypic pattern of segmentation in each animal (Fig. 2.3).

At this point in the development of the fly, the anterior–posterior axis is clearly defined and the embryo is parceled up into domains of gene expression that correspond to the different segments of the animal. The next step in the development of the fly requires a set of genes that will uniquely specify each segment as different from one another. The genes that control the relative identity of the different parts of *Drosophila* were discovered by Edward Lewis (1978). He found mutants of the fly that had two pairs of wings instead of the usual single pair. In normal flies, wings form only on the second thoracic segment;

however, in flies with a mutation in the ultrabithorax gene, another pair of wings forms on the third thoracic segment. These mutations transformed the third segment into another second segment. Mutations in another one of these homeotic genes, *Antennapedia,* cause the transformation of a leg into an another antenna. Elimination of all of the *Hox* genes such as the example shown in Figure 2.4 in the beetle, *Tribolium,* results in an animal in which all of the parts of the animal look identical (Stuart *et al.,* 1991). The analysis of many different types of mutations in this complex have led to the conclusion that in insects the homeotic genes are necessary for a given part of the animal to become morphologically different from another part.

The homeobox genes in *Drosophila* are arranged in a linear array on the chromosome in the order of their expression along the anterior–posterior axis of the animal (Fig. 2.5). A total of eight genes are organized on the chromosome as two complexes, the *Antennapaedia* (ANT-C) and the *Bithorax* (BX-C) clusters (Duboule and Morata, 1994; Gehring, 1993). The *Hox* genes code for proteins of the homeodomain class of transcription factors, and the *Hox* genes were the original members of this very large set of related molecules. All of the *Hox* proteins have a se-

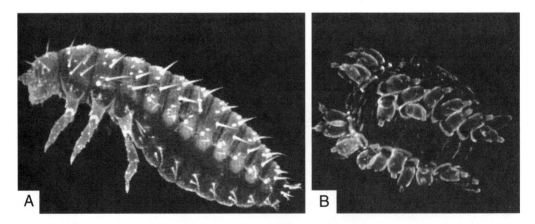

Figure 2.4   Elimination of the *Hox* gene cluster in the *Tribolium* beetle results in all segments developing an identical morphology. (A) Normal appearance of the beetle. (B) An animal without a *Hox* gene cluster. The normal number of segments develop, but all of the segments acquire the morphology of the antennal segment, showing the importance of the *Hox* genes in the development of positional identity in animals. (From Stuart *et al.,* reprinted by permission from *Nature* **350:** 72–74, Copyright 1991 Macmillan Magazines Ltd.)

quence of approximately 60 amino acids that are well conserved among them, and they all bind to a consensus sequence of DNA in the promoters of many other genes, known as the homeobox (Gehring, 1993; Biggin and McGinnis, 1997).

How do these genes control segmental identity in *Drosophila*? A good example is the mechanism by which the BX-C genes control abdominal segment identity. Insects have three pairs of legs, one on each of the thoracic segments, but none on the abdominal segments. The products of the BX-C gene complex are responsible for suppressing the formation of legs on the abdominal segments by the repression of a key regulatory gene necessary for leg formation, the *distal-less* gene. Although this kind of simple regulatory

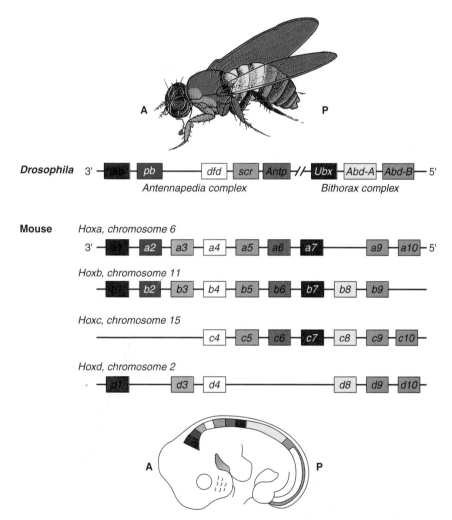

Figure 2.5 *Hox* gene clusters in arthropods (*Drosophila*) and vertebrates (mouse embryo) have a similar spatial organization and similar order along the chromosomes. In *Drosophila*, the *Hox* gene cluster is aligned on the chromosome such that the anterior-most expressed gene is 3', and the posterior-most gene is 5'. In the mouse, there are four separate *Hox* gene clusters on four different chromosomes, but the overall order is similar to that in arthropods: the anterior to posterior order of gene expression is ordered in a 3' to 5' order on the chromosomes.

interaction occurs for some aspects of segmental identity, the *Hox* gene products bind to a rather short core DNA sequence of just four bases, and there are likely to be many genes that contain the sequence in their promoters and thus be potentially regulated by *Hox* genes. In fact, any change in the morphology of a particular segment is likely to require the coordinated activation and suppression of numerous genes. For example, it has been estimated that between 85 and 170 genes are likely regulated by the *Ubx* gene (Gerhart and Kirschner, 1997).

Another striking feature about the *Hox* genes is their remarkable degree of conservation throughout the phyla. Organized *Hox* clusters similar to those found in *Drosophila* have been identified in nearly all the major classes of animals, including Cnidarians, nematodes, arthropods, annelids, and chordates. Figure 2.5 shows the relationship between the *Drosophila Hox* genes and those of the mouse. There have been two duplications of the ancestral *Hox* clusters to produce the A, B, C, and D complexes. In addition, there have also been many duplications of individual members of the cluster to produce the 13 members of each complex. In mammalian embryos, the *Hox* genes are expressed in specific domains. As in *Drosophila,* the *Hox* gene position on the chromosome is correlated with its expression along the anterior–posterior axis. By aligning the mammalian *Hox* genes with their *Drosophila* counterparts, it is possible to infer the organization of the *Hox* clusters in the common ancestor between the phyla.

Hox Gene Function

To determine whether the *Hox* genes of vertebrates control the identity of the different regions of the body in a manner analogous to *Drosophila,* several experimental manipulations of these genes have been carried out in mice. To eliminate the function of a single gene, an inactivated copy of the gene is exchanged for the good copy, producing experimental animals that have come to be known as "knockout" mice (Thomas and Capecchi, 1986). In one method, a gene for neomycin resistance is inserted into the gene of interest, thus inactivating it (Fig. 2.6). Embryonic stem (ES) cells are then cultured with copies of the mutated DNA, and some of the cells incorporate it through homologous recombination. By adding neomycin to the culture, one selects for ES cells that contain the mutated DNA, including the neomycin resistance gene. The ES cells are then injected into a mouse blastocyst and implanted in an adult female. The offspring are chimeric animals. That is, only some of their cells derive from the ES cells that were injected into the blastocyst. The animals that have one copy of the mutated DNA in their germ cells are bred to control animals, producing heterozygote carriers. Finally, heterozygotes are bred to one another to obtain homozygotes.

Some of the most dramatic initial phenotypic changes that were identified as a result of *Hox* gene deletion were found in tissues outside the nervous system. This was expected since these genes are expressed in nonneural cells in a

---

Figure 2.6   The production of knockout mice by gene targeting has allowed for the generation of specific gene deletions. The gene of interest is first inactivated by inserting a sequence for neomycin resistance (for selection of the mutants) into the coding sequence. The mutant gene is then transfected into embryonic stem cells (ES cells) from the inner cell mass of a mouse embryo, and those ES cells that contain the mutant gene (and hence the neomycin resistance gene) will survive when the cells are cultured in a medium that contains the neomycin antibiotic. The ES cells containing the mutant gene are then injected into a blastocyst of another embryo, and, remarkably, the ES cells contribute to the tissues of the embryo. Thus, many of the cells in the resulting "chimeric" mouse will contain a mutant version of the gene of interest. Some of the chimeric animals will have a copy of the mutant gene in the germline cells, and these animals can be bred to generate heterozygous carriers of the defective gene (light red). When the mice that are heterozygous for the mutant gene are then bred together, a quarter of their embryos will have both alleles of the gene of interest (dark red). Therefore the phenotype of these animals will show the affect of eliminating the gene.

Inactivate gene by inserting the neomycin resistence gene

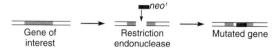

Gene of interest → Restriction endonuclease → Mutated gene

Culture embryonic stem cells

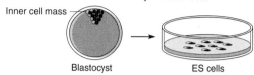

Inner cell mass

Blastocyst   ES cells

Electroporation and homologous recombination

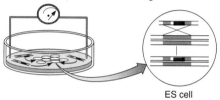

ES cell

Select for neomycin resistance and inject heterozygotic ES cells

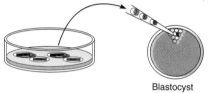

Blastocyst

Inject blastocyst and obtain chimeric offspring

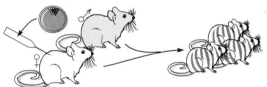

Breed chimeric to wild type

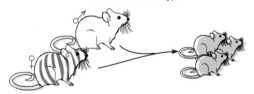

Breed heterozygotes

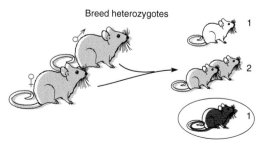

particular region of the body, not just in the neural cells. There is normally a graduated expression of the members of the *Hox4* group in the cervical vertebrae. The second cervical vertebra, has a bony protrusion from the posterior pole. In the *Hox4* knockout animals, more caudal vertebrae partly take on this morphology. Thus, the *Hox* genes are critical for the development of regional differences in the vertebrae. In addition to these effects on the vertebrae, deletion of *Hox* genes also has effects on many other regions of the body. For example the major blood vessels in the neck are also malformed in the animals with deletions in the *Hox4* group genes. Therefore, these genes can be thought of as important in defining the region of the animal's body throughout all of the various tissues.

The nervous system, like the rest of the body, requires the *Hox* genes for the regional differences in the neurons and glial cells. The function of the *Hox* genes in controlling the regional identity of the vertebrate nervous system has been most clearly investigated in the hindbrain. The vertebrate hindbrain provides the innervation for the muscles of the head through a set of cranial nerves. Like the spinal nerves that innervate the rest of the body, some of the cranial nerves contain axons from motor neurons located in the hindbrain, as well as sensory axons from neurons in the dorsal root ganglia. However, we will primarily be concerned with the motor neurons for the time being. The cranial nerves of an embryo are shown in Fig. 2.7. During embryonic development, the hindbrain undergoes a pattern of segment formation that bears some resemblance to that of *Drosophila*. These segments are called rhombomeres (Fig. 2.7) and relate to a segmentally repeated pattern of differentiation of intrinsic "reticular" neurons and the motor neurons that project into the cranial nerves (Lumsden and Keynes, 1989). The reticular neurons can be classified into eight different types, and each rhombomere contains a complete set. The motor neurons are grouped into three classes: somatic motor neurons that innervate the muscles of the eye, visceral or branchiomotor neurons that innervate the mus-

cles derived from the branchial arches (including most of the muscles of the head and neck aside from the eye muscles), and vestibulocochlear motor neurons that innervate the hair cells of the hearing and balance organs. The figure shows how these different classes of motor neurons correspond to the different rhombomeres and give each rhombomere a specific segmental identity. The trigeminal nerve collects axons from motor nerve nuclei in r1, r2, and r3 and innervates the first branchial arch (2.7). The facial nerve contains the axons of motoneurons from nuclei in r4 and r5 and innervates the second branchial arch. The glossopharyngeal nerve contains axons from r6 which innervate the third branchial arch (Clarke and Lumsden, 1993).

The pattern of expression of the hox genes coincides with the rhombomere boundaries (Fig. 2.7) and in fact the expression of these genes precedes the formation of obvious morphological rhombomeric boundaries. *Hox1* through *Hox4* genes are expressed in the rhombomeres. *Hox* genes of the number 4 class are expressed up to the anterior boundary of the 7th rhombomere, *Hox* genes of the number 3 class are expressed up to and including rhombomere 5, and Hox genes of the number 2 class are primarily expressed up to and including rhombomere 3. These patterns are comparable in birds and mammals. As discussed below, loss of a single *Hox* gene in mice usually does not produce the sort of dramatic phenotypes seen in *Drosophila*. This is probably because of overlapping patterns of Hox gene expression from members of the four families, called paralogous groups. When two or more members of a paralogous group are deleted, say *Hoxa4* and *Hoxb4*, then the severity of the deficits increase. The deficits that are observed are consistent with the *Hox* genes acting similarly to their functions in arthropods. That is, they control the relative identity of a region of the body.

As noted above, the studies of *Hox* genes in neural development have concentrated on the hindbrain. Several studies have either deleted specific *Hox* genes or misexpressed them in other regions of the CNS and examined the effect on hindbrain development; we give only a

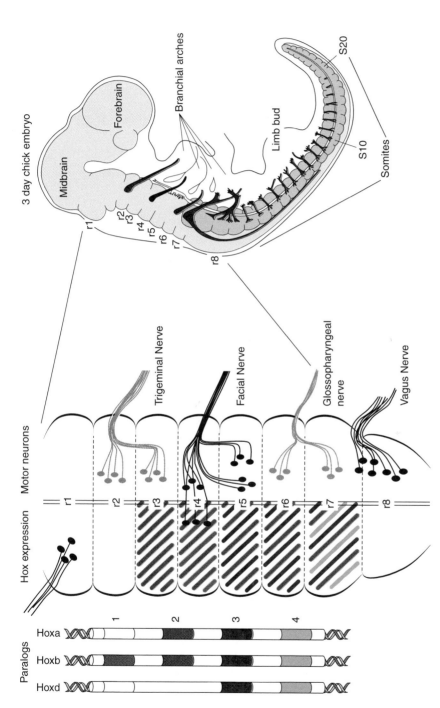

Figure 2.7 Rhombomeres are repeated morphological subdivisions of the hindbrain. The rhombomeres are numbered from the anterior-most unit, r1, just posterior to the midbrain (mesencephalon), to the posterior-most unit, r7, at the junction of the hindbrain with the spinal cord. The members of the *Hox* gene cluster are expressed in a 3′ to 5′ order in the rhombomeres. The segmentation in this region of the embryo is also observed in the cranial nerves, and the motoneurons send their axons through defined points at alternating rhombomeres.

few examples. Deletion of the *Hoxa1* gene in mice causes the fusion of r5 and r6 and a reduction of r4; these are the most anterior rhombomeres with expression of this gene (Figs. 2.7 and 2.8). The motor nerve nuclei that normally develop from r4 and r5, such as the neurons innervating the extraocular muscles, are largely missing. In addition, other neurons that form brain structures in this region of the hindbrain, such as the superior olivary complex, are also completely missing.

Are these defects due to a failure of the rhombomeres to form or do they result from massive cell death? To answer this question, the expression of a rhombomere 4/5-specific gene known as *Krox20* was studied in the *Hoxa1* mutants; *Hoxa1* null mice apparently never contain rhombomeres that express this *Krox20*. Although slightly larger, the adjacent rhombomeres are not twice their normal size, which would occur if the loss of *Hoxa1* caused a posterior transformation of the segmental identity of the rhombomeres, as is the case in *Drosophila*. Therefore, it appears that in the vertebrate CNS the *Hox* genes are important for the initial formation of segment founder cells. When a *Hox* gene is eliminated, the cells fail to progress in their developmental program, rather than being transformed to a different segment. In addition to these defects on r5, the *Hoxa1* knockout also shows changes in the motoneurons of the facial nucleus (Fig. 2.8). When the neurons of this nucleus are labeled with the application of a retrogradely transported dye to the nerve, the pattern of neurons can be easily visualized. The normal and knockout patterns are shown in the figure. The number of facial motoneurons is reduced in the knockout animals, and the axons of the motoneurons fail to converge to a single exit point from r4.

In other *Hox* knockout animals, while there may be no clear abnormalities in the initial patterning of the rhombomeres, examination of the

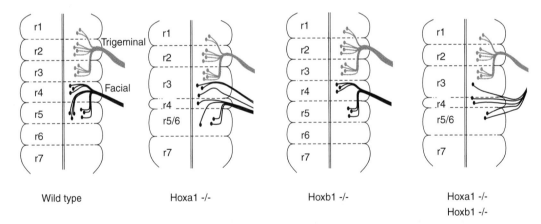

Wild type   Hoxa1 -/-   Hoxb1 -/-   Hoxa1 -/-
                                                         Hoxb1 -/-

Figure 2.8 Rhombomere identity is determined by the *Hox* code. *Hox* gene knockouts in mice affect the development of specific rhombomeres. Wild type animals have a stereotypic pattern of motoneurons in the hindbrain. The trigeminal (V) cranial nerve motoneurons exit from r2, while the facial nerve motoneurons exit from r4. Deletion of the *Hoxa1* gene in mice causes the fusion of r5 and r6 and a reduction of r4. The number of facial motoneurons is reduced in the knockout animals, and the axons of the motoneurons fail to converge to a single exit point from r4. The *Hoxb1* -/- mice also have some abnormalities in rhombomere development, though these changes are more subtle. While r4 appears basically normal in the *Hoxb1* knockout animals, these mice lack some of the facial motor neurons. Some fraction of the facial motoneurons are generated in r4 and then migrate caudally to r5. The *Hoxb1* knockout animals lack the facial motor neurons that are generated normally in r4. Double-mutant animals, of both *Hoxb1* and *Hoxa1,* show a combined, more severe defect, where nearly all of the facial motoneurons are lost.

nervous system at later stages of development can reveal specific defects. For example, *Hoxb1* -/- mice display no abnormalities in the initial formation of r4, where *Hoxb1* is specifically expressed. *Krox20*, which is expressed in both r3 and r5, is also normal in the mutants, and *sek2* (expressed specifically in r4) is also normal in the knockout animals. However, there is a very important defect in the mice: they lack the facial motor neurons that are normally derived from r4. Many of the facial motoneurons are generated in r4 and then some of these migrate caudally to r5. In the *Hoxb1* knockout animals, the facial motor neurons are generated normally; however, they fail to migrate caudally to r5 and the neurons subsequently die (Fig. 2.8). The failure of caudal migration in the mutants may be due to a failure of the cells to "recognize" their position and perhaps can be explained by changes in the expression of genes necessary for the normal patterns of cell migration.

Thus the deletion of two different members of the paralogous groups have different phenotypes. In one sense one can think of the members of the paralogous groups as contributing somewhat different aspects of the positional identity of a given segment of the brain. In addition, more recent double-knockout animals have been generated that lack both *Hoxb1* and *Hoxa1*. These animals display even more defects than would be expected by the simple addition of the two. In the double-knockout animals, there are many fewer facial motoneurons than in either of the single-knockout animals (Fig. 2.8) (Gavalas *et al.*, 1998).

In summary, *Hox* genes are important in establishing and maintaining the regional identity of cells and tissues along the anterior–posterior axis of vertebrates throughout the hindbrain and likely the spinal cord. There are up to four members of each paralogous group and these appear to be partly redundant, though not completely interchangeable. They control many aspects of the development of the regional identity of the hindbrain, particularly the rhombomeres, and thus they can influence and control the many different processes that are required for the production, migration, differentiation, and survival of the particular types of neurons and glia characteristic of a particular CNS region.

Signaling Molecules That Pattern the Anterior–Posterior Axis in Vertebrates

In *Drosophila*, the transcriptional regulators expressed just prior to the *Hox* genes are necessary and sufficient to restrict their domains of expression, and hence the identity of each segment. In vertebrates, it is not at all clear what controls the expression of the *Hox* genes, making it difficult to determine what factors are responsible for controlling the anterior–posterior axis of the nervous system. However, two candidate molecules have been identified that probably play a role in anterior–posterior patterning. Although these two factors are discussed below, it is likely that key elements of the mechanisms have yet to be found.

One way to determine how the anterior–posterior axis of the nervous system arises is to identify the genes that regulate the precise pattern of *Hox* gene expression. There are four known types of transcription factors that have been shown to directly regulate *Hox* gene expression in the vertebrate embryo: retinoic acid receptors, *Krox20*, members of the Pbx/exd family, and the *Hox* genes themselves. Of particular interest are the retinoic acid receptors, since it has been known for some time that retinoic acid (RA) has powerful teratogenic affects during embryogenesis (i.e., causing malformations). RA crosses the cell membrane to bind a cytoplasmic receptor (Fig. 2.9). The retinoic acid receptor (RAR) translocates into the nucleus where it can regulate gene expression through interaction with retinoic acid response element (RARE). Normally, RA levels are about 10 times higher in the posterior region of *Xenopus* embryos, and RA-treated embryos typically show defects in the anterior parts of the nervous system. In experiments where embryos are exposed to increasing concentrations of RA, they fail to develop head structures (Fig. 2.9) and the

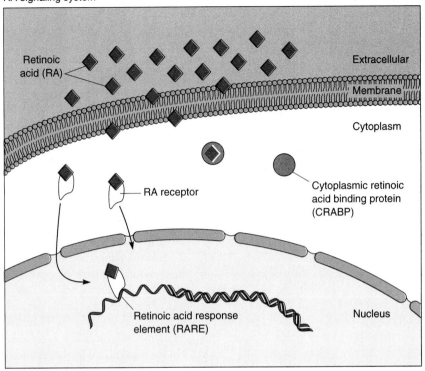

RA signaling system

Retinoic acid (RA)

Extracellular

Membrane

Cytoplasm

RA receptor

Cytoplasmic retinoic acid binding protein (CRABP)

Retinoic acid response element (RARE)

Nucleus

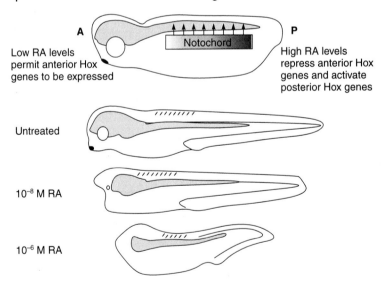

RA in posterior mesoderm at neurula stage

A

Notochord

P

Low RA levels permit anterior Hox genes to be expressed

High RA levels repress anterior Hox genes and activate posterior Hox genes

Untreated

10^{-8} M RA

10^{-6} M RA

Figure 2.9 Retinoic acid signaling is important for the anterior–posterior pattern of *Hox* gene expression. RA crosses the cell membrane to bind to a cytoplasmic receptor. The retinoic acid receptor (RAR) translocates into the nucleus where it can regulate gene expression through interaction with retinoic acid response element (RARE). RA levels are about 10 times higher in the posterior region of *Xenopus* embryos, and RA-treated embryos typically show defects in the anterior parts of the nervous system. When embryos are exposed to increasing concentrations of RA, they fail to develop head structures and the expression of anterior genes is inhibited.

expression of anterior genes is inhibited (Durston *et al.,* 1989).

Do the teratogenic affects of RA have anything to do with the control of regional identity in the CNS? In fact, it has been known for some time that retinoic acid can induce the expression of *Hox* genes when added to embryonic stem cells. With low concentrations of RA added to the ES cells, only those *Hox* genes normally expressed in the anterior embryo are expressed, while at progressively higher concentrations of RA more posteriorly expressed *Hox* genes are expressed in the cell line (Simeone *et al.,* 1991). Targeted deletion of the RARs produces defects similar to those observed from pharmacological manipulation of this pathway (Chambon, 1996). Finally, both the *Hoxa1* and the *Hoxb1* promoters have RAREs, and these elements are both necessary and to some extent sufficient for the rhombomere-specific pattern of expression of these genes (Marshall *et al.,* 1992, 1994; Sruder *et al.,* 1994.).

The results obtained with RA fit nicely into a popular model of neural patterning known as the activator–transformer hypothesis. Experiments in frog embryos have long suggested that the anterior nervous system is the "default" state of the nervous tissue induced by the organizer. This conclusion was initially based on a classic experiment by Nieuwkoop (see Chapter 1). He transplanted small pieces of ectodermal tissue from one embryo into a host at various positions along the anterior–posterior axis. In all cases, the transplanted cells developed anterior neural structures. However, when the cells were transplanted in the caudal neural plate, posterior structures, such as the spinal cord, also developed. Therefore, the initial signal provided by the organizer, known as the "activator," causes ectodermal cells to develop anterior characteristics. A second signal, known as the "transformer," is required to transform a portion of this neural tissue into hindbrain and spinal cord. Consistent with this idea, the neural inducers that have been identified (e.g., noggin, chordin, follistatin) produce primarily anterior brain structures when added to animal caps (see Chapter 1).

Thus the following model has been proposed to bring all of these facts together: First,

the neural inducers enable anterior neural tissue to form in the ectoderm by blocking the BMP signaling. Then, a gradient of RA from the caudal pole of the embryo acts as the transformer to promote more posterior *Hox* gene expression in progressively more posterior positions in the embryo.

A second class of candidate transformer molecules are members of the FGF family of peptide factors. Initially identified as a mitogen for fibroblast cells *in vitro,* FGF has also been shown to play a role in mesoderm induction. Interestingly, FGF is able to posteriorize more anterior neural tissue when coinjected into *Xenopus* blastomeres with other neural inducers or when added to animal caps along with one of the other neural inducers (Doniach, 1995). In addition, when a dominant-negative FGF receptor is expressed in *Xenopus* embryos, spinal neural tissue fails to develop, indicating that FGF may be both necessary and sufficient to posteriorize the nervous system. It is not yet clear whether FGF is actually expressed at the right time and place to act as the posteriorizing signal. However, one member of the family, eFGF, is the best candidate because it is strongly expressed in posterior mesodermal cells in *Xenopus* neurulas. Another interesting aspect of FGF is that it may have both activating and transforming potential. Under some conditions, FGF can induce posterior neural tissue without an additional activator (Kengaku and Okamoto, 1995). Thus, it is possible that some of the transformers also have a level of neural activator activity. This would explain data from experiments by Holtfreter and others where different parts of the organizer could induce head or trunk independently of other regions of the nervous system.

Organizing Centers in the Developing Brain

In addition to the rhombomeres, several other boundaries separate regions of the developing brain. The boundary between the midbrain (mesencephalon) and hindbrain (metencephalon and rhombencephalon) has been recognized as a special domain for some time. This boundary is a major neuroanatomical division of the mature brain, with the metencephalon giving rise to the cerebellum and the mesencephalon giving rise to the midbrain (superior and inferior colliculi). This region also has an important organizing influence on the development of the adjacent regions of the neuroepithelium as highlighted by an experiment by Alvarado-Mallart *et al.* (1993).

In a series of experiments designed to test the state of commitment of this part of the neural tube, Alvarado-Mallart and colleagues transplanted small pieces of the neuroepithelium in this region from chick embryos to quail embryos. Grafting between these two species allows the investigator to follow the fate of the transplanted cells because, although the chick and quail cells behave similarly and integrate

well in the tissues, there are molecular and histological markers that can be used to tell them apart after histological processing. When the presumptive metencephalon region was transplanted from a quail embryo to the same region in a chick embryo, the cells developed as cerebellum, while when a region of the neural plate just anterior to this (the mesencephalon) was transplanted to a corresponding region of the chick embryo the cells developed into midbrain structures, like the optic tectum (or superior colliculus). To determine whether these parts of the neural tube were restricted in their potential at this time in development Alvarado-Mallart *et al.* transplanted the metencephalon to the forebrain. They found that cerebellum still developed from the metencephalon transplants (Fig. 2.10). Remarkably, the

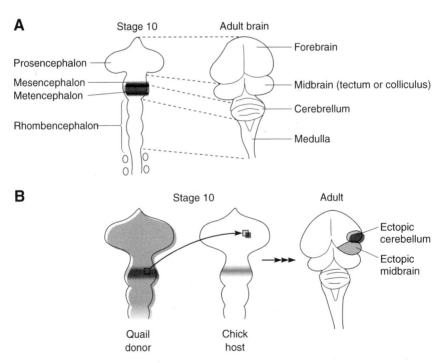

Figure 2.10 A signaling center at the midbrain–hindbrain (mesencephalon–metencephalon) boundary organizes this region of the brain. (A) During normal development, the region of the midbrain–hindbrain junction expresses the homeodomain transcription factor engrailed (red) and this region of the neural tube contains the progenitors of the midbrain (tectum) and the cerebellum. (B) To determine whether these parts of the neural tube were restricted in their potential at this time in development, Alvarado-Mallart *et al.* (1993) transplanted a small piece of the quail metencephalon (red) to the forebrain of a similarly staged chick embryo. Cerebellum still developed from the metencephalon transplants but, in addition, the transplanted tissue induced a new mesencephalon to develop from the adjacent forebrain neural tube cells.

transplanted tissue induced a new mesencephalon to develop from the adjacent forebrain neural tube cells. In other words, the small piece of hindbrain neural tube was able to repattern the more anterior regions of the neural tube to adopt more posterior identities. This experiment is reminiscent of the organizer transplant of Spemann, in which a small region of specialized tissue is able to repattern the surrounding neuroepithelium when transplanted.

In addition to these studies, several important signaling molecules have been localized to this region and shown to have a key role in these patterning activities. For example, a signaling protein known as *Wnt1* is expressed in this region (Fig. 2.11), and when this gene is deleted in mice the animals lose most of the midbrain and cerebellum (McMahon and Bradley, 1990). One of the earliest observed defects in these animals is the loss of expression of a homeobox transcription factor, *engrailed-1* (or En1), which is normally expressed in the region of the mesencephalon–metencephalon boundary. The expression of *engrailed* in this region has also been shown to be critical for normal development of midbrain and hindbrain structures. Mice homozygous for a targeted deletion in the *En1* gene are missing most of the cerebellum and the colliculi (Wurst *et al.*, 1994). These two genes were first identified in *Drosophila* segmentation mutants; when either of these genes is defective in flies, the animals have defects in segmentation. Moreover, in *Drosophila* the orthologous gene for *Wnt1, wingless,* is required for maintaining the expression of the *Drosophila* engrailed gene at the segment boundaries. Thus, the midbrain–hindbrain boundary is one of the places in the vertebrate brain that appears to use the same basic mechanism that is involved in segmentation in invertebrates.

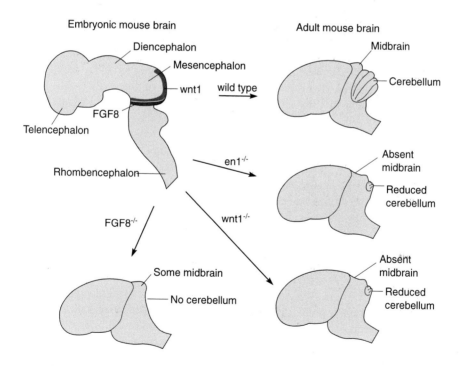

Figure 2.11 Several important signaling molecules have been localized to the midbrain–hindbrain boundary, a key signaling center in the brain. Wnt1, engrailed-1, and FGF8 form an interconnected network that specifies this boundary and is necessary for the growth of the midbrain and the cerebellum. Knockout mice in any of these genes have phenotypes that are similar, in which there are defects in midbrain and cerebellar growth.

In addition to the *Wnt* and *engrailed* patterning system, the midbrain/hindbrain junction also expresses another key signaling molecule, FGF8, a receptor tyrosine kinase ligand. FGF8 is also necessary for either setting up this boundary or maintaining it, since mice deficient in *FGF8* also show defects in cerebellar and midbrain development similar to those of the *Wnt* or *engrailed* knockout animals. *FGF8, engrailed,* and *Wnt1* seem to be in an interconnected network, since deleting any one of them affects the expression of the other two. However, FGF8 may actually be the most critical for the effects of this region in patterning the surrounding neuroepithelium. In a remarkable experiment, Crossley *et al.* (1996) placed a bead coated with FGF8 onto the more rostral region of the neural tube and found that this molecule was sufficient to induce the repatterning of this anterior tissue into midbrain and hindbrain structures.

The unique signaling characteristics of the midbrain/hindbrain boundary suggest that such localized organizing centers may be a basic mechanism of brain patterning. There is evidence that another key organizing region may exist between the dorsal and the ventral thalamus. The expression patterns of several signaling molecules are consistent with this idea, since Sonic hedgehog (see below), other Wnt proteins, and FGFs are also localized to a strip of cells between these two brain regions. However, it is not yet known whether this region has the same type of organizing activity as the midbrain–hindbrain region.

Forebrain Development, Prosomeres, and Pax Genes

To this point, we have explored how *Hox* genes control the specification of anterior–posterior position in the nervous system. However, *Hox* gene expression stops at the anterior boundary of the metencephalon. What are the factors that control positional identity in the rest of the brain? Many other types of homeodomain proteins are expressed in these more anterior

regions of both vertebrate and invertebrate embryos, and they perform a role similar to that of *Hox* gene clusters in more caudal segments. Below, we examine the evidence that homeodomain proteins specify the structures that compose the head and brain.

The most widely held view is that different parts of the brain are generated through the progressive subdivision of initially similar domains. The neural plate begins to show regional differences in the anterior–posterior direction at its formation. Tracing studies with vital dyes show that particular regions of the neural plate normally contribute to a particular part of the nervous system. Many embryologists have also used transplantation between species to define the contributions to the mature brain of particular regions of the neural tube. One particularly useful interspecific transplantation paradigm that was developed by Nicole LeDourin is to transplant tissues between chick embryos and quail embryos. Since these species are similar enough at early stages of development, the transplanted cells integrate with the host and continue developing along with them. The chick and quail cells can later be distinguished since the quail cells contain a more prominent nucleolus, which can be identified following histological sectioning and processing of the chimeric tissue. More recently, antibodies specific for quail cells have been generated and these are also useful for identifying the transplanted cells. Fate maps for other vertebrate neural plate tissue have been derived using other methods, such as vital dye labeling of small numbers of cells or intracellular injections (see Chapter 1). Figure 2.12 shows the fate maps for amphibian, (Eagleson and Harris, 1990) avian, and mammalian neural tubes, particularly the forebrain regions that have been derived from such fate mapping studies. The basic pattern has been elaborated upon to generate the wide diversity of brains that are found in vertebrates.

Although fate mapping studies provide information about the fate of the different neural tube regions, it is important to know when they become uniquely specified. When pieces of the neural plate are transplanted to ectopic locations

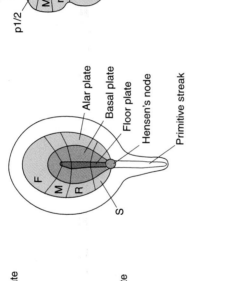

Figure 2.12 The fate maps for amphibian, avian, and mammalian neural plates. The basic forebrain regions are common to all vertebrates; however, the basic pattern has been elaborated upon to generate the wide diversity of brains that are found in vertebrates. The floor plate is shown in red; the basal plate, from which ventral motoneurons are derived, is shown in light red; and the alar plate, from which sensory neurons and most of the forebrain are derived, is pink. The segmental organization (rhombomeres and prosomeres) of the mouse brain can already be recognized at this early stage by the pattern of expression of certain genes.

in the embryo, the cells tend to give rise to particular brain regions. For example, a piece of the anterior neural plate, near the eye, is transplanted to the presumptive flank of another embryo (Fig. 2.13). After sufficient developmental time has passed, the embryos are analyzed for the type of neural tissue that developed from the graft. In this case the finding is that, as early as late gastrula, a particular region of the neural plate will always give rise to anterior brain, including the eye. This occurs regardless of where the tissue is placed in the host animal. A number of embryologists have carried out these types of experiments using various regions of the neural plate as the donor tissue, and the results consistently demonstrate that at some point in early development the cells of the neural plate take on a regional identity.

The fact that different regions of the neural plate are already committed to a particular fate has been extended in recent years by the observations that a number of genes are expressed in highly specific regions of the developing nervous system and in many cases even in the neural plate. In many cases the domain of expression of a particular transcription factor corresponds to that region of the neural tube that will ultimately give rise to one of the five brain vesicles, and the gene may continue to be expressed in that brain vesicle throughout its development.

Many embryologists have taken advantage of the patterns of gene expression in the forebrain to gain insight into the basis of its organization. In what has become known as the prosomeric model of forebrain development, it is proposed that there are longitudinal and transverse patterns of gene expression that subdivide the neural tube into a grid of different regional identities (Puelles and Rubenstein, 1993). The expression of some of these genes is shown for the mouse embryo at two different stages of development (Fig. 2.14). In many cases, the boundary of expression of a particular gene corresponds closely to the apparent morphological distinctions between regions known as prosomeres. Two genes of the emx class are expressed in the

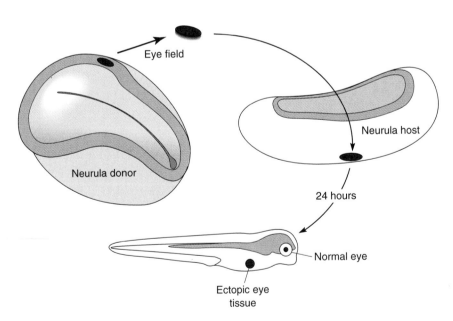

Figure 2.13 The cells of the neural plate take on a regional identity around the time of neurulation. For example, when the presumptive eye-forming region of the neural plate was transplanted to the flank of a different embryo, and the embryos were analyzed for the type of neural tissue that developed from the graft, it was found that an eye would develop from that tissue even in this ectopic location.

telencephalon, one in the anterior half of the cerebral hemisphere (*emx1*) and the other in the posterior half of the hemisphere (*emx2*). Thus, the telencephalic lobes can also be divided into anterior and posterior segments on the basis of the pattern of expression of these two genes. Analysis of the expression patterns of additional genes has led to the conclusion that the prosencephalon can be subdivided into six prosomeres (Fig. 2.14). They are numbered from caudal to rostral, and so prosomere 1 is adjacent to the mesencephalon; p2 and p3 subdivide what is traditionally known as the diencephalon; and p4, p5, and p6 subdivide the telencephalon.

While the studies of regional expression of transcription factors presents a model of brain organization and evolution, the functional analyses of homeodomain factors have yielded re-

markable evidence that these molecules are critically involved in defining the regional identity of the anterior brain. There are now many examples of regionally expressed transcription factors that have essential roles in brain development, but only a few will be mentioned. However, one principle that emerges is that several different classes of transcription factors are likely to be important in specifying the positional identity of cells in any particular region of the brain.

Once again, insight into vertebrate development has profited from studies of the insect brain. The brain of *Drosophila* is derived from each of three regions, called neuromeres. The anterior-most neuromere expresses a gene called *orthodenticle* (otd), a homeodomain gene related to bicoid (see above). Deletion of the otd

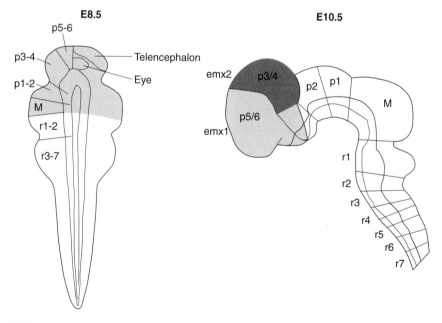

Figure 2.14 Prosomeric model of forebrain development: longitudinal and transverse patterns of gene expression that subdivide the neural tube into a grid of regional identities. The expression of some of these genes is shown for the mouse embryo at two different stages of development. Two genes of the emx class are expressed in the telencephalon, one in the anterior half of the cerebral hemispheres (*emx1*), and the other in the posterior half of the hemispheres (*emx2*). Analysis of the expression patterns of additional genes has led to the conclusion that the prosencephalon can be subdivided into six prosomeres. They are numbered from caudal to rostral, and so the prosomere 1 is adjacent to the mesencephalon (M); p2 and p3 subdivide what is traditionally known as the diencephalon; and p4, p5, and p6 subdivide the telencephalon.

gene causes the loss of both the preantennal and antennal segments of the fly, which essentially results in the absence of the head structures derived from these segments. Homologous genes have been found in a variety of different organisms, and two mammalian homologs have been discovered, *otx-1* and *otx-2*. *Otx-2* is initially expressed widely in the embryo. During the course of development, its expression becomes progressively restricted to the anterior end of the embryo (Fig. 2.14). Mice homozygous for a deletion in the homeobox domain of this gene show severe defects in the development of the anterior nervous system (Acampora *et al.*, 1995).

Another class of transcription factors that is critical for specifying regional differences in the nervous system is the *Pax* genes. These genes have a homeodomain region as well as a second conserved domain known as the paired box (named for its sequence homology with the *Drosophila* segmentation gene *paired*). There are nine different *Pax* genes, and all but two, *Pax1* and *Pax9,* are expressed in the developing nervous system (Chalepakis *et al.*, 1993). Several of these genes are also disrupted in naturally occurring mouse mutations and human congenital syndromes, and the defects observed in these conditions generally correspond to the areas of gene expression. *Pax2,* for example, is expressed in the developing optic stalk and the otic vesicle of the embryo. Mutations in *Pax2* in mice and humans cause optic nerve abnormalities, known as colobomas.

Perhaps the most striking example of *Pax* gene regulation of regional differentiation in the nervous system comes from the studies of *Pax6*. This gene is expressed early in the development of the eye, at the time when this region of the neural plate is committed to giving rise to retinal tissue. Humans with a heterozygous disruption of this gene exhibit abnormalities in eye development, causing a condition known as aniridia (a lack of formation of the iris). In mice and humans with a homozygous disruption of this gene, the eyes fail to develop past the initial optic vesicle stage. A homologous gene has also been identified in *Drosophila* (as well as many other organisms) and mutations in this gene also disrupt eye formation in flies. And even more

surprising, when this gene is misexpressed at inappropriate positions in the embryo, ectopic eyes are induced (Halder *et al.*, 1995). The ability of a single gene to direct the development of an entire sensory organ like the eye is striking; the *Pax* genes act as if they are at the top of a hierarchy and can be thought of as coordinating the signals and genes necessary to organize a "field" or region of the embryo (Fig. 2.15).

Dorsal–Ventral Polarity in the Neural Tube

The early neural tube consists only of undifferentiated neural and glial progenitor cells. The neural tube is essentially a closed system, and the brain vesicles and developing spinal cord are fluid-filled chambers. The surface of the tube, adjacent to the lumen, is known as the ventricular surface, since eventually the lumen of the neural tube goes on to form the ventricular system of the mature brain. The progenitor cells for neurons and glia of the CNS have a simple bipolar morphology and initially span the width of the neural tube. As these cells undergo mitotic divisions, they typically go through the M-phase of the cell cycle at the ventricular surface. The postmitotic immature neurons generated from the progenitor cells migrate away from the ventricular zone toward the margin of the spinal cord to form the mantle layer (see Chapter 3).

At the neural plate stage, several mechanisms are set in motion that will define the overall organization of the neural tube. First, the most ventral part of the neural tube becomes flattened into a distinct floor plate. Second, the most dorsal aspect of the neural tube develops into a tissue known as the roof plate. Third, a distinct fissure, the sulcus limitans, forms between the dorsal and ventral parts of the neural tube along most of its length (Fig. 2.16). These structures are an early sign that the neural tube is differentiating along the dorsal–ventral axis. These structures arise largely due to the interaction between the surrounding nonneural tissue and the neural tube.

Experiments by Holtfreter demonstrated that a significant amount of differentiation in the

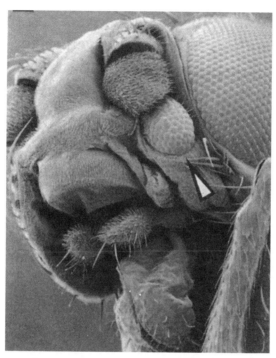

Figure 2.15 Ectopic eyes are formed when the *Drosophila Pax6* gene *eyeless* is misexpressed in other imaginal discs. Halder *et al.* (1995) misexpressed the *eyeless* gene in the antenna disc in the developing fly and found that an ectopic eye was formed in the antenna (arrow). This remarkable experiment argues for the concept that master control genes organize entire fields, or structures, during embryogenesis, possibly by activating tissue-specific cascades of transcription factors. (Reprinted with permission from Halder *et al.*, Induction of ectopic eyes by targeted expression of the eyeless gene in Drosophila, *Science* **267**: 1788–1792. Copyright 1995 American Association for the Advancement of Science.)

neural tube was dependent on factors derived from adjacent, nonneural tissues. Isolation of the neural tube from the surrounding tissues resulted in an undifferentiated tube, without obvious motoneuronal differentiation. Furthermore, by transplanting the notochord to ectopic locations, he was able to induce a second floor plate (Fig. 2.17). Thus, the notochord is both necessary and sufficient for the development of the dorsal–ventral axis of the spinal cord.

Molecular Basis of Dorsal–Ventral Polarity

The studies that led to the identification of the signals that control dorsal–ventral polarity in the developing spinal cord relied on the use of many molecular markers of cell identity that were obviously not around at the time Harrison was doing his experiments. These genes include the *Pax* class of transcription factors discussed in the previous section, as well as a variety of other genes that are restricted to particular populations of both differentiated and/or undifferentiated cells within the spinal cord. The expression of some of the critical genes that define the dorsal–ventral polarity of the spinal cord is summarized in Fig. 2.18.

To track down the polarity signal released by mesoderm, a cell culture system was devised in which the notochord and the neural tube were cocultured in collagen gels. The signal was first shown to be diffusible since pieces of notochord could induce floor plate without touching the neural tube. In addition, the expression of motoneuron-specific genes, such as choline

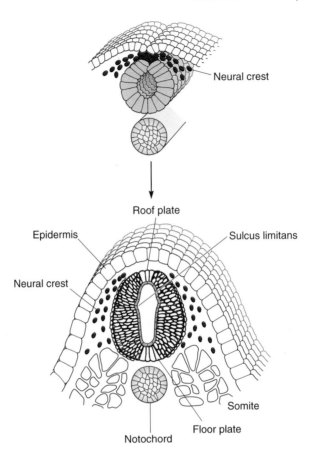

Figure 2.16   The overall organization of the neural tube emerges soon after closure. The most ventral part of the neural tube becomes flattened into a distinct floor plate. The most dorsal aspect of the neural tube develops into a tissue known as the roof plate. A distinct fissure, the sulcus limitans, forms between the dorsal and ventral parts of the neural tube along most of its length.

acetyltransferase was also shown to depend on the notochord. A clue to the identity of the factor was uncovered in a rather roundabout manner. A crucial clue to the identity of the notochord signal again came from *Drosophila*. During a large screen for developmental mutants in the fruit fly (Nusslein-Volhard and Wieschaus, 1980), a severely deformed mutant was found, named hedgehog for its truncated appearance. Through a number of subsequent genetic steps, hedgehog was found to act in a cell nonautonomous manner in fly development, and subsequent cloning of the gene showed that this molecule indeed resembled a secreted protein.

The link between hedgehog and the notochord signaling molecule began with the identification of the mammalian homolog, called Sonic hedgehog (Shh). Sonic hedgehog is expressed initially in the notochord at the time when the dorsal–ventral axis of the neural tube is being specified (Roelink *et al.*, 1994). Shortly after this time, the expression of Sonic hedgehog begins in the differentiating ventral neural tube, leading to the floor plate. This expression pattern of a potential signaling molecule is consistent with the experiments of Harrison (1904, 1907, 1910) and more recently of Jessel and co-workers (1989). Both found that initially the ventralizing

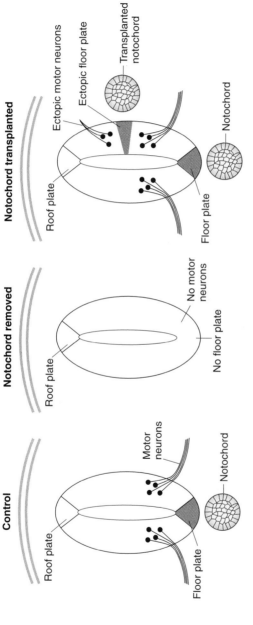

Figure 2.17 Differentiation in the neural tube is dependent on factors derived from adjacent, nonneural tissues. If the notochord, a mesodermally derived structure, is removed prior to neural tube closure, the neural tube fails to display characteristics of ventral differentiation, such as the development of the floor plate and the spinal motoneurons. This shows that the notochord is necessary for the development of ventral neural tube fates. If an additional notochord is transplanted to the lateral part of the neural tube at this same time in embryogenesis, a new floor plate is induced adjacent to the transplanted notochord. New motoneurons are also induced to form adjacent to the ectopic floor plate. Thus, the notochord is sufficient to specify ventral cell fates.

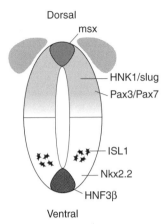

Figure 2.18   Several genes are expressed in restricted domains in the developing spinal cord, and these have served as useful markers for positional identity of cells in this region of the nervous system. The floor plate cells express transcription factors, Nkx2.2 and HNF3β, which are essential for their development; if these genes are eliminated by gene targeting in mice, the animals fail to develop a floor plate. Islet-1 (ISL1) is an early marker of motoneurons; *Pax3,* a transcription factor of the *paired*-homeodomain class, is expressed in more dorsal regions of the neural tube; and *msx1* is expressed in the most dorsal region of the tube and in the neural crest, along with HNK1 and *slug.*

signal arises from the notochord but soon after it is also found in the floor plate.

To determine whether Shh was, indeed, the inducer of dorsal–ventral polarity in the spinal cord, a small aggregate of Shh-expressing Cos cells was placed next to the neural tube. The Shh released from these cells was sufficient to induce a second floor plate, as well as other genes normally expressed in the ventral neural tube. In further experiments, simply adding recombinant sonic hedgehog protein to explants of neural tube was sufficient to induce them to differentiate as ventral neural tissues, including floor plate and motor neurons (Fig. 2.19). These experiments thus show that Shh is sufficient to ventralize the neural tube during development. Two additional results show that Sonic hedgehog is the major, if not the only, signal to specify ventral neural tube. First, antibodies raised against Shh block the differentiation of floor plate and motor neurons when added to neural tube explants. Second, targeted deletion of the *Sonic hedgehog* gene in mice results in the failure of the development of the ventral cell types in the spinal cord.

In addition to its role in the ventralization of the neural tube, Shh is also expressed in the more anterior regions of the body axis immediately subjacent to the neural tube, in what is known as the prechordal mesoderm. Here the function of Shh is similar to that of the notochord and floor plate; it serves to induce ventral differentiation in the forebrain. In the forebrain, the growth of the different brain vesicles gives rise to complex anatomy, and so the induction of ventral forebrain is critical for a number of subsequent morphogenetic events. Consequently, the loss of Shh signaling in the prechordal mesoderm produces dramatic phenotypic changes in embryos and the resulting animals. One particularly striking phenotype that arises from the disruption of Shh in embryogenesis is cyclopia (Roessler *et al.,* 1996). The eyes normally form from paired evaginations of the ventral diencephalon (see above). However, in the neural plate, the eye field is initially continuous across the midline and is split into two by the inhibition of eye forming potential by Shh from the prechordal mesoderm. When this signal is interrupted, the eye field remains continuous and a single eye forms in the midline. The subsequent elaboration of the forebrain depends on the correct midline development, and so the lack

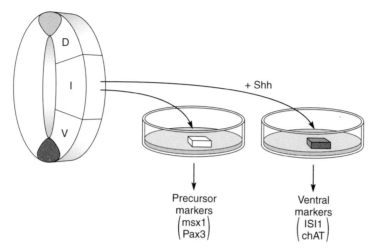

Figure 2.19 A cell culture system in which the notochord and the neural tube were cocultured in collagen gels was used to find the polarity signal released by mesoderm. The signal was first shown to be diffusible since pieces of notochord could induce floor plate without touching the neural tube. Simply adding recombinant Sonic hedgehog protein to explants of neural tube was sufficient to induce them to differentiate as ventral neural tissues, including floor plate and motor neurons.

of Shh also disrupts later stages of brain development as well, leading to a condition known as holoprosencephaly.

The mechanism by which Shh induces ventral differentiation of the neural tube involves several interesting signaling steps. In both *Drosophila* and vertebrates, the hedgehog proteins undergo autoproteolysis to generate an amino-terminal fragment that is associated with the cell surface and a freely diffusible carboxyl-terminal fragment. The amino-terminal fragment is sufficient to elicit ventral differentiation as evidenced by floor plate and motoneuron differentiation. Since floor plate differentiation occurs at higher doses of recombinant Shh and motoneuron differentiation at lower doses of Shh, it has been proposed that a gradient of Shh from the notochord and floor plate patterns the neural tube into these two alternate fates (Ericson *et al.*, 1997).

Dorsal Neural Tube and Neural Crest

The experiments of Harrison and others showed that removal of the notochord resulted in a neural tube without much polarity. This implies that the dorsal neural tube is in some way the default condition, while the ventral structures require an additional signal to develop their fates. However, in the past few years it has also become apparent that the dorsal neural tube also requires signals for its appropriate development. Before the neural tube closes, the future dorsal neural tube is continuous with the adjacent ectodermal cells. As the dorsal neural tube closes, the neural crest forms at the point of fusion of the neural tube margins. Thus, the neural crest is, in some sense, the most dorsal derivative of the neural tube and has often been used as an indicator of dorsal differentiation. In addition, there are several genes specifically expressed in the dorsal neural tube at these early stages of development, and ultimately the dorsal neural tube goes on to differentiate into specific types of sensory neurons.

After extensive migration, the neural crest gives rise to an array of different tissues. In the trunk, the neural crest gives rise to the cells of the peripheral nervous system, including the neurons and glia of the sensory and autonomic ganglia, the Schwann cells surrounding all peripheral nerves, and the neurons of the gastric mucosal plexi. Several other cell types, including pigment cells, chromatophores, and smooth muscle cells are known to arise from the trunk neural crest. Neural crest also forms in the cranial regions, and here it contributes to most of the structures in the head (see Box, Chapter 3). Most of the mesenchyme in the head, including that which forms the visceral skeleton and the bones of the skull, is derived from neural crest. The neurons and glia of several cranial ganglia, like the trigeminal sensory ganglia, the vestibulo-cochlear ganglia, and the autonomic ganglia in the head, are also derived largely from the progeny of the neural crest. Ectodermal placodes separate from the neural plate to produce the olfactory epithelium, the lens, the otocyst, and additional neurons and glia of the cranial ganglia.

Because of the extensive migration of the neural crest cells and the great diversity of the tissues and cell types to which neural crest cells can contribute, the neural crest has been studied extensively as a model for these aspects of nervous system development. In the next section we review what is known about the origin of the neural crest and the factors that control the initial aspects of its differentiation. Later chapters detail additional studies of the factors that control neural crest migration and tissue-specific differentiation.

Classically the neural crest has been thought to arise from the cells that form at the fusion of the neural folds when they become the neural tube. Vogt (1925) used vital dyes to fate map the different parts of the amphibian embryo and found that most of the neural crest forms from a narrow strip of ectodermal cells at the junction between the neural plate and the epidermis. Though this is the typical pattern, there are important exceptions to the classical picture that give a broader picture of the conditions required for neural crest formation. Bronner-Fraser *et al.* (1991) used single cell injections to track the lineages of individual crest cells prior to their migration. The injected cells went on to divide and retained their lineage marker for several cell divisions. Many of the labeled cells went on to contribute to the tissues described above as the normal neural crest derivatives; however, some of the labeled cells that contributed to the neural

crest also had progeny that populated the neural tube and the epidermis. Thus, although most of the cells in the neural crest field at the neural plate stage of development normally develop into neural crest, they are not restricted to this lineage. In addition, although in many embryos the neural crest develops at the fusion of the neural folds, there are regions of the neuraxis in some species that do not form by the rolling of the neural plate. For example, in the fish, the neural tube forms first as a thickening of the neurectoderm, known as the neural keel, and tube formation occurs later by a process of cavitation, but the neural crest still forms from the lateral edges of the plate. Additional recent studies have also shown that while most of the neural crest normally arises from the lateral edges of the neural plate, there is a late migrating population of crest cells that is derived from the neural tube.

As described above, a number of the molecules that are involved in the process of neural induction and the patterning of the developing neural tube have recently been identified. These experiments have also shed some light on the factors that control neural crest formation. The recent studies are nicely consistent with the classical experimental embryology on neural crest formation. Some of the first experimental evidence to indicate that the induction of the neural crest may involve some of the same factors as those responsible for neural induction is that of Raven and Kloos (1945). They found that neural crest can be induced from ectoderm by lateral pieces of the archenteron roof, whereas neural tube was induced by medial pieces, such as the presumptive notochord. Similar results led Dalq to propose that a concentration gradient of a particular organizing substance originating in the midline tissue of the archenteron roof could set up medial–lateral distinctions across the neural plate: "the median strip of the archenteron roof, supposedly rich in organisine, would induce neural structures, while the more lateral parts which elaborate it in smaller quantities, would induce neural crest," (Holtfreter and Hamburger, 1955). Since the cells that will ultimately develop into dorsal neural tube are initially immediately adjacent to the nonneural ectodermal cells, these could provide a signal for dorsal differentiation similar to the notochord-derived Shh for ventralization of the neural tube. This idea has been postulated for a number of years in various forms but has only recently been tested with perturbations of specific candidate-inducing molecules.

Several lines of evidence now support the hypothesis that the ectoderm provides the molecular signals to promote the dorsal differentiation in the lateral regions of the spinal cord and likely more anterior regions of the neuraxis. Moury and Jacobson (1990) first tested whether interactions between the neural plate and the surrounding ectoderm were responsible for the induction of neural crest by transplanting a small piece of the neural plate from a pigmented animal to the ventral surface of the embryo (Fig. 2.20). As shown in the figure, when the embryo

was allowed to develop further, the transplant rolled into a small tube, and at the margins gave rise to neural crest cells, as evidenced by the pigmented melanocytes that migrated from the ectopic neural tissue. These results were extended by similar experiments of Selleck and Bronner-Fraser (1995) in the chick embryo, and in addition they used an explant culture system in which neural plate and epidermis were cocultured and analyzed for proteins and genes normally expressed by neural crest. They found that the neural crest was induced to form from the neural tube when placed adjacent to the epidermis.

Progress toward the identification of the inducing substance has been made by Liem *et al.* (1995). BMPs, discussed in the previous chapter for their role in neural induction, also play important functions in specifying dorsal regional identity in the developing spinal cord. Liem *et al.* used an explant culture system similar to that

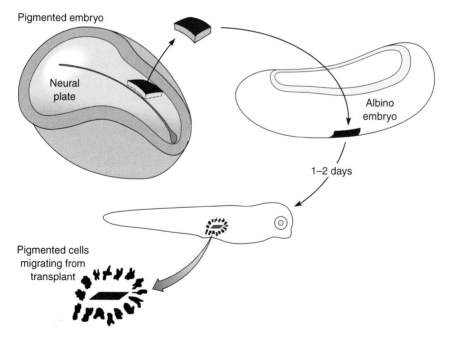

Figure 2.20 Moury and Jacobson (1990) first tested whether interactions between the neural plate and the surrounding ectoderm were responsible for the induction of neural crest by transplanting a small piece of the neural plate from a pigmented animal to the ventral surface of the embryo. As shown in the figure, when the embryo was allowed to develop further, the transplant rolled into a small tube, and at the margins gave rise to neural crest cells, as evidenced by the pigmented melanocytes that migrated from the ectopic neural tissue.

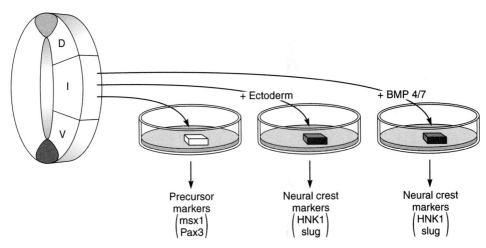

Figure 2.21   Liem *et al.* (1995) used an explant culture system to define the signals that specify dorsal cell fates. The neural tube was dissected into a ventral piece, a dorsal piece, and an intermediate piece. The expression of genes normally restricted to either the dorsal neural tube or the ventral neural tube was examined to determine whether these genes were specifically induced by coculture with the ectoderm. They found that certain dorsally localized genes, like *Pax3* and *msx1,* are initially expressed throughout the neural tube and are progressively restricted from the ventral neural tube by Shh from the notochord and floor plate. However, coculture with the ectoderm was necessary to induce the expression of other, more definitive, dorsal markers, like HNK1 and *slug.* BMPs were found to effectively replace the ectodermally derived signal, since these could also activate HNK1 and *slug,* even from ventral explants.

used for the analysis of Shh effects on ventralization of the neural tube. The neural tube was dissected into a ventral piece, a dorsal piece, and an intermediate piece (Fig. 2.21). They then analyzed the expression of genes normally restricted to either the dorsal neural tube or the ventral neural tube to determine whether these genes were specifically induced by coculture with the ectoderm. They found that certain dorsally localized genes, like *Pax3* and *msx1,* are

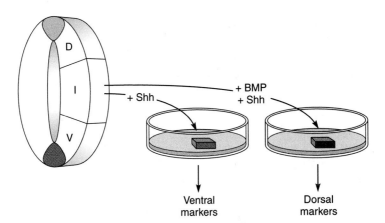

Figure 2.22   When the intermediate neural tube is cultured in the presence of Shh, it expresses markers of a ventral fate. However, when BMP is added along with Shh, the intermediate tube cultures express markers of dorsal neural fate.

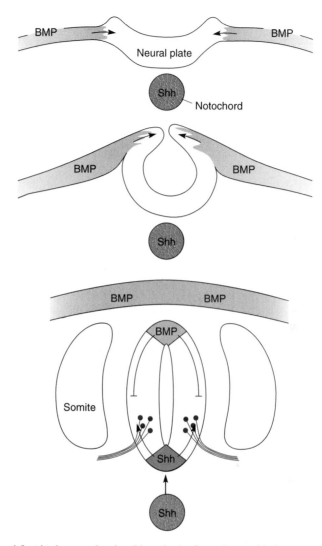

Figure 2.23 Shh is expressed first in the notochord and later in the floor plate and induces ventral differentiation in the neural tube. BMPs are expressed in the ectoderm overlying the neural tube and then in the dorsal neural tube cells later in development. These two signals antagonize one another and through this mutual antagonism they set up opposing gradients that control both the polarity of spinal cord differentiation and the amount of spinal cord tissue that differentiates into dorsal, ventral, and intermediate cell fates.

initially expressed throughout the neural tube and are progressively restricted from the ventral neural tube by Shh from the notochord and floor plate; however, coculture with the ectoderm was necessary to induce the expression of other, more definitive, dorsal markers, like *HNK1* and *slug*. BMPs were found to effectively replace the ectodermally derived signal, since these could also activate *HNK1* and *slug,* even from ventral explants. Thus, there appears to be an antagonism between Shh from the ventral neural tube and BMPs from the dorsal neural tube; when BMP is added along with Shh to the explants, the Shh-induced motoneuron differentiation is suppressed.

Sonic hedgehog, expressed first in the notochord and later in the floor plate induces ventral differentiation in the neural tube. BMP and

Shh antagonize one another and through this mutual antagonism they set up opposing gradients that control both the polarity of spinal cord differentiation and the amount of spinal cord tissue that differentiates into dorsal, ventral, and intermediate cell fates. Thus, when BMP is added along with Shh to a culture of intermediate neural tube, it expresses dorsal markers (Fig. 2.22).

The model of dorsal–ventral polarity in the spinal cord that has emerged from these studies is that the BMP expressed at the margin of the neural plate induces the development of neural crest when it is present at high concentrations. Dorsal neural tube fates occur when BMP is present at lower concentrations (Fig. 2.23). Much more is said about the later stages of development of spinal cord cells in Chapter 4. The understanding of how the basic pattern of the nervous system is established has been put on solid molecular ground in the past decade. One of the basic principles that has emerged from this work is that graded concentrations of antagonizing diffusible molecules are critically involved in setting up these patterns. These diffusible signaling molecules act to restrict the expression of specific transcription factors that go on to regulate the expression of downstream target genes specific for the regional identity of a part of the nervous system (Briscoe et al., 1999). This conceptual framework holds true for vertebrates and invertebrates, and, indeed, many of the molecular systems for generating specific parts of the nervous system have been highly conserved over the millions of years of evolution and considerable morphological diversity of animals.

CHAPTER 3 · · · · · · · · · · · ·

Birth and Migration

· · · · ·

Neurogenesis, or the generation of neurons during development, occurs in many different ways in the various regions of the embryo. As described in the previous sections, both vertebrate and invertebrate embryos have some process that separates the neural progenitor cells from the ectoderm. This section describes the way in which the appropriate numbers of neurons and glia are generated from the neural precursors.

The number of cells generated in the developing nervous system is likely regulated at several levels. In some cases, the production of neurons or glia may be regulated by apparent intrinsic limits to the number of cell divisions a particular progenitor can go through; i.e., a cellular clock. The level of proliferation and ultimately the number of cells generated can also be controlled by extracellular signaling factors, acting as mitogens, promoting progenitor cells to reenter the S phase of the cell cycle. In addition, there is evidence from studies in many tissues, including the nervous system, that factors can act as mitotic inhibitors, which induce progenitor cells to exit from the cell cycle. In this chapter, examples of these mechanisms are reviewed. However, it must also be remembered that the number of neurons and glia in the mature nervous system is not only a function of cell proliferation but also of cell death. There are many examples of neuronal overproduction, and subsequent attrition through programmed cell death. This process is reviewed in Chapter 7.

In the simplest animals, like the nematode, the lineages of the cells directly predict their numbers. Since most of the mitotic divisions are asymmetric, the final number of cells that are produced during embryogenesis depends on the particular pattern of cell divisions and the number of cells that die through programmed cell death. The regulation of these divisions does not appear to depend on interactions with surrounding cells but rather is an intrinsic property of the lineage. As we see in a later section, the lineage of the cells also predicts the particular types of neurons that are generated from a particular precursor, and it appears that the information to define a given type of cell resides largely in factors derived directly from the precursors.

In the *Drosophila* central nervous system, neuronal number is also highly stereotypic. As noted in the previous chapters, the neuroblasts of the insect CNS delaminate from the ventral–lateral ectoderm neurogenic region in successive waves. In *Drosophila*, about 25 neuroblasts delaminate in each segment and they are organized in four columns and six rows. The pattern is basically the same for other insects and other arthropods, but the number of neuroblasts is dependent on the species (Doe *et al.*, 1991). Once the neuroblast has segregated from the ectoderm, the cell undergoes several asymmetric divisions to give rise to approximately 5 smaller ganglion mother cells. Each ganglion mother cell then divides to generate a pair of neurons (see Fig. 3.1). These neurons make up the segmental ganglia of the ventral nerve cord and have stereotypic numbers and types of neurons. The molecular signals that control the number of cell divisions of the neuroblasts are described in the next section, while the mechanisms that de-

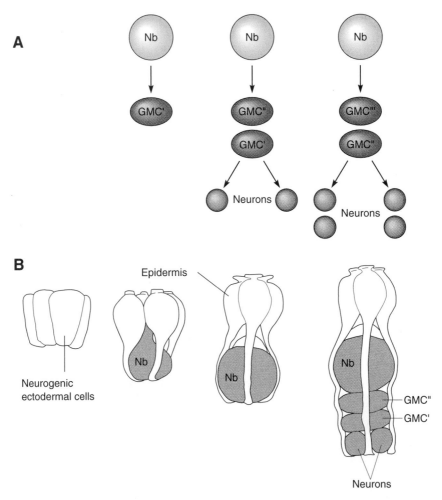

Figure 3.1 *Drosophila* neurogenesis commences soon after neuroblast (Nb) delamination. (A) In the *Drosophila* embryo, the neuroblasts undergo a series of asymmetric divisions to generate ganglion mother cells (GMCs). The GMCs then divide once and so each one produces a pair of neurons. (B) A drawing of the morphological appearance of the process of *Drosophila* neurogenesis. (After Doe, 1992b)

termine what type of neuron is generated by a particular GMC is discussed in the next chapter.

In the vertebrate the situation gets considerably more complex. The neural tube is initially a single layer thick. As neurogenesis proceeds, the progenitor cells undergo a considerable number of cell divisions to produce a much thicker tube with several layers. A section through the developing spinal cord is shown in Fig. 3.2, and this basic structure is present throughout the developing central nervous system. The German developmental biologist His first defined the layers as an ependymal zone (near the ventricle), a mantle zone, and a marginal zone (containing axonal processes). The ependymal zone, the innermost zone of the tube, is where the mitotic figures are located, and His thought these were actually different cells from the more elongate mantle cells (see Jacobson, 1991). Through the work of Sauer and others we know that the nuclei of the progenitor cells undergo a constant migration from the ventricular surface during the M phase to the mantle zone during the S phase (Fig. 3.2).

One of the clearest demonstrations of this constant up-and-down motion of the nuclei of these cells came from the use of [³H]-thymidine to label cells in the S-phase of the cell cycle during the active phase of DNA replication. Figure 3.3 diagrams this type of experiment in a section through the neural tube. If an injection of [³H]-thymidine is made into an embryo and the tissue removed within 1 h, the labeled cells are all found in the outer part of the vetricular zone, away from the ventricle. If the embryo is allowed to survive for 4 h after the injection of thymidine, the labeled cells are all at the ventricular surface undergoing the M phase and can be seen as metaphase nuclei. If the embryo is allowed to survive for 8 h, the labeled cells are in the outer half of the ventricular zone, and by 12 h they are back at the ventricular surface. The thymidine labeling also shows a progressive increase in the number of labeled cells as the cells divide. However, because the thymidine is only available for incorporation into cells for the first hour after injection (before it is cleared from the circulation), the cells labeled in subsequent divisions progressively dilute their label and appear more lightly labeled with each successive division. The function of this interkinetic nuclear migration in unknown. Thus, the mantle zone in the early neural tube is actually composed of the same cells as those at the ventricular surface at a different stage of the cell cycle.

The cells of the ventricular zone are the precursors of differentiated neurons and glia in the central nervous system. These cells undergo between one and two cell cycles per day in homeothermic vertebrates. In the early neural tube, many of the cells undergo symmetric cell divisions, producing two progenitor cells as daughters. However, some of the divisions produce asymmetric daughters, one of which continues to divide and the other of which becomes a postmitotic neuron. In the spinal cord and in most other areas of the developing neural tube, the postmitotic neurons migrate from the ventricular zone to the marginal zone, where they continue their differentiation.

Thymidine labeling also allows one to determine the cell cycle length of a population of mitotically active cells. Since the thymidine is cleared from the circulation of mammalian embryos within 1 h after an injection, a relatively small cohort of S phase cells incorporates the label into their DNA. As described above, these cells then proceed through G2 and in the M phase they are recognizable as mitotic figures. If one counts the number of the mitotic figures at progressively longer intervals after the thymidine injection, their number will continue to increase as a greater proportion of the S phase cells reach the M phase (Fig. 3.3). However, as these cells complete the M phase and proceed into G1 and the next S phase, they are no longer counted as mitotic figures and their number drops. As the first cells finish their second S phase and reenter mitosis the number of labeled mitotic figures once again increases and we see a second peak. The length of time between the first and second peak is therefore the time taken for the cohort of labeled cells to go from one mitosis to another.

In the vertebrate CNS, these types of experiments have been carried out for many regions

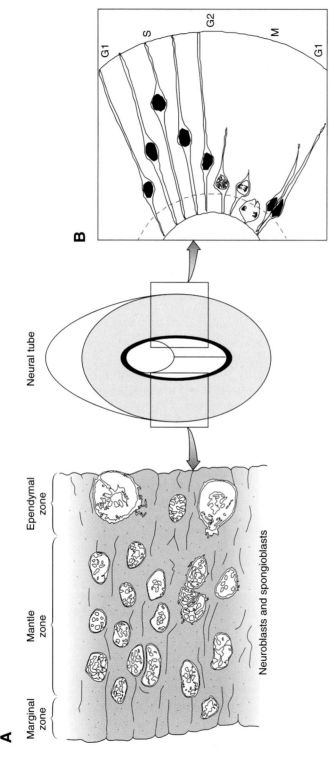

Figure 3.2 The process of neurogenesis in the neural tube. The histological appearance of a section through the neural tube soon after it has formed is shown (A) in a drawing from His and (B) diagramatically. His divided the neural tube into zones: the most central ependymal zone, containing the mitotic figures of the dividing neural progenitor cells; the mantle zone, containing the neuroblasts; and the most peripheral marginal zone, where the axons and postmitotic cells accumulate. His thought the zones were occupied by different cell types, but as shown in panel (B), in the early neural tube the ependymal and mantle zones are occupied by the progenitor cells at different stages of their cell cycle. The progenitor cells span the thickness of the neural tube, and their nuclei translocate to the mantle zone during the S phase of the cell cycle. The nuclei return to the ventricular surface during G2 and the M phase of the cell cycle always occurs at the ventricular surface. Later in development, the mantle zone accumulates postmitotic neurons.

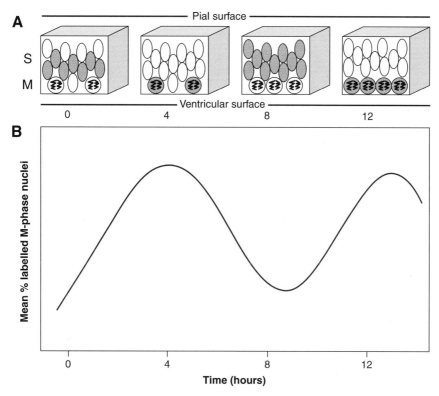

Figure 3.3 Thymidine labeling reveals the cell cycle length of neural progenitor cells. (A) A section of the neural tube is shown at various times after an injection of [³H]-thymidine into a developing embryo. The S phase cells incorporate the label into their DNA (red) and move towards the pial surface. When the labeled cells proceed to the M phase, they are recognizable as mitotic figures at the ventricular surface. (B) A plot of the number of labeled mitotic figures (vertical axis) against the time after the thymidine injection. The number of M-phase cells increases as the S phase cells move through the cell cycle. As these cells complete the M phase and proceed into the G1 phase and the next S phase, they move away from the ventricular surface and are no longer counted as mitotic figures. As the first cells finish their second S phase and reenter mitosis the number of labeled mitotic figures once again increases and we see a second peak at 12 hrs. The length of time between the first and the second peak is the time taken for the labeled cells to go from one mitosis to another, the cell cycle length.

of the brain, and again, some general principles emerge. First, the overall length of the cell cycle increases progressively during embryogenesis. Progenitor cells from the chick optic tectum, for example, have an overall cell cycle time of 8 h on Embryonic Day 3 (E3), but this increases to 15 h by E6. A similar increase in cell cycle period occurs in the mammal as cortical progenitor cells increase their cell cycle time from 11 h in the E12 rat to 19 h at E18. The second generality that can be made is that the increase in the cell cycle period is largely due to increases in the G1 phase. As shown in Fig. 3.4, the M and G2 phases of the cell cycle change little from E10 to E19 in mouse cerebral cortex progenitor cells; however, the G1 phase nearly triples in length. The lengthening of the G1 period likely reflects some regulatory process that restricts or slows reentry of the progenitor cells into the S phase from G1, consistent with the idea that a limiting supply of growth factor controls this step (see next section).

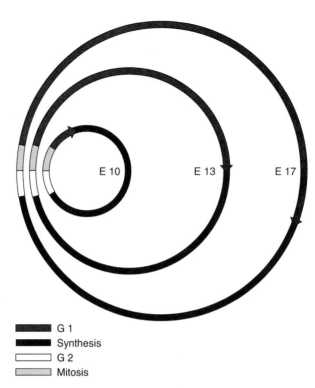

G 1
Synthesis
G 2
Mitosis

Figure 3.4   The overall length of the progenitor cell cycle increases during embryogenesis. The cell cycles of progenitor cells from the mouse cerebral cortex are plotted as circles of increasing size from E10 to E17. The increase in the cell cycle period is largely due to an increase in the G1 phase, which nearly triples in length.

The number of cells generated by a precursor cell in the ventricular zone depends on the stage of development and the region of the nervous system that the progenitor cell comes from. Progenitor cells from the early embryonic CNS must generate a considerably greater number of progeny than those from animals nearing the end of neurogenesis. Likewise, progenitor cells from very large regions of the brain must have given rise to many more cells than those from the spinal cord. The thymidine studies described above show that there are differences in the cell cycle periods of ventricular zone cells of early and late embryos. Thymidine labeling and, more recently, BrDU labeling of the mitotically active ventricular zone cells have given some information as to the number of progeny produced by the entire population of these cells as development proceeds. In the early embryonic cerebral cortex, for example, the number of cells more

than doubles each day. Since it takes approximately a half day for a progenitor cell to generate two daughters, more than half of the progeny must continue to divide; i.e., many of the cell divisions must produce two mitotically active daughters. During this early "expansion phase" of the progenitor cells, most of the cell divisions are symmetric, generating two additional progenitor cells; however, birthdating studies (see below) also show that some neurons are born during these early periods as well, and so some of the divisions must be asymmetric, generating a mitotically active daughter and a postmitotic neuron. As development proceeds, the cell cycle time becomes progressively longer and the increase in cell number is slowed. Fewer cell divisions result in two progenitor cells; rather, a greater number of the progenitor cells differentiate into neurons and glia (Caviness and Takahashi, 1995).

The results from the thymidine and BrDU labeling studies have been nicely complemented by retroviral labeling of individual progenitor cells. Labeling individual progenitor cells from different stages of development has confirmed that the number of progeny generated by a ventricular zone cell declines over the periods of neurogenesis. For example, retroviral labeling of the E15 rat retina results in very large clones of labeled cells while similar labeling of progenitor cell in the retinas of postnatal animals results in much smaller clones. The retroviral labeling technique has also allowed the discrimination of the contributions of neuronal and glial production to the total cell number. In the cerebral cortex, for example, the number of neurons per clone is typically less than 5, while the number of astrocytes and oligodendrocytes may be between 10 and 30 in the same aged embryo. In the chick spinal cord the distribution of clones has been analyzed shortly after injections as well as in the more mature spinal cord. Clonally related cells are typically found in radially oriented arrays when analyzed shortly after the viral infections; however, when similar clones are analyzed in the mature cord, the cells are typically more dispersed. Many of the clones contain both motoneurons and glial cells in the white matter. In the example shown in Fig. 3.5, both astrocytes and oligodendrocytes are derived from the same progenitor cell that gave rise to the motoneurons (Leber *et al.,* 1990).

In addition to the information on the cell cycle that was obtained from the use of [^{3}H]-thymidine, it was also possible to use this isotope to determine the precise time points during embryogenesis when the neurons and glia were generated, i.e., became postmitotic. While the progenitor cells are actively dividing, they are synthesizing DNA and incorporate the [^{3}H]-thymidine. However, as noted above, since the thymidine is available for only a few hours, progenitor cells that continue to divide dilute their label over time. By contrast, those cells that withdraw from the cycle and become postmitotic remain heavily labeled with the radioactive nucleotide. Thus the postmitotic neurons generated (born) within a day after the [^{3}H]-thymidine injection will have heavily labeled nuclei, and neurons generated later in development will be more lightly labeled. This technique, pioneered by Richard Sidman and colleagues (1959) is known as thymidine birthdating and has been applied to virtually all of the areas of the developing mammalian nervous system (eg. Altman and Bayer, 1985; see Jacobson, 1991 for review).

The thymidine birthdating studies revealed that the process of neurogenesis was remarkably well ordered. In many areas of the developing brain, there are spatial and temporal gradients of neuron production (Fig. 3.6). The generation of the cerebral cortex, for example, proceeds from medial to lateral, while the retina is generated in a central to peripheral direction. In general, there are well-conserved and orderly sequences of generation of different types of neurons and glia. For example, in the cerebral cortex, the neurons are arranged in layers or lamina. During neurogenesis, the different lamina are generated in a sequence that is conserved from rats to monkeys (see below). Likewise, in the retina, there are six main types of neurons and one type of glial cell, the Muller cell. Thymidine birthdating of a wide variety of species has shown that the various types of neurons are generated in a well-conserved sequence, even though the period of retinal histogenesis of a monkey takes place for more than a month while that of a frog occurs in less than 2 days.

Several additional generalizations can also be derived from the large number of thymidine birthdating studies that have been carried out in the different regions of the vertebrate CNS. As noted above, it is observed in many areas of the developing CNS that distinct types of neurons originate in a fairly invariant timetable; in addition, the entire population of one type of neuron, like the spinal motoneurons, becomes postmitotic within a relatively short period of development. In general, large neurons are generated before small neurons in the same region. For example, pyramidal cells become postmitotic before granule cells in the hippocampus, cerebral cortex, and olfactory bulb, and in the cerebellum, Purkinje cells are generated prior to granule cells. In addition, the patterns of

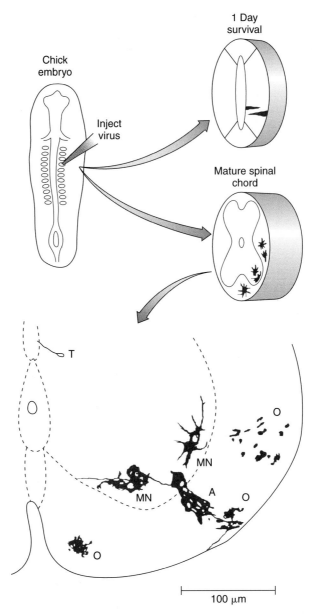

Figure 3.5 Clonal analysis of progenitor cells in the chick neural tube. Injections of a retrovirus with a reporter gene are made into the chick embryo neural tube. After either short or long postinjection survival periods, the spinal cord is sectioned and analyzed for the labeled progeny of the few infected progenitor cells. In the case shown, a single progenitor cell has been infected at this level of the spinal cord, and it has gone through a single cell division to give rise to two daughter cells after 1 day. If the embryo is allowed to survive to a point where the spinal cord is relatively mature and neurons and glial cells can be identified, the labeled cells can be assigned to specific cell classes. In the case shown, the progeny of the infected cell include motoneurons (MN), astrocytes (A), and oligodendrocytes (O) (Leber *et al.,* 1990).

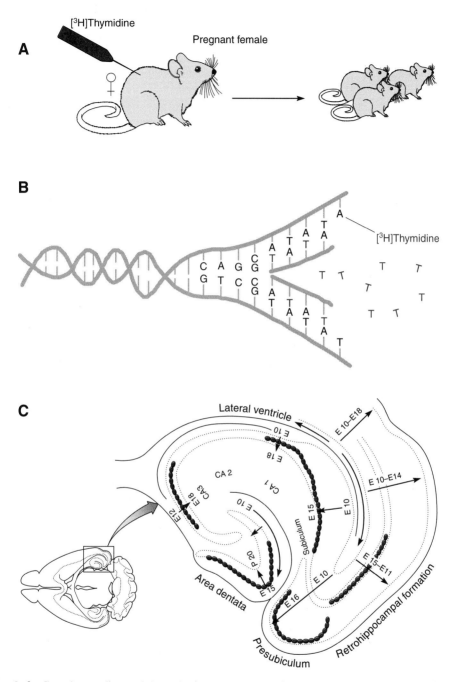

Figure 3.6 Complex gradients of time of origin of neurons in the hippocampus. (A) A pregnant animal is injected with ³H-thymidine, and the offspring are obtained postnatally. (B) ³H-thymidine becomes incorporated into DNA during the synthesis phase (C). Detailed thymidine birthdating analysis of mouse hippocampal formation shows the complex gradients in neuronal production typical of the central nervous system. Pregnant mice were given thymidine injections on the various days indicated (E10–E18). The brains of the pups born from these dams were analyzed for labeled cells. Arrows indicate gradients in time. (From Angevine, 1970)

neuronal generation are also consistent with the hypothesis that phylogenetically older parts of the brain develop before the more recently evolved structures.

Cell Cycle Genes Control the Number of Neurons Generated during Development

The factors that control the number of divisions in both the vertebrate and the invertebrate nervous systems are beginning to be understood. By identifying the gene products of mutations that affect the pattern of neuroblast proliferation in *Drosophila,* several cell cycle proteins are now known to be important in controlling the number of cell divisions of the neuroblasts. Many of these cell cycle genes were initially identified through an analysis of mutations that interfered with the ability of yeast cells to proliferate. Remarkable progress has been made in recent years in understanding the proteins that control the mitotic cell cycle. An intricate sequence of protein interactions control and coordinate the progress of a cell through the stages of cell replication, and there has been a considerable amount of conservation of this molecular mechanism over the millions of years of evolution from the simplest eucaryotic cells, like yeast, to more complex animals and plants (see Box: Cell Cycle).

Cyclins are a group of proteins that show dramatic changes in their expression levels that correlate with specific stages of the cell cycle. The association of cyclins with cyclin-dependent kinases (CDK) results in the activation of these kinases and the subsequent phosphorylation of the substrate proteins necessary for progression to the next phase of the cell cycle. Different cyclin/cdk pairs are required at different stages of the cell cycle; for example, the binding of cyclinB to cdc2 forms an active complex that causes a cell to progress through the M phase of the cycle, while the association of cyclinD and cdk4 or cdk6 causes these kinases to phosphorylate proteins necessary for progression from the G1 phase to the S phase.

Although mutations in several cell cycle genes interfere with the normal pattern of neuroblast proliferation in *Drosophila,* one of the most interesting of these is a gene called *string.* The product of this locus is a cyclin phosphatase, originally discovered as a cell cycle regulator in yeast-cdc25. Bursts of *string* transcription are both required and sufficient to trigger mitosis during the cell cycle. *String* is necessary for the transition of the cell into the M-phase, as it catalyzes the removal of phosphate groups from cdc2, a cyclin-dependent kinase, and thus allows it to form heterodimers with cyclinA and cyclinB.

The *myc* family is also very important in the control of neurogenesis. The *myc* gene was originally identified as an oncogene, and a viral form of the gene was implicated in feline leukemia. The gene product has been known for some time to act as a transcription factor, binding to a particular DNA consensus sequence known as an E-box and activating transcription of several cell cycle genes. The *myc* gene only binds this sequence when it forms a heterodimer with a related protein called Max. Another gene that forms heterodimers with Max is known as *Mad* and this gene is structurally related to *myc;* however, when the *Mad* gene product forms heterodimers with Max, it acts as a transcriptional repressor. *Myc* genes are expressed in nearly all mitotically active cells, including neural precursors, while members of the *Mad* family are expressed in the differentiating neurons. Targeted deletion of these genes has provided evidence for their role in the control of cell proliferation in the nervous system, as well as in other tissues. Elimination of the *myc* gene causes an embryonic lethality in mice and widespread defects in the development of the nervous system. These appear to be defects in the proliferation of the cells in the neural tube, although it is also possible that the loss of *myc* leads to apoptosis in the progenitor cells, since the *myc* gene has also been shown to have an important role in the apoptotic pathway in the hemopoetic lineage (Grandori and Eisenman, 1997).

Since the factors that regulate the cell cycle within the nervous system are largely the same as those involved in cell proliferation in other tissues, targeted deletions of key cell cycle regulator

Cell Cycle

The core of the cell cycle control machine is the cyclin-dependent kinases (CDKs) and their regulatory subunits, the cyclins. The cyclins were originally discovered as proteins that change dramatically in their levels of expression during the stages of the cell cycle. The transcription, translation, and destruction of each of these proteins are tightly tied to a particular stage of the cell cycle. The figure shows the period in the cell cycle when each of the cyclins is expressed.

The cyclins form complexes with specific CDKs, thereby activating the CDK to phosphorylate substrate proteins and consequently drive the cell through the next stage of the cycle. The most well characterized of the cyclin/CDK pairs is that of cyclinB and cdc2, which control the passage of the cell through the M phase of the cycle. In the late 1980s it was found that a cell-free extract of proteins could cause a cell to progress through the M phase of the cell cycle. This activity was called MPF, for mitosis promoting factor. CyclinB and cdc2 were discovered to be the active components of this activity. This complex of two proteins is a key regulator of this transition. Since that time there has been a considerable amount of study of these proteins and the other cyclins and their paired CDKs.

The cyclin/CDK activity is regulated by other proteins as well. For a CDK to be activated it must be phosphorylated at a particualr threonine residue, 161, and at the same time be dephosphorylated on residues threonine 14 and tyrosine 15. The proteins that effect these phosphorylation events are therefore important regulators of the CDK activity in a cell. These reguatory proteins include CAKs (CDK activating kinases) and phosphatases (like *string*). In addition, there are a number of CDK inhibitors, small proteins that act to inhibit CDK activity by binding to them and blocking their catalytic activity. The INK group, p15, p16, p18, and p19, all interact with cdk4 and cdk6, the CDK important in the transition from the G1 phase to the S phase. A second class of these proteins include p21, p27, and p57 and can bind to and inhibit all known CDKs.

A particularly important cell cycle transition is the entry into the S phase, which is the first step in the mitotic cycle. One of the most important regulators of this step is the cyclinD complex with either cdk4 or cdk6. When a cell receives a stimulus to enter the cycle, cyclin D is increased in its expression (see below) and forms a complex with cdk4/6. When this complex is phosphorylated by CAK it can catalyze the phosphorylation of several key substrate proteins necessary for the S phase of the cycle. One of the most important of these is called the retinoblastoma protein, or rb, which was originally identified as linked to a childhood retinal tumor. This protein is also one of a family of genes, known collectively as the pocket proteins, that acts as tumor inhibitors, and when they are absent or inactivated by a mutation, cells undergo unrestricted proliferation. In G1 the rb protein is unphosphorylated and this keeps the cell from entering the S phase; when this protein is phosphorylated by the cyclinD/CDK complex, the cell can then express the proteins necessary to move into the S phase.

The cell cycle control machine shown in the figure is a highly coordinated complex sequence of protein interactions. For the most part, once the sequence is set in motion, it proceeds in an autonomous manner. However, there are a few points where extracellular signals can regulate the progression from one phase of the cycle to another. In mammalian cells, the major checkpoint is in the transition from the G1 phase of the cycle to the S phase. This was first discovered by inducing tissue cultured cells to cease their mitotic activity by

Cell Cycle *continued*

withdrawing critical serum components from their medium. By adding back the serum for brief periods, it was found that once the cycle was started again the serum was not needed until after the cell had completed an entire cycle. In general, it is thought that when growth factors regulate cellular proliferation, they do so by acting at the G1 to S transition, either by promoting cyclinD expression/activity to stimulate entry into the next cycle or alternatively by increasing the expression of a cyclin inhibitor, like p27, to block entry into the next cycle. In *Drosophila* cells, the G2 progression is also frequently the target of control. Cells in the developing eye imaginal disc are held in G2 until they receive an extracellular signal, *hedgehog,* to trigger their progression through the M phase.

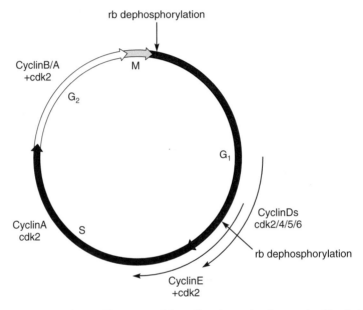

Cell cycle gene expression.   The stages of the cell cycle can be characterized by their expression of unique members of a group of proteins known as cyclins. Cyclic changes in the levels and phosphorylation state of these proteins "drive" the cell through the stages of mitosis. CyclinD for example is expressed in the G1 stage of the cell cycle and, in conjunction with cdk2/4, is necessary for the cell to enter the S phase (red).

genes often cause neural phenotypes. CyclinD1 is a member of a family of proteins termed the D cyclins that together with associated kinases (cdk4) phosphorylate the rb protein, thereby inactivating it and permitting entry of the cells into the S phase (see cell cycle genes above). The *cyclinD1* gene is expressed in mitotically active cells in many regions of the embryo; however, this particular cyclin shows a high level of expression in neural progenitor cells, particularly retinal progenitor cells. As a result, homozygous deletion of the *cyclinD1* gene slows or prevents the entry of neural progenitor cells into the S phase and thereby causes a reduction in the number of cells generated during embryogenesis. Other cell cycle regulators also have predictable effects on neurogenesis. Critical negative regulators of the cyclin-dependent kinases p27 and p21 are also expressed in the nervous system in the differentiating neurons shortly after they have withdrawn from the mitotic cycle. Deletion of the *p27* gene in mice causes a phenotype the opposite of that of the *cyclinD1* knockout; that is, there is an overproduction of cells in animals without the *p27* gene.

Cell Interactions Control the Number of Neurons and Glia Generated

In many tissues in the body, factors have been identified that stimulate or inhibit the progress of mitotically active cells through the cell cycle. These factors are called growth factors or mitogens and were named for the tissue or cell type where they were first found to have mitogenic effects. For example, fibroblast growth factor (FGF) was first found to promote the proliferation of fibroblasts in cell cultures, while epidermal growth factor (EGF) was discovered as a mitogen for epidermal cells *in vitro*. These growth factors most commonly act to control the progression from the G1 to the S phase of the cell cycle, and therefore it is possible that the gradual lengthening of the G1 phase of the cell cycle in neural progenitor cells within the CNS (above) is due to an increasing dependence on these factors for progression through the cell cycle as development proceeds. The factors that have been shown to act as mitogens for the mitotically active cells in the progenitor cells of the vertebrate CNS are primarily those peptides that act on receptor tyrosine kinases, including FGFs, TGF-α, EGF, and insulin-like growth factors (IGF). These studies have been carried out primarily in primary tissue cultures of neural progenitor cells. The cells of embryonic brain, spinal cord, or retina can be enzymatically dissociated and continue to proliferate *in vitro* as long as mitogens are added to the medium (Fig.

3.7). In general, FGFs act on progenitor cells earlier in development, while EGF and TGF-α acts on progenitor cells later in development. In one region of the vertebrate CNS, the retina, sensitivity to EGF or TGF-α only comes about in the latter half of neurogenesis; at early stages of retinal development, the progenitor cells only respond to FGFs. (Lillien and Cepko, 1992)

In addition to factors that act on receptor tyrosine kinases, other types of factors can also act as mitogens. TGF-β can either stimulate or inhibit proliferation in CNS progenitor cells (Anchan and Reh, 1995; Kane *et al.*, 1996). In addition to its function in dorsal–ventral patterning described in the previous chapter, *Sonic hedgehog* is also a mitogen for progenitor cells in the retina (Levine *et al.*, 1997) and the cerebellar external granule layer (Wechsler-Reya and Scott, 1999). Moreover, certain smaller molecules, like neurotransmitters, thyroid hormone, and small peptides, have also been implicated in the regulation of neuronal production in several areas of the brain (see Cameron *et al.*, 1998, for review).

In addition to their function in the regulation of the total numbers of cells produced by the progenitor cells, there is considerable evidence that the relative numbers of neurons and glia that are generated during development depend on growth factors. Early in the development of the CNS, many, if not all, of the progenitor cells have the capacity to generate both neurons and at least one, if not both, type of macroglial cells—the astrocytes and the oligodendrocytes (see above). Retroviral lineage studies have shown that for many regions of the nervous system, all three cell classes can derive from a single infected progenitor cell. At later stages of development, the lineages of these cell classes may become separate, and when cerebral cortical progenitor cells are labeled relatively late in development, the progeny of an infected cell may be restricted to only astrocytes or only neurons (Parnavales *et al.*, 1991; Luskin, 1993). For example, Davis and Temple (1994) have isolated progenitor cells from the embryonic cerebral cortex and cultured them as individual cells. They found that neurons and both classes of

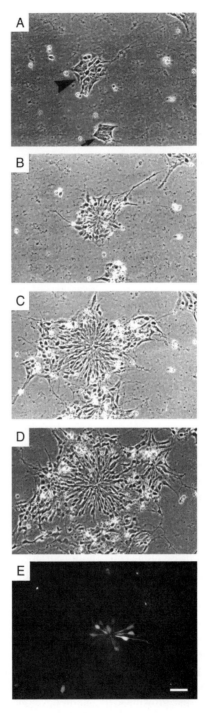

Figure 3.7 Epidermal growth factor stimulates the proliferation of neural progenitor cells grown *in vitro*. The effect of a growth factor is assayed by adding the factor to a dissociated cell culture of retinal progenitor cells. These cells are then followed over the next 4 days in culture by time-lapse microscopy (A–D), and the addition of new cells to the growing cluster can be observed. Under these culture conditions, the retinal progenitor cells form a radial arrangement that is organized similarly to that of the neural tube—the mitotic divisions occur at the center of the cluster as the cells round up to divide. (E) Labeling the cultures with antibodies for specific retinal neurons, in this case photoreceptors, shows that this type of neuron is generated *in vitro*. (A–D from Anchan *et al.*, Copyright 1991 Cell Press; E from Kelley *et al.*, 1994).

macroglia can arise from a single progenitor cell. In general, neurons are generated first in the development of the CNS, while most glial cells are generated later, and the same pattern is found *in vitro*. Several different growth factors can bias the types of cells produced when added to cultures of the progenitor cells. FGF2 and Neurotrophin3 (NT3) cause progenitor cells isolated from brain to develop primarily as neurons (Qian *et al.,* 1997; Ghosh and Greenberg, 1995). By contrast, adding EGF (Kuhn *et al.,* 1997) or CNTF (ciliary neurotrophic factor; Bonni *et al.,* 1997) to the cultures causes the cells to develop as astrocytes.

Members of the TGF-β superfamily of molecules, like BMP2 and BMP4, have also been shown to have effects on the multipotent progenitor cells, causing cells to develop as neurons under some culture conditions and astrocytes in others (Gross *et al.,* 1996). Along these same lines, PDGF (platelet-derived growth factor) promotes oligodendroglial development in some assays (Raff, 1989) and neurons in other assays (Williams *et al.,* 1997). Together, these studies paint a rather complex picture of the progenitor zone (Fig. 3.8). It is possible that these factors act in concert to control the relative numbers of neurons and glia produced by the progenitors, and recent evidence indicates that CNTF and BMP2 act synergistically to activate the promoter of a critical astrocyte gene, GFAP. However, it should also be noted that most of this work has been done *in vitro,* and so it is not known whether all these factors will have the same effects *in vivo,* in the intact ventricular zone. Nevertheless, studies of the effects of EGF and its receptor activation have shown that even *in vivo* this factor acts primarily to promote the production of astrocytes (Kuhn *et al.,* 1997), and biases cells away from neuronal differentiation.

As noted above, the production of the macroglial cells continues after the cessation of neurogenesis in most areas of the brain. Raff and his collegues have taken advantage of the fact that neurons do not develop in the optic nerve to carefully study the glial lineages in restricted glial progenitors (Fig. 3.9). The nerve contains both astrocytes and oligodendrocytes, and *in vitro* studies have shown that a particular type of cell, the O2A progenitor (for oligodendrocyte and type 2 astrocyte), can produce either astrocytes or oligodendrocytes, depending on the culture conditions (Raff, 1989). These O2A progenitor cells thus depend on signals to direct their differentiation. Multiple signals cause these cells to proliferate and develop as oligodendrocytes, including many of the same factors mentioned above: PDGF, NT3, and IGF-1. These factors are all produced by the astrocytes of the optic nerve, and PDGF is also produced by the retinal ganglion cells and present in their axons. In addition to these growth factors, the electrical activity of the axons in the optic nerve is also important for the oligodendrocyte progenitor cells' proliferation; blocking electrical activity results in a decline in the number of oligodendrocytes in the nerve (see Barres and Raff, 1994, for review). Tethering the production of oligodendrocytes to the axons in the nerve may provide a way to ensure that sufficient oligodendrocytes are produced to properly myelinate all the axons.

Cerebral Cortex Histogenesis

In the next section, the histogenesis of two specific regions of the CNS is highlighted. The histogenesis of the cerebral cortex has been a subject of intense study for many years. As noted in the previous chapter, the cerebral hemispheres develop from the wall of the telencephalic vesicle. The neuroepithelial cells initially span the thickness of the wall, and as they continue to undergo cell division the area of the hemispheres expands. At this early stage of development, the progenitor cells are thought to undergo primarily symmetric cell divisions, and their progeny both remain in the cell cycle. Soon, however, a few cells withdraw from the cycle to develop as the first cortical neurons. These neurons migrate a short distance to form a distinct layer, just beneath the pial surface, known as the preplate (Fig. 3.10). The preplate consists of two distinct cell types: a more superficial marginal zone, containing a group of large, stellate-shaped cells, known as Cajal-Retzius cells, and a deeper zone of cells called the subplate cells (Marin-Padilla, 1998; Allendoerfer and Shatz, 1994).

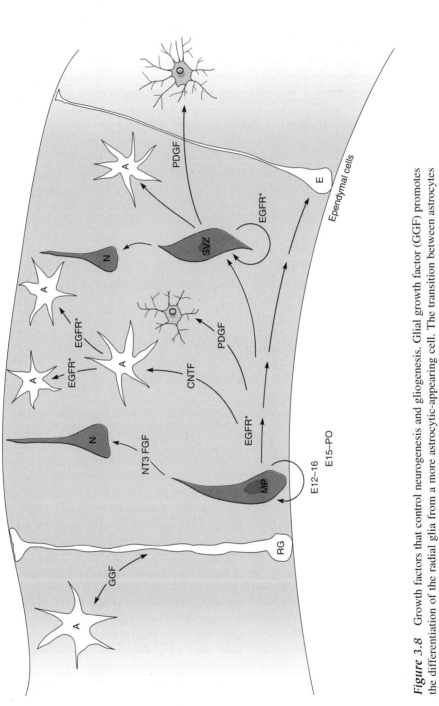

Figure 3.8 Growth factors that control neurogenesis and gliogenesis. Glial growth factor (GGF) promotes the differentiation of the radial glia from a more astrocytic-appearing cell. The transition between astrocytes (A) and radial glia (RG) has been demonstrated to occur both *in vivo* and *in vitro*. The progenitor cells (MP) in the early stages of development normally generate neurons (N). FGF2 stimulates these cells to proliferate and along with NT3 causes them to generate neurons. At later stages of development, the progenitor cells express the receptor for EGF and its related ligand TGF-α, and also begin to produce greater numbers of glial cells. Astrocytes in particular are produced when the EGF receptor is activated; CNTF also induces the progenitors to develop as astrocytes. PDGF causes the cells to develop as oligodendrocytes (o). Cells along the neural

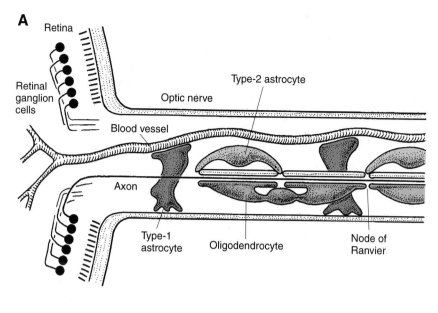

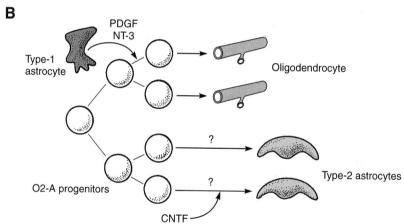

Figure 3.9 Glial diversity in the vertebrate CNS. (A) The optic nerve has three different types of glia, Type 1 and type 2 astrocytes and oligodendrocytes. (B) Culture studies show that Type 1 astrocytes secrete PDGF and NT-3, which causes O2-A progenitors to divide. After a certain number of divisions O2-A progenitors are timed to differentiate as oligodendrocytes, or type 2 astrocytes, if they are exposed to CNTF and other (?) factors. (Adapted from Harris and Hartenstein, 1999)

The next stage of cortical development is characterized by a large accumulation of newly postmitotic neurons within the preplate (Marin-Padilla, 1998). These new neurons form the cortical plate. The cortical plate divides the preplate into the superficial marginal zone, composed primarily of the Cajal–Retzius cells, and the in-termediate zone, composed of the subplate cells and increasing numbers of incoming axons. The developing cortex is thus described as having four layers: the ventricular zone, the intermediate zone, the cortical plate, and the marginal zone. At the very earliest stages of cortical de-velopment, the entire thickness of the cortex is

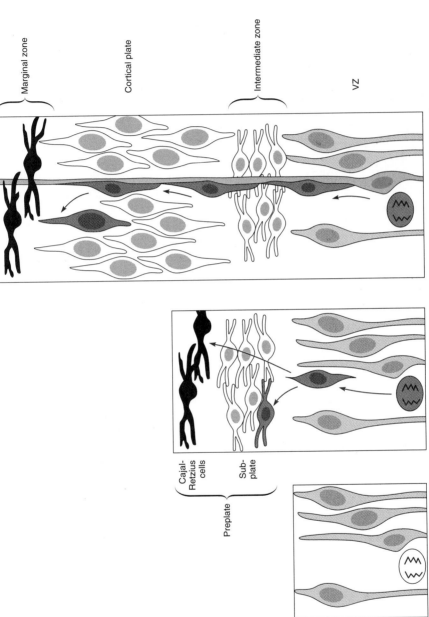

Figure 3.10 Histogenesis in the cerebral cortex proceeds through three stages. In the first stage of histogenesis, the wall of the cerebral cortex is made up of the progenitor cells, which occupy the ventricular zone (VZ). In the next stage of development, the first neurons exit the cell cycle (red) and accumulate in the preplate, adjacent to the pial surface. The neurons of the preplate can be divided into the more superficial Cajal–Retzius cells and the subplate cells. In the next stage of cortical histogenesis, newly generated neurons (red) migrate along radial glial fibers to form a layer between the Cajal–Retzius cells and the subplate. This layer is called the cortical plate, and the majority of the neurons in the cerebral cortex accumulate in this layer.

Marginal zone

Cortical plate

Intermediate zone

VZ

Cajal-Retzius cells

Sub-plate

Preplate

VZ

spanned by the processes of the progenitor cells. The first cortical neurons that are generated use the predominantly radial orientation of their neighboring progenitor cells to guide their mutation. However, the accumulation of neurons within the cortical plate results in a marked increase in cortical thickness. As a result the processes of progenitor cells no longer are able to extend to the external surface of the cortex. Nevertheless, the newly generated cortical neurons still migrate primarily in a radial direction. How is this accomplished?

To guide the newly generated cortical neurons to their destinations, a remarkable set of glial cells, the radial glia, provide a scaffold. These glial cells have long processes that extend from the ventricular zone all the way to the pial surface. They form a scaffold that neurons migrate along. Serial section electron microscopic studies by Pasko Rakic (1971, 1972) first clearly demonstrated the close association of migrating neurons with the radial glial cells in the cerebral cortex (Fig. 3.11). The migrating neurons wrap around the radial glial processes like a person climbing a pole. In recent years, it has been possible to directly observe the process of neuronal migration *in vitro* using dissociated cell cultures (Edmonson and Hatten, 1987) or cortical slices (O'Rourke *et al.,* 1997). These studies have confirmed that newly generated neurons migrate along the glial cells and have shown that the process is saltatory, with migrating neurons frequently starting and stopping along the way.

The next phase of cortical histogenesis is characterized by the gradual appearance of defined layers within the cortical plate. As more and more newly generated neurons migrate from the ventricular zone into the cortical plate, they settle in progressively more peripheral zones. Meanwhile, the earlier generated neurons are differentiating. Thus, later generated neurons migrate past those generated earlier. This results

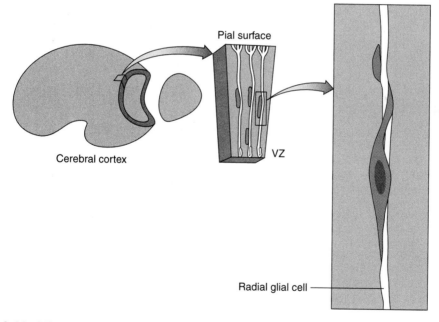

Figure 3.11 Migration of neurons along radial glia. The radial glial fibers extend from the ventricular zone to the pial surface of the cerebral cortex. A section through the cerebral cortex at an intermediate stage of histogenesis shows the relationship of the radial glia and the migrating neurons. The postmitotic neurons (red) wrap around the radial glia on their migration from the ventricular zone to their settling point in the cortical plate. (Adapted from Rakic, *J. Comp. Neurol.,* Copyright 1971, by permission of Wiley–Liss, Inc., a subsidiary of John Wiley & Sons, Inc.)

in an inside-out development of cortical layers (Fig. 3.12). This inside-out pattern of cerebral cortical histogenesis was first demonstrated by Angevine and Sidman using the [³H]-thymidine birthdating technique described above. The neurons labeled in the cortex of pups born from

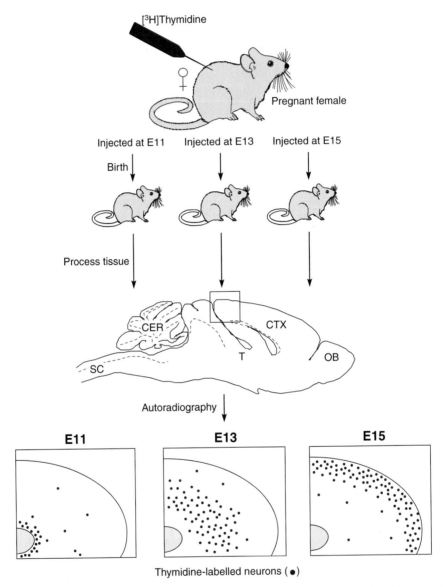

Thymidine-labelled neurons (•)

Figure 3.12   Birthdating studies demonstrate the inside-out pattern of cerebral cortical histogenesis. Pregnant female rats are given injections of [³H]-thymidine at progressively later stages of gestation. When the pups are born, they are allowed to survive to maturity and then their brains are processed to reveal the labeled cells. Neurons that have become postmitotic on E11 are found primarily in the subplate (now in the subcortical white matter), while neurons "born" on E13 are found in deep cortical layers, i.e., V and VI, and neurons generated on E15 are found in more superficial cortical layers, i.e., IV, III, and II. The most superficial layer, layer I, contains only the remnants of the preplate neurons (not shown). (Modified from Angevine and Sidman, 1961)

pregnant female rats injected with thymidine on the 13th day of gestation were located in the deeper layers of cortex, whereas the neurons labeled after a thymidine injection on the 15th day of gestation were found more superficially (Fig. 3.12). This inside-out pattern of cortical neurogenesis is conserved across mammalian species. Figure 3.13 shows the results of similar thymidine birthdating experiments in the monkey, where the process of neurogenesis is much more prolonged than that in the rat. Thymidine injections at progressively later stages of gestation result in progressively more superficial layers of cerebral cortical neurons being labeled. Each cortical layer has a relatively restricted period of developmental time over which it is normally generated (Fig. 3.13).

In mammals, the majority of neurons are generated from the ventricular zone cell divisions prior to birth and migrate radially via the radial glia. In addition to this predominantly medial migration of the newly generated neurons, however, it has been consistently noted that some populations of cortical neurons migrate tangential to the cortical surface. Lineage tracing studies give some indication as to the degree of this dispersion. The progeny of a progenitor cell labeled with a retrovirus can be widely dispersed within the cortex. In addition, chimeric animals expressing reporter genes show that a substantial fraction of the cortical neurons are not associated with nearby radial clusters of similar genotype. Observation of labeled neurons in cortical slice cultures has directly demonstrated this tangential migration of a subpopulation of cells migrating out of the ventricular zone (O'Rourke *et al.*, 1997).

In addition to the intrinsically generated, tangentially migrating neuronal population, at least some of these tangentially migrating cells are not derived from the cortical ventricular zone at all,

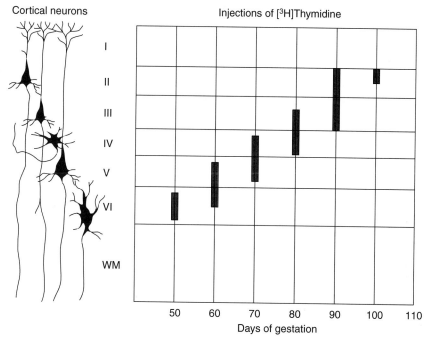

Figure 3.13 Birthdating studies in monkey further demonstrate the inside-out pattern of cerebral cortical histogenesis. In the monkey, where the histogenesis of the cerebral cortex is more protracted than in the rat, the production of the cortical neurons takes place over a 50-day time period. By labeling the pregnant female with [³H]-thymidine at progressively later gestational ages, it is possible to determine the period of embryonic development when each specific cortical layer is generated.

Neural Crest Migration

The neural crest exemplifies the migratory process in embroyology. No other tissue undergoes such extensive migration during development as the cells of the neural crest. As noted previously, the neural crest is a collection of cells that emerges from the dorsal margin of the neural tube, where it intersects with the ectoderm. Although the neural crest was first described by His in the chick embryo in 1868, the migration of the cells of the neural crest was first demonstrated by Detwiler in 1937 by labelling the premigratory cells with vital dye. The neural crest from the trunk takes two basic routes (Weston, 1963) from the neural tube: the ventral stream, along which the cells that will form the sensory, enteric and autonomic ganglia follow, and the dorsal or lateral stream, in which the cells that will form the pigment cells in the epidermis predominate. The route that cells take is to some degree determined by the environment in which they find themselves. There are differences in the types of cells that differentiate from the neural crest at different points along the anterior-posterior axis of the embryo. For example, the neural crest from the most anterior part of the developing spinal cord migrates into the gut to form the enteric nervous system, while the neural crest from somewhat more caudal levels of the spinal cord never migrates into the gut, but instead collects near the aorta and forms the sympathetic ganglion chain. Transplantation of neural crest cells from anterior (enteric ganglion forming) levels of the embryo to more posterior regions results in the anterior crest cells following the posterior pathways and making sympathetic neurons instead of enteric neurons (LeDourin, 1982).

What guides these cells to their proper locations in the embryo? Both permissive and repulsive cues, similar to those that guide growing axons (see Chapter 5), direct the neural crest through these two main routes. There are several large extracellular glycoproteins and sulfated proteoglycans that have been shown to be critical to the migration of many different types of cells. Two of these molecules, laminin and fibronectin, are known to support the migration of neural crest cells when the cells are dissociated from the embryo and plated onto tissue culture dishes. The receptors for these extracellular matrix molecules, heterodimers of integrin proteins, are expressed by the migrating neural crest cells, and purturbation of these receptors also inhibits neural crest migration. If either β1-integrin, or its heterodimeric partner, alpha4-integrin are blocked with specific antibodies, the neural crest migration is blocked (Lallier *et al.,*1994; Kil *et al.,* 1998). These results, and others, have shown that the neural crest of the trunk primarily interacts with the extracellular matrix as the cells migrate to their various destinations.

Another characteristic feature of neural crest cells emerging from the hindbrain and trunk is that they migrate in a segmented manner. Trunk neural crest cells migrate through the rostral half of each somite, but avoid the caudal half. What molecules are responsible for this restriction of their migratory routes. Another family of proteins appears to be necessary for this pattern of migration, the Ephrin receptors and ligands. These molecules were first identified for their roles in repulsive guidance of axonal growth (see Chapter 5). Two of the ligands, Lerk2 and HtkL, are expressed by the caudal halves of the somites, while the receptor, EphB3, is expressed by the migrating neural crest cells (Krull *et al.,* 1997; Wang and Anderson, 1997). If the neural crest cells are given a choice between fibronectin or the ephrin ligand, they avoid the ephrin. Moreover, if the soluble ligand is added to explants of trunk, the normal migratory pattern is disturbed, and the crest cells migrate on both halves of the somite (Krull *et al.,* 1997).

The neural crest that migrates from the cranial regions of the neural tube has many unique features. As noted in Chapter 2, the neural tube has a considerable amount of pattern in the head very early in development. The regions of the brain are dependent on the Hox and Pax gene expression. The neural crest that migrates from the cranial regions of the neural tube also has positional identity which is also dependent on the Hox code. The figure below shows the migration of the neural crest from the rhombomeres. The cranial crest contributes many cells to three tissue bulges known as branchial arches. The neural crest that migrates into these arches will give rise to most of the skeleton and cartilage of the skull and face. Thus, although normally we think of the neural crest as "neural" in the head the bulk of the neural crest cells will develop into non-neural tissues. The unique contribution of the different regions of the cranial neural crest has provided an opportunity to test for the specification of these cells and their migratory patterns. The crest cells from rhombomeres r1 and r2 migrate into the first arch (mandibular), the crest from r4 into the second arch (hyoid), and the crest from r6 and r7 migrates into the third arch (Kontges and Lumsden, 1996). The crest in each of these arches differentiates into specific skeletal elements of the face or jaw (see figure). The neural crest from each rhombomere continues to express the same pattern of hox genes as it migrates from the neural tube, and thus has a unique identity. This unique identity can be demonstrated by transplantation experiments where the crest from one rhombomere is transplanted to the region of another, and its migration and further development are monitored (Noden, 1983). Crest cells that would normally populate the third arch are excised and replaced with first arch crest cells. The transplanted crest cells migrate into the third arch, but instead of making neck cartilage, they form beaklike projections from the neck and form a complete duplicate first arch skeletal system in their new location. Thus it appears that the patterning of branchial arch skeletal and connective tissues is an intrinsic property of the cells of the neural crest prior to their emigration from the neural tube. Though they can use the same cues to migrate through the branchial arches, they will differentiate in accord with the hox code specific for their position or origin.

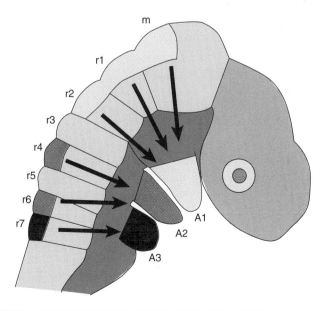

but instead migrate all the way from the ventricular zone in subcortical forebrain regions, the lateral and medial ganglionic eminences (LGE and MGE). Most of the neurons of the cerebral cortex are pyramidal in shape and use the neurotransmitter glutamate. However, there are other populations of neurons in the cerebral cortex, such as a class of stellate-shaped GABA-containing inhibitory interneurons. Single progenitor cells with *lacZ* reporter genes were injected into wild-type mouse embryos, and clones of labeled cells from these progenitors could be clearly identified in the cerebral cortex from very early stages of development. Two patterns of clones were identified: those that were made up primarily of pyramidal neurons, arranged in radial columns or clusters (Fig. 3.14), and those that were more widely dispersed which were GABA-containing stellate cells (Tan *et al.,* 1998). Anderson *et al.* (1997) found that when cortical slices were cultured with the LGE attached, these GABA neurons developed in the cortex. However, when the cortex was isolated from this subcortical region, the number of GABA-containing neurons was greatly reduced (Fig. 3.14). Moreover, they could directly visualize this migration by labeling the premigratory population in the LGE and MGE with a fluorescent dye and track the migration of the GABA-containing neurons to the cerebral cortex. Clearly, the tangentially migrating populations of young neurons within the cortex do not interact with the radial glial cells in the same way as that described for the radially migrating cortical neurons. However, at this time much more is known about the factors that guide neurons along radial glia (see below) than is known about the factors that guide these tangentially migrating populations.

The Subventricular Zone: A Secondary Zone of Neurogenesis

As we have seen, neurons can at times migrate considerable distances from their point of generation in the ventricular zone. Although the cases described so far involve the migration of postmitotic neurons, there are also regions of the brain where the progenitor cells themselves mi-

grate from the ventricular zone and continue to generate neurons in what are known as secondary zones of neurogenesis. There are three well-defined secondary zones of neurogenesis in the mammalian brain: the external granule layer (described in the section on cerebellar histogenesis), the subventricular zone, and the hippocampal granule cell precursors. The subventricular zone is a specialized region of the anterior lateral wall of the lateral ventricle (Fig. 3.15). The SVZ forms as a secondary neurogenic zone in the late embryonic period in rodents and, although most thoroughly studied in mice and rats, is present in all mammals examined to date. In rats, from E11 to E14 mitoses occur exclusively at the ventricular surface; however, at E16, the SVZ forms, subadjacent to the VZ, and the SVZ continues to generate neurons and glia long after the VZ has ceased cell division at E19. The majority of the glial cells of the forebrain is thought to be derived from the SVZ, but this zone also generates neurons. In recent years, the SVZ has become the subject of intense investigation as a potential source of neuronal precursors for neuronal repair, and more is said about this later in this chapter. Less well characterized are the hippocampal granule cell progenitor cells. The progenitor cells of the granule neurons of a region of the hippocampus known as the dentate gyrus originate from the ventricular zone for relatively short periods of embryonic development in the rat prior to E14. These progenitor cells then migrate to the growing dentate gyrus, where they continue to produce neurons for the rest of embryonic development and even into adult life (see below).

Are radial glial cells also important for the migration of neurons and progenitors of neurons in the secondary zones of histogenesis? Studies of the SVZ have been particularly illuminating. After the initial burst of gliogenesis (see above) most of the cells generated in the SVZ during the postnatal period and in mature rodents migrate to the olfactory bulb, in what is known as the rostral migratory stream. The cells migrate in chains, along extended astrocyte networks. These networks are complex (see Fig. 3.15) but in general have rostral–caudal orientation. One might imagine that the association of migrating

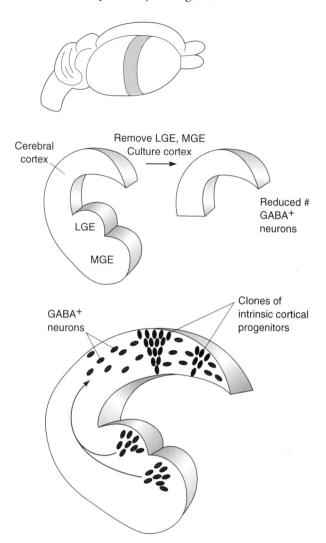

Figure 3.14 The neurons of the cerebral cortex derive from both intrinsic and extrinsic sources. Most of the neurons in the cortex are derived from the ventricular zone cells immediately below their adult location. Clones of cells in the cortex show only a limited amount of radial dispersion when labeled from very early stages of development using chimeric mice. However, the GABA-containing cells in the cortex arise from the lateral and medial ganglionic eminence (LGE), (MGE) subcortical structures that generate the neurons of the basal ganglia. If the cortex is isolated from the LGE and MGE early in its development, and the cortex is allowed to develop further *in vitro,* the number of GABA-containing neurons in the cortex is greatly reduced.

SVZ cells is analogous to the migration of cortical neurons along radial glia; however, the SVZ cells do not appear to require the glia. The migration of the SVZ cells has been termed chain migration and is distinct from the migration of neurons along radial glia. The SVZ cells form a chain *in vitro,* even in cultures devoid of glial cells, and migrate by sliding along one another. Figure 3.15 shows this process of leap-frogging SVZ cells in a time-lapse series. Thus, glia might help to orient SVZ migration, but are not essential for it.

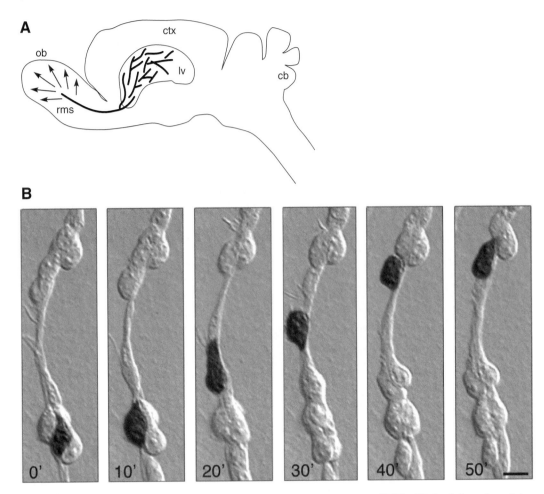

Figure 3.15 The rostral migratory stream from the subventricular zone (SVZ). (A) Sagital section of the mouse brain showing the rostral migratory stream. Cells generated in the SVZ adjacent to the lateral ventricles (lv) of the cerebral cortex (ctx) migrate to the olfactory bulb (ob), in what is known as the rostral migratory stream (rms). The cells normally migrate along complex astrocytic networks that are generally oriented in a rostral–caudal direction. (B) The time-lapse *in vitro* series shows how these cells migrate in chains by sliding along one another, and they can do this without any glia present in the cultures. The darkly labeled neuron migrates along the other unlabeled neurons. (Modified from Garcia-Verdugo *et al.,* 1998)

Cerebellar Cortex Histogenesis

The mature cerebellum is made up of several distinct cell types, each repeated in an almost crystalline array (Fig. 3.16). The two most distinctive of these cell types are the very large Purkinje cells and the very small granule cells. Purkinje cells are the principal neurons of the cerebellar cortex, sending axons out of the cor-

tex to the deep cerebellar nuclei. The cerebellar granule neurons are much more numerous than the Purkinje cells. In the mature cerebellum, they form a layer deep to the Purkinje cells and their axons extend past the Purkinje cell layer into the molecular layer. The axons of the granule cells bifurcate in the molecular layer, into a T shape, and these axons extend in the molecular layer for a considerable distance, synapsing on

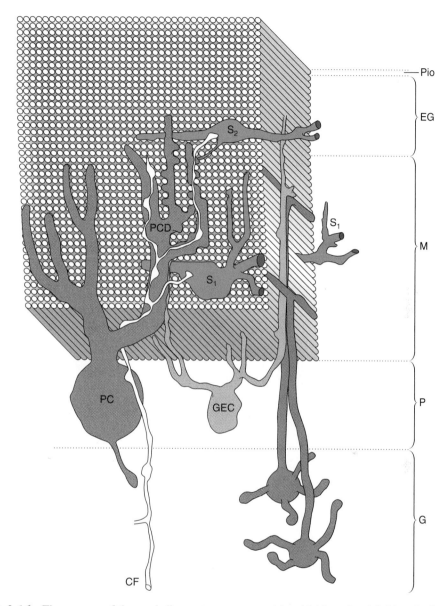

Figure 3.16 The neurons of the cerebellar cortex are arranged in a highly ordered fashion. In the mature cerebellum, the very large Purkinje cells (PC) lie in a single layer (P) and have an extensive dendritic elaboration that lies in a single plane. The granule cells (red) lie deep to the Purkinje cells in the granule cell layer (G) have a T-shaped axon that runs orthogonal to the plane of the Purkinje cell dendrites, like phone wires strung on the Purkinje cell dendritic "poles" in the molecular layer (M). In addition to these distinctive cell types, the cerebellar cortex also contains other cell classes, the stellate cells (S) and the Golgi epithelial cells (GECs). (Modified from Rakic, 1971)

the Purkinje cell dendrites. One can think of the Purkinje cells as telephone poles and the granule cell axons as the telephone wires.

The generation of the intricate cerebellar architecture is a complex process. The large Purkinje neurons are generated from a ventricular zone near the fourth ventricle of the brain stem, in a manner similar to that in which the neurons of the cerebral cortex are produced (as described in the previous section). Once they have finished

their final mitotic division, the Purkinje cells migrate a short distance radially to accumulate as an irregular layer known as the cerebellar plate (Fig. 3.17). As the cerebellum expands, these cells become aligned to form a single, regularly spaced layer. The Purkinje cells then grow their elaborate dendrites. In addition to the Purkinje cells, the ventricular zone generates several other cerebellar interneurons, like the stellate and basket cells.

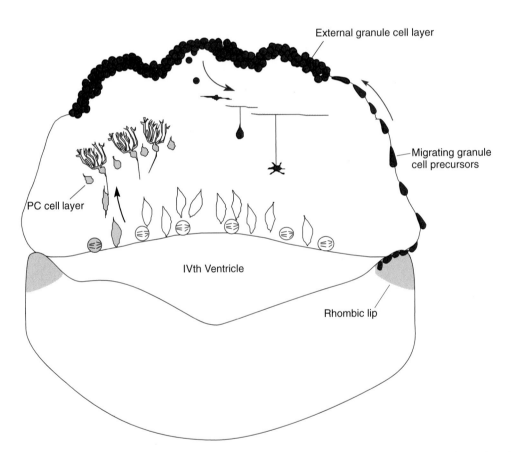

Figure 3.17 The cerebellum is derived from two separate progenitor zones through a complex series of cell migrations. The diagram shows the two sources of cerebellar neurons, but, for clarity, the generation of Purkinje (PC) cells is shown on the left and the generation of granule cells is shown on the right. The Purkinje cells, and some of the cerebellar interneurons, are generated from the ventricular zone in much the same way that most other neurons are generated in the brain. These progeny of these progenitor cells then migrate (arrows) to form a layer of cells known initially as the cerebellar plate and later as the Purkinje cell (PC) layer. The precursors of the granule cells come from a region of the rhombencephalon known as the rhombic lip (arrow). These cells migrate over the surface of the cerebellum and accumulate in a multicellular layer— the external granule cell layer. The cells then migrate into the cerebellum (arrow), trailing long axons as they descend past the Purkinje cell layer.

In contrast to the somewhat standard pattern of neurogenesis of the Purkinje cells, the granule cells arise from a completely separate progenitor zone, known as the rhombic lip. The granule cell precursors are initially generated near the rim of the fourth ventricle, but then migrate away from the ventricular zone, over the top of the developing Purkinje cells (Fig. 3.18) to form a secondary zone of neurogenesis, called the external granule layer. The cells in this layer continue to actively proliferate, generating an enormous number of granule cell progeny, thus increasing the thickness of the external granule layer considerably. The external granular layer persists for a considerable time after birth in most mammals and continues to generate new granule neurons. There are still granule neurons migrating from the external granule layer as late as 2 years after birth in humans (see Jacobson, 1991).

Although the granule neurons are generated superficially in the cerebellar cortex, they come to lie deep to the Purkinje in the mature cerebellum. The developing granule neurons must therefore migrate past the Purkinje cells. Figure 3.19 shows what this process looks like, as originally described by Ramon y Cajal. Soon after their generation, after their final mitotic division, the granule cells change from a very round cell to take on a more horizontally oriented shape as they begin to extend axons tangential to the cortical surface. Next, the cell body extends a large process at right angles to the axon. As this descending process grows deep into the cerebellum, the cell body and nucleus follow, leaving a thin connection to the axon. Meanwhile, the axons have been extending tangentially, and so the cell assumes a T shape. The cell body eventually migrates past the Purkinje cell layer and then begins to sprout dendrites in the granule cell layer.

The migration of the granule cells is another example of the importance of radial glia in CNS histogenesis. As they migrate, the granule cells are guided by a specialized type of radial glia

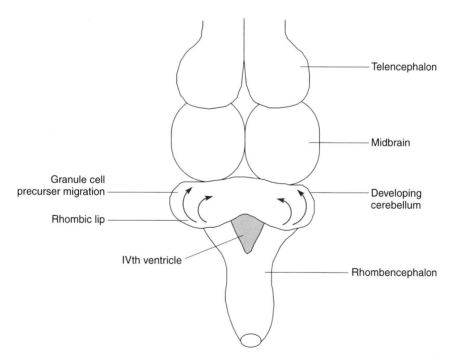

Granule cell precurser migration

Rhombic lip

IVth ventricle

Telencephalon

Midbrain

Developing cerebellum

Rhombencephalon

Figure 3.18 This dorsal view of the developing brain shows the migratory path of the granule cell precursors from the rhombic lip of the rhombencephalon to the surface of the cerebellum.

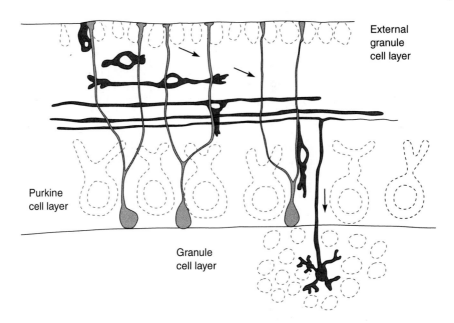

External
granule
cell layer

Purkine
cell layer

Granule
cell layer

Figure 3.19 Granule cell production in the external granule cell layer is followed by the migration of these cells to ultimately lie deep to the Purkinje cell layer. Arrows show the migratory path a single neuron (red) would take from its birth to the granule cell layer. The Bergmann glial cells are shown in gray and function as guides for the migrating neurons. The migration of a granule cell is thought to take place along a single glial fiber, but in the diagram the migrating neuron is shown associated with several glial cells for clarity. (Modified from Ramon y Cajal, 1929).

known as the Bergmann glia. EM studies, similar to those described for the cerebral cortex, first demonstrated the relationship between the migrating granule cells and the Bergmann glia (Rakic, 1971). Throughout the migration of the granule cells, they are closely apposed to the Bergmann glial processes. More recently, Hatten (1985) has been able to demonstrate directly the migration of granule cells on Bergmann glia using a dissociated culture system. When the external granule cell layer is removed from the cerebellum and the cells are cultured along with cerebellar glia, the granule glial cells migrate along the extended glial fibers *in vitro*. Time-lapse video recordings have captured the granule cell migration in action (Fig. 3.20). The *in vitro* systems have also provided a way to explore the molecular basis of neuronal migration on glial cells in the CNS.

Several questions about the molecular mechanisms of neuronal migration have been explored in recent years using the *in vitro* cerebellar micro-culture system developed by Hatten (1993). A particular class of cell surface proteins, known as cell adhesion molecules or CAMs, are known to mediate the adhesion between cells and the migration of cells in many tissues in the embryo. Are these proteins necessary for the migration of granule cells along radial glial fibers? Under control conditions, the granule cells migrate on the radial glial cells in the cultures at about 33 μm/h. To test whether the most abundant CAMs in the nervous system, NCAM, N-cadherin, and L1, are important for granule cell migration, Hatten's group added antibodies that specifically block the function of these molecules in the cerebellar microcultures. They found that none of these antibodies interfered with the migration of the granule cells. However, when they added a polyclonal antiserum that they had raised against cerebellar cells to the cultures, they found a significant inhibition of the granule cell migration (Fig. 3.21). They concluded that some type of adhesion molecule was necessary for the migra-

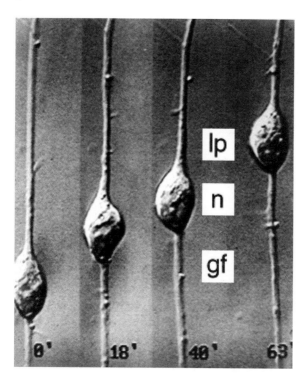

Figure 3.20 Neuronal migration along glial fibers can be observed directly. In cerebellar neuron–glial cocultures the neurons associate with the glial processes and slowly move along them. Using time–lapse microscopy, neuronal migration can be directly observed and quantified. This has provided an excellent assay for investigating the molecular basis for neuronal migration. (lp, leading process; n, neuron; gf, glial fiber) (Reprinted from García-Verdugo, *et al.*, Copyright 1998, by permission of Wiley–Liss, Inc., a subsidiary of John Wiley & Sons, Inc.)

tion of these cells, but that it was not one of the previously known CAMs. To find this new CAM, they used a clever approach—they absorbed the anti-granule cell antiserum with other types of neural cells and cell lines, thus getting rid of those antibodies from the serum that recognize common CAMs. What they were left with was an antiserum that recognized a single protein of approximately 100 kDa, which they named as-trotactin. Subsequent studies showed that astro-tactin is a protein that resembles other CAMs but is in a distinct family (Zheng *et al.,* 1996). It is expressed in the migrating granule cells, and antibodies raised against astrotactin block the migration of the granule neurons along the glial fibers.

In addition to the use of *in vitro* systems for studying migration, advances in our understanding of the molecular mechanisms of cell migration have come about by analysis of naturally occurring mouse mutations that disrupt the normal migration of neurons. One important function of the cerebellum is to maintain an animal's balance. Lesions to the cerebellum in humans frequently produce a syndrome, known as ataxia, that includes unsteady walking. Genetic disruptions of the cerebellum in mice produce a similar syndrome, and therefore they can be identified and studied. By screening large numbers of mice for motor abnormalities, several naturally occurring mutations have been identified that disrupt cerebellar development. Due to the nature of the symptoms, these mutant mouse strains have names like reeler, weaver, and staggerer. The mutant genes that underlie these phenotypes have been identified and one of these mutants, the reeler, has been particularly informative in understanding neuronal migration.

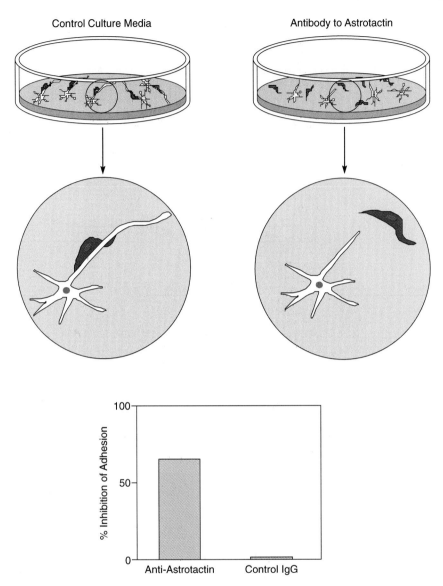

Figure 3.21   *In vitro* assay demonstrates the importance of astrotactin in granule cell migration. When cerebellar glial cells are cocultured with granule cells, the glial cells adopt an elongate morphology and the neurons (red) crawl along the glial processes. When astrotactin antiserum is added to these cultures, the neurons no longer associate with the glial processes and the long processes of the glial cells retract. This *in vitro* assay has also been used to analyze the effects of other molecules, like CAMs and extracellular matrix molecules, on granule cell migration. (Modified from Hatten, 1985)

The reeler mutant mouse has ataxia and a tremor. Histological examination of individually labeled neurons in reeler mutant cerebral and cerebellar cortex revealed gross malpositioning of the cells. In the cerebellar cortex, the Purkinje cells are reduced in number and, instead of forming a single layer, are frequently present as aggregates (Fig. 3.22). There are fewer granule

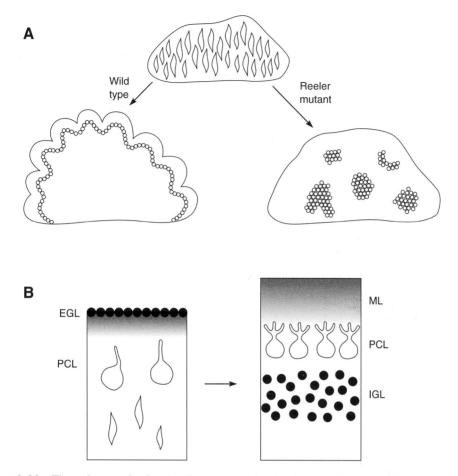

Figure 3.22 The reeler mutation in mice disrupts cerebellar development. (A) In normal mice, the Purkinje cells form a single layer in the cortex. In reeler mice, the Purkinje cells do not form a cortex, but remain in large aggregates. The other cerebellar neurons are also malpositioned in the cerebellar cortex of the reeler mice. As a result, the normal function of the cerebellum in controlling balance is disrupted in the reeler mice and so they "reel." (B) The gene that is disrupted in the reeler mice is known as *reelin*. This gene codes for a large extracellular matrix protein that is produced by the granule cells prior to their migration in the external granule cell layer (EGL). The reelin protein functions to guide Purkinje cells to their proper laminar arrangement (PCL) in the cortex and its distribution is shown in red. One model proposes reelin expressed in the EGL attracts the Purkinje cells to this surface. (Modified from Miyata *et al.,* 1997)

cells and most of them have failed to migrate deep into Purkinje cells. Thus, they lie external to the Purkinje cells. In addition, many other regions of the CNS, including the cerebral cortex, show similar disruptions in normal cellular relationships. In the cerebral cortex of the reeler mouse, instead of the normal inside-out pattern, later generated neurons fail to migrate past those generated earlier, and thus these mice have an outside-in organization.

The defective molecule underlying the reeler phenotype has been identified. It is a large glycoprotein, named reelin, containing over 3,000 amino acids, and bears some similarities with some extracellular matrix proteins (Miyata *et al.,* 1997). The reelin protein is expressed by the granule cells in the external granule cell layer from the very earliest stages of development. Although it is not known what this protein does to ensure the proper migration of the neuroblasts, one attractive hypothesis is that it acts as a chemoattractant signal. Once the new Purkinje cells have begun to migrate out of the ventricular zone, the reelin secreted from the granule cells causes the Purkinje cells to migrate toward them. The originally identified reeler allele contains a mutation that produces a truncated protein. In these mutants, no attractive signal is provided for the migrating neurons and so they do not form a layer, but instead stop once they have left the ventricular zone (Fig. 3.22) and form large aggregates.

In sum, there are clearly many cellular interactions critical for the development of the complex cerebellar architecture. The granule cells appear to play several key roles in orchestrating the development of the cerebellar cortex. Reelin, produced by the granule cells in the external granule cell layer is necessary for the appropriate migration and alignment of the Purkinje cells, while astrotactin, expressed by the migrating granule cells, is important in their migration to the internal granule cell layer. In addition to these molecules, the receptor tyrosine kinase erbB4 and its ligand neuregulin are also important regulators of the granule cell migration (Rio et al., 1997). It has been proposed that neuregulin produced by the granule cells is necessary for the Bergmann glial differentiation. In this way the granule cells may even coordinate the development of the very scaffold upon which they will migrate.

Postembryonic and Adult Neurogenesis

Eventually the process of neurogenesis ceases in most regions of the nervous system. Neurons themselves are terminally differential cells—there are no documented examples of functional neurons reentering the mitotic cycle. However, it has long been appreciated that in most species some new neurons are generated throughout life. There is a considerable remodeling of the nervous system of insects during metamorphosis. Much of this remodeling occurs through cell death, but new neurons are also produced.

Many amphibians also go through a larval stage. Frogs and toads have tadpole stages where a considerable amount of body growth takes place prior to metamorphosis into the adult form. During larval stages, many regions of the frog nervous system continue to undergo neurogenesis similar to that in embryonic stages. One of the most well-studied examples of larval frog neurogenesis is in the retinotectal system. The eye of the tadpole, like that of the fish, increases dramatically in size after embryonic development is complete. During this period, the animal uses its visual system to catch prey and avoid predators.

The growth of the retina, however, does not occur throughout its full extent but, rather, is confined to the periphery (Fig. 3.23) (Hollyfield, 1968). This provides a way for new cell addition to go on at the same time the central retina functions normally. As the new retinal cells are added, they are integrated into the circuitry of the previously differentiated retina, into a seamless structure. At the same time the new cells are added to the peripheral retina, the optic tectum also adds new neurons. The coordination between neurogenesis in these two regions likely involves their interaction via the retinal ganglion cell projection of the tectum. The growth of the optic tectum occurs at its caudal margin, so the axons of the ganglion cell must shift caudally during this time. The rate of new cell addition is comparable to that of the embryo, and there appears to be a true retinal stem cell at the margin capable of generating all the cell types present in the structure.

Fish retinae have an additional means of growth. As the retina grows, the sensitivity to light declines as retinal stretch causes a reduction in the number of rod photoreceptors (Johns and Fernald, 1981). The fish maintains a constant sensitivity by adding new rods to the retina. These cells are generated by a specialized progenitor, the rod progenitor, that under normal circumstances generates new rod photorecep-

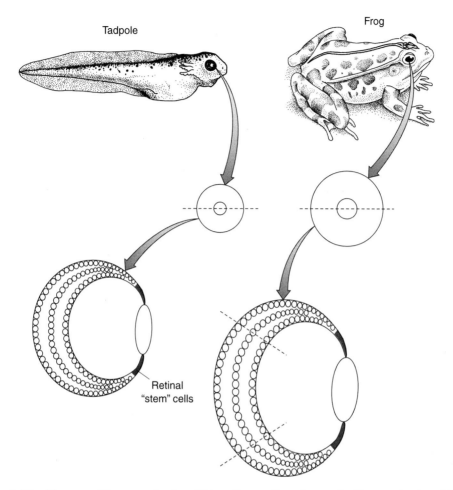

Figure 3.23 The eyes of frogs grow by the addition of new cells to the margin. The neural retina of the frog tadpole is derived from the neural tube, as described in a previous chapter. The initial retinal neurons are generated during embryogenesis. However, as the eye grows, the neural retina grows by means of a specialized ring of retinal stem cells at the peripheral margin of the eye (red). The retinal stem cells generate all the different types of retinal neurons to produce new retina that is indistinguishable from the embryonically generated retina and thoroughly intergrated with it. In the newly postmetamorphic *Rana pipiens* frog, nearly 90% of the retina has been generated during the larval stages; all this time the retina has been fully functional. This process continues even after metamorphosis, but much more slowly.

tors. This specialized progenitor may not be entirely restricted in its potential, however, since, following damage to the retina, these cells are stimulated to generate other retinal cell types as well. Thus, it is possible that the retina of fish has stem cells sprinkled throughout.

One of the most well-studied examples of neurogenesis in mature animals comes from studies of songbirds. In 1980, Fernando Nottebohm reported that there was a seasonal change in the size of one of the brain nuclei important for song production in adult male canaries. In songbirds, there are specific nuclei in the telencephalon of the brain that are critical for the production of the song. The HVC nucleus is of particular importance for both song learning and song production. The HVC is almost twice as large in the spring, when male canaries are generating normal adult song, than in the fall, at which time they no longer sing. Nottebohm initially proposed that this change in size might be due to seasonal changes in the numbers of synapses. In further studies of the HVC in male and female canaries, Nottebohm also noticed that it was larger in males, which learn complex songs, than in female, which do not sing. Moreover, if adult females were given testosterone injections, the HVC nucleus grew by 90% and the female birds acquired male song.

To determine whether new neurons were added to the nucleus in response to the testosterone, female birds were injected with [^{3}H]-thymidine as well as with testosterone, and the animals were sacrificed for analysis 5 months later. They found that in both the testosterone-treated and the control birds there were many thymidine-labeled cells, and many of these had morphological characteristics of neurons. They also analyzed the birds immediately after the injections and found that the new neurons were not produced in the HVC itself, but rather were generated in the subventricular zone (SVZ) of the telencephalon and migrated to the nucleus, in a manner analogous to the way in which the nucleus is initially generated during embryogenesis. Subsequent studies have shown that the newly produced neurons migrate along radially arranged glial processes from the SVZ to the HVC. Thus, neurogenesis is a normally occurring phenomenon in adult canaries (Fig. 3.24). The progeny of the cells produced in the SVZ migrate to the HVC soon after their generation. There they differentiate into neurons, about half of which become local interneurons. The other half differentiate into projection neurons and send axons out of the nucleus to connect with other neurons in the brain to form part of the functional circuit for song learning.

Thus, there appears to be a seasonally regulated turnover of neurons in the HVC and in other song control nuclei in the brain of the adult songbird. The turnover of neurons may correlate with periods of plasticity in song learning. Canaries modify their songs each year; each spring breeding season they incorporate new syllables

into the basic pattern, and then in the late summer and fall they sing much less frequently. Combining thymidine injections with measures of cell death and overall neuronal number in the HVC over a year one can see two distinct periods of cell death, and each one is followed by a burst in the number of new neurons in the nucleus. Both of these periods of high neuronal turnover correlate with peaks in the production of new syllables added to the song. The neurogenesis is balanced by cell death and during periods of new song learning the nucleus adds cells, while during periods when no song is generated the song-related nuclei undergo regression. Is the rate of neurogenesis in the ventricular zone controlled by the seasonal changes in testosterone in the male birds? When the number of labeled cells in the ventricular zone is compared in testosterone-treated and untreated female birds, there are no differences—indicating that the rate of neurogenesis does not change in response to the hormone. However, it appears instead that the survival of the neurons in the HVC is seasonally regulated. Neurons generated in the spring have a much shorter average life span than those generated in the fall. Thus, the seasonal changes in the neuronal number in the songbird HVC are not dependent on changes in the number of newly added cells, but rather on seasonally and hormonally regulated differences in the survival of the newly produced neurons.

Neurogenesis also occurs in the mature mammalian brain. Although for many years this view was regarded as somewhat heretical, it has become well-accepted in recent years. The thymidine birthdating studies of Altman and Bayer, described at the beginning of this chapter, thoroughly documented the time and place of origin of neurons and glia of many regions of the rodent brain. It was found that many brain neurons are generated after birth in rodents. They next extended the labeling period to the second and third postnatal weeks and found that in one particular region thymidine-labeled olfactory cells continued to be found up to 4 weeks postnatally (Altman, 1969). These cells are generated in the subventricular zone in the forebrain and then migrate to the olfactory bulb (Fig. 3.24). In recent years it has been recognized that this neuro-

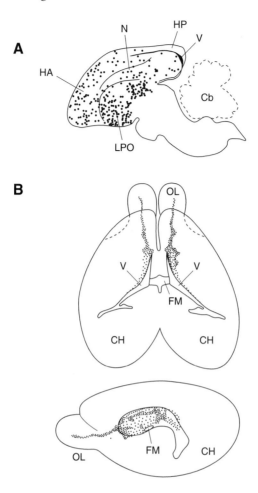

Figure 3.24 Neurogenesis in the brains of adult birds and rodents. (A) Sagittal section of an adult canary brain showing the widespread pattern of newly generated cells, many of which will go on to differentiate as neurons. (Modified from Alvarez-Buylla, 1998). (B) Dorsal and sagittal views of an adult mouse brain showing thymidine labeling of proliferating subventricular zone cells and the rostral migratory stream. (Modified from Smart, 1961; see also Jacobson, 1991).

genesis also occurs in the adult hippocampus, and several studies have now shown that these cells are multipotent, like progenitor cells in the embryonic brain (Lois and Alvarez-Buylla, 1993; Luskin, 1993; Reynolds and Weiss, 1992). Even in some areas of the primate cerebral cortex, these stem cells also produce new neurons.

Why do mammals generate new neurons in these regions? Frogs and fish have eyes that grow; birds learn new songs. What is the advantage to the mammal? While there are no studies of a change in the animals' abilities that correlate with this cellular addition in mammals, several possibilities may be entertained. For example, since both the olfactory bulb and the hippocampus are involved in the formation of olfactory memories, the neuronal turnover in these regions could be important in a seasonal change in nests or mates. Future studies of adult neurogenesis in the mammalian brain will likely lead to new insights in how our brains change and adapt throughout life.

Determination and Differentiation

·   ·   ·   ·   ·

The nervous system is a coral reef of the body where evolution and development have collaborated to produce the most extraordinary diversity of cell types. Within the brain, there is enormous variety in cellular anatomy, physiological function, neurochemistry, and connectivity. For example, the rod photoreceptors in the human retina are short cells that have no axons or dendrites to speak of, are filled with visual pigment, do not fire action potentials, yet release the transmitter glutamate continuously. In contrast cerebellar Purkinje cells are relatively huge, have an impressive electrically active dendritic tree and a long spiking axon, and release the inhibitory neurotransmitter GABA. There are a host of other molecular differences between these cells as well obvious differences in their circuitry and connectivity. In other neurons, differences can be more subtle. Various motor neurons of the spinal cord may share a great deal of morphology, chemistry, physiology, and circuitry yet make connections to different muscles. If one considers the neurochemistry of the brain alone, it becomes clear that this organ must use

a great deal of genetic information. Furthermore, neurons need genetic information to tell them what shape to take on, what axonal pathways to follow, and with what targets to connect. The number of genes used to carry out this task of specification is also impressive. It has been estimated that of all the genes expressed in the body, over 50% of them are expressed exclusively in the nervous system. Most of these are developmentally significant and are involved in various aspects of neuronal differentiation (Shankland and Macagno, 1992; Harris and Hartenstein, 1999; Moody, 1999).

The genetic information that leads a neuron to a particular fate may be expressed in the tissues surrounding that neuron (Fig. 4.1). The environment into which the neuron is born and in which it gradually differentiates provides extrinsic cues in the form of diffusible molecules, as well as cell surface proteins or molecules in the ECM. In addition to these external signals, cells may inherit molecules from their precursors that can affect their fate. Many types of neurons, particularly those of invertebrates, are formed by a

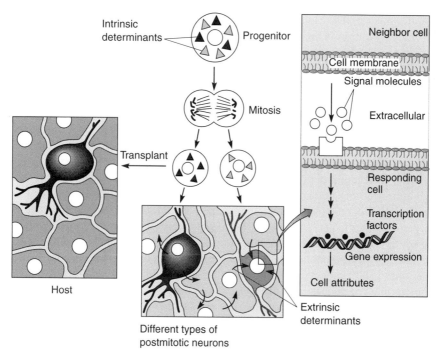

Figure 4.1 Intrinsic and extrinsic determinants of cell fate. The red daughter of the progenitor cell has inherited the intracellular determinants (red triangles). Its fate is determined by these determinants and is not altered when the cell is transplanted to a different host (left). The sister cell has not inherited the determinants and the new host environment changes the fate of the cell by signals coming from neighboring cells that are transduced on a pathway that leads to new genes being activated (right).

lineage-dependent mechanism. Intrinsic factors expressed at various stages during progenitor cell proliferation play an important role in specifying these different cell fates. Sydney Brenner coined a useful metaphor for thinking about the question of the relative importance of these intrinsic and extrinsic influences on cell fate. Cells are either European or American. The fate of a European cell is largely the result of who its parents are. In America, neighbors are more influential than lineage. In real life, both in the world of cells and in the world of people, fates aren't totally controlled by either lineage or environment, but rather by a mixture of the two. The adoption of a particular fate is a multistep sequential process that happens in the context of both. Thus, if a cell has been externally influenced to take a step along a particular fate pathway, the unborn daughter of that cell has also, in a sense,

taken the same step and is through her lineage restricted to a narrower set of fates. The establishment of fate is thus a hierarchical process.

To understand the cues that shape a neuron's fate, experimental analysis is necessary. Cell ablation is a technique that is useful for asking about cell fates in the context of all the other surrounding cells. As noted in Chapter 1, one of the first demonstrations of interactions among the cells of a proneural cluster involved the ablation of the developing neuroblast, which induced a neighboring cell to adopt the ablated cell's fate. Transplantation is a classical technique for finding out whether a cell's fate is an intrinsic (or autonomous) property or whether it is controlled nonautonomously. A progenitor cell from a donor animal is transplanted to another part of a host animal. If the fate of the cell is unaltered by such procedures, then the cell is already determined. If, however, the result is a new fate consistent with the position in the host, then the fate at the time of transplantation is still flexible and can be determined nonautonomously. Putting cells into tissue culture is another valuable technique. By isolating it from the embryo entirely, it is possible to assay a cell's state of determination. Moreover, since the culture medium can be controlled, potential signal molecules can be screened for their effect on cell fate choices. The most powerful technique for studying the events leading to neuronal fate and differentiation are carefully designed genetical manipulations. Mutations in particular genes alter the development of certain types of neurons. With a mutant it is possible to show not only where and when the normal gene product must function but, using molecular techniques, it is also possible to identify the gene product in question.

Transcriptional Control of Invariant Lineages

The nervous system of *C. elegans* affords an opportunity to investigate the generation of cell fates in a system where descriptive studies have shown that there is an almost invariant lineage of every cell in the body and the nervous system (Sulston and Horvitz, 1977; Sulston *et al.,* 1983). Ablating the ancestral mother of a particular set of neurons causes the loss of those neurons in the adult animal (Sulston and White, 1980). Even though nervous system development is highly determinative in this organism, it is generated in a piecemeal fashion. That is, given neural elements may come from a variety of different lineages. For example, some of the motor neurons of *C. elegans* arise during embryogenesis from three separate precursors, while the rest arise postembryonically from 13 different precursors. Each of these precursors gives rise to nonneural cells as well.

Most of our knowledge concerning the generation of different cell types comes from mutants that interfere with cellular determination. These mutants have been used to dissect multi-step processes into hierarchical pathways. Many of the mutations that affect CNS lineages are in genes that code for nuclear transcription factors. One of the best understood examples of neuronal fate is that of the specialized mechanosensory cells in nematodes studied by Martin Chalfie and his colleagues (Chalfie and Au, 1989; Chalfie, 1993). Most nematodes rush forward when touched lightly on the rear and move backward when touched on the front. By prodding mutagenized nematodes with an eyelash hair attached to the end of a stick, Chalfie was able to select a large number of touch-insensitive mutants. These mutants represent a group of genes involved in the specification and function of the mechanosensory cells that are responsible for touch sensitivity. One of the genes identified in this screen was called *unc-86*. Mutations in this gene result in the failure of the mechanosensory neurons or touch cells to form. *Unc-86* encodes a transcription factor of the POU-homeodomain family. It is expressed transiently in many neural precursors and particularly in the lineage produced by a neuroblast called Q. In wild-type animals, Q divides into two daughter cells, Ql.a and Ql.p (Fig. 4.2). Both of these cells continue dividing, giving rise to different progeny: Ql.p produces a touch cell and an interneuron while Ql.a. produces a ciliated sensory neuron. The *unc-86* gene is turned on only in the Ql.p daughter cell and its progeny. A loss of function mutation in *unc-86* results in the "transformation" of Ql.p, the cell in which it is normally expressed, into a stem cell that behaves like the mother. Thus, instead of producing the sensory neurons, the cell continues to divide in the pattern of its mother cell, the Q neuroblast. Thus, mutations in *unc-86* affect the lineage of touch cells in such a way that these cells are never born.

Another gene uncovered in Chalfie's screen of touch mutants was named *mec-3*. Touch cells are born when the *mec-3* gene is mutated, but they do not differentiate into mechanosensory neurons. Instead, they develop into a different sort of neuron. Thus, the *mec3* mutation does not perturb the commitment to a neural fate, but rather the specific neural subtype. It turns out that the *mec-3* gene codes for a transcription factor

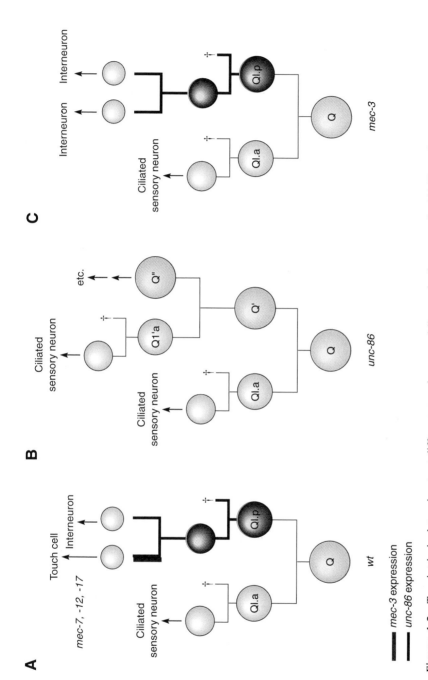

Figure 4.2 Two intrinsic determinants at different steps in a neural lineage in the nematode. (A) Normal lineage. If Q1.p cannot express *unc-86*, it becomes Q' a copy of its mother, Q (B). The result is a repeat of the previous division, which results only in Q progenitors and ciliated sensory neurons. *Mec-3* needs to be expressed in the touch cell. If it isn't, in *mec-3* mutants this cell turns into an interneuron like its sister (C).

of the LIM-homeodomain family. Cells fated to become touch cells all express *unc-86* at first, and this transcription factor binds to and activates the expression of the *mec-3* gene. Thus, when *unc-86* is mutated, the cells will not express *mec-3*. However, when MEC-3 and UNC-86 proteins are expressed in the same cell, they physically interact to make a new heterodimeric transcription factor. This heterodimer maintains *mec-3* expression and turns on a set of up to 15 other genes in the touch differentiation pathway, such as the *mec-7, mec-12,* and *mec-17* genes. These three genes encode structural proteins that are used in the construction of the specialized touch cell cytoskeleton. Thus, in this system we witness a hierarchical cascade of intrinsic transcription factors, one regulating the next, until the last turns on genes that the differentiated cell uses to realize its determined fate.

Another set of neurons that has been studied in detail genetically in *C. elegans* is the hermaophrodite-specific neurons or HSNs (Desai *et al.,* 1988; Desai and Horvitz, 1989). These neurons are crucial for egg laying as shown by mutants that are unable to lay self-fertilized eggs. In a lurid bit of biology, the eggs of these mutant HSN worms hatch into feeding larvae within the worm mother's uterus. The mother is devoured by her progeny from the inside and becomes a bag of wriggling worms that in their hunger eventually eat through her cuticle into the world. Thus mutants defective in HSNs are easy to detect, and a large collection have been gathered by Horvitz and colleagues. Only one of the 20 or so genes that affect HSN development are used in the touch cell development, and this is the *unc-86* gene that we have just discussed. Surprisingly, however, the role of *unc-86* seems entirely different in HSN differentiation, where, instead of regulating lineage, it regulates neurotransmitter expression and axon outgrowth. The fact that there is so little overlap in the genes that are involved in these two heavily studied genetic systems suggests that the molecular cascades of cell determination are genetically complex and highly individualized. However, there are similarities that are worth pointing out. In the case of both the HSNs and the mechanosensory neu-

rons, it is possible to establish a hierarchical pathway, rich in transcription factors. Some of these factors regulate others in a molecular cascade whereby the lineage, the specification, the differentiation, and finally the function of neurons are established through a series of successive stages.

Position and Determination

As described in Chapter 1, the CNS of an insect develops from a set of individual neuroblasts that enlarge within the neurogenic region and then delaminate to the inside, forming a subectodermal neuroblast layer. The neuroblasts arise in three successive waves (SI–SIII) and are arranged in columns and rows (Doe, 1992a). Neuroblasts can thus be identified by their position and time of formation. Each neuroblast divides a characteristic number of times to produce a small set of ganglion mother cells (GMCs). GMCs then divide once more to produce two neurons. A neuroblast in a specific position always generates GMCs that produce the same group of neurons. Thus, each neuroblast, each GMC, and each neuron has a distinct fate (Fig. 4.3). Although these patterns of cell division and determination are invariant from embryo to embryo, position, rather than lineage, plays an important role at the top of the hierarchy. This is suggested by the fact that it is possible to predict the fate of a neuroblast based solely on its position in the neurogenic region. For example, the neuroblast called MP2 always develops in the same position. Experimental support for this hypothesis comes from *Delta* mutants in which the *Notch* signaling cascade is interrupted. In these mutants, several neighbors also assume the MP2 fate. In addition, when a specific neuroblast is ablated, one of the neighboring cells assumes its fate, a process called regulation. Thus several cells, each with different lineages, have the potential to become the MP2 cell, if they end up in the right position and no neighboring cell has already adopted that cell fate (Fig. 4.4).

As we have seen in Chapter 2, the *Drosophila* embryo is finely graded in the anterior

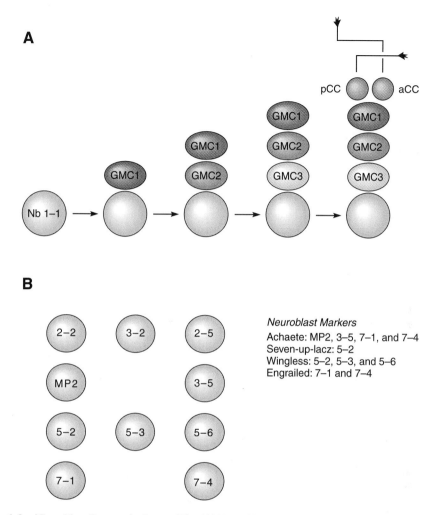

A

B

Neuroblast Markers
Achaete: MP2, 3–5, 7–1, and 7–4
Seven-up-lacz: 5–2
Wingless: 5–2, 5–3, and 5–6
Engrailed: 7–1 and 7–4

Figure 4.3 Neuroblast lineages in *Drosophila*. (A) Neuroblast (Nb) 1.1 giving rise to three ganglion mother cells (GMC) in three divisions. GMC1 then divides to produce the two distinct neurons aCC and pCC. These neurons have different axonal outgrowth pathways, as indicated. (B) Several NBs in a *Drosophila* hemisegment are shown. For simplicity they are shown in rows and columns. Each gives rise to a distinct and reproducible set of neurons, so the NBs have individual names and fates. These fates are in part determined by the different molecules, neuroblast markers, that they express. (Adapted from Doe, 1992a.)

to posterior axis by the expression of stripes of pair-rule and segment polarity genes, some of which are intrinsic transcription factors and others of which are signals and receptors. These positional identity genes play a key role in determining the identity of the neuroblasts. For instance, the *wingless* gene which encodes a Wnt-type signaling molecule is expressed in such stripes. In conditional mutants where *wing-less* has been inactivated at the time of neuroblast determination, the neuroblasts on either side of this stripe may be absent or duplicated. Another set of genes divides the embryo along the dorsoventral axis. Thus a cell in any position can be identified by these markers of latitude and longitude (Fig. 4.3B).

The position of the CNS neuroblast is responsible for regulating genes that are involved

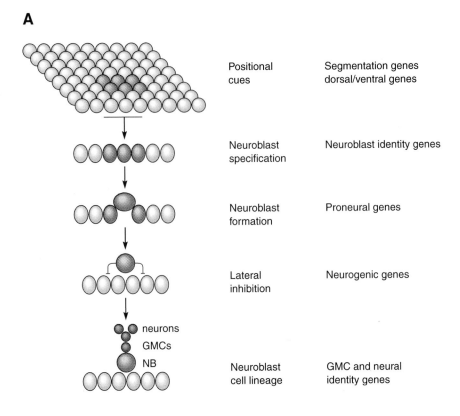

A

Positional cues — Segmentation genes dorsal/ventral genes

Neuroblast specification — Neuroblast identity genes

Neuroblast formation — Proneural genes

Lateral inhibition — Neurogenic genes

neurons
GMCs
NB — Neuroblast cell lineage — GMC and neural identity genes

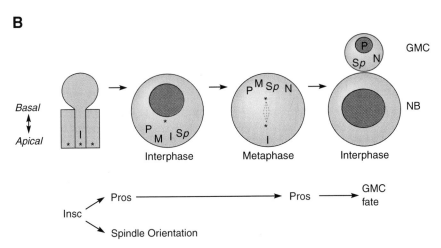

B

Basal ↕ Apical

GMC

Interphase   Metaphase   Interphase

NB

Insc → Pros ——————————→ Pros → GMC fate
Insc → Spindle Orientation

Figure 4.4 Generating diversity. (A) A group of ectodermal cells in the *Drosophila* neurogenic region is shown. This group already expresses several positional identity genes, such as a specific dorsal–ventral gene. The whole group then begins to express the same neuroblast identity and proneural genes (red), but only one neuroblast forms because the most advanced inhibits its neighbors from taking the same fate. The NB then divides characteristically to produce GMCs. The GMCs divide once more to produce neurons. (B) An alternative way of generating diversity by asymmetric cell division in a NB is shown. The NB expresses *prospero* (P), *Miranda* (M), *Inscutable* (I), and *Staufen* (Sp) on its apical side. As the NB divides, P moves to the basal daughter, dragging M and Sp, which in turn drag P to the newly formed GMC. *Numb* in the GMC protects it against lateral inhibition, while P goes to the nucleus and determines the GMC fate.

in neuroblast identity. All neuroblasts express proneural genes of the *achaete scute* type as we have seen in Chapter 1 (Figure 4.4). In addition, each neuroblast also expresses a particular combination of neuroblast identity genes. Mutant analysis has shown that under- or overexpression of these genes alters the fates of whole groups of clonally related cells. The gene called *prospero* was one of the first neuroblast identity genes found (Doe *et al.,* 1991). It is expressed in a subset of neuroblasts. Mutants lacking *prospero* function have the normal complement of neuroblasts. However, the daughters (GMCs) of these neuroblasts do not give rise to a normal complement of central neurons. *Prospero* is therefore thought to be necessary to activate the program of gene expression in GMCs (Fig. 4.4B).

Another example is the control of neuroblast lineage fate by the homeobox gene *gooseberry* (*gsb*). In normal development, *gsb* is expressed in the fifth row of neuroblasts, which includes the neuroblast 5-2. The lineage produced by 5-2 consists of at least 10 neurons with different phenotypes. By contrast, neuroblast MP2 in the third row, which normally does not express *gsb*, exhibits a quite unusual lineage formed by two neurons, MP2d and MP2v. In *gsb* mutants, the fifth row of neuroblasts is converted to the third row, and 5-2 assumes MP2 fates. Experimentally controlled ubiquitous expression of *gooseberry* results in the transformation of rows 3 into row 5. Thus, MP2 is converted into a 5-2 cell. There are at least 20 neuroblast identity genes, too many to discuss individually here. Like *gooseberry* and *prospero,* some are expressed broadly in large subsets of neuroblasts, while others are restricted to just a few neuroblasts. The neuroblast identity genes that have more restricted expression patterns may be controlled by particular combinations of broadly expressed genes.

The progeny of specific neuroblasts (GMCs) also have unique identities and have been found to express genes that specifically control the fate of this next phase of specification (Fig. 4.5). The *Drosophila* homolog of the nematode gene *unc-86,* called *dPOU28,* is an example. It is ex-

pressed in a subset of GMCs and seems to function in a way that is closely related to its function in the mechanosensory pathway in *C. elegans.* In one particular lineage, it is expressed in the first GMC (GMC1) of the neuroblast 4-2 lineage. In wild type animals, GMC1 produces two identified neurons, RP2 and its sibling RP2'. If *dPOU28* is ubiquitously overexpressed by heat shock, the would-be postmitotic neurons in this lineage adopt the fates of their GMC1 mother cell and divide again.

Two other homeodomain transcription factors, *eve* and *ftz,* are also important in defining the identity of the GMCs in this lineage. Soon after it is generated, GMC1, but not GMC2, begins to express *ftz* and *eve*. *Eve* expression is controlled by *ftz* in GMC1: eliminating *ftz* in these cells leads to the absence of *eve* expression. The loss of *eve* alone is sufficient to transform GMC1 into GMC2. Hence the daughter neurons of GMC1 (in the absence of *eve*) generate RP1 and RP3-like neurons, the daughters of GMC2, instead of RP2 and RP2'.

Finally single GMCs often produce two distinct daughters: GMC1 of NB 4-2 produces RP2 and RP2', while GMC1 of NB 1-1 produces aCC and pCC. In both cases the sister neurons are very distinct in terms of the pathways their axons take and the connections they make. The daughters of these GMCs often form miniequivalence groups in which one neuron has a primary fate (RP2 or pCC) while the other (the RP2' or aCC) has a secondary fate. Ablation of the pCC neuron shortly after its birth causes the transformation of the aCC into its dead sister's pCC fate. Similarly killing RP2 soon after its birth leads to replacement by its sibling.

Thus specification of central neurons in the insect CNS is similar in many ways to the specification of neurons in the nematode CNS. A hierarchical and very particular sequence of extrinsic and intrinsic factors expressed at successive stages of cell division is critical for sequentially restricting the fate of each daughter cell. The final postmitotic neuron has a very limited choice of fates. In many vertebrate systems too, the fate of a neuron is not completely determined even at the moment of its birth.

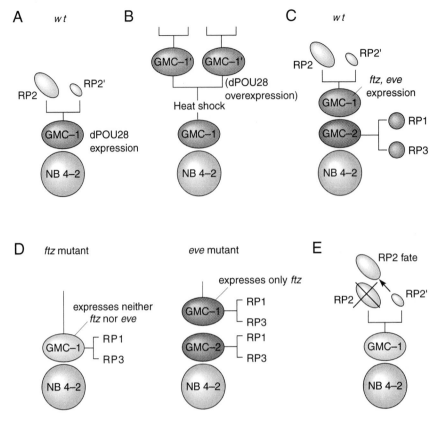

Figure 4.5   Manipulation of the fate of the NB 4-2 lineage. (A) The first division produces GMC1, which expresses *dPOU28* and divides to produce RP2 and RP2'. (B) Overexpression of *dPOU28* leads to a repetition of the GMC1 fate. (C) In wild-type embryos, once GMC2 is generated, GMC1 begins to express *ftz* and *eve*. (D) Loss of either *ftz* or *eve* causes GMC1 to express a GMC2-like fate. (E) The RP2' fate is secondary since killing RP2 causes the RP2' neuron to take over the RP2 fate.

Multiple Interactions in a Lineage-Based System with Asymmetric Cell Division

In the cases discussed above, there are clearly some important nonautonomous events, but many of the determinative steps result from a cascade of transcription factors, which helps explain why lineage plays a dominant role in these systems. The sensilla in the peripheral nervous system of *Drosophila* represent not only a system in which lineage is invariant and intrinsic transcription factors play important roles. It is also a system in which cellular interactions

appear to play a significant role. These sensilla are built of a small number of uniquely identifiable cells that derive from one cell, called the mother cell or sensory organ precursor (SOP). *Drosophila* sensilla are formed by one neuron surrounded by three accessory cells. Several steps lead up to the determination of an individual sensillum. Proneural genes of the AS-C family are initially expressed in a small patch of ectoderm, and these cells are competent to form SOPs (Fig. 4.6). This group of cells is called a proneural cluster (see Chapter 1). The proneural genes activate inhibitory cell–cell interactions, mediated by the neurogenic genes, which together with positional signals help single out one

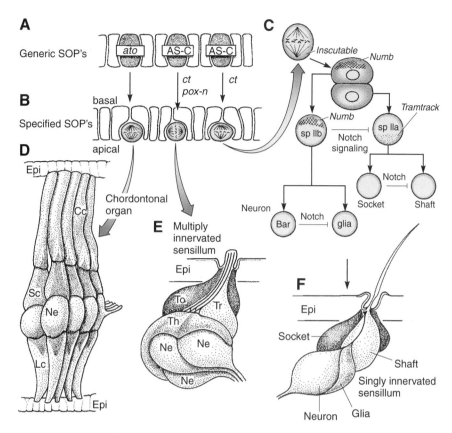

Figure 4.6 Determination of sensillum fate in *Drosophila*. (A) Precursors (SOPs) are selected from the epithelium and express proneural genes: atonal, achaete, and scute. (B) As the specified SOPs delaminate, they begin to express organ-specific genes, such as *ct* and *pox-n*. (C) Asymmetric cell division machinery is coupled with lateral inhibition machinery to produce the different cells of singly innervated sensilla (F) as well as chordotonal organs (D) and the multiply innervated sensilla (E). (Adapted from Harris and Hartenstein, 1999.)

SOP and prompt all other cells of the proneural cluster to abort neural development and follow the secondary fate of epidermis (Hartenstein and Posakony, 1990).

SOPs are specified to produce different sensillum types by the action of intrinsic transcription factors (Ghysen and Dambly-Chaudiere, 1992; Vervoort *et al.*, 1997). SOPs of the external mechanoreceptors express a homeobox-type factor called *ct*. If *ct* is absent, external sensilla do not develop and internal stretch receptors called chordotonal organs appear instead (4.6). The progenitors that give rise to chordotonal organs express a bHLH factor called *atonal* (*ato*). Ectopic expression of *ato* in other SOPs induces

them to produce chordotonal organs instead of external sensilla. Chemoreceptor precursors express a different transcription factor, *Pox neuro* (*poxn*) (4.6). Deletion of poxn causes multiply innervated chemoreceptors to be "transformed" into singly innervated mechanoreceptors.

Although morphologically identical, the early postmitotic sensillum cells are inherently different from one another as a result of a number of intrinsic cues expressed in the SOP and its progeny. The SOPs of the mechanosensilla divide into two inherently different secondary SOPs, spIIa and spIIb (4.6). spIIa has a shorter cell cycle and always produces the outer two accessory cells mentioned above. spIIb divides later than its sibling and forms the neuron and glial support cell. Several genes are involved in controlling the fate of spIIa versus spIIb. Among them are a set of very interesting factors that are involved in the asymmetric cell divisions (Fuerstenberg *et al.,* 1998; Jan and Jan, 1998). *Numb* encodes a membrane-bound protein that starts to appear in the primary precursor but is asymmetrically distributed to only its basal daughter. In the absence of *numb,* neurons do not appear, and spIIb is transformed into a spIIa cell. The expression of the transcription factor *tramtrack* is negatively regulated by *numb,* so the cell that inherits the *numb* protein does not express *tramtrack* which is essential for the separation of the spII fates. Thus, mutations in the *tramtrack* gene lead to the opposite phenotypes as mutations in the *numb* gene. While *tramtrack* is downstream of *numb,* another factor called *inscutable* acts upstream, and collects in the apical or top side of the SOP, and is responsible for the orientation of the cleavage plane and thus the correct segregation of *numb* and activation of *tramtrack.* Asymmetric cell division then contributes to the generation of distinct fates among sibling cells. Homologs of many of the genes described above that control asymmetric cell division in this system have been found in vertebrates and expressed in patterns that suggest they control asymmetric divisions in an evolutionarily conserved manner.

The neurogenic genes mediate a further set of interactions between the SOP progeny (e.g., the spIIa/IIb cells in mechanosensilla), as well as between postmitotic sensillum cells. *Numb* seems to antagonize the action of *Notch,* therefore the spIIb cell that normally inherits most of the *numb* protein does not express as much *Notch* as spIIb. In the absence of *Notch* signaling, both daughters of the spI assume a neural fate (see Chapter 1). *Notch* is used again at the second division shortly after the sensillum cells are born. If *Notch* is also reduced at this stage both spIIb daughters become neurons. Another gene required for interactions among sensillum cells is *Bar,* a putative transcription factor expressed in sensory neurons. Absence of *Bar* function in the neuron leads to changes in shaft cell differentiation, indicating that the neuron

must exert an influence on this cell. This example of cell determination and diversification in what appears to be a rather simple lineage invariant system demonstrates the biological complexity involved in cell fate assignment.

The Dominance of Cellular Interactions in the Determination of Drosophila Retinal Cells

The genetic approach has been particularly powerful in discovering the molecular mechanisms by which cell fates are determined in the *Drosophila* eye. The compound eye of an insect is composed of a large number of identical units, called ommatidia, each with its own lens and each with an identical array of cell types, This system provides a rather different example of how specific cells get their fates. Each of the 800 or so ommatidia in a *Drosophila* eye possesses 8 photoreceptors and 12 accessory cells. The 8 photoreceptors (R1–R8) are specialized sensory neurons (4.7). Among the accessory cells, there are cone cells that form the lens of each ommatidium and pigment cells that surround the photoreceptors and optically shield the ommatidia from one another.

Experimental results have shown that there is no clear clonal relationship among the cells of the ommatidia (Ready *et al.,* 1976). This situation is quite different from the sensilla discussed above or the neuroblasts of the CNS whose cells typically are produced in a fixed lineage. In the eye, cell–cell interactions between the postmitotic photoreceptors and accessory cells are primarily responsible for specifying cell fate (Banerjee and Zipursky, 1990). After proliferation is over, cells in the eye remain temporarily uncommitted to a differentiated fate.

The mechanism controlling retinal cell fate depends on the fact that ommatidial cells do not differentiate all at once, but follow a precise, reproducible temporal sequence. Thus, during late larval life, a wave of differentiation passes over the eye disc in a posterior to anterior direction (Fig. 4.7). The wave front, or the position at

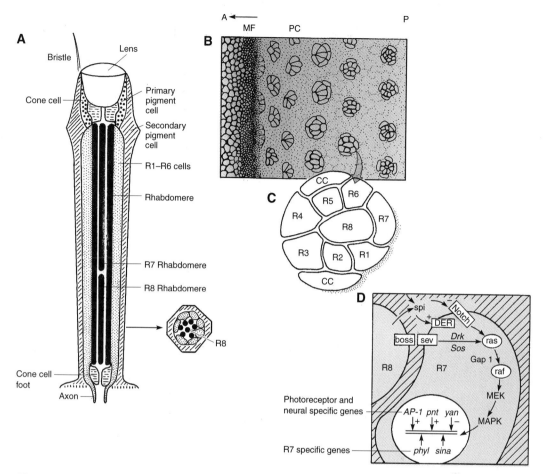

Figure 4.7 Cell determination in the *Drosophila* compound eye. (A) A single facet or ommatidium of an adult fly in longitudinal and cross section views showing the different cell types that compose it. (B) Cellular organization of the eye disc. The morphogenetic furrow (MF) is sweeping to the left (anterior) and leaving in its wake crystallizing clusters of cells (C). The clusters will give rise to the photoreceptors (R1–R8) and cone cells (CC). (D) Transduction pathways that help specify the R7 fate. Three receptors, *sev,* DER, and *Notch,* are all involved, as is the ras pathway that promotes neurogenesis in combination with several transcription factors that drive neural-, photoreceptor-, and R7-specific genes.

which ommatidial differentiation begins, is morphologically visible as a morphogenetic furrow (MF), a narrow groove formed by apical constriction of the eye disc cells. As the furrow advances, cells in its wake aggregate into intricate "rosettes" that foreshadow the regular ommatidial pattern. One cell is then singled out in each rosette. This becomes the R8 photoreceptor.

Both proneural and neurogenic genes play a role in the determination and spacing of R8 pho-

toreceptors. Thus, similar to the function of the *achaete scute* genes in the rest of the nervous system, the proneural gene *atonal* is necessary for the development of the R8 photoreceptors (Jarman *et al.,* 1994) (Fig. 4.8). *Atonal* is expressed in the MF and is subsequently concentrated in the rosettes and particularly in R8. Loss of *atonal* function results in the absence of R8 photoreceptors, and since R8 is necessary for the other photoreceptors to develop, the atonal

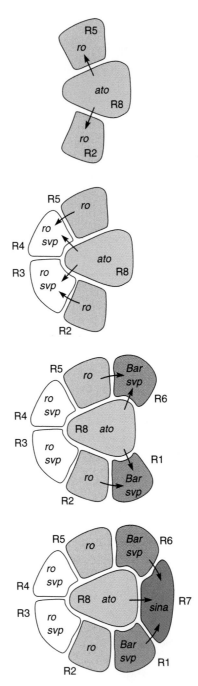

Figure 4.8 Cascade of photoreceptor determination in a developing ommatidial cluster. R8, the first to be determined, expresses *atonal* (ato) and signals neighboring cells to become R2 and R5, which then express *rough* (ro). R2 and R5 in combination with R8 then signal the next set of neighboring cells to join the cluster of five, and become R3 and R4, which express *seven-up* (svp). On the other side, a cluster of seven cells is formed when R1 and R6 are induced to express *Bar* and svp by R2, R5, and R8. Finally R8 in combination with R1 and R6 induce the final photoreceptor R7 (expressing *sevenless-in-absentia*, sina) to join.

mutant has no ommatidia. *Notch* and *Delta* mediate cell–cell interaction within the rosettes, and it is thought that the lateral interactions mediated by these genes allow only a single cell in a cluster to develop as the R8 cell, similar to the delaminating neuroblasts in the *Drosophila* CNS and sensory organs.

R8 cells act as organizers of ommatidium assembly. The first cells that join each R8 cell shortly after its determination become R2 and R5, and the next become R3 and R4. The sixth and seventh cells to join the ommatidial clusters become R1 and R6, and they are followed shortly by R7 and the four cone cells. At this point in time, the photoreceptors segregate from the surface and come to lie beneath the four cone cells. Next, cells surrounding the cone cell–photoreceptor cluster become arranged in two regular layers of pigment cells (Ready, 1989).

All photoreceptors receive a signal in the form of the Spitz (Spi) protein (a member of the TGF-α family of proteins). This tells them to become "generic" neuronal cells. Spi is secreted by R8 and other photoreceptors. It activates the DER receptor (*Drosophila* EGF receptor), a receptor tyrosine kinase that, in turn, triggers a signal transduction cascade inside the cell known as the Ras pathway (Chang *et al.,* 1994). At the end of the Ras pathway are several transcription factors, among them those encoded by the *yan* and *pointed* genes, which activate a program for photoreceptor differentiation. Signaling has been studied in the most detail for photoreceptor R7, which is the last neuronal cell to join the photoreceptor cluster (Zipursky and Rubin, 1994). In R7, the Ras pathway leading up to neuronal determination is activated by another receptor tyrosine kinase, *sevenless* (*sev*). A signaling molecule, encoded by the *bride of sevenless* (*boss*) gene, is expressed specifically by R8 and reacts with sev present on the membrane of the presumptive R7. Boss–sev interaction triggers the Ras pathway, leading up to the activation of *Pnt* and *AP-1,* transcription factors that promote photoreceptor differentiation, as well as the inhibition of the negative regulator of photoreceptor differentiation *yan*. Loss of any member of this signaling pathway results in the transformation of R7 into the next cell type to join the cluster, the cone cell.

There exists a second signaling mechanism that conveys more specific fates to the different photoreceptors. It is believed that this mechanism first emanates from R8 which then signals to the next cells joining the precluster, R2 and R5, and these cells in combination with R8 help give the next cells a specific fate, and so on. The ommatidium incorporates cells somewhat as a growing crystal incorporates molecules. That is, the new cells are added at specific positions and become neighbors of cells that are already incorporated. These neighbors instruct the new cells of their specific fates. Once incorporated, they have the ability to instruct the next cells that join (Fig. 4.8). Thus determination of a specific fate moves as a wave of crystallization across the eye disc and so the developing *Drosophila* eye has been called a neurocrystalline array. In the absence of appropriate signals between cells, particular photoreceptors are missing, whereas overexpression of these molecules may lead to the conversion of other cell types into the corresponding photoreceptors. The homeobox gene *rough* (ro) is only expressed in cells R2 and R5, but in its absence the fates of the R3 and R4 cells are also compromised. Similarly, the transcription factor lozenge, *lz,* activates the expression of transcription factor *Bar1* in R1 and R6 but inhibits the gene called *seven-up* in the forming R7 cell. *Svp,* a member of the nuclear receptor family, is required for the outer photoreceptors R1/6 and R3/4. Absence of *lz* in R1 and R6 gives a phenoptype similar to misexpression of *svp* in the presumptive R7, i.e., the development of this cell as an outer photoreceptor (R1/6 or R3/4) instead of R7.

Vertebrate Retinogenesis Has a Similar Developmental Strategy

The vertebrate retina is also a highly organized structure, with repetitive arrays of neuronal elements not unlike those of the fly. In addition to photoreceptors which include rods and cones, the vertebrate retina contains many types of interneurons. These include horizontal cells, bipolar cells, amacrine cells, amd glial cells.

Finally, retinal ganglion cells project out of the retina and relay the visual image to the brain. Retinal cells develop from a population of pluripotent neuroepithelial progenitors, which produce this diversity of neurons and glia. A single retinoblast will produce a clone of mixed, and rather random, cellular composition (Turner and Cepko, 1987; Holt *et al.*, 1988).

Determination in the retina follows a temporal order just as in the fly (Fig. 4.9). Cells that are born and differentiate early are likely to become retinal ganglion cells, horizontal cells, cones, and some types of amacrine cells. Later born cells include rods, bipolar cells, and Müller cells (Sidman, 1961). Within this general order, there is a great deal of overlap, such that cells of all types may be born within a given time window. For example, cohorts of cells in the chick born within a succession of 5-h intervals between Embryonic Days 4 and 8 all give rise to very heterogeneous populations, indicating that time of cell birth is not a major cell fate determinant. However, the results from retroviral lineage experiments indicate a growing bias in the fates of clonal progenitors to make rods, bipolar cells, and Müller cells (4.9) (Cepko *et al.*, 1996). So, while clonal composition suggests cellular determination by lineage-independent mechanisms, there is strong evidence to suggest a progressive restriction in fate possibilities, just as seen in the *Drosophila* retina. Retinoblast cells certainly exhibit biases toward certain fates, especially late in the clonal progression. This is most clearly seen in the mature fish retina in which the retinal progenitors generate only rod cells (Johns and Fernald, 1981). The progressive change in fate is supported by experiments in which progenitors at various stages of retinal development are forced to differentiate in culture. If progenitor cells are isolated at the time when retinal ganglion cells are born, they tend to turn into ganglion cells in culture, while those isolated at a later stage tend to become rods (Fig. 4.10).

What is the mechanism of this change in fate potential? Is it a restriction imposed externally by a changing environment or internally by a clock? This can be addressed with heterochronic experiments. If retinal cells at the stage

that RGCs are being born (E15) are mixed together into an aggregate and cultured *in vitro,* the labeled cells still differentiate into RGCs. If, however, they are mixed with an excess of retinal cells that are several days older, then they have a higher probability of becoming rods (Watanabe and Raff, 1990) (Fig. 4.11). Similarly, if a particular cohort of cells is allowed to reside within the retina and then is isolated in culture, these cells mimic their *in vivo* fates. If the same temporal cohort is isolated after shorter exposures to the retinal microenvironment, they give rise predominantly to earlier fates. This work shows that the same cells have the capacity to differentiate into different cell types and suggests that fate restrictions of these progenitors are due to changes in the external environment (Fig. 4.12). It is very likely that, as in the *Drosophila* eye, there is a cascade of differentiation, such that earlier differentiating cells influence the fates of later differentiating cells (Reh and Cagan, 1994; Cepko *et al.,* 1996; Harris, 1997). Indeed, there are diffusible signals from ganglion cells that limit the production of further ganglion cells (Waid and McLoon, 1998).

Neurotrophic factors and growth factors have been found in abundance in the developing retina. A variety of explant and dissociated cell culture systems, as well as *in vivo* strategies, have been used to test the effects of such factors on retinogenesis and the determination of cell type. Ciliary neurotrophic factor, CNTF, and its receptor, CNTFR, are expressed during retinogenesis. Addition of CNTF to the postnatal rat retina decreases rod differentiation and increases bipolar differentiation suggesting that the postmitotic cells that would normally differentiate into rods switch their fate and differentiate as bipolar cells instead. As one would predict, retinal explants from mice lacking a functional CNTFR contain more rods. It seems only natural that retinoic acid (RA), whose analogs have such striking effects on the physiology of photoreceptors, might influence their differentiation. Application of RA to zebrafish causes precocious differentiation of rods in postmitotic cells. If its synthesis is inhibited, rod differentiation is impeded. RA treatment of dissociated retinal cell

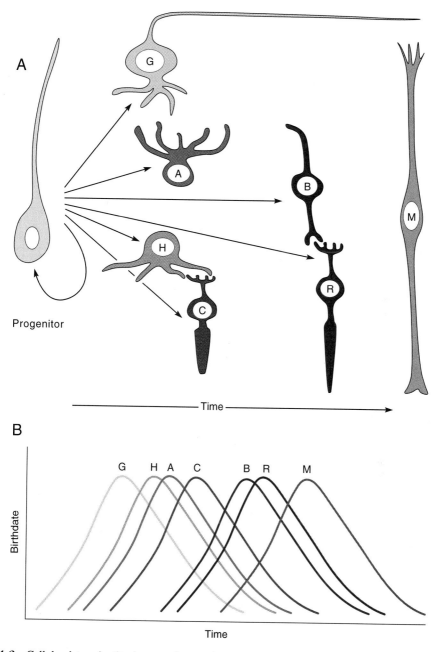

Figure 4.9 Cellular determination in a vertebrate retina. (A) A progenitor cell in the neuroepithelium divides several times and gives rise to clones of cells that contain all the major cell types of the retina, including ganglion cells [G], amacrine cells [A], horizontal cells [H], bipolar cells [B], rods [R], cones [C], and Müller cells [M]. These cells tend to be born at different developmental times, indicating a rough histogenetic order that is shown in (B).

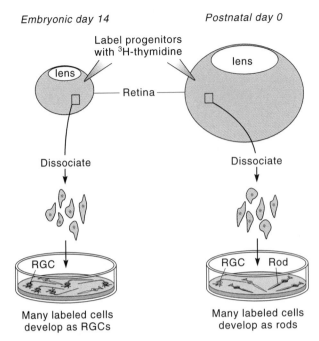

Figure 4.10 Birthdate and cell fate. Cells born on E14, even if dissociated into tissue culture tend to differentiate into retinal ganglion cells (RGCs) while cells born on P0, when dissociated, tend to differentiate into rods. (Watanabe and Raff, 1990.)

cultures also increases the number of progenitors that develop as rods. As expected the retinas of RA receptor mutant mice are thinner than normal and there is a lack of photoreceptor differentiation. These are just a few examples of the factors that influence cellular fate in the retina. A number of growth factors, neurotrophic factors, hormones, and morphogens have been shown to be present in the retina and are capable of influencing the proportions of retinal cells that choose particular fates in culture (Harris, 1997) (Fig. 4.12).

The dogma of developmental induction is that secreted factors activate signal transduction pathways that result in the expression of specific transcription factors. These factors may then intrinsically restrict fate choice. In the retina, we find transcription factors like *Pax6* and the bHLH proneural genes involved in functions common to all retinal cells (Chapter 3) and others that influence the differentiation or determination of distinct classes of retinal cells. The Brain-3 (Brn-3) family of POU domain transcription factors, for example, is expressed in

subsets of retinal ganglion cells. Deletion of one Brn-3 family member that is expressed in all ganglion cells causes the loss of 70% of these cells while not affecting other cell types (Erkman *et al.*, 1996; Gan *et al.*, 1996). Ocular retardation in mice is caused by a mutation in the homeobox region of the *Chx10* gene. *Chx10* is expressed at high levels in bipolar cells and its loss leads to the specific absence of these cells (Burmeister *et al.*, 1996). A related transcription factor, *Crx*, is necessary for the development of photoreceptors, and mutations in this gene cause degenerative diseases of rods and cones (Freund *et al.*, 1997). There are, no doubt, many other transcription factors expressed in the retina that have not been described or discovered, which are also likely to be involved in the sequential restriction of progenitor fates or the explicit expression of molecular characteristics of retinal neurons (Fig. 4.12).

As in the fly eye, *Notch* signaling is clearly active in the developing vertebrate retina, allowing only a certain number of cells to differentiate at any one time. If one imagines a scenario in

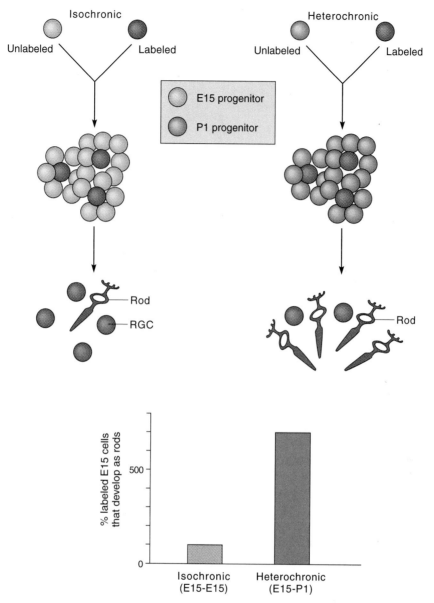

Figure 4.11 Early cell fate in the vertebrate retina is flexible and influenced by extrinsic factors. E15 cells labeled with thymidine and mixed with other E15 cells (isochronic) are not as likely to differentiate as rods. Instead, they primarily make retinal ganglion cells (RGC). If the same cells are mixed with P1 cells (heterochronic), they tend to differentiate as rods (Watanabe and Raff, 1990).

which there is spatiotemporally orchestrated expression of specific factors that affect cell fate, then the changing competence of a cell to respond to its immediate environment will have a dramatic impact upon its fate. Retinal cells can be made to differentiate earlier or later than normal by manipulating the levels of *Notch* and *Delta* signaling. This causes cells to assume fates that appear appropriate for the time at which they differentiate (Dorsky *et al.*, 1997; Henrique *et al.*, 1997) (Fig. 4.12). Imagine if all cells were permitted to respond at the same in-

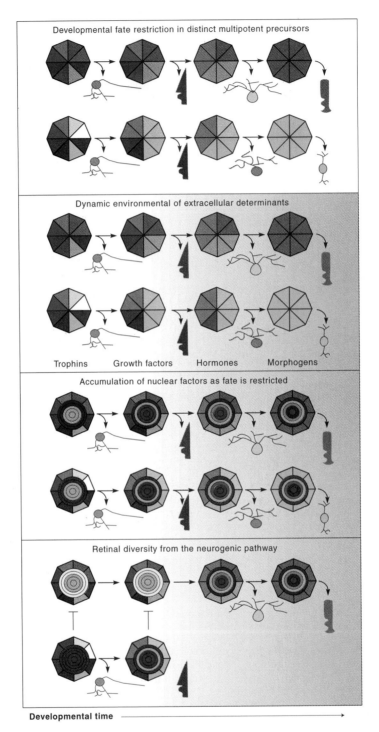

Figure 4.12 Model of fate specification in the vertebrate retina. The different colors in each pinwheel represent different fate potentials. (Top) Different multipotential precursors give rise to early, middle, and late cells. As they do so, there is a progressive restriction in potential fates. (Middle top) Part of what influences these precursors is the changing extracellular environment of trophins, growth factors, hormones, and morphogens. (Middle bottom) As the extrinsic cues are transduced, nuclear transcription factors build up in the nucleus causing the cells to further refine their fates. (Bottom) Lateral inhibitory pathways cause differentiating cells to

stant. They might all choose the same fate! Thus the neurogenic signaling pathway in the vertebrate retina is a basic regulatory mechanism that can be used to generate neuronal diversity by affecting the timing of differentiation in the changing external environment.

Glial Cell Fate

As discussed earlier, the nervous system is composed of two basic types of cells, neurons and glia. In fact, it is estimated that there are about 10 times more glia than neurons in the mammalian brain. Although very different in their structural and functional properties, neurons and glial cells are generally produced by the same progenitors. As described in Chapter 3, many soluble factors act on the progenitor cells to direct them toward neural or glial cell fates. Evidence from *Drosophila* is beginning to elucidate the underlying genetic mechanisms that control neuronal and glial cell fates. One well-studied case in which a progenitor gives rise to both neurons and glia is the median neuroblast (MNB) of segmented insects, such as grasshoppers (Condron and Zinn, 1994) (Fig. 4.13). Each segmental ganglion possesses just one MNB that gives rise to a specific set of neurons and glial cells along the midline. The MNB goes through three phases of proliferation. Neurons are generated during the first phase, glial cells during the second, and neurons again during the third. The switch to produce glial cells requires the expression of the transcription factor *engrailed* (*en*). When the MNB cells are injected with antisense oligonucleotides to *en,* they fail to produce glia and supernumerary neurons appear instead (Condron *et al.,* 1994). Protein kinase A (PKA), part of the cAMP signaling pathway, controls the shift to the third phase. If PKA is inhibited shortly before the onset of the third

phase, the formation of neurons is blocked, and glia cells continue to form instead (Condron and Zinn, 1995) (Fig. 4.13).

Several of the genes required for normal glial development in the *Drosophila* have been determined through an analysis of mutants in which glial cell development is disrupted. One of the most important genes is known as *glial cell missing (gcm)*. This gene codes for a transcription factor that is expressed in nearly all glial cells (Hosoya *et al.,* 1995; Jones *et al.,* 1995). When this gene is absent, the cells that were fated to become glia instead develop as neurons. Moreover, when *gcm* is expressed ectopically in neurons, they express glial-specific genes. Ectopic expression studies in non-neuronal tissue also show that *gcm* is sufficient to direct even mesodermal lineage cells into a glial differentiation path. Thus *gcm* seems to control the glial differentiation pathway in *Drosophila*.

Along with *gcm,* several other genes have been identified in *Drosophila* that are critical regulators of glial development. *Reversed polarity* (or *repo*) encodes a homeodomain protein essential for the differentiation and maintenance of glia. In the embryo, the gene is expressed in all lateral developing glia and closely related cells in both the central and the peripheral nervous systems (Halter *et al.,* 1995). In *repo* mutants, the early stages of glial development are not affected but the later stages of glial differentiation are disrupted. *Tramtrack (ttk)* encodes two zinc-finger proteins, and one of these, called ttkp69, is exptressed in all nonneuronal cells in the *Drosophila* central nervous system (Giesen *et al.,* 1997). Like *repo*, the initial stages of glial development appear to be normal in *ttk* mutants. However, the glia fail to migrate properly and many of them die. One of the main functions of *ttk* seems to be the inhibition of neuronal gene expression in glial cells. Ectopic expression of ttkp69 inhibits neuronal differentiation in the neuroectoderm.

---

inhibit neighboring cells from differentiating at the same time, thereby increasing cellular diversity, by spreading out the time of differentiation and the exposure of progenitors to varied extrinsic environments. (Adapted from Harris, 1997.)

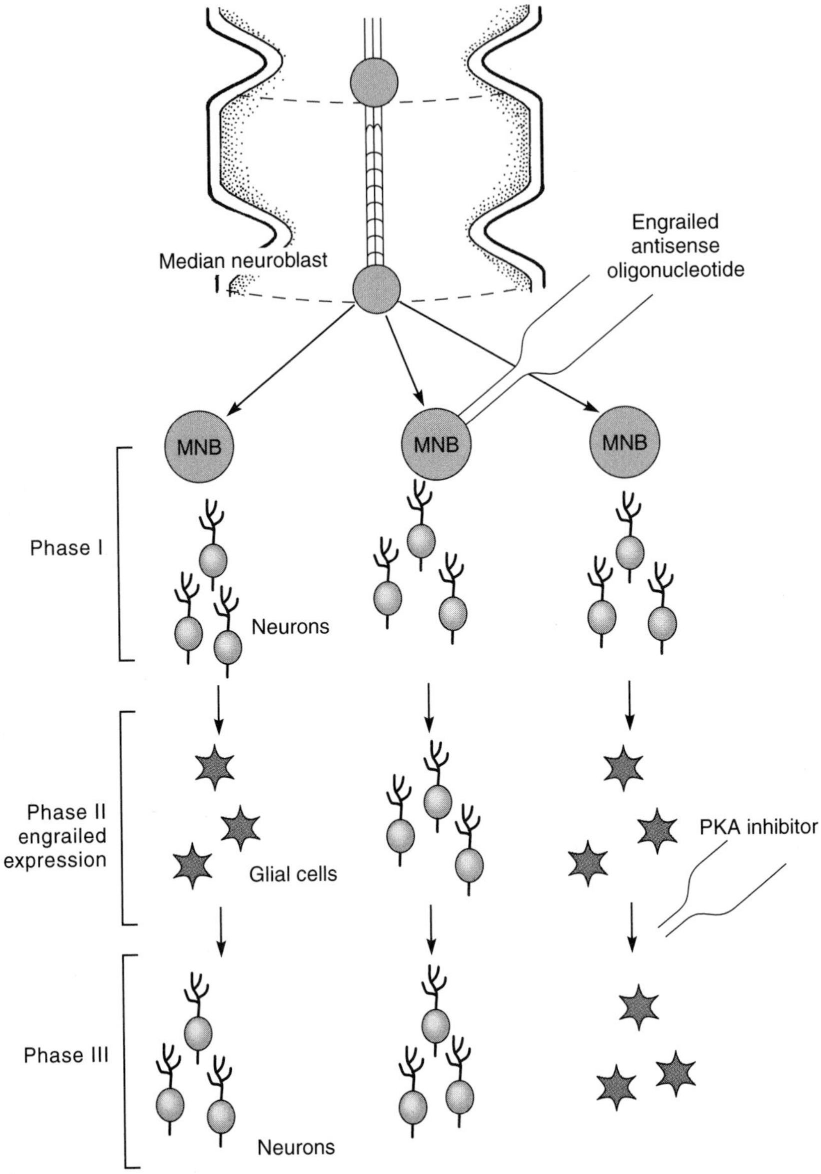

Figure 4.13 Neural and glial lineages in the grasshopper CNS. (Left) The median neuroblasts (MNB) in each segment give rise first to neurons (phase I), then glial cells that express *engrailed* (phase II), and then neurons again (phase III). (Middle) If *engrailed* expression is blocked by antisense, glial cells fail to form in phase II. (Right) If cAMP signaling is blocked at phase III, the transition back to neuron production is blocked and the MNB continues to produce glia (Condron and Zinn, 1994).

On the basis of these and other findings, Giesen *et al.* (1997) have put forward the model shown in (Fig. 4.14). Some of the progeny of the neuroblast lineage begin to express the *gcm* gene and this then acts as a master switch to activate the glial pathway. The *gcm* gene then activates *ttk*, which inhibits neuronal differentiation in these cells, and activates *repo*, which activates the expression of glial-specific genes. Given the high degree of homology in the pathways to neuronal

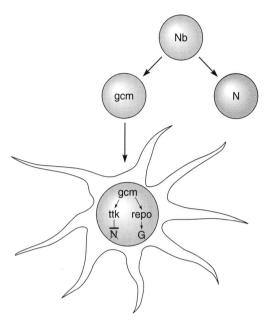

Figure 4.14 The expression of *gcm* in a daughter cell in neuroblast lineage switches the descendents to a glial pathway. *gcm* then activates *ttk* and *repo*, which respectively inhibit neuronal differentiation and promotes the expression of glial specific genes (after Giesen *et al.,* 1997).

differentiation discussed in Chapter 1, we might expect that a similar homologous pathway may control the development of glial cells in vertebrates. Several groups have identified vertebrate homologs to the *gcm* gene, but these have not shown the expected expression in the developing glial cells. Instead, *gcm* is expressed in nonneuronal cells outside the nervous system (Kim *et al.,* 1998). Thus the role of the *gcm* gene has apparently diverged, although it is possible that it still acts to inhibit neural differentiation in nonneural tissues.

Fate Decisons in the Vertebrate Neural Crest

The vertebrate neural crest is a transient stem cell population that arises along the lateral edges of the neural plate due to an interaction between the presumptive epidermis and the neural plate (Chapter 1). Neural crest becomes localized to the dorsal part of the neural tube as it folds up, and the cells then leave the neural tube and migrate along several well-defined pathways. These neural crest progenitors continue to divide as they migrate until they coalesce at each of their final destinations. As described in Chapter 2, crest cells generate a stunning variety of cell types. Not only does the crest produce the entire peripheral nervous system, including the autonomic and sensory ganglia, and the peripheral glia (Schwann cells), it also produces endocrine chromaffin cells of the adrenal medulla, smooth muscle cells of the aorta, melanocytes, cranial cartilage, and a variety of other nonneural components.

Because of the many different cell types that the crest can give rise to, this tissue has been a popular model for testing the molecular mechanisms that generate cell diversity (Le Douarin, 1982). To test whether premigratory crest cells are committed to a particular fate, the cells have been transplanted between different anterior–posterior positions (Fig. 4.15). These experiments took advantage of the chick–quail chimeric system described in Chapter 2. The results generally

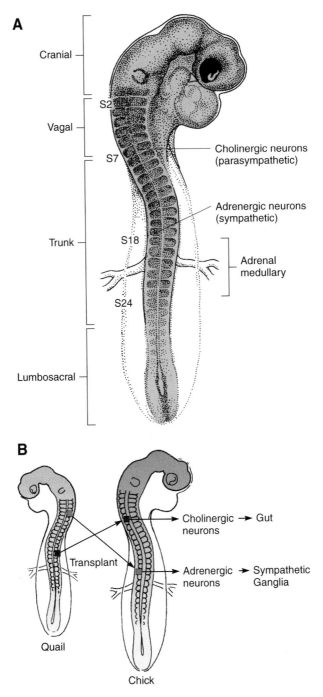

Figure 4.15 The environment influences the fate of neural crest cells. (A) Crest cells from the trunk normally give rise to adrenergic cells of the sympathetic nervous system, whereas the more anterior crest cells give rise to cholinergic parasympathetic neurons that innervate the gut. (B) When anterior crest cells from quail embryos are transplanted into the trunk region of chicken embryos, they differentiate into adrenergic neurons. Similarly, trunk crest cells that are transplanted anteriorly give rise to cholinergic neurons (LeDouarin *et al.*, 1975).

show that crest cells acquire instructions to differentiate during their migration, as well as when they arrive at their final destination. For example, crest cells from the trunk normally give rise to adrenergic cells of the sympathetic nervous system, whereas the more anterior crest cells from the vagal region give rise to cholinergic parasympathetic neurons that innervate the gut. When vagal crest cells from quail embryos were transplanted into the trunk region of chicken embryos, the transplanted vagal crest migrated along the trunk pathways and differentiated into adrenergic neurons in sympathetic ganglia. Similarly, trunk crest cells that were transplanted to the vagal region gave rise to cholinergic neurons of the gut. Thus, crest cells display great flexibility in responding to local environmental cues. The commitment to a particular fate is a multistep process and seems to occur in successive stages of determination. Migrating crest cells become exposed to a sequence of instructive environments, each perhaps with a unique set of factors, and the migrating cells respond to these factors by successively limiting their potential.

Initially neural crest cells are pluripotent, and labeling of single progenitors at the earliest stage of migration shows that such cells can give rise to a wide variety of derivatives (Bronner-Fraser *et al.,* 1991) (Fig. 4.16). But as the cells migrate along particular routes, they segregate into several classes of more specialized progenitors. As development proceeds they lose their pluripotency. Thus an early decision separates the cells that will become the ectomesenchymal progenitors, which give rise to skeletal and connective tissue, from the NGM progenitors (those that still have the capacity to produce neurons, glia, and melanocytes). Transplantation studies with these two types of progenitors shows they can no longer make the full array of cell types. Sympathoadrenal (SA) progenitors arise from the NGM group at a subsequent stage of restriction. Each of these progenitor classes is still not committed to a single fate. For example, SA progenitors can give rise to adrenergic and cholinergic neurons, as well as to endocrine cells.

The specification of different progenitor classes takes place during the migration of neu-

ral crest cells and experiments with purified populations of neural crest cells in culture suggest that different factors seem to be involved in these restrictions (Groves and Anderson, 1996; Anderson, 1997). Thus, glial growth factor (GGF) is capable of driving neural crest cells toward a glial fate, while BMP2, a member of the TGF-β family, turns on a program of neurogenesis (Fig. 4.17). TGF-β1 drives the same population of crest stem cells to assume smooth muscle fates. It turns out that where cells encounter such factors on their migration route is very important in shaping appropriate destinies. BMP2 is expressed in the dorsal aorta, where sympathetic ganglia form. The SA progenitors, which can be isolated from the adrenal gland primordium of embryonic mammals and raised in culture, give rise to two very different types of cells, the adrenergic sympathetic neurons and the endocrine chromaffin cells. Prior to differentiation, all SA progenitors express markers for both cell types. When SA progenitors are exposed to glucocorticoid hormone *in vitro,* which normally is produced in the adrenal gland, they develop as chromaffin cells.

As cells of the crest become sequentially acted upon by different environmental signals they turn on a successive set of transcription factors that act as intrinsic determinants and restrict cellular fate by activating and repressing particular genetic programs. The *MASH1* gene is induced by BMP2 and is involved in promoting neuronal identity. The *Phox2* gene, a paired-like transcription factor, is also induced in those neurons that are going to be adrenergic and may be responsible for controlling the expression of tyrosine hydroxylase, a key member of the synthetic pathway for this transmitter. Glucocorticoids are steroid hormones that act on cytoplasmic receptors. After binding to the hormone (ligand) the receptor–ligand complex is transported to the nucleus where it acts as a transcription factor, binding to DNA and activating or repressing certain genes. In the case of the SA progenitor, glucocorticoids evoke two different responses in sequence. First, they inhibit neuronal differentiation by suppressing the transcription of neuron-specific genes and then

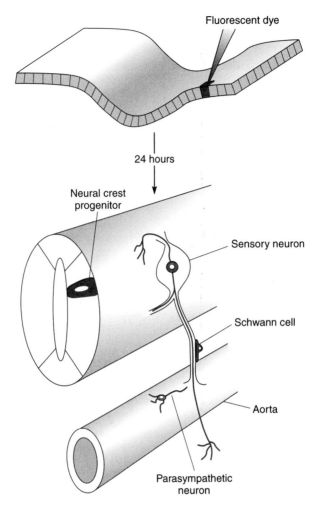

Figure 4.16 Fates and migration of neural crest cells. A single progenitor cell is injected with a lineage tracer and its progeny are followed as they migrate out of the neural tube. Some cells may become sensory neurons while others become Schwann cells or neurons of the autonomic nervous system. Environments these cells pass through on their migration routes influence their fate choice (Bronner-Fraser *et al.,* 1991).

they activate transcription of chromaffin cell-specific genes.

GGF influences the progeny of neural crest progenitors to become glial (Jessen and Mirsky, 1994; Shah *et al.,* 1994). GGF is a member of the epidermal growth factor/TGF-α family of ligands. GGF is expressed in neural crest cells once they have migrated peripherally and coalesced into distinct ganglionic masses. Specifically, it is expressed in those cells that have

already started to express a neuronal phenotype. The GGF receptor is already expressed by migrating neural crest cells, so cells are sensitive to GGF as soon as they arrive at their destination. In the absence of added GGF, the majority of clones obtained from cultured neural crest cells contain both neurons and glial cells, but if GGF is applied, then most cells in each clone develop as pure glia (4.17). Since the overall number of clones remains unchanged, it appears that cell

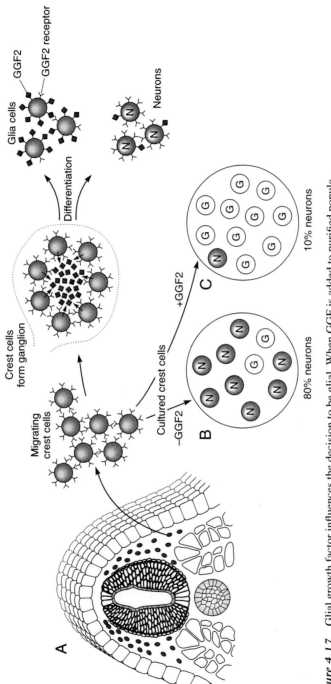

Figure 4.17 Glial growth factor influences the decision to be glial. When GGF is added to purified populations of migrating neural crest cells, it drives them toward a glial fate. The GGF receptor is expressed in all crest cells while GGF2 is expressed by cells that become neural in the forming peripheral ganglion. When new crest cells enter the ganglion, they are exposed to the GGF2 signal and adopt a glial fate.

division is not affected and the suggestion is that GGF suppresses the expression of a neuronal phenotype so that all cells become glial cells.

Neuronal Fate in the Vertebrate Spinal Cord

The vertebrate spinal cord is responsible for local reflexes, relaying signals from the periphery to the brain and activating organized movements. It is composed of a variety of cell types including different classes of motor neurons, local interneurons, and projection neurons. The embryonic spinal cord even contains a set of sensory neurons, called Rohon–Beard cells, that send processes to the periphery. During the course of development, Rohon–Beard cells die and sensory input to the spinal cord is supplied by dorsal root ganglion neurons. The spinal cord starts to develop at the caudal end of the neural plate, along a sheet of neuroepithelium centered above the notochord. Lineage tracing experiments show that cells in the lateral neural plate tend to give rise to Rohon–Beard cells and dorsal interneurons, while cells in the medial plate tend to give rise to motor neurons and ventral interneurons (Hartenstein, 1989) (Fig. 4.18). Since clones in the spinal cord are not restricted to a single class of cell, it is assumed that local position, rather than lineage mechanisms, is involved in the generation of neuronal diversity here (Chapter 2).

The notochord plays a key role in early development, being involved in neural induction, along the rostrocaudal extension of the embryo. As the cells in the spinal cord begin to differentiate, the notochord plays another important role by acting as an organizing center for the induction of cell fate in the spinal cord (Jessell *et al.,* 1989). At the lateral parts of the neural plate which become dorsal during the formation of the neural tube, cells are less exposed to the actions of the ventral organizing center and more exposed to dorsal organizing factors which seem to emanate from the epidermis above the developing spinal cord (Fig. 4.19).

As described in Chapter 2, the dorsal–ventral polarity of the developing spinal cord is set up through opposing gradients of two molecules: *Sonic hedgehog* (Shh), secreted by the notochord and subsequently the floor plate, defines the ventral cell fates, and BMPs, secreted from the ectoderm and dorsal spinal cord, define the dorsal cell identities. Several studies have also shown that once the floor plate has been induced in the ventral spinal cord, the Shh released by this tissue induces adjacent cells in the spinal cord to differentiate into spinal motoneurons (Ericson *et al.,* 1997). The floor plate is close to the notochord and is exposed to high levels of Shh. Further from the notochord, the cells fated to become motor neurons, are exposed to lower concentrations of Shh. *In* vitro, high levels of Shh are able to induce the expression of a floor plate-specific transcription factor (HNF3b) in neural plate explants, while lower levels of Shh induce the expression of motoneuron-specific biochemical markers (e.g., the transcription factor Islet1) in similar explants. Conversely, antibodies against Shh can block the development of motorneurons in explants of neural tubes.

In recent years, much progress has also been made in identifying the specific downstream targets of the Shh signal that define the motoneuron cell identity. A differential screen of a cDNA library derived from single Shh-induced motor neurons was used to identify a novel homeobox gene called *MNR2* (Tanabe and Jessell, 1996). This transcription factor is expressed by motor neuron progenitors and may initiate the cascade of expression of the different transcription factors leading to the motoneuronal phenotype. To test this possibility, *MNR2* was ectopically expressed in the dorsal neural tube of chick embryos (Fig. 4.20). This initiated a program of motoneuronal development, in which motoneuron-specific genes were expressed and dorsal-specific genes were suppressed (Tanabe *et al.,* 1998). In addition, some of the cells in the dorsal spinal cord were actually induced by the gene to send axons out into the motor nerve. Thus, it appears that *MNR2* is sufficient to define the motoneuronal cell fate in the spinal cord.

Another gene that is specifically expressed by developing motoneurons after receiving the Shh signal is the LIM homeodomain transcription

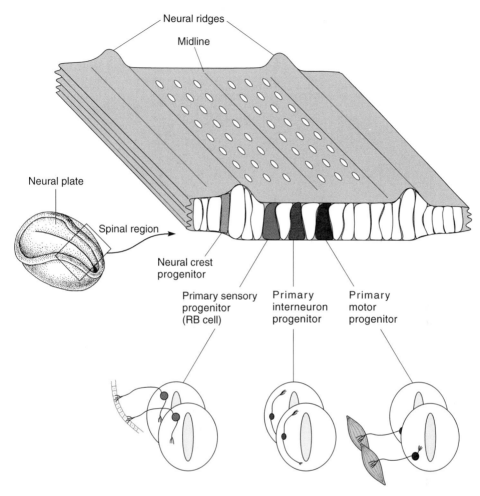

Figure 4.18 Rows of primary neurons in the neural plate. The most lateral row gives rise to sensory neurons (Rohon–Beard cells), the middle row gives rise to interneurons, and the most medial row gives rise to primary motor neurons (Hartenstein, 1989).

factor Islet1 (ISL1). LIM homeodomain factors also play a role in defining motorneuron identity, just as the *mec-3* gene, another member of the LIM family has an important role in mechanosensory cell identity in *C. elegans*. Disruption of ISL1 expression through knoockouts or antisense techniques caused a loss of the spinal motoneurons. These results indicate that motoneuronal identity in the vertebrate, like mechanosensory neuronal identity in the worm, is dependent on a key chain of transcriptional regulators. In additional to a function in specifying the overall fate

of motoneurons, there is also some evidence that more subtle aspects of the motoneuronal fate may also involve these genes. The motoneurons in the spinal cord are organized into functional columns that project to different muscle groups in the mature animal. Several lines of evidence indicate that there may be a combinatorial code of different LIM/homeodomain transcription factors. In addition to ISL1, motor neurons also express four additional LIM homeobox genes: ISl2, *Lim3, Gsh4,* and *Lim1.* The expression of these genes uniquely defines the different motor

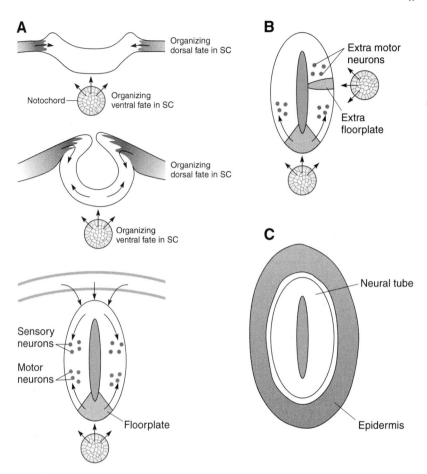

Figure 4.19 Dorsal and ventral fates in the neural tube are induced by nearby tissues. (A) The notochord, lying below the medial neural plate, induces the floor plate and motor neurons of the ventral neural tube by a *Sonic hedgehog* signal. The epidermis that lies lateral to the neural plate represses ventral fates through a BMP signal. (B) Transplantation of an extra notochord laterally induces an ectopic floor plate and motor neurons. (C) Wrapping the neural tube in epidermis suppresses the formation of ventral neurons.

columns (Tsuchida *et al.,* 1994). These motor columns can be further divided into pools that innervate specific muscles. These pools are distinguished by the expression of distinct members of the ETS family of transcription factors (Lin *et al.,* 1998). For example the ETS gene *ER81* is expressed in the motor neurons that innervate the limb adductor muscle in chicks, while a second group of motor neurons express the ETS gene, PEA3. We will come back to these ETS genes in the last part of this chapter where we discuss target influences on the development of neuronal phenotype.

Laminar Fate in the Cerebral Cortex

The cells of the cerebral cortex are, as most neuronal cells in vertebrates, generated at the ventricular zone. From there, the cells migrate

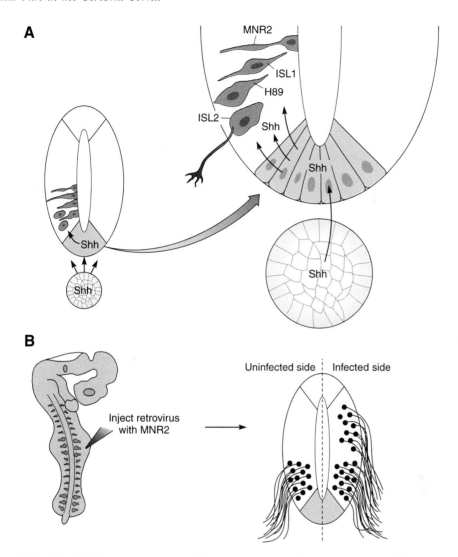

Figure 4.20 The LIM homeodomain is sufficient to transform cells to motoneurons. (A) *Sonic hedgehog* (Shh) released from the floor plate in response to a Shh signal from the notochord induces motorneurons that express LIM homeodomain transcription factors such as Islet1, Islet2, H89, and *MNR2*. (B) Injection of *MNR2*-expressing retrovirus into the dorsal spinal cord transforms cells in this region to motoneurons as seen by their ventral root projection patterns and neurochemistry (Tanabe *et al.,* 1998).

radially outward and coalesce just under the pial surface of the brain forming the cortical plate (Fig. 4.21). Migrating progenitors use a scaffolding of early generated radial glial cells that stretch from the ventricular to the pial surface as substrate on which to migrate. The first cells to migrate to the surface become the Cajal–Retzius cells of layer I and the deep ephemeral cells of the subplate (Fig. 4.21). It is not known exactly what role subplate cells have in the embryo, but some experiments suggest they are involved in developing the thalamocortical connections. In

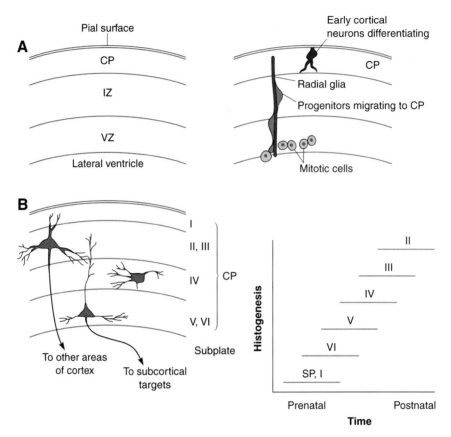

Figure 4.21   Histogenesis of the cerebral cortex. (A) In the embryo, the region of the CNS giving rise to the cortex is divided into three main zones: the ventricular zone (VZ), where mitosis occurs, the intermediate zone (IZ), through which newly born cells migrate on glial scaffolds to the cortical plate (CP), where they leave the scoffold and begin to differentiate. (B) Cells in different layers of the cortical plate (CP) in the adult animal are distinct in terms of morphology (pyramidal cells in layers II/III and V/VI and stellate cells in layer IV) and projection pattern (II/III neurons project to other cortical targets, V/VI cells project to subcortical targets). Cells in the different layers are also born in a histogenetic order, with cells of the subplate and layer I being generated first, followed by cells in layers VI through II in an inside to outside pattern.

many mammalian species, these cells die post-embryonically. The Cajal–Retzius cells, as we shall see, have an import role in cortical lamination (Del Rio *et al.,* 1997).

A normal cortex is made up of six cellular layers distinguishable by size, shape, and packing density. Each layer is composed of many cell types but different layers tend to have layer-specific projection patterns (McConnell, 1995). Thus in primary visual cortex, layers 2 and 3, neurons are large pyramidal cells that project to other cortical areas; layer 4 cells are small stel-

late local interneurons; and layer 5 and 6 cells are largely pyramidal and project to subcortical targets. Birthdating studies show that the cortical layers are generated in an inside-out manner, with the cells of layer 6, the deepest layer, being born before the cells in layer 5, which are born before the cells in layer 4, etc. (Fig. 4.21). In the reeler mutant mouse, an extracellular protein called reelin, which expressed specifically on Cajal–Retzius cells, is defective and the result is aberrant cortical layering. Without a functional reelin protein, which may serve to help unload migrating cortical progenitors from their radial migrations, the first cells climb all the way to the pial surface and the next cells pile up underneath. Thus in the reeler mutant, there is an inversion of laminar histogenesis, and deeper cells are born after superficial ones.

In the ferret, layer 6 cells are born at E29 and layer 2 and 3 cells are born at P1. Cells born at P1, fated for layers 2 and 3, must migrate through layers 6, 5, and 4 which have already formed. Cortical cells could be determined with respect to layer as soon as they are generated, or they might get their fate from the position they migrate into. To test when cortical cells get their laminar identity, cells generated in the ventricular zone of E29 ferrets were transplanted into older P1 hosts (Fig. 4.22). Although their time of birth would have fated them for a deep layer, the experiments showed that many of the transplanted cells switched their fates and ended up in layers 2 and 3, suggesting that these young cortical neurons were flexible with regard to fate (McConnell, 1988). Further studies showed that cell interactions are involved in this commitment since if the E29 cells are removed and cultured with other E29 cells for a number of hours their deep layer fate is determined even when challenged by transplantation to an older environment (Fig. 4.22). This type of experiment is useful for addressing exactly when with respect to birthdate these cells become committed to their laminar fate. If the E29 cells were allowed to complete their final division amongst similarly aged donor cells they retained a deep layer fate, while if they were transplanted to an older host to complete their final division they switched to a layer 2/3 fate. Thus, cell fate, according to layer, is decided by precursor cells in the environment of the germinal zone, and not in the cortical plate. This is supported by studies of reeler mice, which show that though the lamination is defective the cortex is composed of the right type of cells born in the appropriate order. As in the retina, this germinal environment will change with time in a way that influences the prospective fates of the progenitors that are produced there. Thus, as in the retina, one might expect later progenitors to have a more restricted set of fate choices. Indeed, when P1 precursor cells were transplanted into younger brains, these cells no longer showed the capacity to differentiate as deep layer cells (Fig. 4.22). These results argue that the pluripotency of cortical precursors is restricted over time, perhaps by environmental factors controlling intrinsic competence or else by an intrinsic clock.

Positional Cues Determine Axonal Projection Patterns

In this section, examples are given to demonstrate how the position of a neuron influences one key aspect of its fate, i.e., the connections it makes. We discuss how positional cues influence the orderly projection of a set of neighboring neurons onto a set of neighboring target cells in Chapter 6. In the present examples, the neuron's basic phenotype does not change. The cells remain motor or sensory independent of where they arise, yet the local environment at the cell body region influences the pathway and postsynaptic target choices that axons of these neurons make. These wiring decisions, in turn, have fundamental significance for the behavior of the organism.

In the nematode, all the touch-sensitive cells express *mec-3* and downstream genes are activated by *mec-3*. Although all touch cells have a similar morphology and chemistry, they are not equivalent in the connections they make. For example, the anterior and posterior ventral mechanosensory cells (AVM and PVM) are born from parent cells Q1 and Q2 that are originally close together in the posterior of the animal (Fig. 4.23). The Q2 cell migrates anteriorly and gives rise to the AVM which receives touch information from the anterior part of the animal and leads to rearward movement when the animal is touched on the nose. Q1 migrates posteriorly and gives rise to PVM which receives touch information from the posterior of the animal and leads to forward movement. Thus, these two very similar cells must contact different motor pathways. In a mutant for the gene encoding a

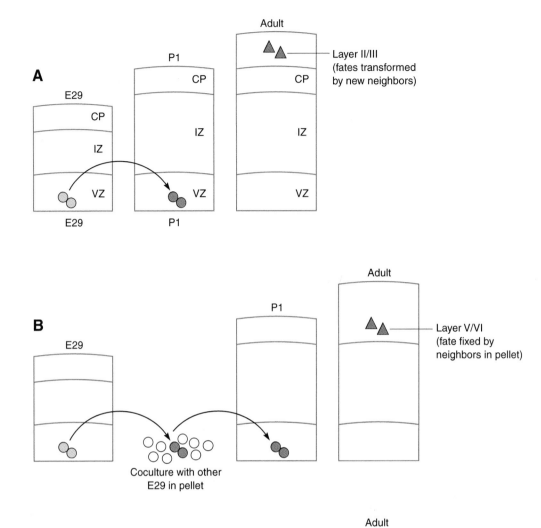

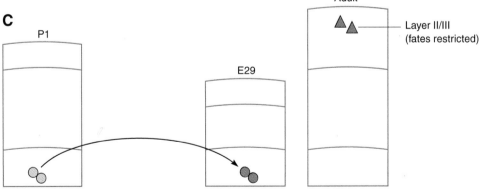

Figure 4.22 Laminar fate determination in the cerebral cortex. (A) Transplantation of cells from the VZ of an E29 ferret to a P1 ferret leads these cells to change from a deep layer (early) to a superficial layer (late) fate. The fates of transplanted cells are transformed by the surrounding tissue. (B) When the same transplantation is done after culturing the cells with their normal neighbors for a few hours, they retain their deep layer fates. (C) Late generated cells are restricted and do not assume deep layer (early) fates even when transplanted to the VZ of E29 animals. (Adapted from Harris and Hartenstein, 1998.)

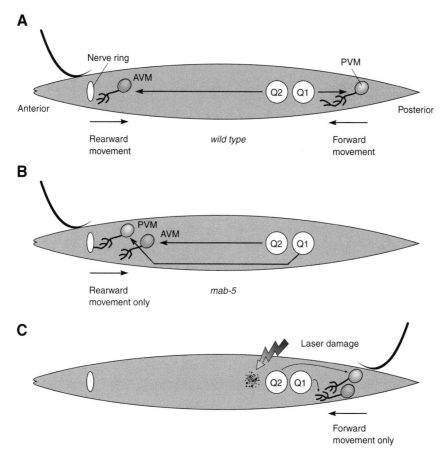

Figure 4.23 Position determines mechanosensory cell fate differences in a nematode. (A) In a wild-type worm, AVM, which mediates rearward movement to a touch on the head, and PVM, which mediates forward movement to a touch on the tail, arise from Q2 and Q1, respectively. Q2 migrates anteriorly; Q1 migrates posteriorly. (B) *Mab-5* mutants only respond to head touches. In this mutant, Q1 also migrates anteriorly, resulting in a duplication of the AVM fate. (C) Damage to Q2's migration route with a laser leads to a lack of anterior migration, both Qs give rise to PVMs, and the worm can only respond by moving forward to a tail touch (Chalfie, 1993).

homeobox called, called *mab-5,* Q1 moves anteriorly instead of posteriorly and the PVM that it gives rise to is now more anterior than usual. This cell makes connections just like the AVM, and like the AVM mediates rearward movement to anterior touch. Alternatively, when a laser is used to block the forward migration of Q2, the AVM it generates is more posterior than usual and now this cells takes on the characteristics of the PVM and mediates the forward reflex to touch on the rear. From these studies, it appears

that the position of the AVM or the PVM is critical for the appropriate connections that it makes in the nervous system (Chalfie and Au, 1989).

In the chick, specific muscles of the limb are innervated by motor neurons from different positions along the anterior–posterior axis of the spinal cord. When a length of the embryonic spinal cord of the chick is rotated, the motoneurons still establish connections to their normal target muscles although axons now have to navigate along novel pathways. This establishes that the position of the cell body along the anterior–posterior axis is an important determinant in the specification of a motor neuron's target choice. In zebrafish, this issue has been approached on a single cell level since each spinal segment has just three primary motor neurons named RoP, MiP, and CaP (for rostral, middle and caudal primary) (Eisen, 1991a) (Fig. 4.24). Each neuron extends an axon out of the spinal cord to the same choice point. However, RoP grows to innervate central muscle, MiP grows up to the dorsal muscle, and CaP grows down to the ventral muscle (Fig. 4.24). Transplantion of a CaP cell to the MiP position before axonogenesis results in CaP developing MiP axonal characteristics: It innervates dorsal muscles (Eisen, 1991a). Similar results are found when other switches are made. These results suggest that the position of the soma along the rostrocaudal axis of the segment specifies the axonal projection of the different primary neurons. One possible molecular determinant of the projection of these motoneurons is the pattern of the LIM transcription factors they express. As we have seen above, different LIM genes are expressed in different motor columns, and a key question is how these different motor fates arise? The transplantation experiments demonstrate that when primary motoneurons change their projection pattern, they initiate a new program of LIM homeobox gene expression (Appel *et al.,* 1995). Transplantion of these neurons after axonogenesis has begun, however, does not lead to a switch in fate and each one maintains its original projection pattern. Thus, each cell becomes committed to a particular fate dependent on its position at a particular time in development and thereafter differentiates autonomously.

Regulation of Phenotype by the Target

A neuron's fate may be completely determined in many respects at the time it is born or shortly thereafter. For some neuronal properties, the final fate choice comes only after the cell has migrated or established connections with its target. Thus, decisions about cell fate begin during early embryogenesis and extend through later stages of development. Final fate choice may be between survival and death and depend on trophic factors produced by the target (Chapter 7). Neural crest cells that become sympathetic neurons receive a signal to express noradrenalin as they migrate, and by the time these neurons aggregate as a ganglion they are all adrenergic. Most of these sympathetic neurons send axons out to smooth muscle targets, and these cells remain adrenergic throughout life. Several signals have been identified that bias transmitter phenotype toward the adrenergic state (Landis, 1992; Schotzinger *et al.,* 1994). When neural crest cells are cultured with pieces of the aorta, the cells express noradrenalin. It has since been found that dorsal aorta releases the TGF-β family member, BMP7, and this molecule is also able to induce crest cells to assume the adrenergic phenotype *in vitro* (Fig. 4.25).

It is interesting that a few sympathetic neurons, such as those that innervate sweat glands, switch their neurotransmitter phenotype late in development and become cholinergic. Neurotransmitter phenotype in these cells is an extremely late cell fate choice that is regulated by the target. In fact, sweat gland innervation begins as adrenergic, and all the enzymes and transmitter machinery for noradrenalin are found in the sympathetic neurons that first innervate the sweat glands. During the second postnatal week in the rat, these neurons begin to turn off tyrosine hydroxylase and other adrenergic enzymes and begin to make choline acetyltransferase, the synthetic enzyme for ACh production. Ablating the early adrenergic fibers with the neurotoxin 6-hydroxydopamine also abolishes the later cholinergic innervation showing that the two transmitters come from a single set of fibers that switch transmitter phenotype, rather than from distinct populations of cholinergic fibers that arrive at a later time.

A direct role for the sweat glands as an inducing signal for the switch in transmitter phenotype comes from transplant and explant experiments (Fig. 4.26). Coculturing young sympathetic neurons with sweat gland tissue caused the neurons

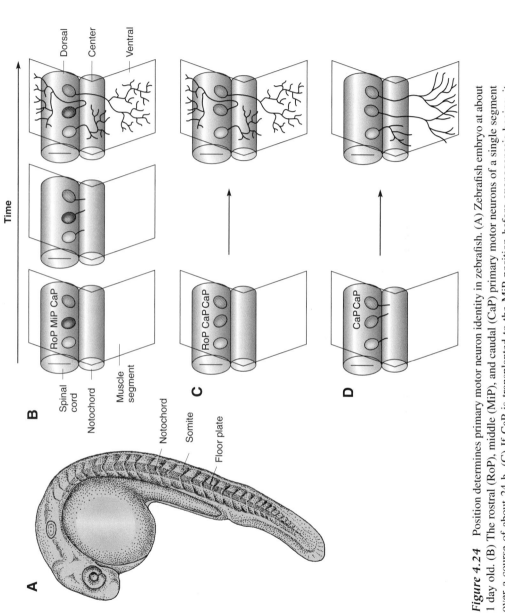

Figure 4.24 Position determines primary motor neuron identity in zebrafish. (A) Zebrafish embryo at about 1 day old. (B) The rostral (RoP), middle (MiP), and caudal (CaP) primary motor neurons of a single segment over a course of about 24 h. (C) If CaP is transplanted to the MiP position before axonogenesis begins, it develops a MiP axonal projection. (D) However, if the transplant is done several hours later after the axons have begun to grow, the neuronal fates are fixed.

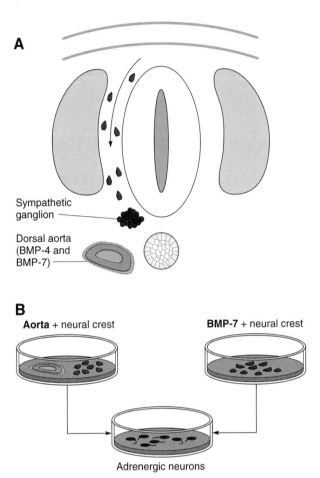

A

Sympathetic
ganglion

Dorsal aorta
(BMP-4 and
BMP-7)

B

Aorta + neural crest   **BMP-7** + neural crest

Adrenergic neurons

Figure 4.25   Control of transmitter phenotype by the aorta. (A) Neural crest cells that migrate close to the aorta often become sympathetic ganglia with adrenergic neurons. The dorsal aorta is a source of BMP4 and BMP7. (B) When neural crest cells are cultured with aorta or BMP7, they become adrenergic neurons (Reissmann *et al.,* 1996).

to become cholinergic. When cultured with pineal gland, a normal adrenergic target, the cells expressed noradrenalin. Transplanting foot pad tissue rich in sweat glands to areas of the body that usually receive adrenergic sympathetic innervation, such as the hairy skin of the thorax, led to the production of unusual cholinergic sympathetic neurons in the ganglia that innervate this skin. Similarly, replacing the footpad tissue with parotid gland, another adrenergic target, led the population of sympathetic neurons that usually become cholinergic, to remain adrenergic. Although factors such as interleukin-6

that are capable of causing an adrenergic to cholinergic switch in phenotype have been purified from culture media, the actual factor that operates in the sweat glands to produce this effect has not been definitively identified. Nevertheless, these experiments make it clear that targets can retrogradely determine that transmitter type of the innervating neurons.

The Retzius neuron of the leech is a serotonergic interneuron in each ganglion involved in swimming and other behaviors. Retzius neurons in each of the leech's midbody segments start life identically to Retzius cells in all other segments.

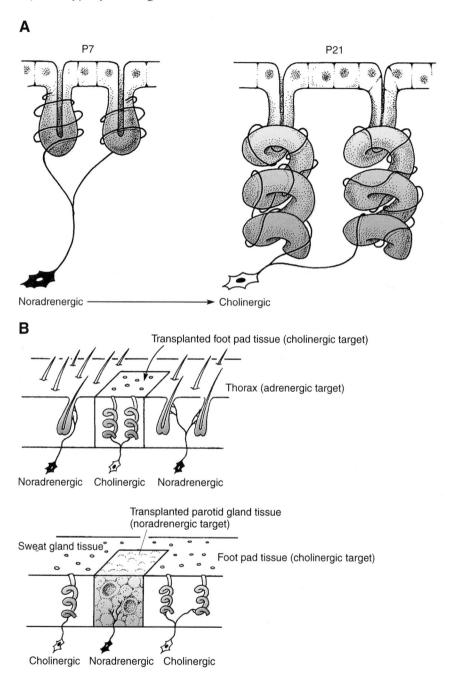

Figure 4.26 Control of transmitter phenotype by sweat glands in the footpad. (A) A noradrenergic neuron begins to innervate developing sweat glands. As it does so, it switches and becomes cholinergic. (B) Neurons that innervate hair follicles are noradrenergic, yet when a piece of footpad containing sweat glands is transplanted into hairy skin, the local neurons that innervate the transplanted sweat glands become cholinergic. Conversely, when a piece of parotid gland tissue, which is normally innervated by adrenergic neurons, is transplanted to the footpad, the local neurons that innervate it are noradrenergic (Landis, 1992).

They begin to make serotonin and send projections laterally into the body wall and longitudinally along the interganglionic connectives (French and Kristan, 1992). At Embryonic Day 10, however, Retzius neurons in ganglia 5 and 6 begin to differ from the Retzius neurons in all the other ganglia. Instead of continuing their growth laterally into the body wall, these axons change direction and head toward the midline genital tissues which they innervate. The interganglionic connectives R5 and R6 retract, and the cells change their physiological responsiveness to neurotransmitters and rearrarange their central connectivity within the ganglion. Interaction of the Retzius cell axons with the reproductive tissue appears to control the fate choice, as transplantation experiments have shown. If moved into a nonsex segment early enough, gonadal tissue from segments 5 and 6 causes the Retzius cells of that segment to innervate the transplanted reproductive tissue. These cells are transformed, physiologically and anatomically, into Retzius neurons typical of the sex ganglia. Similarly ablation of the reproductive tissue in segments 5 and 6 causes the transformation of the Retzius cells in the sex ganglia toward those of the standard midbody ganglia. Contact with the reproductive tissue is critical for the transformation because in ablation or transplantation experiments only the Retzius neurons that successfully make contact with the reproductive tissue show the sex ganglion Retzius cell characteristics.

As a final example, we consider how vertebrate sensory neurons can distinguish the correct motor neurons to innervate. Sensory neurons called spindle afferents carry information from the stretch receptors of individual muscles. Each spindle afferent has a dendritic process in the muscle, a cell body in a dorsal root ganglion, and an axon in the spinal cord that terminates specifically on motor neurons that project back to that same muscle, the so-called homonymous motor neurons. We know that sensory afferents are not programmed to recognize these motoneurons because if the sensory fibers are forced to innervate other muscles they choose new synaptic partners, namely, the motor neurons innervating those other muscles (Frank and Wenner,

1993). One could imagine a mechanism by which this synaptic match up was made on the basis of synchronized activity patterns, but blockade of activity during the period when these connections are made does not alter the specificity. Rather, it seems that molecular cues from the periphery are transmitted to the sensory axons, and the sensory axons use this information to find the appropriate synaptic partners centrally. This is demonstrated by an experiment in which ventral limb muscles were replaced with dorsal muscles (Fig. 4.27). The sensory and motor neurons that normally innervate the ventral muscles were thus forced to innervate ectopic dorsal muscle, but in this case these sensory neurons did not make contact with these "ventral" motor neurons but rather with the motor neurons that were originally specified to innervate the dorsal musculature. Interestingly, after sensory neurons innervate muscles, they start to express the same ETS gene as the motor neurons that innervate that muscle (Lin *et al.,* 1998). Limb ablation studies show that signals from the periphery, perhaps from the muscles themselves, help establish the coordinated pattern of ETS gene expression in the motor and sensory neurons that innervate particular muscles, so peripherally coordinated gene expression may hold part of the secret to this synaptic specificity (Fig. 4.27).

Conclusions

One of the main conclusions of this chapter is that there is no single mechanism by which neurons get their specific identities. There are common themes such as successive restrictions in potency and potential as progenitor cells develop and divide, but the molecular basis of such restrictions varies from system to system. In fact, it seems that almost every neuron has its own set of molecular restrictions and hierarchy of determinative events. Clearly there is immense variation in the role of lineage versus environment in neuronal determination. In some systems, lineage is exceedingly important. In others, it means little, and unrelated cells have an equal chance to assume a particular fate.

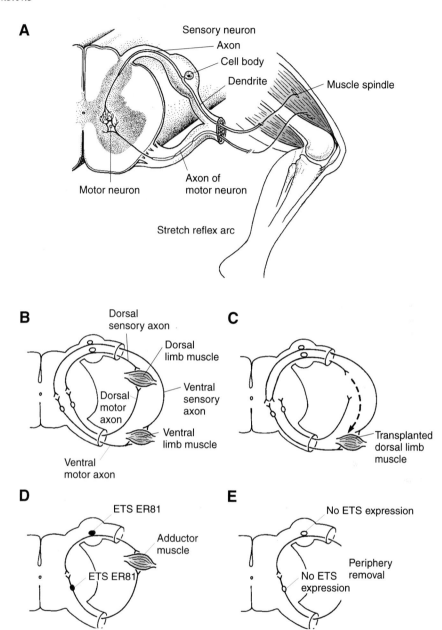

Figure 4.27   Matching sensory motor connectivity determined by muscles. (A, B) Spindle afferents terminate on homonymous motor neurons. (C) If the sensory fibers that normally innervate ventral muscles are
forced to innervate dorsal muscles, they switch synaptic partners to the motor neurons innervating dorsal
muscles. (D) Different muscles seem to induce the particular ETS molecules on both the motor and the sensory
neurons that innervate it. Thus the motor and sensory neurons that innervate the adductor muscle express the
ETS *ER81* molecule. (E) If the peripheral muscles are removed, the motor and sensory neurons no longer
express ETS molecules (Lin *et al.*, 1998).

There is a general rule that representatives of more ancestral invertebrates are dominated by lineage mechanisms through a succession of intrinsic transcription factors and cytoplasmic inheritance, while more "advanced" species and vertebrates are dominated by lineage-independent mechanisms such as diffusible signals and cellular interactions. In truth, this rule, while predictive, does not bear close scrutiny at the cellular level. In nematodes there are many cases where signaling molecules and cellular interactions play powerful roles in cellular determination while in the vertebrates the successive restriction of fates among some mitotic progenitors implies a dominant role for lineage. In truth, each determination pathway brings its own mix of lineage-dependent intrinsic and lineage-independent nonautonomous mechanisms. One could only fairly say that the successive determination of cells in the nervous system usually happens as an interplay between extrinsic signaling molecules that induce the expression of intrinsic transcription factors. Some of the targets of these transcription factors are other signaling molecules that induce other transcription factors and so on.

Each part of the nervous system seems to depend on its own particular set of molecular determinants, and so one almost wonders if there are more neuronal determination factors than there are kinds of neurons. It nevertheless appears, however, that common molecular themes run through the determination of neurons in various systems. Thus, of the transcription factors, bHLH genes of the proneural class help tell cells to become neurons, while homeobox and paired domain transcription factors are often used to restrict neurons to certain broad classes. Finally, POU domain and LIM domain transcription factors may restrict cellular phenotypes even further. Of the signaling molecules, we find important roles for *Delta,* TGF-β type molecules, *hedgehog* and other morpogens like retinoic acid, and various growth factors in many systems—both vertebrate and invertebrate. It is not clear how many new kinds of signaling molecules and transcription factors have yet to be discovered. We imagine the list is far from complete. Yet it is somehow reassuring to see the same types of molecules used for these purposes over and over again.

One final general comment concerns the last phases of neuronal determination, which include wiring up and interaction with synaptic targets. In many systems, these phenotypic traits are regulated by extrinsic features such as the position of the neuron in the body and the accessibility of particular targets. Eventually, the neuron becomes an individual cell with its own set of synaptic inputs and outputs. These features make a particular neuron of a given class uniquely equipped to deal with certain situations in processing neural information. These aspects of phenotype, as we have begun to see here, are the product of the further differentiation of neurons as the nervous system continues to wire up and begins to function. The activity electrical pattern of the developing nervous system plays an increasingly important role as the brain matures. These are aspects of neural determination that we deal with in subsequent chapters.

Axon Growth and Guidance

· · · · ·

After it stops dividing, but before it begins its life as a functioning element of the nervous system, a neuron must change in many ways. It must not only develop the biophysical and biochemical machinery of a neuron; it must also connect up to other neurons. Some neurons have short axons and make local connections to cells in their immediate vicinity, while others send long axons to distant central or peripheral targets. Axons extend by adding components to the distal end, which is the growing zone. At the tip of a growing axon, there is a specialized structure, called the growth cone (Landis, 1983; Kater and Letourneau, 1985; Letourneau *et al.,* 1991), which we discuss in detail in this chapter.

When the embryonic phase of an animal's life has ended, many of the brain's connections have been made, and the nervous system looks like a weave of axon tracts, with different origins and destinations. In the visual system, for example, retinal ganglion cell axons from the eye enter the brain at the junction of the optic nerve and diverge to about 10 different target nuclei, including the tectum and the lateral geniculate

nucleus. Each of these targets contains neurons that also diverge again to various targets of their own, and so on. Tracing pathways retrogradely on the motor side starting from a single muscle soon yields a similar complexity in convergence. Thus, with thousands of target nuclei and billions of axons, the interweaving of axonal pathways is remarkably rich. When looking at an adult brain, it is difficult to imagine how such precise patterns of connections are made. But by looking at early embryonic brains when the first pioneering pathways are forming, there is the possibility of seeing the first axons on their way (Wilson *et al.,* 1990; Ross *et al.,* 1992; Easter *et al.,* 1994). As more axons are added, they navigate through an increasingly complex environment, but are aided by pathways laid down by pioneering axons (Fig. 5.1).

Axonal Navigation

If the brain region in which a neuron is born is a like city or village, then its growing axon is

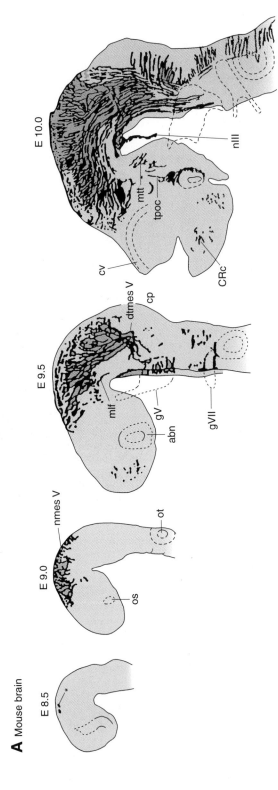

Figure 5.1 The increasing complexity of fiber tracts in the developing vertebrate brain. (A) Antibodies against axons in the embryonic mouse brain at E8.5, E9.0, E9.5, and E10 reveal a variety of new axons added at each stage. (B) Similarly, in the fast developing zebrafish, new axon tracts are added over the course of just 20 h. (After Ross *et al.*, 1992; Easter *et al.*, 1994, with permission.)

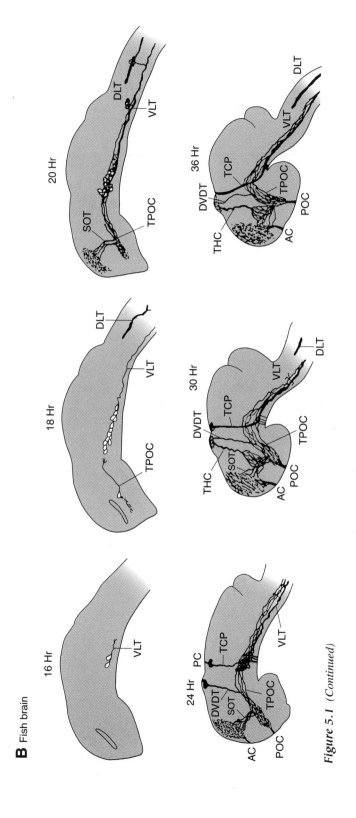

B Fish brain

16 Hr

18 Hr

20 Hr

24 Hr

30 Hr

36 Hr

Figure 5.1 *(Continued)*

147

like a driver on his way to another place (Fig. 5.2). As he pulls out from his home on a particular street, the driver knows which turns to make, which highway to get on, which exit to take, and which smaller roads to follow on the way to his destination. Unlike humans, most axons make these long journeys for the first (and only) time without errors. Growing axons are able to recognize various molecules on the surfaces of and diffusing away from other axons

A

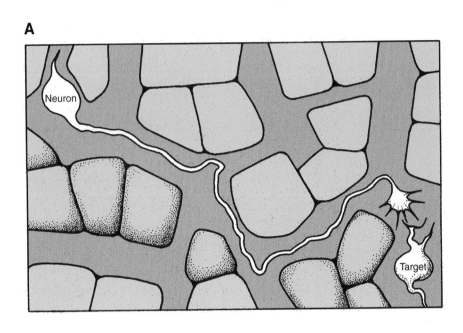

B

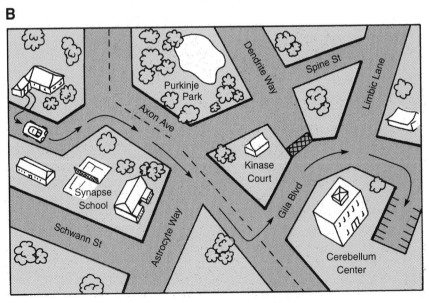

Figure 5.2   An axon growing to its target (A) is like a driver navigating through city streets (B). See text for details.

and cells and to use these as cues to navigate the circuitous pathway to their particular destinations. They need sensory abilities to perceive this guidance information that distinguishes the correct pathways from the incorrect ones. They must read the landmarks and signs and sometimes integrate conflicting information. In addition, they need to be able to move forward, sometimes rapidly, make turns, avoid obstacles, and stop when they reach their target. This means they need a motor, a mechanism to change directions, and a mechanism for changing speed. These functions, the sensory, the motor, and the integrative, are all contained within the specialized tip of a growing axon, the growth cone. This highly dynamic cellular structure, as we shall see, is responsible for many aspects of axon growth and guidance. That growth cones are capable of all these functions is demonstrated in experiments in which growth cones cut off from their cell bodies continue to navigate appropriately in the brain (Harris *et al.,* 1987). When the axon of a retinal ganglion cell is cut off from its cell body, the growth cone is still able to detect cues in its environment and extend toward the optic tectum (Fig. 5.3).

In 1965, Hibbard rotated a piece of the embryonic salamander hindbrain. In this tissue arises a pair of giant neurons called Mauthner cells that are responsible for a rapid escape response. These neurons send large diameter axons, easily visible with silver staining, caudally down the spinal cord. In the rotated piece of hindbrain, Hibbard saw that the axons of Mauthner cells initially grew rostrally instead of caudally, as though they were guided by local cues within the transplant (Hibbard, 1965). However, when the axons of these rotated neurons reached the rostral boundary of the transplant and entered unrotated neural tissue, they made dramatic U-turns and headed caudally down toward the spinal cord, proving that the growing axons were being guided by external cues (Fig. 5.4).

Another particularly illustrative example of axonal navigation is that of the sensory neurons that arise in the distal part of a grasshopper leg (Keshishian and Bentley, 1983b). These cells, called Ti's, pioneer the axonal tract that later de-

veloping sensory axons will follow to their targets in the central nervous system. Pioneer fibers were first recognized by Harrison (Harrison, 1910) as those axons that establish the highway that later axons will follow. If these Ti pioneers are ablated with a laser, then the later axons cannot find their way into the CNS (Keshishian and Bentley, 1983b). But how, then do the Ti's find their way? Part of the answer is that the Ti's use local cues on their journey. Spaced at short distances from one another are a series of well-spaced "guidepost" cells for which the Ti growth cones show a particular affinity (Caudy and Bentley, 1986). In fact, the distances between guideposts are small enough that a growth cone can reach out to a new guidepost while still contacting the previous one. Ti axons use these guidepost cells as stepping-stones into the CNS (Fig. 5.5). Some of guideposts are critical for pathfinding because when they are obliterated with a laser microbeam the Ti axons get stuck and are unable to make it from one segment to the next (Bentley and Caudy, 1983). In addition to guidepost cells, there are also patterns of adhesive molecules (see Box: Dendrite Formation) on the epithelium that help direct the growth cone from one guidepost cell to the next and a set of growth-inhibitory molecules that prevent the growing axons from traveling in inappropriate directions (Singer *et al.,* 1995). Analysis of live preparations of the embryonic grasshopper limb shows that the growth cone is a very active participant in this process. It explores the environment relentlessly by means of long rapidly moving filopodia. A single touch of one filopodium to a guidepost cell can dramatically reorient the direction of the axon's growth (O'Connor *et al.,* 1990).

The Growth Cone

Growth cones were recognized more than a hundred years ago by the famous Spanish neuroanatomist, Ramon y Cajal, as expansions at the tips of axons in fixed embryonic material. He imagined the growth cone as a sort of soft battering ram that extending axons used to force their

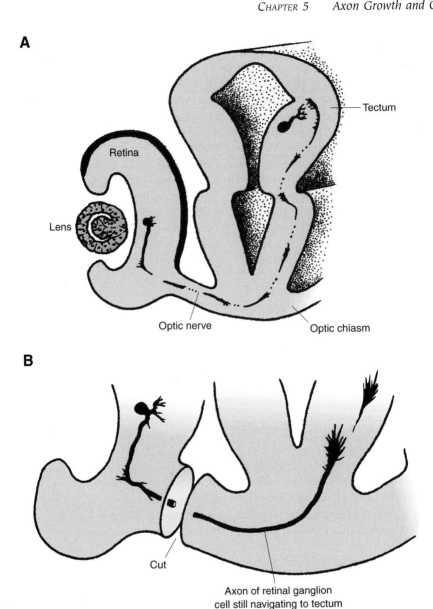

A

Retina

Lens

Optic nerve

Optic chiasm

Tectum

B

Cut

Axon of retinal ganglion
cell still navigating to tectum

***Figure* 5.3**   Axons grow from the retina to the tectum using their growth cones to guide them. (A) Time-lapse images of single retinal ganglion cell axons shows that they grow rather directly to the tectum, and are always tipped by active growth cones. (B) When the axon is separated from the cell body by cutting the optic stalk, the growth cone still grows along the correct pathway (Harris *et al.*, 1987).

way through the packed cells of the embryonic brain (Ramon y Cajal, 1890, 1937). In 1910, Ross Harrison took pieces of embryonic neural tube and put them into culture. From these pieces axons tipped with growth cones grew along a glass microscope coverslip (Harrison, 1910). As he looked at these live, he was astounded to see the growth cones move and wiggle in real time. They send out long thin filopodia and form lamellipodial veils between

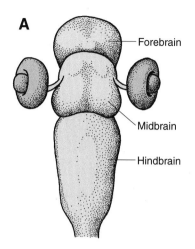

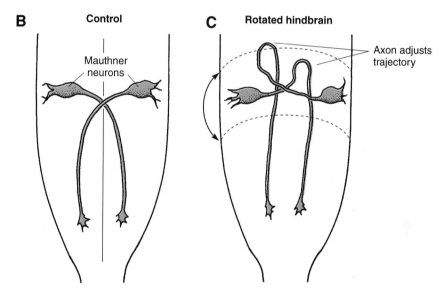

Figure 5.4 Mauthner cells grow posteriorly in the hindbrain due to local cues. (A) A dorsal view of a larval amphibian brain. (B) The bilaterally symmetric giant Mauthner neurons. (C) What happens to the growth of these axons when in an embryo the segment of the hindbrain containing the Mauthner primordia is rotated (Hibbard, 1965).

the filopodia (Fig. 5.6). They also retract these processes rapidly as the growth cone feels its way along the surface of the culture dish. In the 1930s Spiedel observed these active structures at the ends of growing sensory axons *in vivo* in the transparent growing tail fin of a frog (Spiedel, 1941). He followed single growth cones over days and even weeks, and he watched how they responded to obstacles, injuries, and various drugs. He was impressed with the ability of growing nerve fibers to change directions, branch, and respond to mechanical and chemical stimulation. These very active structures have now also been observed using sophisticated imaging techniques in the living embryonic central nervous system (Fig. 5.7).

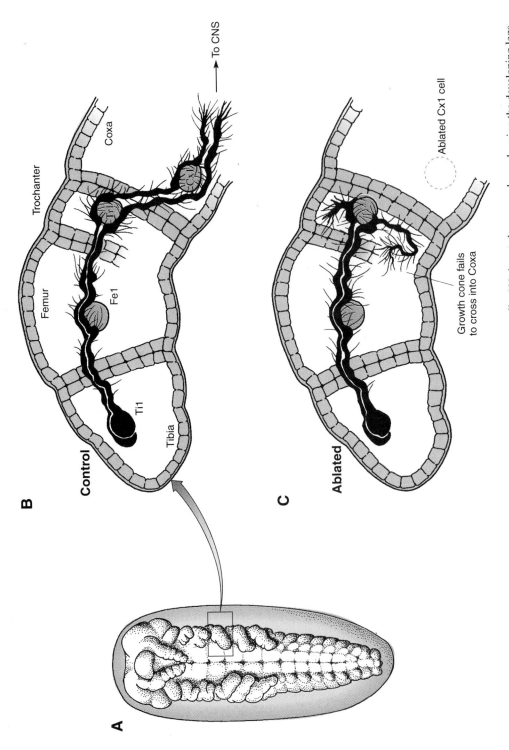

Figure 5.5 The growth of the Ti1 pioneers is aided by guidepost or stepping stone cells. (A) A grasshopper embryo showing the developing legs. Protoleg is identified by the box. (B) The Ti1 pioneers (black) reach from one guidepost neuron to the next, successively contacting Fe1, Tr1, and Cx1 on their way to the CNS. (C) When the Cx1 cells are ablated, the Ti1 cells lose their way and do not cross into the coxal segment of the embryonic leg (Bentley and Caudy, 1983).

Dendrite Formation

Dendrites, the neuritic processes that are the main receivers of synaptic input, are perhaps the most distinctive features of neuronal morphology. Dendritic trees differ from axonal arbors in a variety of ways, the most obvious being that dendrites have more postsynaptic specializations while axons have more presynaptic specializations. The cytoskeleton of a dendrite is also different than that of an axon, usually having a higher ratio of microtubules to actin filaments and more rough endoplasmic reticulum and polyribosomes. Axonal microtubules have their plus ends pointed distally while the dendritic microtubules have a mixture of plus and minus ends leading. Microtubule-associated proteins are also differentially distributed in axons and dendrites. For example MAP2 is located in dendrites while Tau is located mainly in axons. Treatment of cultured neurons with antisense constructs that reduce MAP2 or Tau expression have the expected specific effects on the formation of dendrites or axons, indicating that these proteins are particularly critical in the formation or stabilization of these structures. Certain membrane proteins are also differentially distributed among axons and dendrites; for instance, transmitter receptors are more common on dendrites while certain cell adhesion molecules are found mainly on axons (Craig and Banker, 1994). This polarity implies a sorting mechanism, but the molecular basis of sorting different proteins to different neuronal processes is not understood.

Just as the axon may stretch over long distances according to a cell-specific stereotyped pathway to connect with postsynaptic targets, each type of neuron has a characteristic dendritic tree. In some neurons, like the Purkinje cell, the dendritic tree is enormously complex and supports synaptic input from thousands of presynaptic fibers. In other neurons, the dendritic tree may be very simple, consisting of a single postsynaptic process. In the cortex, different neurons have dendritic trees in different layers. In the central nervous system of a cockroach or a leech, the dendritic trees of each identified cell has a unique signature branching pattern recognizable from individual to individual. Compared to what is known of pathfinding in axons, little is understood about how dendrites grow to their appropriate destinations.

Dendrites, like axons, grow out of the soma, usually lagging behind. Hippocampal cells in culture initially put out several short neurites. One of these then begins to extend more rapidly and gather axonal-specific markers. If the emerging axon is selectively cut off, the longest of the short processes starts to grow faster than the others and it becomes the axon. The remaining processes then begin to grow and accumulate dendritic markers. Thus neurons have an axon versus dendrite polarity that is not only intrinsic but to a certain extent internally regulated through a feedback mechanism by which the axon inhibits the other neurites from assuming the axonal identity they would attain by default (Goslin and Banker, 1989). In some cases, growing dendrites are tipped with dendritic growth cones that appear as miniature equivalents to axonal growth cones.

It has been thought that mature dendrite formation is somehow dependent on the axon making proper connections to its target. The situation, however, may be the more the reverse. If, for example, embryonic frog retinal ganglion cells are prevented from sending axons to target structures by transplanting the developing eye bud to the belly region, the different classes of retinal ganglion cells develop dendritic arbors that resemble those of normal ganglion cells (Sakaguchi, 1989). Axonal connections with the tectum seem more important to whether the retinal ganglion cells survive or not, as they pick up trophic factor

Dendrite Formation *continued*

from the target (see Chapter 8). Rather active axonal connections of RGCs with the tectal cells are important in the development of the dendritic arbors later (see Nedivi *et al.,* 1998; Rajan and Cline, 1998; and Chapter 7). So, in general, it seems that it is the input onto the dendrites themselves that helps shape their development. The complexity of the dendritic tree is, in many systems, proportional to the amount of innervation. Thus, for example, the dendritic trees of the principle sympathetic neurons of the superior cervical ganglion are larger and more complex in larger mammals that have more inputs onto these cells. Moreover, if inputs to the SCG are reduced or silenced this causes a concomitant decrease in the complexity of the dendritic tree that develops (Purves and Lichtman, 1985; Voyvodic, 1989).

Even though the final shape and complexity of the tree is sensitive to innervation, it would not be fair to consider dendrite development as completely dependent on synaptic input. One of the interesting examples of the independence of dendritic growth from innervation is the case of the Purkinje cells in weaver mutant mice. In these mice, the granule cells do not migrate properly into the cortex of the cerebellum and thus fail to make synapses on the Purkinje cells. The Purkinje cells nevertheless make a dendritic tree that, although smaller and less well formed than the trees of properly innervated Purkinje cells, is still characteristically complex (Bradley and Berry, 1978). The most dramatic demonstrations of the ability of neurons in the absence of synaptic input to produce dendritic trees come from culture experiments. Conditions have been worked out in which pyramidal neurons from the hippocampus, principle neurons of the SCG, and even cerebellar Purkinje cells are able to develop a characteristic dendritic tree in dissociated cell culture.

While there are intrinsic tendencies, dendritic growth-promoting factors can be found in the environment. Dendritic outgrowth from mouse cortical neurons was specifically enhanced by astrocytes derived from the forebrain (Le Roux and Reh, 1994). Similar results were obtained with glial-conditioned medium. Embryonic astrocytes were a particularly good source of such dendritic growth factors, as were reactive astrocytes even though the latter appear to inhibit axon growth (Le Roux and Reh, 1996). Superior cervical ganglion neurons grown in serum-free medium in the absence of nonneuronal cells were unipolar and only grew axons. When the same neurons were exposed to serum, they became multipolar and developed processes that could be categorized as dendrites by morphological and antigenic criteria (Bruckenstein and Higgins, 1988). Thus, serum contains factors that stimulate dendritic extension. The bone morphogenetic proteins, BMP2 and BMP6, and the osteogenic protein, OP-1, were subsequently found to selectively induce the formation of dendrites and the expression of MAP2 in sympathetic neurons in a concentration-dependent manner (Lein *et al.,* 1995; Guo *et al.,* 1998). Dermatin sulfate also specifically enhances dendritic growth. Dendritic retraction occurs in many regions of the developing brain. Leukemia inhibitory factor (LIF) and ciliary neurotrophic factor (CNTF) specifically cause dendritic retraction in SCG cells (Guo *et al.,* 1997, 1999). Axon growth is unaffected by these factors. Taken together, these results suggest separate but extensive molecular mechanisms for promoting and inhibiting dendrite outgrowth that parallel the growth-promoting and collapsing mechanisms known to be involved in axonogenesis.

Many dendritic trees, like axonal arbors, are dynamic throughout the life of the animal. The plasticity of these branches in response to experience and neuronal activity is discussed in Chapter 9.

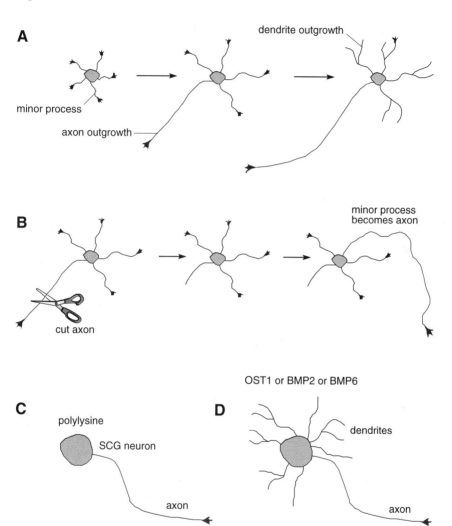

A

dendrite outgrowth

minor process

axon outgrowth

B

minor process becomes axon

cut axon

C

polylysine

SCG neuron

axon

D

OST1 or BMP2 or BMP6

dendrites

axon

Dendritic growth. (A) In tissue culture, a hippocampal neuron begins by putting out several minor processes that are basically equivalent. One of these, the future axon, then begins to grow faster than the other processes and expresses axon-specific components such as GAP43 and tau. After the axon has elongated, dendrites begin to grow and express dendrite-specific components such as MAP2. (B) When the emerging axon of a hippocampal cell is cut, a minor process, which would have become a dendrite, begins to grow more rapidly and becomes the axon. This suggests that all processes are initially capable of forming an axon. (C) When a superior cervical ganglion (SCG) neuron is plated on a polylysine substrate, only an axon grows out. (D) However, when a SCG neuron is grown on polylysine in the presence of OST-1 or BMP2 or BMP6, dendrite growth is specifically promoted (Goslin and Banker, 1989; Guo *et al.* 1998).

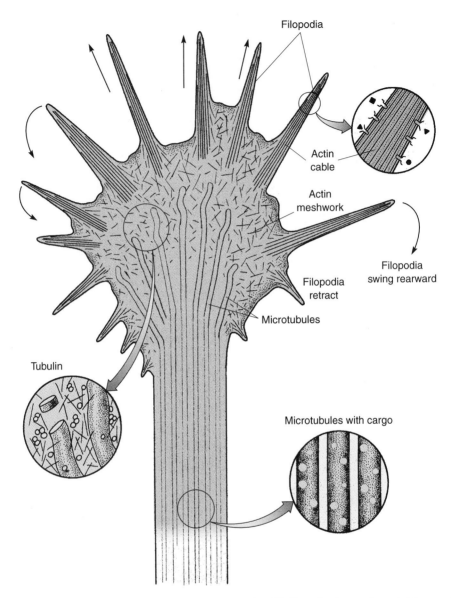

Filopodia

Actin
cable

Actin
meshwork

Filopodia
swing rearward

Filopodia
retract

Microtubules

Tubulin

Microtubules with cargo

Figure 5.6 The structure of the growth cone. Actin bundles fill filopodia that are bounded by membranes containing cell adhesion molecules and various receptors. The filopodia poke out at the advancing edge and are retracted at the trailing edge of the growth cone. Between the filopodia are sheets of lamellipodia that extend forward. They are filled with an actin meshwork that is continuous with that in the main body of the growth cone. Here also microtubules push forward and carry cargo to and from the cell body along the axon shaft as they enter the growth cone and fan out toward the filopodia.

As axons traverse the pathway to their target, they generally assume one of two morphologies (Tosney and Landmesser, 1985; Bovolenta and Mason, 1987; O'Connor *et al.*, 1990). The axons of later growing axons often fasciculate with earlier pioneering axons, and their growth cones assume a bullet-shaped appearance with few filopodia (Fig. 5.8A). But, as they approach

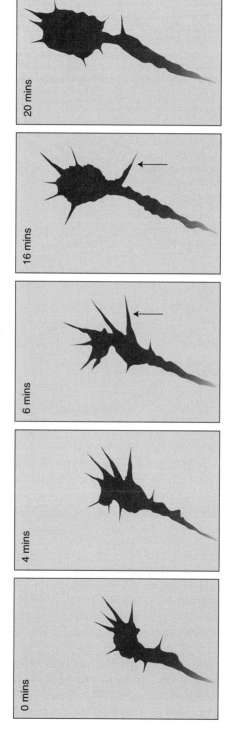

Figure 5.7 Growth cone of a retinal ganglion cell in the optic tract of a frog embryo. The activity of this fluorescently labeled growth cone is seen over the 20-min recording interval. The arrow points to a filopodium that at first extends forward but then swings rearward as the growth cone advances in the CNS (Harris *et al.*, 1987).

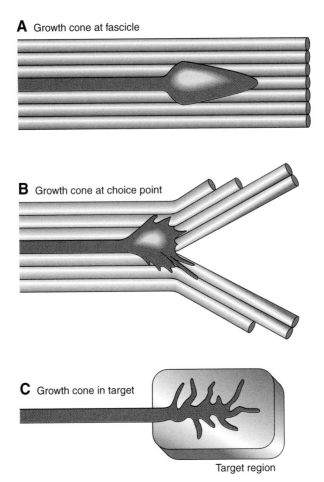

A Growth cone at fascicle

B Growth cone at choice point

C Growth cone in target

Target region

Figure 5.8 The different shapes that a growth cone can assume. (A) Growth cones that are fasciculating with other axons tend to be simple and have few filopodia. (B) Growth cones at choice points are complex with filopodia and lammelipodia. (C) Growth cones in the target region become even more complex and sprout backbranches along the axon shaft.

regions where they defasciculate, change direction, or decide to follow other axons, they assume a broad veil-like appearance and often generate several filopodia. These changes in cell behavior suggest that the growth cone has entered a novel environment and that it now must make choices based upon interactions with this environment (Fig. 5.8B). Upon reaching an appropriate target of innervation, growth cones once again alter their shape and rate of growth. Horseradish peroxidase was used to label chick motor axons (Tosney and Landmesser, 1985) and mouse retinal ganglion axons (Bovolenta and Mason, 1987) at the age when they first contact the myotome or lateral geniculate, respectively. Growth cones at the target border once again assume a broad lamellipodial shape, consistent with a decision-making process. But after crossing the target border and entering the postsynaptic neuropil, growth cones display thin, branched terminals with small tapered growth cones (Fig. 5.8C). A similar transformation is observed for motoneuron terminals in the body wall musculature of *Drosophila* as they contact their appropriate muscle fiber (Halpern *et al.,* 1991).

While static observations from fixed tissue are quite accurate, they provide neither the rate of growth nor the local sampling strategy that single growth cones employ as they make decisions. Speidel had initially described sporadic growth that occurred at a maximum rate of about 40 μm/h in the transparent tail fin of immobilized frog tadpoles. The resting growth cone assumed a smooth contour and acquired a number of delicate processes when it advanced in an amoeboid fashion, consistent with Harrison's earlier *in vitro* observations. The advent of high-resolution video microscopy and fluorescent tracer techniques have provided a new set of answers to these questions in the form of magnificent time-lapse movies of axonal pathfinding and target invasion (see Box: The TV Age: Advances in Vital Dyes and Video Microscopy).

The Growing Zone

As a growth cone crawls forward, it leaves an axon behind it, and this means that new material must be incorporated continually into the axon. In culture, when a particle is attached to a growing axon, it generally remains stationary while the distal tip of the axon elongates. This suggests that membrane associated material is assembled distally, at the growth cone. Indeed, labeled glycoproteins are added preferentially at the distal tips of axons in the growth cone region (Hollenbeck and Bray, 1987). Other studies using labeled lectins show that new unlabeled membrane glycoproteins appear predominantly at the distal growing tip. The production of this new membrane material is calcium dependent, suggesting that new membrane is added by the fusion of internal vesicles, often a calcium-dependent process, to the membrane of the growth cone's surface. There appears to be a supply of these vesicles in the central region of the growth cone. Recent experiments have attached tiny beads to membrane proteins or lipids at various places along the length of a growing axon in culture (Dai and Sheetz, 1995). The beads then move

slowly toward the cell body, proving that membrane is being added at the growing tip and flowing back. Traction force can be applied to these beads with a laser beam focused through a microscope; a process called laser tweezering. When attached beads are pulled away from the axon with laser tweezers, they drag a bit of membrane with them until it is stretched so thin that it snaps off. Beads attached near the growth cone are able to pull out a longer piece of membrane than those attached near the soma. This indicates that the membrane is much looser near the growth cone, presumably because this is where the majority of it is added.

The addition of cytoskeletal components also takes place primarily at the tip of the growing process. This was shown with a fluorescent bleaching technique. Neurons were injected with fluorescent tubulin and actin monomers, which are incorporated into the cytoskeleton. Part of the axon was then illuminated with a bright spot to bleach the fluorescence at a particular location (Fig. 5.9). The result is that the bleached spot stays relatively still as the growth cone continues to advance, suggesting that cytoskeletal components are not pushed forward, but assembled distally. This distal assembly can be directly observed, also with fluorescent techniques. If different areas of an axon are bleached, recovery of fluorescence in these areas should result from the addition of new fluorescent monomers, which are not visible until they are part of the cytoskeleton. The recovery of fluorescence occurs first in the growth cones, suggesting that this is where they are first assembled into microtubules. Furthermore, pools of unassembled, tubulin are concentrated in the growth cone. It turns out that this is the most sensitive part of the axon to the effects of microtubule depolymerizing agents such as nocodozole (Brown *et al.,* 1992). Natural microtubule stabilizing proteins, such as tau, are also highly concentrated near the growth cone, suggesting that this is where unpolymerized tubulin is fashioned into microtubules and stabilized.

These results suggest that most axonal growth takes place at the growth cone. Yet there is clearly some forward transport of assembled

The TV Age: Advances in Vital Dyes and Video Microscopy

Most biological questions eventually demand an answer in the form of a picture. Questions concerning the manner in which axons grow and innervate their target have been transformed by the most spellbinding modern picture, the TV image. While Cajal's remarkable visual memory and artistry allowed him to produce accurate drawings of growth cones nearly a century ago, simple video microscopy systems now permit most laboratories to view and measure the growing axon. Over the past 20 years, the standard compound microscope has been embellished with a number of technical wonders. These advances include low light-sensitive video cameras, scanning laser illumination, and specialized image-processing software (Allen *et al.,* 1981; Inoué, 1981, 1989). Coupled with the recent introduction of fluorescent labels that are rapidly transported along living axons, one is now able to produce time-lapse movies of process outgrowth and innervation (Honig and Hume, 1986; Glover *et al.,* 1986).

There are at least three kinds of vital axon tracers that are commonly used to observe living processes. The first type of tracer, called DiI and DiO, is lipophilic. They diffuse rapidly down neuronal processes when small crystals placed in close apposition to the neurons of interest, and are visualized with epifluorescent illumination. The second type of tracer, called dextran-amines, is water soluble. They are transported rapidly down an axon when introduced within the neuron's cytoplasm. Dextran-amines are typically coupled to fluorescent molecules, such as fluorescein. Once labeled with one of these methods, axonal processes may be visualized by shining light onto the tissue and observing the fluorescence emitted by the tracer. Unfortunately, the exciting wavelength of light is not as benign as one might hope, and tissue can be easily damaged. Therefore, the fluorescent emissions are best observed for brief intervals with very sensitive photon detectors. Since a full video image can be acquired within 30 ms, it is possible to average several video frames without compromising tissue viability, thus enhancing the signal-to-noise ratio. The third type of tracer, now growing in use, is a green fluorescent protein (GFP) that is a natural protein found in certain types of jellyfish. The gene for this protein has been cloned and various genetically engineered forms of genes coding for proteins with different spectral characteristics are available. When a growing neuron is transfected with such a GFP gene, it creates its own fluorescent protein. By genetically engineering chimeric genes, combining GFP with a protein potentially involved in axon growth, one can test the effect of misexpressing the protein of interest in live axons. By putting the GFP gene under the control of a promoter that is active in a subset of developmental nerve cells in a transgenic animal, it is possible to monitor a whole class of growing axons.

One problem, often encountered in thick specimens, is the excessive level of out-of-focus fluorescence. The confocal laser microscope overcomes this obstacle and allows one to observe sharp fluorescent images in a limited depth of field (0.5–1.5 µm), called optical sectioning. This is accomplished by scanning a focused laser beam across the specimen in a point-by-point fashion. The emitted light from each "point" is acquired and used to reconstruct an image of the specimen. Using a combination of these techniques, it has become possible to watch axons growth out and innervate their target in living animals in great detail.

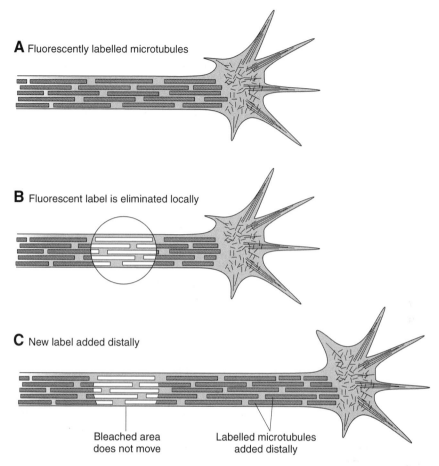

A Fluorescently labelled microtubules

B Fluorescent label is eliminated locally

C New label added distally

Bleached area does not move

Labelled microtubules added distally

Figure 5.9 Microtubules are added at the growing end of an axon. A growing axon (A) is labeled with fluorescent tubulin and then some of this fluorescence is bleached by a beam of light (circle in (B)) focused on the axon near the growth cone. As the axon elongates distally, the bleached spot stays in approximately the same place (C) implying that the microtubules along the axon shaft do not move forward but rather new microtubules are assembled at the distal tip.

microtubules. By looking at the growing separation of two beads or two dye spots on a growing axon, it is also clear that some membrane is also added along the axon. Such growth is presumably crucial as the brain or body enlarges and after initial connections are made, or if branches off the main axon are to form. Nevertheless, it is obvious from these studies that the bulk of axon growth and the assembly of its parts takes place at the growth cone and an important function of the growth cone is that of organizing the insertion of new components.

The Dynamic Cytoskeleton

The cytoskeleton of a growth cone is filled with molecules that can be mobilized for cell movement (Reinsch *et al.,* 1991; Bentley and O'Connor, 1994; Heidemann *et al.,* 1995; Heidemann, 1996; Letourneau, 1996). Among these molecules are actin and tubulin, along with several actin- and microtubule-associated proteins. Tubulin polymerizes at the distal tip to form microtubules and actin polymerizes to form microfilaments. Actin-associated proteins such as myosin may be involved in generating vectorial force in the growth cone by pulling on the actin filaments, similar to the role it plays during muscle cell contraction. Other associated proteins anchor actin and microtubules to the cell membrane or to other cytoskeletal components. They also participate in the assembly, disassembly, and stabilization of actin and tubulin. The rapid assembly of actin filaments at the tips of growing filopodia is probably responsible for the jutting out of new filopodia, whereas microtubule assembly may push the whole growth cone forward.

Drugs such as cytochalasin that depolymerize actin have been shown to prevent filopodia formation, and axons with growth cones lacking filopodia due to such treatments either stop growing altogether or slow down dramatically. The fact that they are able to move at all was a surprising finding at first because it was previously thought that the filopodia did all of the work in terms of axonal growth. Clearly filopodia are important for the progress of a growth cone *in vitro* and *in vivo,* but other factors such as microtubule polymerization contribute to the forward advancement of growth cones. Interestingly, filopodia-deprived growth cones often lose their way in the developing organism, failing to make critical turns or making turns where they should not. Thus, when the growth cone of the Ti1 pioneer neuron in the grasshopper limb is treated with cytochalasin, the axons meander off course and often do not make the turns necessary to grow into the CNS (Bentley and Toroian-Raymond, 1986) (Fig. 5.10A). In the amphibian brain, retinal axons must make a posterior turn in the diencephalon to get to their targets in the midbrain. If these growing axons are treated with cytochalasin, they grow past the turning point and fail to find their targets (Chien et al., 1993). (Fig. 5.10B). These results demonstrate that filopodia are also critical for steering the growth cone, either by acting as sensors that compare one direction with another or by acting as differential motors that exert directional tension.

The actin filaments in filopodia are bundled and oriented so that their fast growing barbed ends are pointing away from the growth cone.

Thus, filopodia appear to grow from their distal tips. In the lamellipodia, the actin filaments appear to be short and branched and are highly cross-linked to form a meshwork. This actin meshwork may offer some resistance to the material pushing and squeezing forward from the central region. When cytochalasin is added to disrupt actin filaments, engorgement of lamellipodia with material from the central core occurs rapidly. In a normally extending growth cone, tension is generated by the filopodia that appear to move backward from their base, somewhat like the oars in a rowboat boat. The actin filaments within each filopodium are probably attached to the network of cortical actin at their base. If the membranes of the filopodia attach to the extracellular environment, then as the filopodia move rearward they pull the growth cone forward. This tension can be observed by the way a single filopodia that contacts an axon lying in its path can pull the axon toward the advancing growth cone (Bray, 1979) (Fig. 5.11A).

Single filopodia that make contact with a more adhesive substrate in tissue culture are able to steer the entire growth cone by pulling it toward the adhesive substrate (Letourneau, 1996). When the filopodia on one side of the growth cone stick strongly enough to a surface, then they provide a relatively stronger tension that steers the growth cone in that direction, especially if the filopodia on the other side are unattached at the time (Fig. 5.11B). This idea of steering is consistent with experiments in culture using growth cones with several filopodia. When one filopodium is detached using a fine glass needle, the growth cone virtually snaps into a new direction, consistent with the release of tension on one side (Wesells and Nuttall, 1978) (Fig. 5.11C). It has also been shown that single filopodia that have been detached from their parental growth cone are able to respond to putative guidance factors by becoming shorter (Davenport et al., 1996), demonstrating that individual filopodia have both sensory machinery and responsive cytoskeletal components (Fig. 5.11D).

How do filopodia generate tension? One possibility is that the actin filaments are pulled centrally by myosin molecules located at the

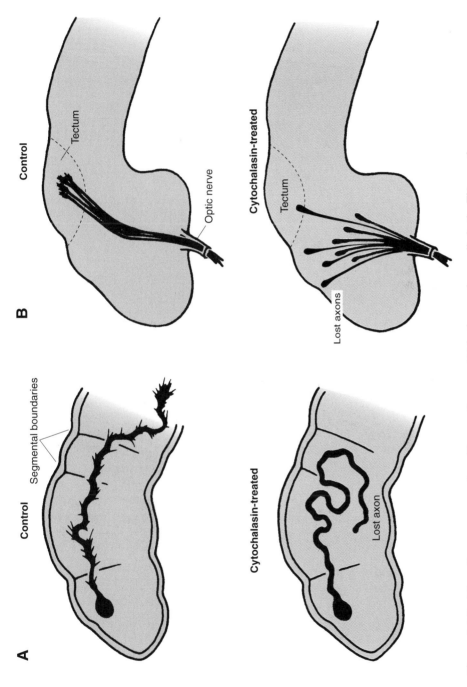

Figure 5.10 Filopodia are necessary to guide growth cones. (A) in the grasshopper limb, the Ti1 growth cones are hairy with active filopodia (top). If the filopodia are removed with the actin-depolymerizing agent cytochalasin, the axon fails to navigate to its target (bottom). (B) In the vertebrate visual system, axons enter the brain from the optic nerve and grow toward the tectum by growing dorsally and turning posteriorly (top). When the filopodia of these axons are removed with cytochalasin, the axons fail to make the appropriate posterior turn and most axons miss the tectum (bottom) (Bentley and Toroian-Raymond, 1986; Chien *et al.*, 1993).

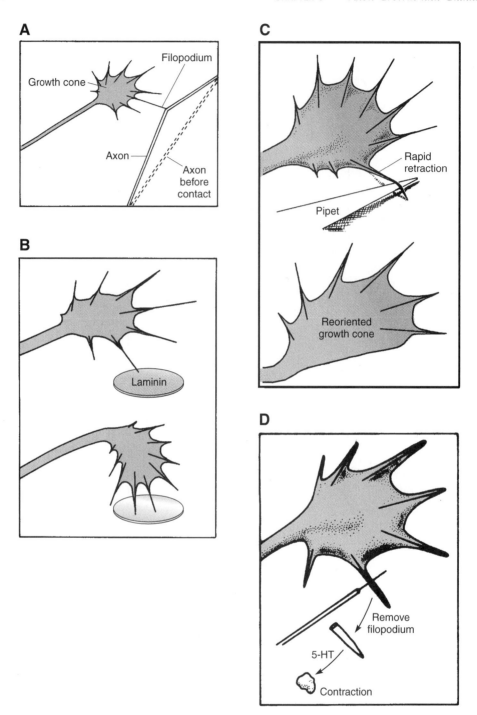

Figure 5.11   Single filopodia direct growth cones. (A) A single filopodium from a growth cone exerts tension and pulls on an axon it contacts in culture. (B) A single filopodium touches a laminin-coated spot in a culture dish and reorients. (C) A single filopodium is detached from a culture dish and the growth cone reorients in the opposite direction. (D) A single isolated filopodium contracts when exposed to serotonin (5-HT). (E) A single filopodium of a Ti1 cell contacts a guidepost cell and by the process of microtubule invasion becomes the new leading edge.

E

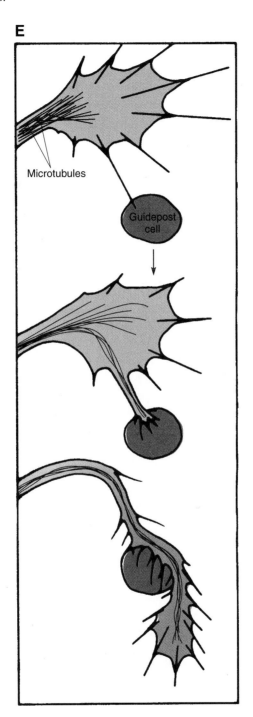

Figure 5.11 *(Continued)*

base of the filopodia. Indeed, blocking myosin function in growth cones retards forward progress, establishing that myosin is involved. However, filopodia themselves tend to lengthen in these cases, as if a force that restrained them was gone (Lin *et al.,* 1996). Actin assembly mediated by actin-polymerizing factors, when combined with molecules that anchor the cytoskeleton to the substrate, can also generate tension. For example, it is thought that filopodial actin might get anchored to the substrate as it is assembled distally and generate tension against the load of the large growth cone which cannot advance as rapidly as a single filopodia.

The importance of filopodia as cytoskeletal elements that direct growth cones *in vivo* has been demonstrated in the pioneer axons of the grasshopper limb. Here it can be seen that when a single filopodium of a Ti1 neuron makes contact with a guidepost cell that signals the correct direction of movement, then it remains in close contact while other filopodia retract (Fig. 5.11E). The filopodium in contact with the guidepost cell becomes engorged and is invaded by microtubules, eventually becoming the shaft of the growing axon (Sabry *et al.,* 1991).

Microtubules run straight and parallel inside of the axon, but when they enter the base of the growth cone they splay out and bend like the soft spokes on a fan (Fig. 5.6). Like the actin filaments in the filopodia, the microtubules of the axons have a "plus" end where polymerization takes place, and this is positioned at the growing tip. In fact, axons that have been deprived of filopodia by treatment with actin-depolymerizing agents, such as cytochalasin B, continue to grow, and this is probably due to the addition of tubulin at the distal process. Depolymerization of microtubules at the distal tip, which is the most sensitive region of the growing axon to these drugs, completely inhibits axon elongation. The control of microtubule assembly may be partially controlled by post-translational modifications. A carboxyterminal tyrosine is added to α-tubulin by the enzyme tubulin tyrosine ligase inside of the growth cone. The tyrosinated form of tubulin is quite dynamic, and it is also more sensitive to depolymerizing agents. In contrast, tubulin loses the tyrosine group and becomes acetylated when it enters the axonal pool of microtubules, making them more stable and insensitive to depolymerization (Brown *et al.,* 1992).

Several microtubule-associated proteins (MAPs) are found in growing neurites, and these proteins may regulate the growth process. For example, MAP1B and Tau are dramatically upregulated in PC12 cells that are induced to put out neurites by the addition of NGF, particularly in the growth cones. When developing neurons are incubated in Tau antisense mRNA, and the expression of this MAP is reduced, the outgrowth of neurites is disrupted. Thus, Tau probably has a fundamental role in process outgrowth (Letourneau, 1996).

What is the force that causes axons to add microtubules and grow? Apparently, the growth cone generates tension as its filopodia attach to the substrate. This tension acts as a signal that leads to the polymerization of tubulin. If a neuron is lifted onto a thin glass needle while its growth cone grows along the substrate, one can observe the needle bend and thus measure the force that the growth cone can exert on the axon (Bray and Hollenbeck, 1988). Apparently this force is enough to initiate growth because if the axon is mechanically stretched by the investigator at the same tension, then the axon fills with polymerizing microtubules and elongates so that its ultrastructure remains rather normal looking.

These studies suggest a functional association between actin and microtubules. Tension generated by actin and its accessory molecules is the intermediary step in microtubule polymerization. But there are suggestions for a more direct link between actin and microtubules. For instance, in the steering of a growth cone by filopodia, the bending and movement of microtubules toward and even into that filopodia, which can be blocked by agents that stabilize microtubules, suggest that the actin network must be pulling directly on the microtubules (Letourneau, 1996; Williamson *et al.,* 1996) (Fig. 5.12). Indeed, some of the MAPs may also bind actin and provide mechanical links between these two structural components. It is clear from this discussion that we are still in the early stages of understanding

A Control

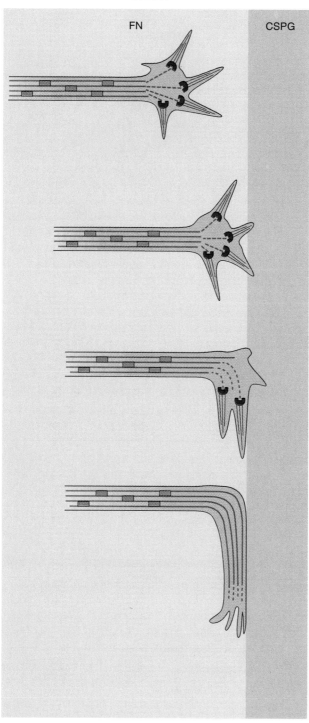

Figure 5.12 Growth cones need dynamic microtubules to turn. (A) Growth cones from chick spinal cords on a fibronectin (FN) substrate turn abruptly when they encounter a chondroitin sulfate proteoglycan (CSPG) border. It is thought that actin bundles in the filopodia reorient the dynamic microtubules. (B) When treated with taxol, a microtubule stabilizing agent, the axons do not turn when they confront the border but seem to be stuck pointing straight ahead (Williamson *et al.*, 1996).

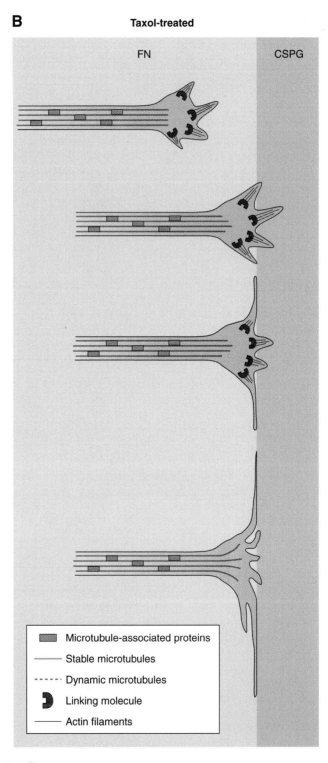

Figure 5.12 (Continued)

the mechanism by which growth cones advance and the molecular constituents of the motor. There is much to learn about how these components transduce the sensory stimuli that attract a growth cone, how they interact with each other in the cytoplasm, and how they generate tension to move the system forward.

Growth Cone Guidance

Growth cones have the ability to sense their environment and make choices based on extracellular information. These choices are made as the growth cone passes through a complex environment of physical and chemical factors. In the brain, growth cones are exposed to a variety of substrates: the cell membranes of other neurons, glial cells, undifferentiated neuroepithelial cells, a variety of axons traveling in different directions, extracellular matrix proteins, glycoproteins, cell adhesion molecules, and various diffusible growth-promoting or growth-inhibiting factors. To discover the biochemical nature of the guidance mechanisms, reagents have been tested in tissue culture experiments to see whether they influence the rate and direction of axonal growth. Many such molecules have been identified in this way. Genetic approaches in *Drosophila* and nematodes have also led to the identification of dozens of genes that, when disrupted, lead to growth and pathfinding errors. These molecules and the genes that code for them are discussed in some detail throughout the remainder of this chapter.

Mechanical Guidance

Growth cones also confront a mechanical environment, where sometimes the going is easy and there are few obstacles and other times the going is hard and there is no clear pathway ahead. In one simple set of experiments, growth cones in culture were found to respond to artificial mechanical pathways. When axons are grown on a surface with parallel scratches carved in it, they tend to grow on the smooth surfaces between the scratches where the growth cones can spread out. On a dried cracked collagen surface, they often follow the pattern of the stress fractures (Fig. 5.13A). *In vivo,* a plastic barrier can be placed as an obstacle in the path of growing axons, and the axons will grow around it (Fig. 5.13B). When tracts or commissures are absent or experimentally severed, axons may be physically impeded from growing as they normally would. In such cases, it is sometimes possible to provide axons with an artificial mechanical pathway across the wound (Silver and Ogawa, 1983) (Fig. 5.13C). All these pieces of evidence suggest that growth cones can sense and be guided by physical features in their environment. Indeed, some of the first theories of growth cone guidance were centered solely on steric or mechanical guidance, and examination of embryonic tissues seemed to confirm that growth cones grow in grooves or spaces between cells (Carney and Silver, 1983; Silver, 1984) (Fig. 5.13D). Certain axons appear to grow through channels that open up in front of them, and so it appears that these channels lead growth cones along their correct path.

A number of direct experiments, however, made it clear that there is much more to axonal pathfinding than mechanical guidance. Dennis Bray observed that, if growth cones were led by all of the objects they encounter (blood vessel, folds of tissue), then axons would never find their targets. In fact, axons have little trouble finding their targets when they are transplanted into regions of the brain where such channels do not exist. A variety of different transplant experiments in different tissues show the remarkable ability of axons to traverse unusual paths to get to their appropriate targets. For example, when optic nerves are forced to enter the brain at a variety of different locations they nevertheless travel directly to the tectum (Harris, 1986). Such results reveal that there is obviously more to pathfinding than following preformed mechanical trails. Growth cones also blaze a trail themselves. If neurons are grown on protein-coated nitrocellulose that is then stained to reveal protein, it is found that there are protein-free trails that the growth cones have made as they wander

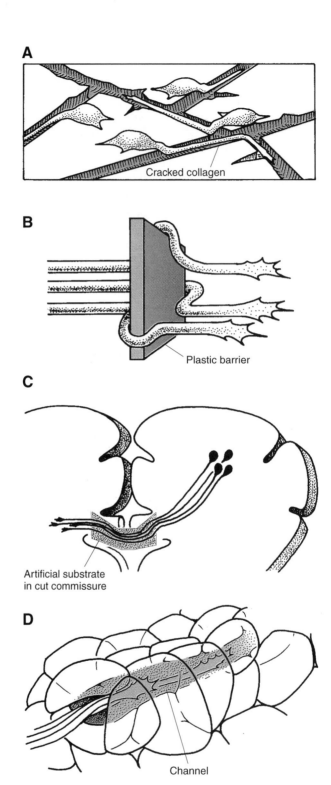

Figure 5.13 Axons may follow mechanical pathways. (A) The axons of neurons on a dried collagen matrix growing through the cracks. (B) Axons growing around barriers in culture or in the brain. (C) Axons of the corpus callosum using an artificial sling to grow from one side of the brain to the other. (D) Axons growing through intercellular channels in the embryonic brain.

over the surface. They form these trails by secreting proteases, such as plasminogen activator (Pittman, 1985). Therefore, the channels seen in front of growth cones may be due to the fact that growth cones digest away extracellular matrix material that may impede their progress.

Adhesive Guidance

Some of the original experiments exploring growth cone behavior in a culture dish focused on the growth of axons across various adhesive substrates. When neurons are plated on plain glass or tissue culture plastic, the cells often attach, but they rarely put out long neurites with active growth cones. However, when they are plated on polycationic substrates, such as polyornithine or polylysine, that stick well to negatively charged biological membranes, the neurons are much more likely to initiate outgrowth. The growth cones of such neurons look flattened against the substrate as though they adhere very strongly to it (Fig. 5.14A). When axons are

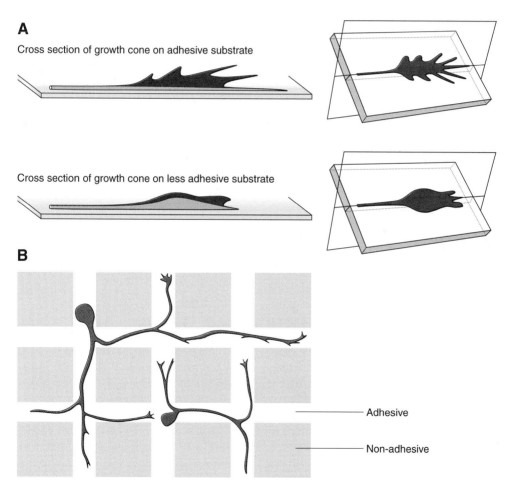

Figure 5.14 Growth cones and adhesion. (A) On a very adhesive substrate, growth cones are flattened, have lots of filopodia, and do not move rapidly (top). On a less adhesive substrate, growth cones are more compact, are rounded, have fewer processes, and often move more quickly. (B) Neurites in culture given a choice between an adhesive and a nonadhesive substrate will tend to follow the adhesive trails.

grown on a patterned dish that offers them the choice between a nonadhesive substrate like palladium, versus an adhesive substrate such as polyornithine, the growth cones follow the adhesive trail (Letourneau, 1975; Hammarback *et al.,* 1985) (Fig. 5.14B). Thus, axon outgrowth and direction can be stimulated or affected by differences in the adhesive properties of the substrate.

These findings led to the idea that growth cones might simply follow gradients of adhesion in the developing organism. In fact, this may be the case for some neurons. In the wing of the moth, sensory axons of the wing grow in the distal to proximal direction along a basal lamina of epithelial cells (Nardi and Vernon, 1990). Examination of this epithelium microscopically shows that it becomes increasing complex toward the base. Transplantation of the epithelium suggests that this change corresponds to an adhesive gradient. Axons readily cross onto a transplant that has been moved in the proximal to distal direction, but avoid distal transplants that have been moved proximally, suggesting that axons readily grow onto more adhesive membranes but will not onto less adhesive ones (Nardi, 1983).

To measure growth cone attachment to various cell adhesion molecules, a pipet can be positioned in a culture dish containing growing axons and culture media squirted at the growth cones in an attempt to "blast" them off the substrate (Fig. 5.15). The longer the growth cone stays attached to the surface, the stronger its adhesion must be. Neurite growth rate can then be measured on these same substrates for comparison (Lemmon *et al.,* 1992). Surprisingly, these experiments indicate that there is *not* a relationship between adhesion and the rate of growth (Fig. 5.15). Moreover, when axons are given a choice between pairs of naturally occurring cell adhesion molecules, they do not grow preferentially on the more adhesive substrate.

Another way to visualize adhesion is to use interference contrast microscopy, which shows zones of close apposition between the membrane of the growth cone and the surface upon which it is growing. Interestingly, it turns out that the most adhesive substrates, such as Con-

canavalin A, are not good supporters of axon outgrowth. In fact, growth cones tend to get stuck on such a surface. They become flattened, fail to retract their filopodia efficiently, and grow slowly, taking tortuous courses. As is the case for invasive cancer cells, the ability to detach is critical to migration. Thus, when axons are given choices of surfaces to grow on, they do not necessarily choose the more adherent substrate.

Direct tests of growth cone guidance by gradients of adhesive molecules *in vitro* have shown that even steep gradients of the extracellular matrix molecule, laminin, which serves as an attachment factor and growth promoter, are incapable of directing axon growth (Fig. 5.16). Rather, it appears that above a certain threshold concentration laminin will support neurite outgrowth, and below it, it will not (McKenna and Raper, 1988). The implication is that axons *in vivo* grow on concentrations of adhesive substrates that permit growth, but these substrates are not necessarily instructive, as the axons do not necessarily grow up or down a concentration gradient of these substrates. Nevertheless, as with mechanical guidance, it is clear that growth cones are influenced by adhesive differences and probably encounter such differences *in vivo.*

Extracellular Matrix and Axon Outgrowth

Many molecules have been isolated from the extracellular matrix (ECM) and found to be very good at supporting neurite outgrowth in tissue culture (Bixby and Harris, 1991). These factors were initially purified from culture media that were conditioned by cells known to support axonal outgrowth. Several of the most abundant proteins in ECM, such as laminin, fibronectin, vitronectin, and various forms of collagen, all promote outgrowth. Many of the native ECM proteins are large and have many different functional domains for cell attachment, for collagen attachment, and for protein interaction. For example, studies with antibodies and various

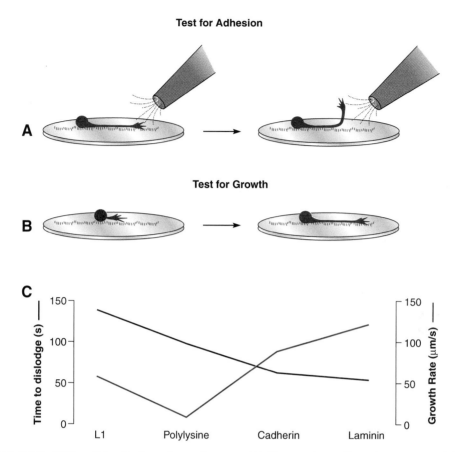

Test for Adhesion

A

Test for Growth

B

C

Figure 5.15 Differential adhesion of growth cones. (A) To quantitate adhesivity, a measured "blast" of culture medium is directed at the growth cone. At a particular time the growth cone becomes detached. (B) The neuron (red) grows at a certain rate along a particular substrate. (C) Using such tests it can be shown that neurons have different adhesion and growth profiles which depend on the substrate molecules (Lemmon *et al.*, 1992).

peptide inhibitors reveal that there appear to be several distinct neurite outgrowth-promoting domains in the laminin protein.

Different neurons seem to show a preference for particular ECM molecules. Vertebrate CNS cells grow particularly well on laminin, while some peripheral neurons seem to grow better on fibronectin. In experiments where retinal neurons are given a choice between laminin and fibronectin laid down in alternate stripes, retinal axons clearly prefer laminin, though they will grow on either substrate if given no choice. Thus, specific ECM molecules may promote the growth of specific axons.

Integrin is a receptor for many different extracellular matrix proteins, and it is composed of two subunits, an α and a β (Fig. 5.17). The extracellular matrix molecules that an axon will respond to are largely a matter of which integrin molecules are found at the growth cone. The specificity of integrin for particular ECM proteins depends on the combination of α and β subunits that is expressed (McKerracher *et al.*, 1996). There are at least 10 different α subunits and 5 different β subunits, and it is clear that different tissues, including different neural tissues, use several subunit combinations. The α5 subunit is particularly good at binding fibronectin

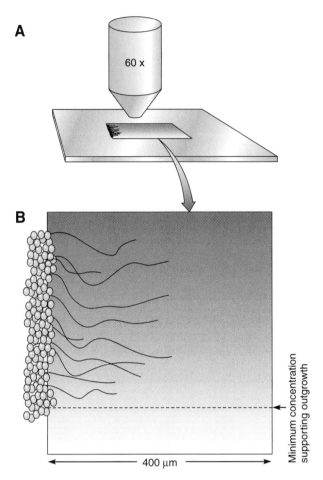

Figure 5.16 Adhesive gradients do not direct growth cones. In this experiment, CNS cells are plated on a laminin gradient (red). The axons paths are examined microscopically. (A) High laminin concentrations support axon growth (dark red), whereas low laminin concentrations (light red) do not support growth. (B) Axons do not tend to grow from low to high laminin concentrations (McKenna and Raper, 1988).

while the α6 subunit is better at binding with laminin. Over the course of development, axons may change which integrin subunits they express and thus change their sensitivity to a particular ECM molecule. For instance chick retinal ganglion cells express α6 and grow well on laminin when they are young. As they mature, they stop expressing this subunit and lose their ability to respond to laminin as their axons make contact with the tectum (Cohen and Johnson, 1991).

The functional activity of ECMs can be modified by their association with other proteins and carbohydrate groups, such as the glycosaminoglycans, which include heparin sulfate, keratin sulfate, and chondroitin sulfate. Some axons prefer to grow on a laminin–heparin sulfate proteoglycan and an antibody directed against this complex prevents growth, whereas antibodies to laminin alone do not. There are a host of extracellular matrix molecules that growing axons come in contact with, but not all promote growth (Lander *et al.,* 1983). Some like tenascin and or chondroitin sulfate may even retard or inhibit axon growth.

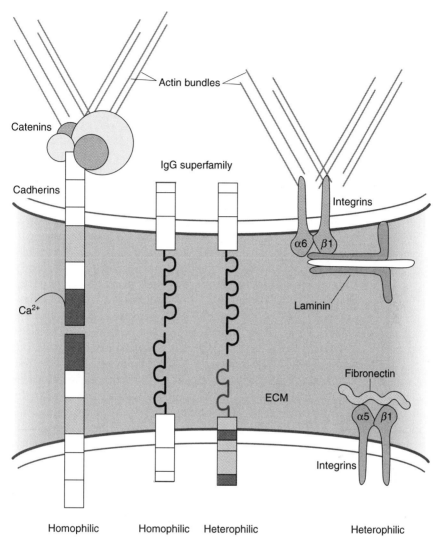

Figure 5.17 A few of the classes of adhesion molecules expressed on the growth cone. Cadherins are calcium dependent homophilic adhesion molecules. Some members of the IgG superfamily of adhesion molecules can bind homophilically; others are heterophilic. Integrins composed of various α and β subunits bind to a variety of different extracellular matrix (ECM) components with distinct affinity profiles. They are also connected to intracellular cytoskeletal elements. Extracellular space is gray. The type of interaction between molecules (heterophilic or homophilic) is shown at the bottom.

Cell Adhesion Molecules

Most growth cones, especially those in the CNS, grow along the surfaces of other cells and axons. In this function, they are supported largely by class of growth-promoting molecules that are expressed on cell surfaces and known as cell adhesion molecules (CAMs) (Walsh and Doherty, 1997). There are a host of such molecules and they come in several classes (Fig.

5.17). The most prominent class known is the IgG superfamily. These are molecules that have a set of extracellular repeat domains similar to those found in antibodies, which may reflect an ancient adhesive function for the IgG superfamily. One property that many of these molecules share is their ability to bind homophilically. Homophilic binding means that proteins of the same type bind to each other. Thus, if two cells are expressing the same CAM on their surfaces, the CAMs on the one cell will act as receptors for the CAMS on the other cell and vice versa. To test whether a particular CAM binds homophilically, nonadherent cells are transfected with the CAM of interest. If the cells then form aggregates with each other, this suggests a homophilic interaction. Homophilic adhesion in the developing nervous system may have several functions. During organogenesis or subdivision of the nervous system, particular CAMs may keep certain tissue types together. During outgrowth, axons expressing the same CAM may fasciculate with one another, allowing the early growing axons to guide those that grow later.

Monoclonal antibodies raised against axonal membranes have been used to search for cell adhesion and axonal guidance molecules that are expressed on particular fascicles of fibers during neural pathway formation. Several molecules were discovered in this manner, and many turned out to be CAMs with homophilic activity. Neural cell adhesion molecule (NCAM), the most extensively studied of the CAMs, appears to be expressed on all neurons and glia. Because of its broad distribution in the nervous system, NCAM may act as a generally permissive neurite outgrowth-promoting factor (Edelman, 1984). Interestingly, NCAM exists in many different forms, some with an intracellular domain that may interact with the cytoskeleton, and some without. The extracellular portion of NCAM can be highly modified by the addition of carbohydrates, particularly sialic acid residues. Desialylated forms are very adhesive compared to the sialylated forms. In the course of a neuron's development, there may be changes in the sialylation state of its NCAM, thus adjusting its adhesion (Walsh and Doherty, 1997). For ex-

ample, developing motor neurons of the chick grow out of the spinal cord and enter a complicated plexus region, where they cross in many directions and eventually segregate into distinct nerve roots leading to their appropriate muscles. These motor neurons show an amazing capacity to find their way in the plexus region, which must be loaded with cues that many different motor neurons can recognize. During the time when these axons are growing in the plexus, the NCAM they express is highly sialylated. Apparently, this keeps the axons that are headed toward many different muscles from fasciculating indiscriminately with one another. If the sialic acid is digested away with endoneuraminidase (Endo-N), errors in pathfinding occur in the plexus region, and motor axons exit into the wrong peripheral nerves (Tang et al., 1994) (Fig. 5.18).

In addition to its various sialylation states, NCAM comes in different splice forms that are expressed in specific regions of the brain. Therefore, it was very surprising when the gene for NCAM, including all its splice forms, was removed by homologous recombination and the resulting NCAM-deficient mice appeared to grow almost normally (Tomasiewicz et al., 1993). At a gross level, their brains are a bit smaller than normal, especially the olfactory bulb. These mutants also show a deficiency in learning ability associated with the hippocampus, an area of the brain associated with learning and memory. Olfactory and hippocampal defects are also seen in mice in which the sialylation state of NCAM has been compromised.

Another particularly heavily studied family of CAMs are the cadherins (Fig. 5.17). N-cadherin is one such member of these calcium-dependent adhesion factors (Muller and Kypta, 1995; Redies, 1997). When embryonic cadherin function is disrupted, cells tend to separate from one another or fall out of the developing epithelium, suggesting that they play a critical role in maintaining tissue integrity. Like NCAM, N-cadherin is expressed on almost all cells of the vertebrate nervous system, and it facilitates neurite outgrowth. When cadherin function is blocked in retinal ganglion cells *in vivo* by transfecting them with a dominant negative mutant, the ability of these

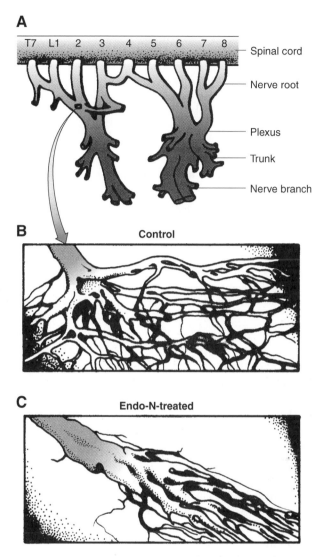

Figure 5.18 Homophilic adhesion is regulated by polysialic acid. (A) The brachial plexus region in the chick where motor axons destined for particular muscles sort out into their correct nerve roots. (B) Higher magnification of the plexus region showing fascicles breaking up and axons regrouping with other axons. (C) After treatment with Endo-N to remove sialic acid residues from N-CAM, the axons do not defasciculate properly and stay in large fascicles. As a result, innervation errors are made (Tang *et al.,* 1994).

neurons to put out axons is compromised. Blocking cadherin function does not, however, interfere with pathfinding in those axons that are able to extend (Riehl *et al.,* 1996). This result suggests that cadherins may be permissive factors that facilitate outgrowth, but are not guidance molecules. When the N-cadherin gene is knocked out in mice, they die at early embryonic stages and show a variety of defects in several tissues, suggesting a broad role for this molecule during development.

Some CAMs show a particularly restricted expression and result in very specific defects in axon growth. For example, a *Drosophila* homolog

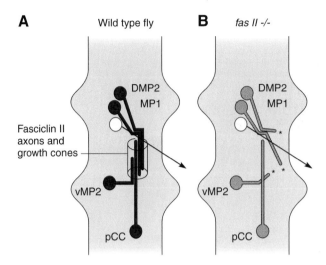

Figure 5.19 A homophilic mutant in flies. (A) In normal *Drosophila* embryos, DMP2, MP1, vMP2, and pCC axons fasciculate in a longitudinal bundle in which all axons express fasII. (B) In a fasII mutant, these axons do not fasciculate normally (Grenningloh *et al.,* 1991).

of NCAM, called fasciclin II (fasII), is expressed on a subset of axon longitudinal tracts or fascicles in the CNS (Bastiani *et al.,* 1987). FasII mutants cause the CNS axons that normally express this gene to defasciculate and their longitudinal tracts to become disorganized (Grenningloh *et al.,* 1991) (Fig. 5.19). When fasII is transgenically misexpressed on CNS neurons that would not normally express fasII, their axons tend to join together abnormally. Another CAM in *Drosophila,* called IrreC, leads to the miswiring of the optic pathway when the gene is knocked out in mutants or expressed globally in transgenic flies (Ramos *et al.,* 1993). The vertebrate homolog of IrreC, (called BEN, DM-GRASP, or SC-1) has been implicated in the formation of specific tracts in the spinal cord and cerebellum. In mammals, limbic-associated membrane protein, LAMP, is an IgCAM expressed by neurons throughout the limbic system, a cortical and subcortical area of the brain that functions in emotion and memory. Administration of LAMP antibodies to developing mouse brains results in abnormal growth of the fiber projections in the limbic system, suggesting that LAMP is an essential recognition molecule for the formation of limbic connections (Pimenta *et al.,* 1995).

Not all CAMs are homophilic. Some are involved in heterophilic interactions with other CAMs. For example, *axonin-1* binds to a different CAM, called NrCAM. NrCAM is expressed on glial cells in the periphery and in the floorplate of the spinal cord (Stoeckli and Landmesser, 1995). Commissural interneurons, which express axonin-1, are attracted to the floor plate by a mechanism that we discuss later in this chapter. Antibodies to NrCAM or axonin-1 can be used to perturb the heterophilic interaction between these two CAMs, and the result is that commissural interneurons are much less likely to cross through the floor plate and instead remain ipsilateral (Stoeckli *et al.,* 1997) (Fig. 5.20). A similar phenotype is seen in *commissureless,* a *Drosophila* mutant for a membrane protein expressed in the ventral midline (Seeger *et al.,* 1993; Tear *et al.,* 1993). In these mutants commissural neurons seem unable to cross the midline and remain ipsilateral, suggesting that *commissureless* might play a role in *Drosophila* similar to that which NrCAM does in vertebrates (Fig. 5.21). Interestingly, there is another class of mutant in *Drosophila* that has the opposite phenotype. Instead of being unable to cross the midline, commissural axons in roundabout (robo) mutants

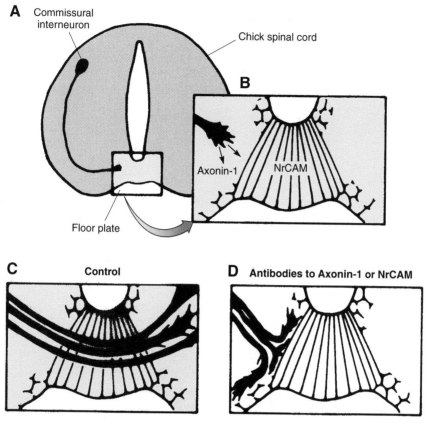

Figure 5.20 Crossing the midline of the vertebrate spinal cord. (A) A commissural interneuron, sends an axon toward the floor plate. (B) At higher magnification we see that the growth cone of the commissural neurons express the heterophilic CAM, axonin-1, while the floor plate cells express a CAM partner, NrCAM. (C) In a normal animal these commissural axons cross the midline. (D) If either axonin-1 or NrCAM function is perturbed with antibodies, the axons do not cross the midline (Stoeckli *et al.,* 1997).

cross the midline and then recross it at the next commissure. They do this over and over, going in circles (Fig. 5.21). Robo is a multi-Ig-domain transmembrane protein that is expressed on either side of the midline and is a receptor for an inhibitory factor called "slit" expressed by cells of the midline (Kidd *et al.,* 1999). Commissure-less downregulates the expression of the robo protein on the growth cones of commissural axons as they cross the midline (Kidd *et al.,* 1998). Once they have crossed, robo levels rise again and the axons do not recross the midline.

Because growing axons are responding to a variety of cues as they navigate, the loss of just one of these may only slightly increase the probability that errors are made. There is some redundancy in the cues that help axons navigate. In many gene deletion studies in *Drosophila,* there is a significant increase in pathfinding errors, but the majority of axons usually grow along the correct pathway. For instance, in fasII mutants, although some longitudinal tracts are defasciculated, the axons are still able to grow in the correct directions. This idea of molecular redundancy for pathfinding in the developing nervous system is supported by the finding that sometimes doubly mutant embryos, which have deletions of more than one particular adhesion

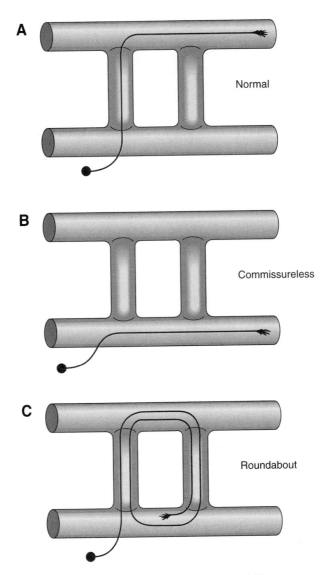

A   Normal

B   Commissureless

C   Roundabout

Figure 5.21   Midline crossing mutants in *Drosophila*. (A) In normal flies many neurons cross the midline once in a commissure and then travel in longitudinal fascicles on the other side. (B) In commissureless mutants, the axons do not cross but rather travel in the longitudinal tracts on the same side. (C) In roundabout mutants, the longitudinal tracts do not form properly because the axons keep crossing back and forth (Seeger *et al.,* 1993).

molecule, exhibit severe axonal growth defects, whereas the single mutants are relatively normal. For example, *Drosophila* that lack fasciclin I, a CAM that is expressed in commissural fascicles, have a normal looking CNS at all stages examined, indicating that the molecule is not essential for either growth or guidance. To test whether *fasI* is part of a redundant system, a series of double mutants were made with *fasI* and several other putative guidance or growth cone function mutants, each of which also had no striking phenotype on its own. Only one of the several double mutants tested showed neural defects in combination with *fasI*. This was the *fasI/abl* double mutant (Elkins *et al.,* 1990). *abl* codes for a tyrosine kinase, which may function in a signal transduction pathway in the growth cone (see below). Since both genes had to be knocked out to achieve axon disorientation, the two genes are probably part of two distinct molecular pathways, either of which may suffice for axon guidance. Similarly, in vertebrate tissue culture, motor axon growth over muscle fibers is not seriously impaired unless two or more adhesion molecules are simultaneously disabled with functional antibodies (Tomaselli *et al.,* 1986; Bixby *et al.,* 1987). Axonal growth is such an important part of building an organism that such fail-safe molecular mechanisms operate to help ensure that the nervous system is properly wired.

Labeled Pathways and Global Guidance

The fact that some CAMs are expressed on specific cell surfaces and axon tracts makes them attractive candidates for axonal navigation. This has led to an important hypothesis about axon guidance, referred to as the labeled pathways hypothesis. According to this idea, the first axons to grow out, the pioneer axons, lay down the original tracts in the nervous system. In the case of the grasshopper central nervous system, for example, the axon of the G neuron extends across the posterior commissure along a pathway pioneered by the Q1 and Q2 neurons (Goodman *et al.,* 1983, 1984). Once it has crossed, the growth cone of the G neuron pauses for a few hours while its filopodia seem to explore a number of different longitudinal fascicles in the near vicinity. Upon reconstruction of these growth cones in the electron microscope, it is clear that filopodia from the G neuron preferentially stick to the P axons in the A/P fascicle. After the pause, the G growth cone joins the A/P fascicle and follows it anteriorly to the brain. If the P axons are ablated before the G growth cone crosses the midline, the G growth cone

acts confused upon reaching the other side (Fig. 5.22). It does not show a high affinity for any other longitudinal bundle or even the A axons. As a result, it often stalls and does not turn at all, and sometimes it grows posteriorly instead of anteriorly. Thus the P axons seem to have an important label on their surface that the G growth cone can recognize, possibly because of a specific receptor on the G cell membrane.

These early axon tracts can be thought of as subway lines: the orange line, the red line, and the green line. As the pioneer axons grow, they express particular CAMs on their surfaces, creating a labeled "line" that other growth cones can follow. When a new neuron sends out its axon, the growth cone is able to distinguish and grow along specific pioneer axons because it expresses complementary CAMs on its surface. Examination of fasciclin expression with the electron microscope confirms that it is distributed on the surface of axons in particular fascicles (Bastiani *et al.,* 1987; Goodman, 1996). Just as you may have to change lines at a subway stop to reach your final destination, so an axon may have to change pathways. To do so, it must change the cell surface adhesion or growth-promoting molecule on its surface. Such a change in the expression of particular CAMs has now been seen in a number of systems at places where axons switch directions. For example, when axons in the central nervous system of *Drosophila* travel on a longitudinal tract, they express fasciclin II, but when they leave the longitudinal tract and turn onto a horizontal commissure, they stop expressing fasciclin II and express fasciclin I (Fig. 5.23).

In addition to following a scaffold of CAM-expressing axons, a new axon may also pioneer a new route during the last leg of its journey and add a new CAM to help future axons reach the same site. Thus, the simple scaffold of the first pioneers with a small number of CAMs becomes increasingly complex as more axons and more CAMs are added to the network. In vertebrates, there is an indication that some axons in the spinal cord and brain use a labeled pathway mechanism. The tract of the postoptic commissure (TPOC), for example, is a pioneering tract for

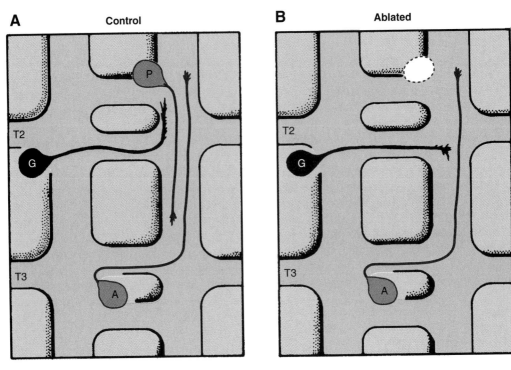

A   Control   **B**   Ablated

Figure 5.22   An experiment supporting the labeled pathways hypothesis. (A) In a control embryo, the G growth cone, fasciculates with P axons and not A axons. (B) When the P neuron is ablated, the G growth cone stalls and does not fasciculate with the A axons (Raper *et al.*, 1984).

axons from the pineal. The pineal axons fascic-ulate with the TPOC as they turn posteriorly at the boundary between forebrain and midbrain. If the TPOC is ablated, pineal axons often fail to make the appropriate turns (Chitnis *et al.*, 1992).

How do the pioneer axons, themselves, find the correct path to their target? In some cases, as in the insect nervous system, glial cells with particular growth-promoting molecules are pre-arranged in a geometry that supports directed outgrowth by the pioneer axons. One could then ask what sets up the arrangement of these glial cells (Bastiani and Goodman, 1986). Unfortu-nately, our understanding becomes less explicit at this stage. One possibility is that early mo-lecular events in the formation of the embryo, such as the patterned expression of homeobox genes, provide the information that sets the placement of the developing glial cells (see Chapter 2).

The optic tract from the retina to the tectum presents an example of guidance different from that suggested by the labeled pathways hypoth-esis. Retinal axons enter the optic tract in the ventral diencephalon and grow dorsally in close association with the TPOC, although they do not fasciculate with it. The transplantation of eyes from older embryos to younger ones has been used to force retinal axons to enter the brain be-fore the TPOC forms. In these instances, retinal axons grow in virgin, axonless neuroepithelium as true pioneers, yet they can navigate correctly to the tectum (Cornel and Holt, 1992) (Fig. 5.24A). Eyes can also be transplanted so that the optic nerve enters the brain at abnormal locations, far away from the TPOC, and the axons still grow directly to the tectum (Harris, 1986) (Fig. 5.25). Examination of retinal axons in the electron mi-croscope shows that even in normal animals there is no direct fasciculation with the pioneers

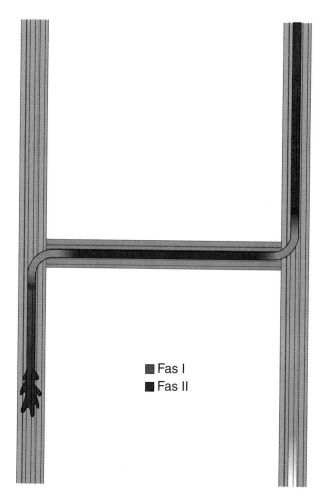

Figure 5.23 Axons express different CAMs on different segments. A commissural axon in an embryonic *Drosophila* CNS. This axon expresses fasII in the longitudinal pathway to help it fasciculate with other fasII-expressing axons. It switches to fasI while it is in the commissure and fasciculates with other fasI-expressing axons, but switches back again to fasII once it has reached the other side (Goodman *et al.*, 1983).

of the TPOC, so the retinal axons are themselves pioneers even though they grow out in a brain already populated by other axons (Burrill and Easter, 1995).

One possible explanation for this result is that the target releases a diffusible molecule that attracts retinal axons. However, no direct evidence for such an attractant has been found so far. In fact, if the tectum is removed, retinal axons grow toward the missing tissue. This suggests that optic axons use local cues as they grow along the optic tract. Furthermore, if a small

piece of the optic tract neuroepithelium is rotated 90° before the axons enter it, then they become misoriented when they enter the rotated neuroepithelium (Harris, 1989) (Fig. 5.24B). They only correct their course of growth when they exit. This suggests that the entire neuroepithelium contains local information to which growing axons respond in order to arrive at their appropriate targets. It is not clear what the cues in the epithelium are. It is suspected that the positional information encoded by homeobox genes (see Chapter 2) may also be used

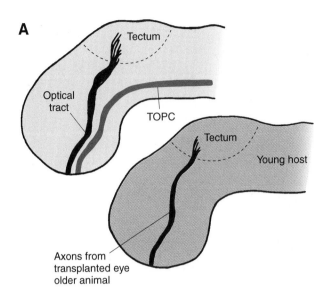

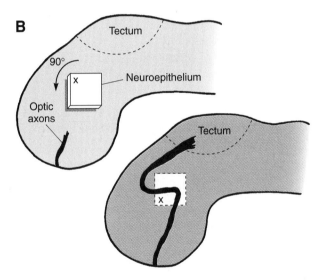

Figure 5.24 Retinal axons follow local guidance cues in the neuroepithelium. (A) When the retinal axons first grow into the brain they grow alongside the previously formed tract of the postoptic commissure (TPOC) (top). When an eye from an older animal is transplanted to a young host in which the TPOC is not yet formed, the axons still grow correctly to the tectum (bottom), showing that they do not need TPOC fibers to guide them. (B) A piece of neuroepithelium in front of the retinal axons is rotated 90° (top). When the retinal axons enter the rotated piece, they are deflected in the direction of the rotation, but correct their trajectories when they exit the rotated piece, showing that these axons pay attention to localized cues within the neuroepithelium (Harris, 1989; Cornel and Holt, 1992).

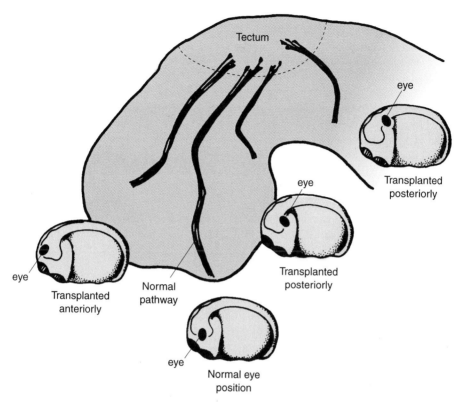

Figure 5.25 Global guidance mechanisms. When the eye primordium is transplanted to different regions of the head, as shown in each embryo below. The optic nerve innervates the brain from unusual locations. Nevertheless, the retinal axons grow rather directly to the tectum (Harris, 1986).

to control the expression of regionally specific CAMs or other guidance molecules in the neuroepithelium. In support of this idea, axonal tracts in embryonic brains exhibit unusual patterns when the expression of homeobox genes is perturbed and pioneer axons are often found at the boundaries of brain territories that express different homeobox positional markers (Wilson *et al.,* 1997).

Gradients of Diffusible Tropic Factors

Axons may be guided by diffusible molecules. In a process termed chemotaxis, growth cones claw their way up concentration gradients of diffusible attractants to their source. The idea

of chemotactic guidance has been in and out of favor since it was first proposed at the beginning of this century. During the past decade, however, tissue culture experiments and genetic evidence have provided strong support for chemotaxis during axon guidance.

In chemotaxis, an axon turns toward a source of an attractant if the growth cone is positioned in the gradient such that one side is exposed to a higher level of the factor than the other side. What is the evidence that growth cones can make this kind of comparison and respond with directed outgrowth? Gradients of different molecules have been produced by ejecting solution from the tip of an electrode (see Box: The Tissue Culture Advantage), and allowing the concentration to dissipate as it spreads out into the tissue culture medium. Using this method, it was

The Tissue Culture Advantage

The tissue culture technique, a mainstay of all biological research in this century, has continuously embraced innovative solutions to address neurobiological questions (Bunge, 1975; Banker and Goslin, 1991). Ross Harrison's (1907, 1910) original preparation consisted of pieces of tissue, now termed organotypic cultures. Such cultures may now be obtained from vibratome sections of neural tissue and grown under conditions that promote thinning to a monolayer, thus providing greater access and visibility of individual neurons (reviewed by Gähwiler *et al.,* 1991). Slices are attached to a coverglass and placed in rotating tissue culture tubes (hence the term "roller-tube culture") such that the tissue culture medium transiently washes over them. If one requires a slice of tissue with somewhat greater depth, then the cultures can be grown statically at the gas/liquid interface by using tissue culture plate inserts that provide a porous stage for the tissue and a reserve of medium below (Stoppini *et al.,* 1991). The relative simplicity of modern organotypic preparations has resulted in a wealth of data on the interaction between afferent and target populations, as described in the text.

In the arena of primary dissociated cell cultures, it has become feasible to isolate particular cell types. This may be performed by an immunoselection technique in which a cell-specific antibody is adsorbed to a plastic petri dish, creating a surface on which one cell type will selectively attach. This approach has led to a 99% pure retinal ganglion cell preparation (Barres *et al.,* 1988). A different means of separating cells relies upon selective prelabeling with a fluorescent dye and subsequently performing fluorescent-activated cell sorting (FACS). When passed through such a device, single cells are sequentially monitored for fluorescence and then selectively diverted to a receiver tube if they are labeled. This approach led to the isolation of retrogradely labeled spinal motor and preganglionic neurons (Calof and Reichardt, 1984; Clendening and Hume, 1990). Finally, it is possible to isolate large and small cell fractions following centrifugation on a Percoll density gradient and then further enrich the cells with a short duration plating step, that allows the more adhesive cells (e.g., astrocytes) to be retained on a treated surface. This approach led to the isolation of a >95% pure granule cell population from cerebellar tissue (Hatten, 1985). Once specific cell types have been isolated, they may be mixed together in known ratios or plated on two surfaces that are subsequently grown opposite one another as a sandwich (Banker and Goslin, 1991). This technique allows one to produce a "feeder layer" of astrocytes on one surface that promotes survival of low-density neuronal cultures. It may also allow the experimenter to discriminate between contact-dependent and -independent phenomena.

Having obtained the neurons and glia of interest, tissue culture offers the opportunity to perform insightful manipulations. For example, it is possible to produce nonuniform distribution growth substrates to test the role of specific molecules in axon guidance (Letourneau, 1975). The technique has been extended to create gradients of laminin or neuronal membrane on a surface that subsequently serves as the tissue culture substrate (McKenna and Raper, 1988; Baier and Bonhoeffer, 1992). The gradients can be visualized and quantified by including a fluorescent or radioactive marker along with the intended substrate. Gradients of soluble molecules can be produced *in vitro* with repetitive pulsatile ejection of pl volumes from a micropipet tip into the tissue culture medium, an "infinite" sink (Lohof *et al.,* 1992). The concentration gradient is quantified by ejecting a fluorescein-conjugated dextran and measuring the fluorescent signal at increasing distances from the pipet tip.

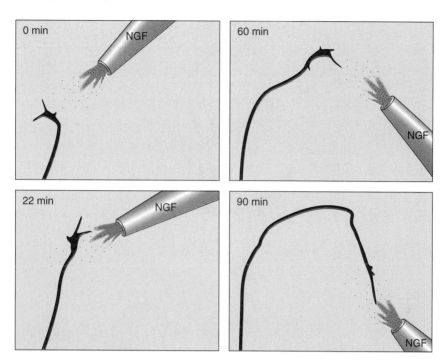

Figure 5.26 Growth cones can rely on chemotaxis to orient their growth. Time lapse video recordings of a sensory neuron turns toward a pipet that is ejecting nerve growth factor (NGF) and produces a diffusable gradient. Each time the pipet is moved, the axon reorients its growth (Gundersen and Barrett, 1979).

demonstrated that chick dorsal root axons turn toward a source of nerve growth factor (NGF) (Fig. 5.26) and that *Xenopus* spinal neurites turn toward an extracellular source of dibutyryl-cAMP or ACh (Gundersen and Barrett, 1979; Zheng *et al.*, 1994).

These experiments indicate that growing processes have a mechanism for recognizing small concentration differences across a relatively small distance. In the case of NGF, the growth cones were growing forward at a reasonable pace and turned toward the pipet without speeding up, suggesting that NGF was not simply acting as a general growth-promoting substance, but as a directional cue. Other clues from these tissue culture experiments provide some insight into the biological basis of this tracking. For example, growth cones exposed to NGF become significantly more adherent to the substrate. Growth cones that turn toward neurotransmitters also send out more filopodia on the side where

the concentration is higher, presumably creating greater traction force on that side.

Do axons *in vivo* use similar mechanisms of growth cone guidance? There are at least three good examples of chemoattraction to a distant target by a diffusible substance. In the first situation, the trigeminal ganglion of the mouse sends tens of thousands of sensory axons to the maxillary pad epithelium at the base of the whiskers between the mouth and the nose, making it the most heavily innervated skin in the entire body. When the maxillary pad and the trigeminal ganglion are removed and placed near each other in a three-dimensional collagen gel, the trigeminal axons preferentially grow toward the explant of whisker pad, even when there are competing targets explants of neighboring pieces of epidermis equally distant or even closer (Lumsden and Davies, 1986) (Fig. 5.27). Thus, it was hypothesized that the maxillary pad emits a tropic agent for axon growth. This factor was named "max

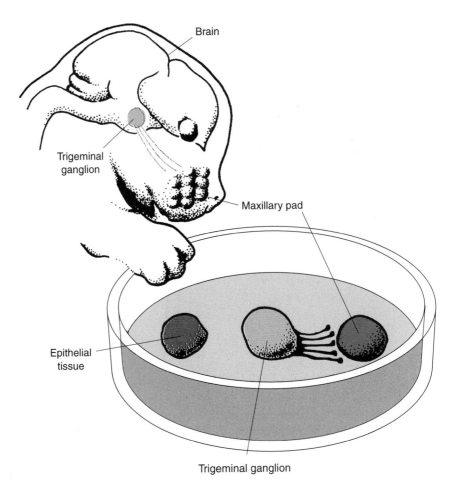

Figure 5.27   Chemotactic agents from target tissues. Sensory axons from the trigeminal ganglion heavily innervate the maxillary pad of the mouse face, the site of the whisker field. When the trigeminal ganglion is placed into a three-dimensional collagen gel with the maxillary pad tissue and another piece of epithelium, the axons leaving the ganglion grow toward their appropriate target, suggesting that it is releasing a chemotropic agent (Lumsden and Davies, 1986).

factor.'' The maxillary pad makes NGF, which attracts sympathetic axons, but it does not transcribe mRNA for NGF until after the trigeminal fibers have reached the target, indicating that NGF is not the chemoattractant (Lumsden and Davis, 1983). The job of NGF at that time may be a survival factor or trophic factor as opposed to a tropic agent (see Chapter 7). However, ''Max factor'' has recently been identified as 2 neurotrophins (see Chapter 7). Interestingly, these molecules promote outgrowth of trigeminal axons, but they apparently do not direct these

axons to the target because the projection is normal in mice deficient for both neurotrophins (O'Connor and Tessier-Levigne, 1999).

Similar experiments have been done using a region of developing hindbrain, the pons, which attracts collateral axons of corticospinal fibers *in vivo*. Most corticospinal axons make a connection with the pons, but developing fibers first grow right through the hindbrain and toward the spinal cord without sending a branch into the pons. Only later do these axons form small interstitial branches with growth cones that navigate into the pons. These observations suggest that at a certain stage of development, the pons puts out a soluble factor that evokes a side branch to form and directs its growth. This hypothesis has been tested *in vitro* with cocultures of pons and cortex (O'Leary *et al.,* 1991). The presence of nearby pons, but not other pieces of the CNS, causes the cortical explant to put out more axons, many of which appear to grow and turn toward the pontine explants. The "pons factor" remains unidentified.

The final example concerns the guidance of dorsal commissural in the spinal to the ventral midline and the circumferential guidance of axons in the nematode. Two factors were biochemically purified from embryonic chick brains using a bioassay that caused outgrowth from commissural neurons in explants of dorsal spinal cord. They were partially sequenced, and the genes encoding these proteins were pulled out of a cDNA library (Kennedy *et al.,* 1994; Serafini *et al.,* 1994). They were called netrin-1 and netrin-2 after the Sanskrit "netr," meaning "one who guides." In the spinal cord netrin-1 is expressed in the floor plate (Fig. 5.28). The netrins are found largely attached to cell membranes, but are somewhat diffusible and can clearly reorient growing commissural axons toward a local source of netrin over a distance of hundreds of micrometers (Colamarino and Tessier-Lavigne, 1995) (Fig. 5.28).

In netrin-1 knockout mice, the growth of many axons is disoriented. For example, the dorsal commissural interneurons of the spinal cord fail to grow toward the ventral midline. Netrins have also been found in *Drosophila* where they serve a similar role in guiding commissural axons to the ventral midline. A single gene mutation in nematodes, called *unc-6,* also exhibits defects in the circumferential guidance of certain cells and axons (Culotti, 1994). In null mutants, both dorsal and ventral migrations are affected. Interestingly, certain partial loss of function alleles affect only dorsal migration while others effect only ventral migration, suggesting that the molecule may have more than one functional domain. Perhaps one domain attracts fibers in one direction while a different domain repels

them in the other direction. More information about repulsive guidance cues is presented in the next section.

Nematodes with a deletion of the *unc-40* gene show defects in the migration of cells and neuronal processes toward the ventral midline, the source of *unc-6.* Unlike *unc-6* mutants, the *unc-40* phenotype is cell autonomous, suggesting that the *unc-40* gene product must be present in the migrating cells. In fact, *unc-40* is a receptor to *unc-6,* and this led directly to the mammalian receptor for netrin. Cloning of the *unc-40* gene showed it to be a homolog of the mammalian protein known as DCC or neogenin (Chan *et al.,* 1996). The DCC protein has the characteristics of a transmembrane receptor. In vertebrates, DCC binds netrin, is expressed in commissural interneurons, and is essential for the attraction of their axons to the floor plate (Keino-Masu, Masu *et al.,* 1996). A mutation in the *Drosophila* netrin receptor homolog, called *frazzled,* shows similar defects in commissural guidance (Kolodziej *et al.,* 1996). These results suggest a strongly conserved function of netrins and netrin receptors in chemoattraction.

There are clear limits on the contribution of chemotropism to selective outgrowth, or at least limits on what tissue culture experiments can tell us. For example, when pieces of rat embryonic lateral geniculate nucleus (LGN) are cultured between pieces of occipital cortex (i.e., their normal target) and pieces of frontal cortex (i.e., a CNS structure that they never innervate), the axons display no preference for one region over the other (Molnar and Blakemore, 1991).

Repulsive Factors

In addition to adhesion molecules and extracellular matrix molecules that promote neurite attachment and growth, there are a different set of factors that do just the opposite. These are the inhibitory or repulsive factors (Kolodkin, 1996). Tissue culture experiments have indicated that neural tissue produces diffusible substances that serve to repel axons. In these sorts of experiments, the trajectories of axons are observed

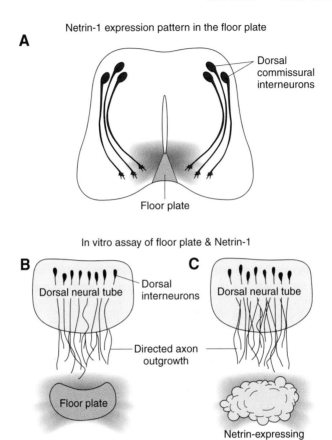

Figure 5.28 Dorsal commissural interneurons are attracted by a gradient of netrin. (A) Dorsal commissural interneurons grow directly to the ventral midline of the spinal cord along a gradient of netrin that is released by floor plate neurons. (B) When dorsal neural tube and floor plate tissue are explanted into a collagen gel, the dorsal interneurons are attracted at a distance to the floor plate. (C) The dorsal interneurons are also attracted to netrin that is released from a pellet of COS cells that have been transfected with the netrin gene (Kennedy *et al.,* 1994).

when they are cultured in the presence of tissues they normally avoid. For example, *in vivo,* the axons of dorsal root ganglia (DRG) generally innervate dorsal spinal cord and do not enter the ventral region of the spinal cord. When these DRGs are grown alongside pieces of dorsal and ventral spinal cord in tissue culture, the DRG axons preferentially invade their normal target, the dorsal cord (Peterson and Crain, 1981). Surprisingly, most of the DRG axons are deflected from pieces of ventral spinal cord and will avoid this tissue even if, as a result, they have to grow in a circuitous fashion to reach the dorsal spinal cord (Figs. 5.29A and 5.29B). These data provided the first indication that a chemorepulsive mechanism could play a role in target selection. However, sequential short latency observations were not performed on these cocultures, leaving open the possibility that DRG neurites transiently contacted and withdrew from ventral spinal cord pieces. Similar results were obtained by coculturing pieces of olfactory bulb with septum, a structure that olfactory tract axons initially grow away from

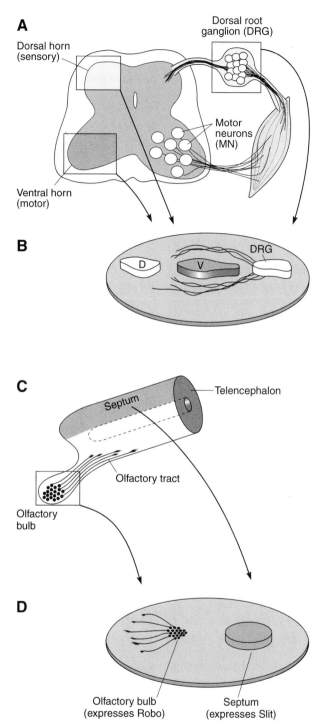

Figure 5.29 Repulsive guidance. (A) The central projections of most DRG axons do not enter the ventral horn of the spinal cord, but rather make synapses in the dorsal horn. (B) When cultured together, DRG neurons avoid ventral spinal cord explants to grow to dorsal targets. (C) A cross section through the telencephalon shows olfactory tract fibers originating from the olfactory bulb traveling in the lateral region, far away from the medial septum. (D) When cultured together, olfactory bulb axons travel away from the septum indicating the existence of a diffusible chemorepellent (Peterson and Crain, 1981; Pini, 1993).

in vivo (Pini, 1993). When the explant of bulb tissue was placed near the explant of septal tissue, the olfactory axons emerged from the side of the explant opposite the septum (Figs. 5.29C and 5.29D).

In recent years, there has been much progress in determining the chemical nature of growth-inhibitory mechanisms. The repulsive factor responsible for the guidance of olfactory tract axons away from the septum has recently been putatively identified as the vertebrate homolog of the previously mentioned *Drosophila* slit protein, the ligand for robo (Li *et al.*, 1999). The olfactory bulb axons express the vertebrate homolog of robo. Motoneurons of the vertebrate spinal cord also express robo and grow away from the ventral midline, which expresses slit (Brose *et al.*, 1999). The axons of motoneurons and olfactory bulb neurons also grow away from cells transfected with slit in culture, proving that slit is a secreted repulsive guidance factor.

Growth cone repulsion to a membrane bound factor was first demonstrated in explant cultures of retinal and sympathetic neurons grown together. Often, when two explants are cocultured, there is intermingling of the axons, but in this case the retinal and the sympathetic axons appeared to avoid one another. Time-lapse video films made of growth cones from one explant as they approached the axons of the other show that these growth cones collapse when they first make contact with a foreign axon. They lose their filopodia, retract, and become temporarily paralyzed (Kapfhammer and Raper, 1987a) (Fig. 5.30). Often, after a few minutes, a new growth cone is formed that advances once more until it again encounters the unlike axon in its path and again collapses. These time-lapse studies demonstrate that just the briefest contact from a single filopodium is necessary to elicit this aversive behavior, strongly suggesting that growth cones sense a repulsive signal on the surface of the other axon.

By pairing different types of explants in such cultures and observing the growth cone interactions, a variety of collapsing activities effective on different types of growth cones were discovered (Kapfhammer and Raper, 1987b).

For example, peripheral axons, such as those from the dorsal root ganglion, ciliary ganglia, and sympathetic ganglia all collapsed when they confronted CNS axons and CNS axons tended to collapse when they encountered peripheral axons. There is a rich heterogeneity of repulsive interactions between neurons. For instance, fibers from the nasal retina show no preference for growing over nasal or temporal fibers of the same retina, whereas temporal fibers clearly prefer temporal axons and collapse when confronted with nasal ones in tissue culture. Thus, it appears that nasal fibers have a collapsing activity to which temporal but not nasal growth cones are sensitive. Such specificity may aid in topographic map formation *in vivo,* since the temporal fibers remain restricted in their growth to the anterior tectum (see Chapter 6).

Attempts to purify collapsing factors biochemically were aided by a bioassay in which reconstituted membrane vesicles containing repulsive factors were added to cultures of axons growing on laminin substrates. When vesicles enriched in collapsing activity from the CNS were added to cultures, they caused the immediate collapse and paralysis of all the sensory ganglion cell growth cones on the plate. A 100-kDa glycoprotein that could cause growth cone collapse, called collapsin, was eventually purified sufficiently to obtain a partial protein sequence (Luo *et al.,* 1993). Using the sequence data, the gene was obtained. Collapsin 1 turns out to be a member of a large molecular family called the semaphorins. Semaphorin I was the first member of this family to be identified in grasshoppers (Kolodkin *et al.,* 1993). It was originally named fasciclin IV because it is expressed on particular axon fascicles and in stripes near segment borders on the limb bud epithelium. Antibodies that neutralize semaI function in the limb allow the Ti1 pioneers to cross the segment border, suggesting that this molecule normally serves a repellent function. Conversely, if a single filopodium from a growth cone of a DRG neuron in culture touches a bead coated with collapsin 1, the growth cone is inhibited from putting out lamellipodia on that side and turns away from the bead, definitively demonstrating that

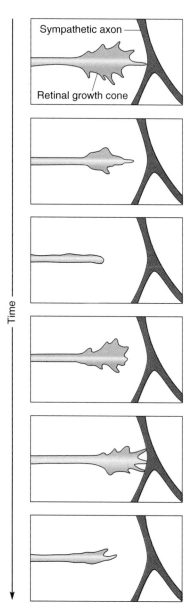

Figure 5.30 Growth cone collapse. A time-lapse series of a growth cone from a retinal ganglion cell encountering an axon of a sympathetic neuron in culture. Upon first contact the growth cone retracts and collapses. After several minutes, the growth cone reforms, but when it encounters the sympathetic fiber again, it collapses once more (Kapfhammer and Raper, 1987a).

guidance by repulsion is possible (Fan and Raper, 1995) (Fig. 5.31).

The mouse homolog of collapsin 1, called semaphorin III, is expressed in the ventral spinal cord. Sensory neurons that carry information from pain receptors to the CNS grow into dorsal roots of the spinal cord and synapse locally with dorsal interneurons, avoiding the more ventral

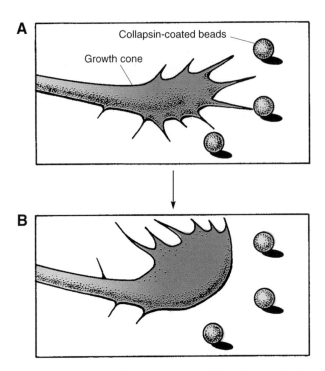

A Collapsin-coated beads
Growth cone

B

Figure 5.31 Collapsin can influence growth cone steering. (A) Beads coated with collapsin are sprinkled into the culture dish. (B) When a single filopodium of a growth cone that is sensitive to collapsin touches a bead, the growth cone turns away without collapsing and travels in a new direction (Fan and Raper, 1995).

spinal cord. Both ventral spinal cord and COS cells made to express SemaIII are able to repel these pain neurons (Messersmith *et al.,* 1995). In contrast, afferents from stretch receptors that also enter the spinal cord through the dorsal root and dive ventrally to synapse on motor neurons are not repelled by semaIII. Together, these results suggest that the family of collapsin/semaphorin signals is specifically arranged in the CNS to repel specific axons, presumably those that have receptors to particular family members, but not others. The ectoderm, dermomyotome, and notochord, it turns out, also repel DRG axons (Fig. 5.32). If a DRG is placed between a dermomyotome and a piece of notochord in a collagen gel, the result is bipolar axon growth that mimics the *in vivo* trajectory of these neurons and suggests that "surround repulsion" may be a dominant guidance mechanism for the developing nervous system (Keynes *et al.,* 1997).

The spinal nerves that define the segments of the vertebrate spinal column arise first from the sensory and motor neurons that exit the spinal cord in a segmented pattern. This pattern is actually imposed upon the spinal column by the primitive somites, for if the somites from a particular region are removed before the axons grow out the axons in this region show no segregation into segmental nerves. Apparently, the outgrowing axons and the neural crest cells grow only through the anterior portion of each somite. When individual somites are flipped, reversing the anterior–posterior order, the segmental nerves of the spinal cord respond to the new position of the transplanted somite (Keynes and Stern, 1984).

Are the axons and neural crest cells attracted into the anterior half of the somite or repelled by the posterior half? A series of biochemical experiments was performed with a lectin called peanut agglutinin, which bound only to the posterior half of somites. The peanut lec-

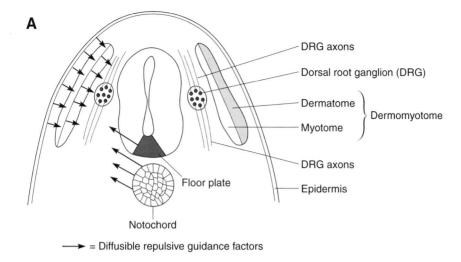

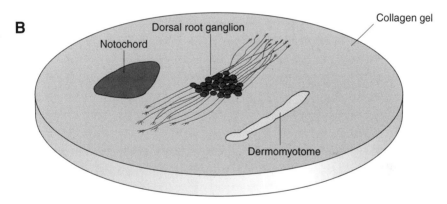

Figure 5.32 Surround repulsion. (A) DRG axons outside the spinal cord elongate in a bipolar fashion between the dermomyotome and the ventral spinal cord and notochord. Many surrounding tissues including the epidermis, the dermomyototome, the floor plate, and the notochord secrete diffusible repellents. (B) When placed in a collagen gel between a piece of notochord and dermomyotome, DRG axons extend in a bipolar fashion, similar to their pattern *in vivo*. These results suggest that the orientation of the DRG axons is due to repellant molecular cues (Keynes *et al.,* 1997).

tin was used to partially purify a collapsing factor from the somites. Whether the ability of this factor to cause axons to collapse is related to the core protein or to a glycosaminoglycan attached to the protein core is still uncertain.

Another putative avoidance molecule, T-cadherin, is a member of the cadherin family, but lacks the functionally important cytoplasmic domain. Also expressed in the posterior half of somites, it inhibits motor axon outgrowth *in vitro* (Fredette *et al.,* 1996). Finally, Lerk2 and HtkL, ligands for Eph receptors (see Chapter 6) are also expressed on caudal somites and repel the axons of motor neurons (Wang and Anderson, 1997). Based on the trajectories of motor axons as they first head out of the spinal cord, it seems very likely that they are actually attracted to anterior halves (Oakley and Tosney, 1993). Thus,

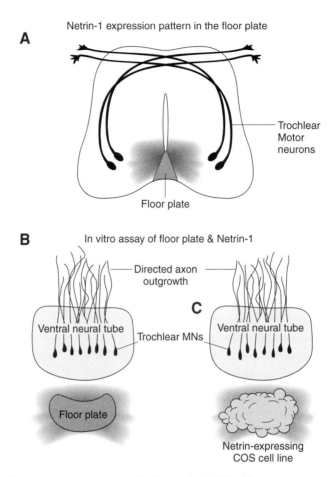

A　Netrin-1 expression pattern in the floor plate

Trochlear Motor neurons

Floor plate

B　In vitro assay of floor plate & Netrin-1

Directed axon outgrowth

Ventral neural tube

Trochlear MNs

C

Ventral neural tube

Floor plate

Netrin-expressing COS cell line

Figure 5.33　Trochlear motor neurons are repelled by netrin. (A) Trochlear motor neurons arise in the ventral neural tube at the midbrain/hindbrain region. They grow away from the ventral midline to decussate and leave the brain dorsally. Trochlear neurons in a collagen gel explant culture grow away from the floor plate (B) and from COS cells expressing netrin (C) (Colamarino and Tessier-Lavigne, 1995a).

the segmental patterning of spinal roots may be a complex mixture of attractive factors pulling motor axons to the anterior half of somites and repellent ones pushing them away from the posterior halves.

Some tropic factors, like netrin, turn out to have both attractive and repellent activity (Fig. 5.33). In the nematode, the *unc-5* mutant has disrupted dorsal migrations (Culotti, 1994). Interestingly, when neurons whose axons normally grow laterally or ventrally are made to misexpress *unc-5*, these axons now grow dorsally, but depend on the normal expression of *unc-6* to do

so. Thus *unc-5*, which like *unc-40* codes for a transmembrane protein, is possibly another *unc-6* receptor, but is involved in chemorepulsion rather than chemoattraction. If so, this means that netrins could act as chemorepulsive agents for neurons that express *unc-5* type receptors and chemoattactive factors for neurons that express *unc-40*- or DCC-type netrin receptors. That netrin can act as a long-range chemorepulsive factor in vertebrates has been demonstrated in trochlear motor neurons whose axons grow dorsally away from the ventral midline (Colamarino and Tessier-Lavigne, 1995a). In collagen gels, these axons grow away from explanted floor plate tissues or from cells transfected with a netrin-1 expressing gene. Netrin is unlikely to be the only repulsive factor that guides these axons away from the ventral midline since the trajectories of trochlear motor neurons and some other dorsally directed axons appear normal in netrin knockout mice.

Axon Regeneration

In the adult mammalian CNS, neurons fail to regenerate axonal processes following injury (Ramon y Cajal, 1928; Aguayo et al., 1990). In contrast, retinal ganglion cells in fish and amphibia are fully capable of such regrowth (Piatt, 1955). The capacity of central axons to regenerate is lost during the early stages of mammalian development (Kalil and Reh, 1982). Moreover, axons that are able to regenerate following a pyramidal tract lesion in neonatal hamsters or cats are found to grow *around* the lesion site and are not able to penetrate the injury site (Bregman and Goldberger, 1983). Even though axon regeneration is absent in adult mammals, axons can grow for a short distance (<500 μm) in many central locations (Liu and Chambers, 1958; Raisman and Field, 1973a). Furthermore, *in vitro* experiments have shown that adult rat retinal ganglion cells are able to extend axonal processes on a growth-promoting substrate when they are kept alive with neurotrophins (Ford-Holevinski et al., 1986; Bahr et al., 1988). The growth of very young neurons does not appear to be so restricted when they are transplanted into an adult nervous system. Human neuroblasts are able to form long axon pathways when transplanted into excitotoxin-lesioned adult rat striatum (Wictorin et al., 1990). Similarly, mouse embryonic retinal ganglion cells are able to grow long distances within the rostral midbrain of neonatal rats and selectively innervate some normal targets (Radel et al., 1990).

The failure of mammalian central neurons to regenerate axonal projections may stem from the absence of growth-permissive signals or the presence of obstructions at the sight of injury.

The importance of extracellular cues *in vivo* are clearly illustrated by the ability of peripheral nerve grafts to support central axonal regrowth (Richardson et al., 1980; David and Aguayo, 1981; Aguayo et al., 1990). In a set of classic studies, it was shown that transected central axons that were unable to grow within the CNS were able to grow for many centimeters when they were provided with a sheath of nonneuronal cells that ordinarily provide insulation to motor axons in the periphery (Fig. 5.34).

While embryonic glial cells support neurite outgrowth, others, particularly adult astrocytes and oligodendrocytes, appear to inhibit neurite outgrowth. When a central nerve bundle is injured in a mammal, the axons are usually unable to regrow across the wound and thereby reestablish connections they had lost. Part of the problem, it appears, is the invasion of the wound site with various glia that produce repulsive cues that the axons cannot navigate around. By X-irradiating mouse spinal cords during neonatal development, it was possible to create mice that were deficient in glial cells. In these animals, spinal axons regenerated past a transection point, a behavior that they never display in normal animals.

Cultured CNS neurons stop, and sometimes collapse, when they touch oligodendrocytes. Liposomes from these cells and preparations of myelin were used to identify two neurite inhibitory factors, NI-35 and NI-250, that caused CNS growth cones to collapse. A monoclonal antibody to NI-35 was then made and tested in culture for its ability to block the collapsing activity. In the presence of antibody, axons grew over oligodendrocytes without stopping or collapsing. The antibody was then tested *in vivo*, using mice with partially severed spinal cords. In the presence of antibody, spinal tracts regenerated beyond the crush, suggesting that NI-35 is a critical component of the failure of spinal regeneration (Bregman et al., 1995). This regeneration in the presence of the NI-35 antibody can be further enhanced by neurotrophin-3, NT-3, a trophic factor for CNS neurons (Chapter 7). Although fish do have oligodendrocytes in their optic nerves, these cells apparently do not have

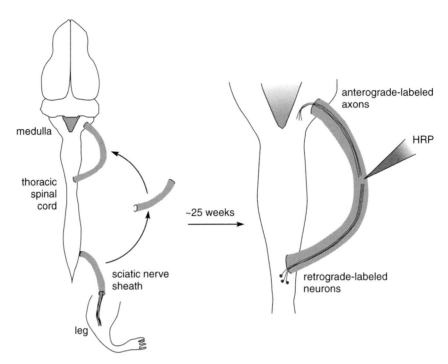

Figure 5.34   Peripheral nerve sheath permits cut central axons to regrow. (Left) A piece of peripheral sciatic motor nerve root is obtained (the axons die away, but the non-neuronal tissue survives. This tube of non-neuronal tissue is inserted into the central nervous system in two locations. This manipulation injures the nervous tissue locally, and also provides a path for injured neurons to growth through. (Right) To determine whether central axons do, in fact, regenerate through the sciatic nerve sheath, an anatomical tracer (HRP) is injected into the center of the sheath after a 25 week survival period. Central axons can regrow over substantial distances through the nerve sheath (David and Aguayo 1981).

an active form of the NI-35 avoidance molecule. In fact, mammalian oligodendrocytes can cause a collapse or avoidance response in fish optic axons in culture, and this repulsion can be overcome by the application of the NI-35 antibody. In contrast, glia from fish do not inhibit the growth of mammalian axons (Bastmeyer *et al.,* 1993). Thus, this avoidance factor may be in part responsible for the inability of mammalian CNS, as opposed to that of lower vertebrates, to regenerate successfully following injury.

Astrocytes often accumulate around CNS wounds, forming complex scars. These cells produce an extracellular matrix that is inhibitory to axon regeneration even on laminin. In culture, the inhibitory component can be digested away with chondroitinase, rendering the matrix more permissive to axon growth and regeneration. More knowledge of the biochemistry of avoidance factors may prove useful in medical treatments of damage to the CNS (Fawcett, 1997).

Stop Factors

When a growth cone finally nears or encounters its target, it must slow down and eventually stop altogether in order to form a synapse (Chapter 8). In certain cases, growth factors may be involved in these functions (Holt and Harris, 1998). Retinal axons grow toward their target on a pathway that is rich in FGF, and this molecule has been found to accelerate axonal growth in the tract and *in vitro*. As retinal axons enter the tectum, they encounter a sudden drop in external FGF, because the tectum expresses very little of it (McFarlane *et al.,* 1995). Therefore, one cue that decreases growth rate of retinal axons at their target is a drop in FGF levels (see Chapter 6).

Some growth cones are also sensitive to neurotransmitters, not as attractive factors, but as stop factors. In the snail, *Heliosoma,* particular CNS neurons send out axons that stop and preferentially form synapses on serotonergic cells. To test the idea that the growth cones are sensitive to neurotransmitter released from their targets, serotonin was applied to cultured neurons (Haydon *et al.,* 1984). In this case, growth cones became completely immobilized. Other neurons synapse with dopaminergic cells and their axons are immobilized when dopamine is applied (McCobb *et al.,* 1988). All axons seem programmed to find their targets and stop growing, and there are probably a variety of stop factors, not all of them neurotransmitters. In making neuromuscular connections, for example, the growth cones of motor neurons stop and stick to a special form of laminin at the site of the future synapse (see Chapter 8).

Thus, growth cones are sensitive to a variety of external molecules: adhesion molecules that help attach growth cones to their substrates, growth-promoting molecules, substrate attached and diffusible cues that a growth cone can use to orient and turn, repulsive molecules, and stop signals. How many different cues a single growth cone can respond to is not known. Moreover, we have seen that as an axon grows and encounters different environments it may express different molecules on the growth cone membrane, dynamically changing its sensitivity to the environment.

Signal Transduction

The final aspect of outgrowth that we explore concerns how the environmental cues are able to influence growth cone behavior, referred to as signal transduction. Because filopodia are relatively long and motile, they are able to sample and compare different parts of their local environment. The also have a very high surface-to-volume ratio, which can convert membrane signals into large changes in intracellular messengers. Thus, growth cone filopodia have been thought of as sensory antennae, as well as tension-generating devices. We have seen how the entire behavior of a growth cone can change upon the interaction of a single filopodium with a particular substrate. If a growth cone is going to move when the filopodium contacts a particular signal, it must be able to amplify a membrane signal from the filopodium to the cytoskeleton, leading to the depolymerization of actin or the release of forward tension. When a growth cone chooses among substrates, it must be able to integrate different signals, stabilize certain filopodia, reorient microtubules, and bias lamellipodial extension and retraction on one side versus the other. It is thought that signals spread through the growth cone, perhaps in gradients, so that one side may act differently than the other. When an axon changes the CAMs or the receptors that it expresses on its surface after leaving a particular tract, it may stop advancing, transform into a terminal arbor, and begin accumulating synapse-specific molecules (see Chapter 8).

Cellular signaling pathways that make use of CAMs, integrins, repulsive factors, attractive factors, and growth factors are received by receptors on the surface of the growth cone. Many of these receptors have enzymatic activity and can immediately amplify the signal (Strittmatter and Fishman, 1991). For example, receptors that have intracellular tyrosine kinase (RTK) or tyrosine phosphatase (RTP) activity have been found in abundance on growth cones (Goldberg and Wu, 1996; Goodman, 1996). Tyrosine kinase activity seems to be involved in axon growth, because neurite outgrowth can be enhanced or inhibited when kinase activity is blocked pharmacologically. In *Drosophila,* a RTK called *derailed* is expressed on particular fascicles in the nervous system, and *derailed* mutants exhibit striking defasciculation and pathway errors (Callahan *et al.,* 1995). Some homophilic CAMs, such as NCAM, do not possess intracellular tyrosine kinase domains. However, they are able to recruit other RTKs, such as the FGF receptor, to do the work. Thus, there is a CAM-binding site on the FGF receptor, and CAM binding can stimulate phosphorylation of growth cone proteins via FGF receptor activity.

There are a number of RTPs that are found predominantly in growth cones, such as DLAR, which is expressed in *Drosophila* motor axons. Mutants in these genes can also lead to growth and pathfinding defects (Desai *et al.,* 1996). Unfortunately, it is not yet clear what the natural ligands for many of these RTKs and RTPs are. In addition to RTKs, some receptors are thought to signal through cytosolic tyrosine kinases and phosphatases. Among the non-receptor tyrosine kinases (NRTK) are *src, yes* and *fyn,* small molecules that might act downstream of specific CAMs. Neurons from single gene mouse knockouts that have no *src* are specifically unable to grow on L1, while neurons from single gene knockout mice that have no *fyn* are unable to grow on NCAM (Beggs *et al.,* 1994). It is not known what the critical targets of phosphorylation and dephosphorylation are in the growth cone for any of the (N)RTKs or the RTPs. However, it is likely that cytoskeletal components or associated proteins such as tubulin and MAPs are phosphorylated in response to neurite outgrowth.

Calcium, which may be released from internal stores in response to a signal from the cell surface or enter the growth through calcium channels, may stimulate or inhibit neurite outgrowth. Growth cones of the snail *Heliosoma* stop advancing when the level of intracellular of calcium is either too high or too low (Chapter 8). Serotonin, which stops growth cone advancement in certain neurons, appears to work by increasing calcium levels locally, as even isolated filopodia from these growth cones react to the application of serotonin by showing a marked increase in calcium along with a shortening response (Kater and Mills, 1991). This stopping behavior of *Heliosoma* growth cones can be mimicked using calcium ionophores.

Not all growth cones use calcium in the same way. For example, vertebrate spinal neurons collapse in response to the neurite-inhibiting factor from oligodendrocytes, particularly in response to a molecule called NI-35. This collapse

appears to be mediated by calcium released from internal stores, immediately before the growth cone withdraws. If the drug thapsigargin is used to inhibit this calcium release, then growth cone collapse is prevented. In contrast, the CNS-derived factor that is repulsive to peripheral nerves, collapsin or Sema III, causes growth cone withdrawal without an increase in intracellular calcium. Thus, calcium is not involved in the avoidance responses of neurons to all repulsive factors. In other neurons, calcium appears to stimulate neurite outgrowth and growth cones will grow in the direction of agents that increase intracellular calcium on one side of the neuron over the other. It is not yet clear how calcium triggers this response. One possibility is that calcium activates cytoplasmic enzymes, such as CAM kinase II or PKC, which then phosphorylate cytoskeletal components. Calcium is involved in so many aspects of intracellular function, it would be surprising if calcium had no influence on neurite growth. The challenge is to see how calcium is used in the normal pathway of signal transduction in the growth cone.

cAMP is another small molecule that is used in signal transduction in many cell types including growth cones (Chapter 8). Some growth cones are stimulated to grow by increasing intracellular cAMP and will turn toward permeant analogs of cAMP, while in others growth motility is inhibited. The level of cAMP is controlled by two enzymes: adenylate cyclase synthesizes cAMP, while phosphodiesterase breaks it down. Both of these enzymes may be modulated by various receptor-activated processes. cAMP goes on to activate protein kinase A (PKA), a serine threonine kinase that may modulate the activity of cytoskeletal elements. As with calcium, the response of a growth cone to various levels of internal cAMP depends on the concentration of cAMP. In fact, the level of cAMP can bias a neuron's response to other factors in its environment (Ming *et al.,* 1997; Song *et al.,* 1997). Whether a growth cone turns toward or away from a diffusible tropic agent is sometimes a matter of the internal state of the growth cone rather than a difference in the receptors it expresses. Thus, if the cAMP level inside the growth cone is lowered, a positive tropic response to netrin and the neurotrophin BDNF can be rapidly changed into a negative one. Moreover, the repulsive effect of collapsin I/semaphorin III can be changed to an attractive one by altering the level of cGMP inside the growth cone (Song *et al.,* 1998).

Most growth cones studied have high levels of G_o, a G protein that couples various transmembrane receptors to enzymatic signaling cascades within cells. Recently it has been shown that the growth cones of DRG axons are particularly sensitive to mastoparan, a wasp venom peptide that stimulates G proteins directly by a receptor-like mechanism. Mastoparan, like brain membrane extracts, can lead to the collapse of these growth cones, and both effects can be blocked by the application of pertussis toxin (PTX), which blocks receptor-stimulated activation of G_o (Igarashi *et al.,* 1993). Mutants in G_o that are constitutively active may, however, increase neurite outgrowth in some cells, suggesting that like phosphorylation levels, calcium levels, and cAMP levels, the response of the growth cone to a particular transduction cascade depends on the levels of G_o activity. One imagines that in the extension mode growth cones are poised to slow down, speed up, retract, stop, or turn, based on a number of signaling cascades that may be working independently but converging on the same cytoskeletal components.

GAP-43, a growth-associated protein in axons, is highly enriched in growth cones of growing and regenerating axons (Skene *et al.,* 1986). It is an internal protein that is associated with the cytoplasmic membrane and various cytoskeletal proteins. The function of GAP-43 has been tested by overexpressing it in cultured neurons and in transgenic mice and by inhibiting its expression. The results show that extra GAP-43 enhances axon outgrowth, while inhibiting GAP-43 compromises growth and leads to stalling (Fishman, 1996). In GAP-43 knockout mice, retinal axons stall and then take random courses when they reach the optic chiasm (Strittmatter *et al.,* 1995). When GAP-43 is overexpressed in transgenic mice, exuberant growth occurs and pathfinding errors are also made. These results suggest that regulated levels of GAP-43 are essential for the normal responses of axons to external cues. The activity of GAP-43 is regulated, in part, by phosphorylation through PKC and dephosphorylation through a phosphatase. The phosphorylated form of GAP-43 seems to stimulate its activity and promote outgrowth, while the dephosphorylated form is less active. It is not yet known how GAP-43 regulates axon growth, but it is proposed that increases in PKC activity lead to the phosphorylation of GAP-43 which then can interact directly with the cytoskeleton and enhance growth cone motility.

Closer to the cytoskeleton, a series of small GTP-binding proteins play major roles in signal transduction through a variety of receptors (Luo *et al.,* 1996). This Ras superfamily of proteins has also been implicated in oncogenesis cellular determination, and apoptosis. Three additional members of the Ras superfamily seem to have a unique role in affecting the actin cytoskeleton of the growth cone. These are rac, rho, and cdc42. Their function was first elucidated by injecting them into fibroblasts. From these studies, it appeared that rac regulates the formation of lamellipodia, rho regulates the formation of stress fibers, and cdc42 regulates the formation of filopodia. When a mutant form of *Drosophila* rac was misexpressed in neurons, axons did not grow properly, presumably because actin filaments could not polymerize and depolimerize normally. Mutations of cdc42 affect both axon and dendritic growth, suggesting a differential role for these proteins in process outgrowth. The rho protein activates a rho kinase which in turn inactivates a myosin phosphatase. This leads to increased phosphorylation and activity of myosin, and this is important in growth cone extension. Thus, these three proteins are all very closely associated with different aspects of the cytoskeleton and may serve as sites for the integration of signals that promote extension, turning, and retraction of growth cones.

Summary

We began this chapter by comparing axonal navigation with human navigation. We mentioned the need for a motor, and we have seen that the growth cone by virtue of its ability to incorporate new membrane and protein and its dynamic cytoskeleton is able to locomote forward, turn, stop, and even retract. We mentioned the need for guidance cues, and we have seen a variety of cues: some that are attached to the extracellular matrix and cell surfaces and some that act as diffusive gradients of guidance molecules. Some of these factors are positive: they attract axons, promote their growth, or promote adhesion. Some are negative: they are repulsive, inhibit growth, or lead to defasciculation. In addition there appears to be a variety of stop factors. We suggested that these various signals had to be integrated and communicated to the motor, and we have seen a variety of intracellular agents in the growth cone that can be regulated in response to external cues and communicated to the active cytoskeleton. We are, however, still a long way from understanding how axons grow to their targets. The molecules mentioned in this chapter are known to be used in some neurons only, and it is fair to say that, for even the best-studied neurons, we understand only small parts of their navigation, but not their entire route. There are many more guidance factors to be discovered and there is still much to be learned about the inner workings of the growth cone.

Target Selection

· · · · ·

Axons navigate along commissures and tracts in the CNS and nerves in the periphery. As they near their targets, they tend to branch off. In Chapter 5, we learned that changes in cell adhesion enable axons to pathfind along these tracts and commissures and exit at the correct points. How is it that axons recognize their particular targets? For motor neurons innervating the body wall muscles of a fly larva, the correct target may consist of a single muscle fiber. In the vertebrate brain, the target may have millions of cells and the axon terminals must find a particular complement of neighboring postsynaptic neurons within the target. In such cases, the axons of presynaptic neurons map isomorphically onto the postsynaptic neurons of the target structure. For example, the nasal retina maps onto the caudal midbrain and the temporal retina maps onto the rostral midbrain. Philosophers such as Immanuel Kant noted that the world outside appears to be organized along intuitively continuous dimensions of space and time. The maps we investigate in this chapter are topographic neural representations of the world, raising the possibility that the ability of humans and other animals to perceive these continua is simply a reflection of systematically ordered projections in their nervous systems.

Cellular Target Recognition

When growth cones from motor neurons reach the body wall muscles of a *Drosophila* embryo, they slow down but continue to form broadened lamellipodia, presumably to sample the local environment for topographic information. In each segment of a *Drosophila* larva, the growth cones of about 40 motor neurons touch about 30 different muscles, both appropriate and inappropriate, before they select those onto which they will synapse (Nose *et al.,* 1992; Broadie *et al.,* 1993). This is a simple example of targeting at the level of single cells. Differences between the motor neurons and muscles may be subtle since muscle cells are, by and large, similar to one another. Each muscle has a variety of adhesion, growth-promoting, and repulsive molecules on its surface, which are shared with all its neighbors. But these muscles also express cell surface molecules that are shared only with some of their neighbors or they may express the same molecules but at different concentrations (Winberg *et al.*, 1998).

Netrin genes (see Chapter 5) are expressed by subsets of muscles. Axons of the intersegmental nerve (ISN) normally innervate the netrin-expressing dorsal muscles. Embryos in which netrin is not expressed by the muscles, or mutants in which the netrin receptor (frazzled) is not expressed on the ISN axons, exhibit targeting defects in which axons grow past their appropriate targets and innervate inappropriate targets (Mitchell *et al.*, 1996; Winberg *et al.*, 1998). However, other muscle cells in these mutants are innervated correctly suggesting that additional recognition molecules must be involved.

Connectin is second molecule that could play a role in nerve–muscle specificity. It is a homophilic cell adhesion molecule that is expressed under the direct control of a homeotic gene on the surface of a subset of motor neurons and the muscle cells that they innervate (Nose *et al.*, 1992; Meadows *et al.*, 1994; Nose *et al.*, 1994; Raghavan and White, 1997). Unlike netrin mutants, the loss of connectin leads to few neuromuscular innervation defects. Such results certainly suggest that connectin does not act alone in specifying the appropriate connections between the expressing motor neurons and muscles. However, when connectin is expressed ectopically on all muscles in transgenic flies, motor axons frequently make targeting errors and invade nontarget muscles adjacent to their normal targets. The defects seen with connectin overexpression may be attributed to increased adhesion between different muscles that do not normally adhere to each other, making it difficult for the axon to take its usual pathway through the muscle field.

Yet a third candidate for neuromuscular specificity is fasII, a homophilic adhesion molecule that is expressed differentially on subsets of muscle fibers (Schuster *et al.*, 1996a). In the case of fasII, a more subtle experiment was done. The relative levels of FasII expressed on specific

muscles was altered. The result is that extra synapses form on muscles that express higher levels of fasII at the expense of synapses formed on neighboring muscles that do no not have increased fasII. This is true over a range of fasII levels, and it appears that the relative, and not the absolute, level of fasII is important.

FasIII, another homophilic adhesion molecule, and semaII, a secreted growth cone repulsive factor, are also expressed on overlapping specific muscle subsets in *Drosophila*. As with connectin mutants, loss of function mutants in these molecules display no serious effects on neuromuscular targeting (Winberg *et al.*, 1998). But as for the other molecules described, misexpression of fasIII or semaII in inappropriate muscles leads to dramatic targeting effects. The change in probability of particular motor neurons targeting particular muscles caused by experimentally changing the levels of a single cell adhesion molecule is consistent with the idea that growth cones are able to distinguish targets by relative changes in the concentrations of a number of such molecules. Furthermore, targeting errors caused by the increase in an attractive or adhesive factor can be compensated by a simultaneous increase in a repulsive factor, showing that indeed the combination or balance of various factors is what counts. In summary, the results with fasII, fasIII, connectin, semaII, and netrin suggest that in *Drosophila* neuromuscular targeting is based on a combinatorial code involving at least these molecules, and probably others (Fig. 6.1).

There are many other examples of single cell targeting in the central nervous systems of invertebrates with identified neurons. The ganglia of the leech and *Aplysia* are full of identified neurons whose connectivity is relatively well understood. When the interganglionic connectives are crushed in a leech and then allowed to regenerate, specific cellular connections are often precisely reestablished (von Bernhardi and Muller, 1995). Similarly, if identified neurons that make chemical synapses with each other are plucked from the ganglion and then cultured together, they often make similar synapses, while neurons that do not synapse together *in vivo*,

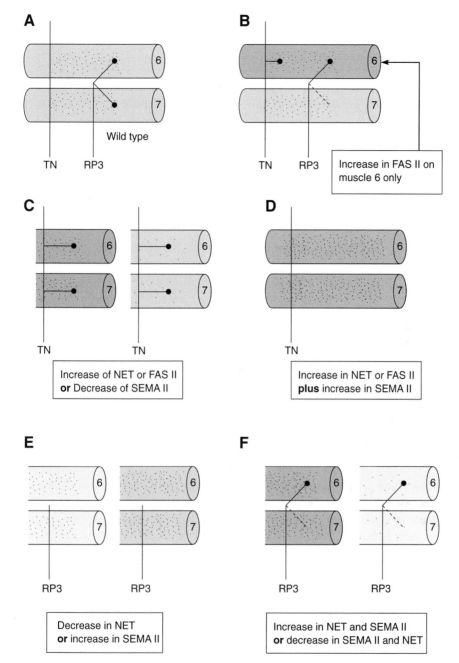

Figure 6.1 Combinatorial coding of targeting at a single cell level. (A) In wild-type *Drosophila* larva, the TN nerve does not innervate muscle fibers 6 and 7, whereas the RP3 nerve innervates both. (B) When fasII (red) is increased on muscle fiber 6 only, both the TN nerve and the RP3 nerve innervate this muscle differentially. (C) When netrin expression or fasII expression is increased on both muscles or when semaII is decreased, the TN nerve innervates both muscle fibers 6 and 7. (D) When netrin or fasII are increased but semaII is also increased simultaneously, then the TN nerve does not innervate muscle fibers 6 and 7. (E) When there is a decrease in netrin or an increase semaII, the RP3 nerve does not innervate muscle fibers 6 and 7. (F) However, when there is either an increase or a decrease in both semaII and netrin, the RP3 nerve innervates as normal (Winberg *et al.*, 1998).

also tend not to *in vitro* (Nicholls and Hernandez, 1989). There is even specificity among the specific dendritic branches of a single postsynaptic target cell. For example, an inhibitory motor neuron in the leech has a powerful inhibitory connection to an excitatory motor neuron. The anatomical location of this synapse was revealed by the photoablation of the postsynaptic dendrites. The majority of the inhibitory responses were abolished by the elimination of a single dendrite called d1, yet only a minority from a second dendrite called d2 (Lytton and Kristan, 1989). Furthermore, when leech cells are cultured together the type and strength of synapses between them depends upon the parts of the neurons that are in contact with each other, so that synapses made on the soma region are different in character from those made on the growing neurite stump, also suggesting subcellular localization of synaptogenic properties (Nicholls and Hernandez, 1989).

Multicellular Targets

The advent of high-resolution video microscopy and fluorescent tracer techniques has provided informative time-lapse movies of target invasion. After entering the postsynaptic neuropil, growth cones in many systems display thinly branched terminals with small tapered growth cones. For example, retinal ganglion cell axons in *Xenopus* embryos grow at a rate of about 60 μm/h in the optic tract, but slow to about 16 μm/h when they enter the optic tectum (Harris *et al.*, 1987) (Fig. 6.2). Once within the optic tectum, these terminals may advance in a saltatory manner, by momentarily attaining rates of over 100 μm/h or halting their growth entirely. At the same time, these transformed axon terminals emit wormlike side-branches and backbranches that continue to grow and extend over the tectal surface as if they are searching for a target.

Recent evidence suggests that growth factors and neurotrophic factors may play a critical role in this type of target recognition. For example, sympathetic axons fail to enter the pineal gland and the external ear in mice that lack the neurotrophin NT-3. When NT-3 is administered to the ears of mutant mice, target invasion is restored (ElShamy *et al.*, 1996) (Fig. 6.3). Sympathetic neurons are known to orient to gradients of NGF, (Chapter 5) which may also serve as a target recognition factor for sympathetic neurons in the pancreas. However, in transgenic mice, sympathetic axons that ectopically express NGF fail to innervate the pancreas. The problem in target recognition appears to be that the growth cone senses its own NGF and cannot respond to the increased concentration of this factor in the pancreas. The normal phenotype can be rescued by causing the pancreas to express higher than normal levels of NGF (Hoyle *et al.*, 1993). A similar situation is found in the retinotectal system. Here, fibroblast growth factor 2 (FGF2) seems to be involved in target entry. FGF2 is heavily expressed in the optic pathway, but the levels decline abruptly at the tectal border. When ectopic FGF2 is exogenously applied to the developing pathway so that differences in FGF2 levels between the pathway and the target are abolished, or when retinal axons express a dominant negative receptor so that they can no longer sense FGF2 gradients, these axons fail to invade the optic tectum (McFarlane *et al.*, 1995, 1996) (Fig. 6.2).

Once they have recognized and entered a target area, axons may be prevented from exiting a large target area by repulsive cues at the perimeters. For example, semaIII/collapsin1, which was discussed earlier, repels the growth cones of cutaneous sensory neurons from dorsal root ganglion. Analysis of knockout mice provides additional evidence that collapsin1 serves as an exclusion factor which confines the peripheral terminals, to the correct areas of the skin (Taniguchi *et al.*, 1997). In these mice, axons that are normally restricted from innervating collapsin-1-expressing skin now enter these territories. Sema III/collapsin1 is also expressed at the posterior boundary of the olfactory bulb and is hypothesized to act as a stop signal that restricts olfactory axons to the bulb and prevents them from entering the telencephalon (Kobayashi *et al.*, 1997). The repulsive molecule ephrin A5, which will be discussed in more detail below, reaches

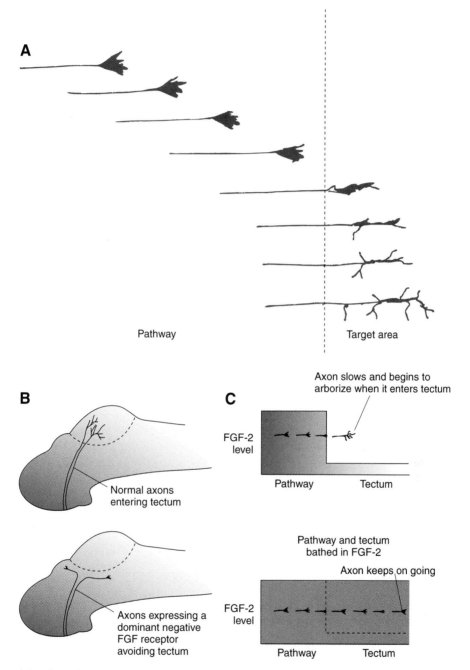

Pathway

Target area

Axon slows and begins to arborize when it enters tectum

FGF-2 level

Pathway

Tectum

Normal axons entering tectum

Pathway and tectum bathed in FGF-2

Axon keeps on going

FGF-2 level

Axons expressing a dominant negative FGF receptor avoiding tectum

Pathway

Tectum

Figure 6.2 Growth cones change when they enter their target zones. (A) Images from a time-lapse movie of a retinal ganglion cell growing in the optic tract and then crossing (at the dotted line) into the tectum. The simple growth cone becomes much more complex and slows down dramatically as it enters the target. (B) Tectal innervation by control retinal axons (top) and tectal avoidance by retinal axons that misexpress a dominant negative FGF receptor. (C) Retinal axons slow down and branch when they reach the tectum in control animals (top), but when the pathway is exposed to high levels of FGF2, the axons keep going and do not innervate the tectum (Harris *et al.,* 1987; McFarlane *et al.,* 1995, 1996).

A

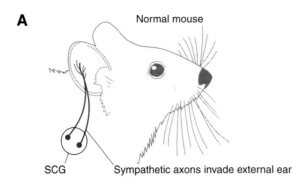

Normal mouse

SCG   Sympathetic axons invade external ear

B

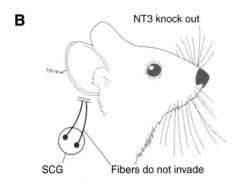

NT3 knock out

SCG   Fibers do not invade

C

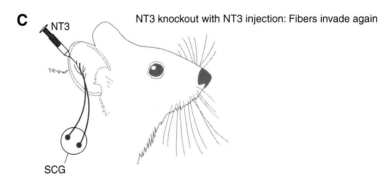

NT3   NT3 knockout with NT3 injection: Fibers invade again

SCG

Figure 6.3   Some sympathetic neurons use a change in NT-3 expression to innervate their targets in the ear. (A) Some SCG neurons project to and arborize in the pinna of a normal mouse. (B) In NT-3 knockout mice, these fibers do not invade the pinna. (C) Restoration of targeting by injection of NT-3 into the ear (ElShamy *et al.,* 1996).

its highest concentrations at the posterior aspect of the superior colliculus (tectum) a target of retinal axons, suggesting that this ligand may also serve to confine these axons to the target. Indeed, recent studies show that retinal axons extend freely beyond the posterior border of the superior colliculus in ephrin A5 knockout mice (Frisen *et al.,* 1998).

Secondary Targets

Reinnervation and cross-innervation experiments show that when the normal targets of axons have been moved or removed, functional synapses can be made on the wrong target. Deliberate misinnervation of limb muscles can be accomplished by crushing the normal nerve and moving a foreign nerve onto the denervated muscle. The foreign nerve quickly innervates the denervated muscle, which produce sprout-inducing factors. These factors, combined with the ability of peripheral axons to regenerate, allow the original crushed axons to innervate their targets again, thus restoring function. The ability of axons to innervate local foreign targets is a common theme in brain damage, whereby inappropriate connections are made to otherwise denervated dendrites. As in the periphery, denervated CNS neurons often induce local axonal arbors to sprout new connections.

To test how promiscuous axons are and whom they will synapse with if given the chance, one can test a variety of foreign targets with different axonal populations. For example, to know whether retinal ganglion cell axons are determined to invade a specific target, one of their normal targets (i.e., the lateral geniculate nucleus) was ablated and a neighboring nonvisual region (i.e., somatosensory thalamus) was denervated (Metin and Frost, 1989). In this case, retinal axons permanently innervate the somatosensory thalamus (Fig. 6.4). In a similar experiment, retinal ganglion cell axons innervated the medial geniculate nucleus the normal site of auditory input (Roe *et al.,* 1992). The thalamocortical connections are basically normal in these animals, giving rise to the possibility that the animals could feel or hear the visual world (Fig. 6.4).

There are many experimental examples where axons can be induced to form synapses with unusual synaptic partners. For instance, as we see later in the chapter, preganglionic neurons of the spinal cord usually innervate neurons of the sympathetic chain, but if a sympathetic ganglion is removed and a skeletal muscle is transplanted in its place, the cholinergic preganglionic fibers functionally innervate the muscle (Wigston and Sanes, 1985). It may be that the axons which use glutamate as a neurotransmitter are not able to make effective synapses with cells that have only acetylcholine receptors. Barring such neurotransmitter mismatches, the possibilities for secondary target innervation, combined with the results suggesting combinatorial coding of target muscles in the fly, suggest that target-derived molecular cues may be more subtle than a lock and key mechanism that would only allow particular axons to make connections with particular targets.

Targeting to the Correct Layer

Many targets in the nervous system are layered structures like the tectum and the cortex. Therefore, invading axons must find the appropriate layer. Central terminals of DRG sensory fibers enter the spinal cord and make synapses in various laminae of the dorsal horn or ventral gray matter depending on their modality. For instance, stretch receptors make monosynaptic contact with motor neurons in the ventral horn. In contrast, pain and temperature sensory fibers innervate neurons in dorsal laminae of the spinal cord (Fig. 6.5). The result of this laminar arrangement by different types of input is that somatosensory modalities sort out in the spinal cord and thus make a multilayered registered map, such that a column of cells in the spinal cord represents one area of the body with different modalities at different depths. Multimodal, layered maps are used in several places in the nervous system.

Why do only stretch receptors penetrate the more ventral layers of the spinal neuropil? In the chapter (Chapter 5) on axon growth guidance, we described the varying sensitivity of different classes of neurons to the repulsive effects of semaphorin. Semaphorin repels pain and thermoreceptive neurons, which are dependent on NGF for their survival. Stretch receptive neurons, which are responsive to NT-3, ignore semaphorin (Messersmith *et al.,* 1995). In mice in which the semaphorin III gene is knocked out, the pain and thermoreceptive axonal terminal appear to extend into the ventral regions of the spinal

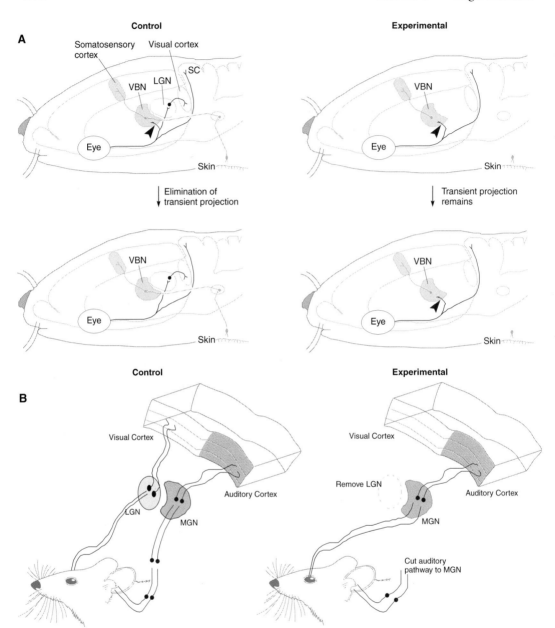

Figure 6.4 Aberrant innervation of sensory areas. (A) A transient projection from retinal ganglion cells to the somatosensory thalamus (red arrow) is eliminated during normal development (left). When the retinal ganglion cell target (LGN) is ablated and the somatosensory thalamus is denervated, then retinal axons permanently innervate the somatosensory thalamus (right) which relay visual signals to the somatosensory cortex. Visual signals to the auditory cortex. (B) In a normal ferret the auditory input goes indirectly to the medial geniculate nucleus of the thalamus and from there to the auditory cortex. Retinal input is to the LGN and then on to the visual cortex. When the auditory pathway is cut and the LGN removed, the visual input sprouts into the MGN which projects as usual giving visual physiological properties to the auditory cortex (Roe *et al.*, 1992).

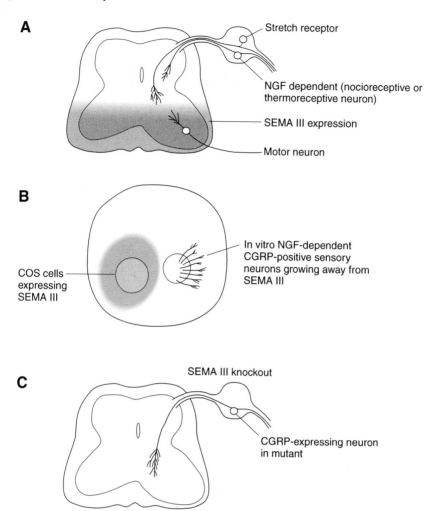

Figure 6.5 The role of sema in keeping some axons out of a target region. (A) Stretch receptors project their central axons into the ventral horn of the spinal cord where they synapse on motor neuron dendrites. Nocio-receptive and thermoreceptive axons that are NGF dependent and cGRP positive, however, terminate in the dorsal gray matter of the spinal cord. SemaIII is expressed only in the ventral cord. (B) Cos cells in culture repel nocioceptive and thermoreceptive axons from DRG cultures. (C) In semaIII knockout mice, these sensory neurons extend into the ventral horn (Messersmith *et al.*, 1995).

cord, similar to the stretch receptors (Taniguchi *et al.,* 1997; Catalano *et al.,* 1998) (Fig. 6.5).

As is the case for target recognition and topographic mapping, a variety of molecules seem to be involved in the process of layer-specific projections. For example, in the hippocampus, entorhinal afferents innervate two layers while commissural afferents innervate three other layers. The entorhinal cortex afferents grow into their specific target layers from the beginning of the innervation process which indicates that the lamina-specific cues are present early in embryogenesis in this system (Super and Soriano, 1994). When entorhinal axons first grow into the hippocampus, they make synaptic contacts with specialized cells called the Cajal–Retzius (CR) cells, a transient population of early generated neurons (see Chapter 4). When CR cells are selectively ablated, very few entorhinal afferents innervate the hippocampus whereas commissural axons innervate their specific layers normally (Del Rio *et al.,* 1997). When Reelin, a molecule on the surface of CR cells, is functionally inhibited (by antibody blocking) or absent (in reeler mutant mice) entorhinal axons also fail to make robust connections within appropriate layers. Thus, the Reelin protein appears to provide layer-specific innervation information in the hippocampus. Layering abnormalities in the cortex and the cerebellum of reeler mice suggests that Reelin may have a more widespread role in laminar-specific innervation (see Chapter 4).

The cerebral cortex is a highly laminated structure, composed of different types, sizes, and densities of neurons in different layers. In addition, the different layers of the cortex are innervated by different inputs and send axons to different targets. Some of these targeting characteristics are preserved in explant cultures. Axons branch preferentially on the layers in cortical slices (or even on membranes from the layers) that they would target *in vivo*. When given a choice to grow on membranes from either their target or nontarget layers, they show a clear preference for the target layers (Castellani and Bolz, 1997). This indicates that membrane-associated targeting cues are confined to individual layers. Heat inactivation studies with these membranes suggest that there are both attractive and inhibitory factors in specific layers. Some molecules, like ephrin A5 (see below), are expressed in specific laminae of the cortex, and when tested on membrane stripes *in vitro,* these molecules increase the extent of branching from the axons that normally innervate these layers and at the same time inhibit the growth of neurons that innervate neighboring layers (Castellani *et al.,* 1998) (Fig. 6.6).

Laminar-selective growth also occurs in the highly laminated chick optic tectum where the terminals of retinal axons are confined to 3 of the 15 laminae (Sanes and Yamagata, 1999). Several different cadherin molecules, such as N-cadherin, R-cadherin, and T-cadherin, are ex-

pressed in different combinations within these laminae. For example, N-cadherin is selectively present in the three retinorecipient layers and possibly as many as 20 different genes of the cadherin superfamily are expressed in a restricted pattern in the tectum during synaptogenesis (Miskevich *et al.,* 1998). When the function of N-cadherin is disrupted by function-blocking antibodies, retinal axons have reduced branching and an increase in laminar-specific errors (Inoue and Sanes, 1997).

Single postsynaptic cells may have dendritic branches that extend through several laminae; the process of laminar targeting is thus sometimes a question of where on a single post-synaptic cell to make a synapse. Recent experiments suggest that cadherins are involved in the selection of specific synapses (Fannon and Colman, 1996). Several different types of cadherins are expressed in the developing CNS and found localized at particular synapses (Redies and Takeichi, 1996). Antibodies to N- and E-cadherin have been used to show that these two cadherins are distributed at synaptic junctions in a mutually exclusive pattern along the dendritic shafts of pyramidal neurons in the cerebellum. Ultrastructural examination of double-immunolabeled material revealed the existence of many unlabeled synapses, raising the possibility that synapses in other layers are linked by other cadherins. Multiple cadherins that are differentially distributed along the dendritic shaft may be responsible for "locking in" synapses appropriately by homophilic adhesion.

Topographic Mapping

Topographic maps in the brain are orderly representations of some physical property of the world. Some topographic maps preserve anatomical axes. For example, in the visual system, the retina is basically a curved two-dimensional sheet of cells. Cells in a particular position in this retina are maximally stimulated from a sector of the visual world. Neurons in neighboring retinal positions send projections to neighboring regions in the visual target to which they project.

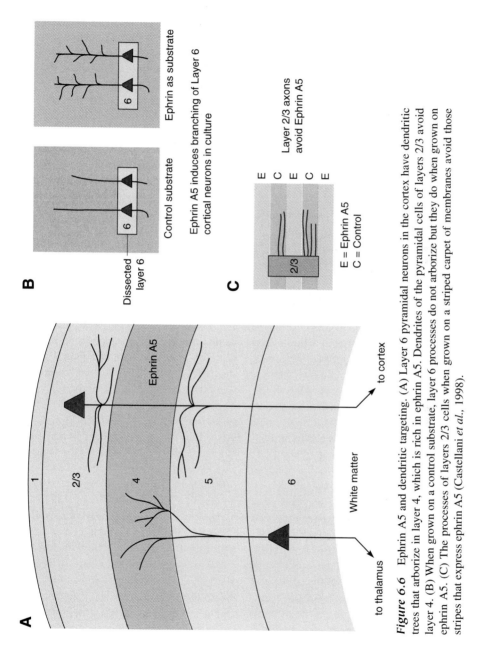

Figure 6.6 Ephrin A5 and dendritic targeting. (A) Layer 6 pyramidal neurons in the cortex have dendritic trees that arborize in layer 4, which is rich in ephrin A5. Dendrites of the pyramidal cells of layers 2/3 avoid layer 4. (B) When grown on a control substrate, layer 6 processes do not arborize but they do when grown on ephrin A5. (C) The processes of layers 2/3 cells when grown on a striped carpet of membranes avoid those stripes that express ephrin A5 (Castellani *et al.*, 1998).

This orderly projection preserves retinal topography in the brain and provides a neuroanatomical basis for the contiguity of perceived visual space. Similarly, most central auditory nuclei have a representation of the cochlea's frequency axis. Such maps may be referred to by the anatomical substrates that they preserve (e.g., retinotopic, cochleotopic). Furthermore, orderly topographic projections often preserve such features of contiguity from one brain nucleus to another. Even simple animals like the nematode, with only 301 neurons, have ordered arrays of sensory receptors that make somatopically organized central projections. These help them respond appropriately to stimuli that strike the animal from different directions (see Chapter 4).

There is a second type of neural map, a computational map, which can be revealed by recording from neighboring single nerve cells *in vivo*. What is represented in such maps is not obvious from the anatomy of the connections, yet these maps may also display orderly representations of a physical parameter. For example, in the auditory system we find nuclei that display a topography of sound source location, even though the ear contains only a one-dimensional array of neurons representing sound frequency. Another example is the echo delay map in the cortex of an echolocating bat. Such maps are constructed from many overlapping afferent projections and are referred to by the functional characteristic that they encode (e.g., map of auditory space or distance), rather than a piece of tissue. There are also stranger maps, such as maps of taste and smell that we discuss below.

Rather remarkably, there is a consistency of topographic maps between animals. For example, in the mammalian primary visual cortex, the representation of the center of gaze is always near the extreme occipital pole of the cortex and the vertical meridian separating the left and right visual fields runs along the border of primary visual cortex. The cochleotopic map of pitch and the somatosensory map of the body are also arranged along the same axes in different animals. The preservation of neural topography strongly suggests a development program for orienting the maps and making sure the axons find their appropriate targets within them.

Mapping the Body

In the late 1800s John Langley, a great contributor to our understanding of the autonomic nervous system, discovered that superior cervical ganglion (SCG) neurons mediate reflexes in a topographic manner (Langley, 1895, 1897). When Langley stimulated the first or top thoracic root to the ganglion in the rat, this activated ganglion cells that caused dilation of the pupil. When he stimulated the fourth thoracic root to the ganglion, blood vessels of the ear constricted. This suggested that there was some sort of topographical organization within the SCG. All reflexes were immediately lost when the preganglionic nerve to the SCG was cut, but the fibers reinnervated the SCG in several weeks, as peripheral nerves often do in mammals, and the autonomic reflexes recovered. The surprising discovery was that the connections reformed with such precision that all reflexes were reestablished accurately (Fig. 6.7). This result suggested that individual SCG neurons have some possibly topographic mechanism that enables the regenerating preganglionic fibers to distinguish one SCG neuron from the another.

The sympathetic chain ganglia provide a simple system in which to examine somatotopic specificity because each ganglion is selectively innervated by afferents from a limited number of spinal cord segments. Thus, the SCG is primarily innervated by preganglionic afferents from thoracic segments T1–T4, whereas the more caudally located fifth thoracic ganglion (T5) is primarily innervated by afferents from spinal thoracic segments T4–T7 (Nja and Purves, 1977). In one experiment, a T5 ganglion was transplanted to different locations along the sympathetic chain exposing this target to afferents from a large range of spinal cord segments (Purves *et al.*, 1981). Selective reinnervation was then assessed electrophysiologically. The sympathetic chain ganglia were dissected out along with the ventral nerve roots through which all preganglionic fibers course from the ventral spinal cord. Stimulating electrodes were then placed on the ventral roots from each spinal cord segment, and an intracellular recording was obtained from the reinnervated T5 ganglion. The spinal segments that innervate each T5 neuron were then recorded.

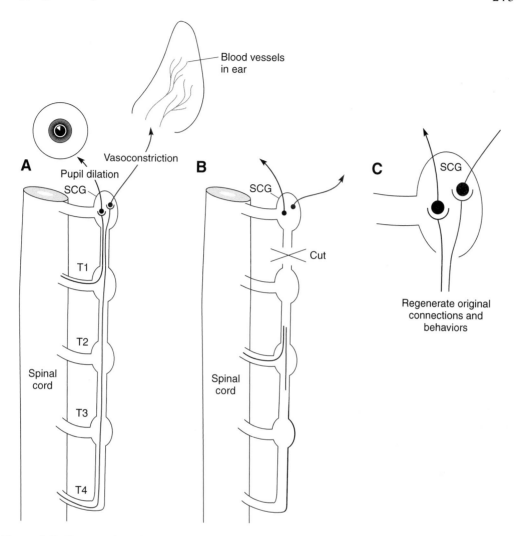

Figure 6.7 Regeneration of topographic specificity. (A) Langley's classic study showed that stimulation of preganglionic root T4 activated ganglion cells in the SCG causing vasoconstriction of the ear pinna vessels, whereas stimulation of root T1 excited other SCG neurons causing dilation of the pupil. (B) When he cut the sympathetic tract above T1, all these sympathetic reflexes were abolished, but with time they recovered. (C) Specificity associated with this regeneration, such that the axons that enter the chain at T4 reinnervate the SCG cells that cause ear vasoconstriction, and the axons that enter at T1 reinnervate the cells that cause pupil dilation (Langley, 1897).

The results clearly indicated that T5 neurons were selectively reinnervated by their original spinal segments regardless of their aberrant position (6.8). This was not merely an artifact of the host explantation site because when the SCG was placed in the same location it too became reinnervated by its original set of afferents. These experiments strongly suggest that axons from different rostrocaudal levels can distinguish individual sympathetic ganglion cells, which must also carry some label of their rostrocaudal origin.

In an analogous situation motor cortex is topographically connected to motor neuron targets in the spinal cord: The forelimb cortex innervates the cervical cord while the hindlimb cortex innervates the lumbar cord (Fig. 6.9).

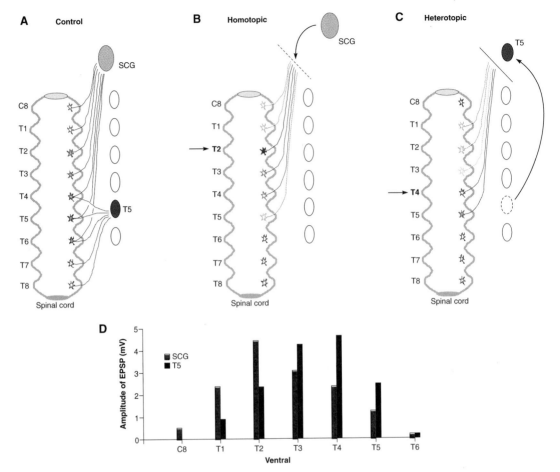

Figure 6.8 Topographic input into the sympathetic chain. (A) Electrophysiological studies show that the SCG receives input from many roots but primarily the more anterior ones. The ganglion at T5 receives its primary inputs from more posterior roots. (B) When the SCG is removed and replaced with another SCG, the axons that reinnervate it tend to be from more anterior roots. (C) When a T5 ganglion is put in place of the SCG, its neurons still tend to get innervated by more posterior roots even though the ganglion is in an anterior position. (D) This topographic specificity of reinnervation is reflected in the shape of the histogram of EPSP amplitudes as a function of nerve root stimulation for the homotopic and heterotopic transplants (Purves *et al.,* 1981).

When challenged *in vitro* with explants from cervical and lumbar enlargements of the early postnatal spinal cord, sensorimotor cortical explants from newborn hamsters made target selection choices that were topographically appropriate (Kuang *et al.,* 1994). Forelimb cortex axons grew selectively to cervical cord and hindlimb cortex grew selectively to lumbar cord. Matching presynaptic axons to postsynaptic targets on the basis of position is part of the process of selective topographic innervation among cells that are otherwise similar.

The idea that there are positional labels along the rostrocaudal axis of the nervous system is inviting since there is a rather simple relationship between the rostrocaudal axis of the spinal cord and its peripheral targets. Thus, muscles of a particular body segment are generally

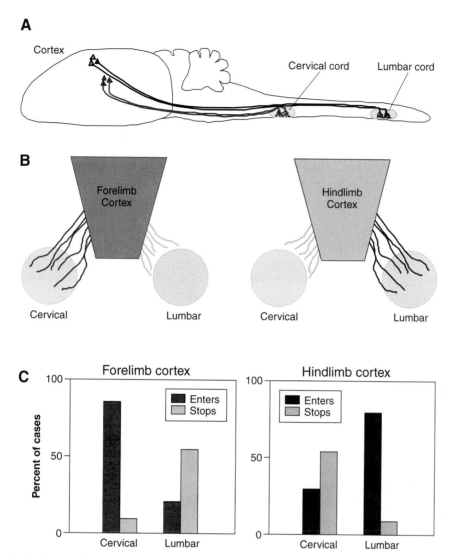

Figure 6.9 Somotopic specificity in corticospinal projections. (A) The motor cortex is topographically arrayed such that the cortical area that sends axons to the lumbar cord controlling the hindlimbs is located at a distinct site from the area that sends axons to the forelimb motor neurons in the cervical cord. (B, C) In cultured explants of forelimb cortex, cells prefer to send axons into explants of cervical cord, while explants of hindlimb cortex prefer to send axons into lumbar cord (Kuang *et al.*, 1994).

innervated by motor neurons of similar segments. It has even been shown that there is innervation topography within a single muscle, such that axons originating from a particular spinal cord level of that muscle's motor pool innervate one part of the muscle. The topographic specificity develops crudely at first, but is refined by synapse elimination of topographically inappropriate connections. As we shall see, this is very similar to map refinement in the visual system (Chapter 9).

Support for a rostrocaudal positional specification of the muscles comes from experiments in which intercostal muscles are transplanted so that they become innervated by cholinergic preganglionic fibers of the sympathetic trunk (Wigston and Sanes, 1985). The result is that the most rostral muscles are preferentially innervated by the most rostral preganglionic axons (Fig. 6.10). These kinds of transplant experiments also show that the topographic maps formed are unlikely to be due to timing, since the reinnervation process is rather synchronous, or fiber–fiber interactions that maintain order since in a cut or crushed nerve there is a severe disruption of fiber ordering. Thus, these studies imply that there are chemically coded positional cues on axons and their targets along the rostrocaudal axis.

A search for molecules whose expression in neuronal cells is graded along the rostrocaudal axis of the sympathetic chain was undertaken using the technique of immunosuppression (Suzue *et al.*, 1990). Mice were immunized to membranes from rostral ganglia but their immune response was suppressed to antigens presented on the membranes of caudal ganglia. Thus the immunized mice preferentially made antibodies to epitopes that were expressed rostrally. One of these monoclonal antibodies, called ROCA1 (rostrocaudal 1), strongly stained the rostral ganglia and nerves but the intensity diminished in more caudal ganglia. This staining was due to an epitope on a protein called CD9, a membrane protein used in adhesion-dependent signaling in the hematopoietic system (Kaprielian *et al.*, 1995). In the nervous system, CD9 is associated with integrins, and it is known to influence the outgrowth of sympathetic neurites. Another antibody that was raised to rostral CNS membranes, using a different procedure, recognizes a high-molecular-weight proteoglycan from the earliest stages, even prior to neural tube closure (Kaprielian and Patterson, 1993). This work shows that there appears to be at least two molecular correlates of rostrocaudal positional identity in the CNS, both of which are candidates for mediating topographic connections.

How are different levels of protein produced along the rostrocaudal axis? An insight into the expression of such positional markers came from work in transgenic mice (Donoghue *et al.*, 1991). When a transgene containing a myosin light chain kinase promoter plus a downstream enhancer driving a bacterial reporter was placed in the genome, expression of the reporter was approximately 100-fold higher in rostral axial muscles than in caudal ones. Truncations of the promoter showed there to be distinct regions that repress transgene activity in neck muscles and promote it in intercostal muscles. This gradient of expression across a large fraction of the body may reflect the activities of positionally restricted sets of transcription factors, such as homeobox genes.

Rostrocaudal positional information along the body axis is also seen in insects. When wind-sensitive sensilli are transplanted from one location to another in the locust, it is found that axons from the sensory cells reestablished connections with their central targets based on their original position on the body wall (Anderson and Bacon, 1979; Anderson, 1985). This occurs even though the sensory axons may enter the CNS from an abnormally rostral position. Transcription factors that determine positional identity (Chapter 2) with respect to somatotopic mapping may affect other aspects of pattern as well. In *Drosophila*, a transcription factor called *iroquois* is responsible for positioning mechanosensory hairs along the side of the thorax (Grillenzoni *et al.*, 1998). In the absence of *iroquois,* these side hairs are gone leaving only a tuft of hairs running down the middle of the dorsum. In a normal fly, neurons of the side hairs project more laterally in the thoracic ganglion than the neurons from the central hairs, establishing a somatotopic representation. Could it be that *iroquois* is involved in this mapping? To answer this question, the effects of eliminating *iroquois* on hair formation was overcome by driving the *achaete* gene, which is usually under the control of *iroquois* in this region, under another promoter in transgenic flies. These flies have side bristles but no *iroquois.* The projections of these side hairs, however, were similar to the central hairs (Fig. 6.11). Similarly, if *iroquois* is misexpressed in central hairs, the effect is to transform their CNS projections to those of side hairs. These experiments establish that *iroquois* is involved in somatotopic mapping at a transcriptional level and

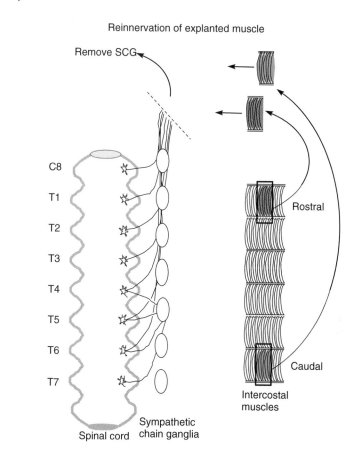

A

Reinnervation of explanted muscle

Remove SCG

C8
T1
T2
T3
T4
T5
T6
T7

Rostral

Caudal

Intercostal muscles

Spinal cord

Sympathetic chain ganglia

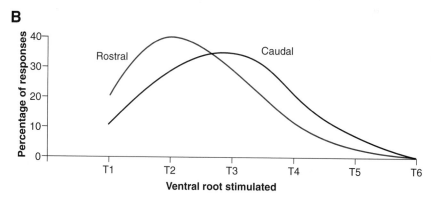

B

Rostral

Caudal

Percentage of responses

40
30
20
10
0

T1   T2   T3   T4   T5   T6

Ventral root stimulated

Figure 6.10 Somatotopic specificity as a whole body phenomenon. (A) When intercostal ribcage muscles from different regions are transplanted in place of SCGs, they become reinnervated by cholinergic preganglionic axons of the sympathetic chain. (B) Like the sympathetic ganglia themselves, the more anterior muscles attract innervation from more anterior roots while the more posterior muscles tend to receive more innervation from more posterior roots (Wigston and Sanes, 1985).

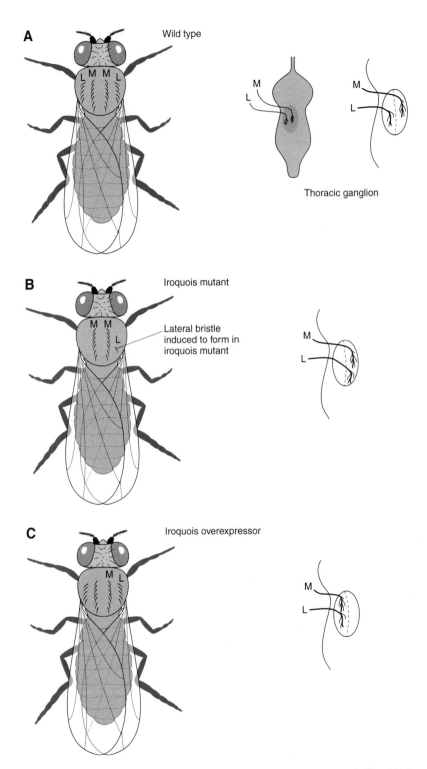

Figure 6.11 *Iroquois* gives topographic information to external sensory receptors in flies. (A) In a wild-type fly, axons of lateral thoracic sensory bristles project to the lateral part of the thoracic ganglion in the CNS, and axons from medial bristles project more medially. (B) The *iroquois* mutant lacks lateral bristles. If an ectopic lateral bristle is induced to form, it projects medially. (C) Similarly, if the *iroquois* gene is misexpressed in both medial and lateral bristles, then both bristle types project laterally (Grillenzoni *et al.,* 1998).

raise the interesting question of what the targets of *iroquois* regulation are, especially, among, the membrane receptors that are more directly involved with target recognition.

Somatotopy: Maps in the Brain and Their Modification

Somatosensory neurons in the spinal cord that respond to distinct stimuli (e.g., touch, kinesthesia, pressure, and pain) project to the hindbrain where they form topographic representations of the body surface. These brain stem somatosensory neurons project to the ventrobasal thalamus, and the thalamic neurons project to the somatosensory cortex. At each level of the CNS (cord, hindbrain, thalamus, cortex), a representation of the body surface remains intact. The discovery of a somatosensory representation of the body, a homunculus in the case of humans, was discovered by the neurosurgeon Wilder Penfield (Penfield, 1954). While performing operations to remove epileptic foci in the brains of fully conscious patients, Penfield took the opportunity to study the organization of the cortex by locally stimulating different regions with an electrode.

When he stimulated points in the postcentral gyrus, patients reported the sensation of touch in specific areas of their bodies. Stimulation of neighboring points caused the patients to experience sensations in neighboring parts of their body surface although there were occasional jumps, such as between the hand and the face. By mapping these sensations on the cortex of different patients, Penfield was able to come up with a consistent somatosensory homunculus (Fig. 6.12).

One striking feature of the homunculus that Penfield noticed immediately is the relative magnification of parts of the map. This appears to be a consistent feature of many maps in the CNS. The largest features of the human homunculus are the lips, tongue, and tips of the fingers. In contrast, the representation of the upper back is quite small. In other animals, the somatosensory cortex has an expanded representation of different body parts: the hands of the raccoon, the snout of a star nose mole, and the whiskers of the mouse, for example, are particularly enlarged. The differential magnification of certain body parts in the cortical representation is probably due to the density of peripheral innervation. Thus, in humans, each finger tip has almost as many sensor receptors as the whole of the upper

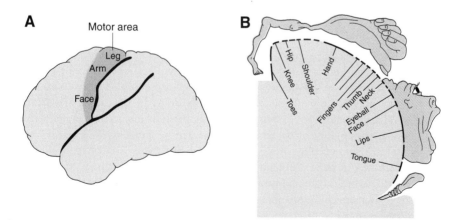

Figure 6.12 Somatosensory representation in the motor cortex. (A) The motor area of the precentral gyrus of the right cerebral cortex was stimulated electrically in human patients during neurosurgery. (B) A "homunculus" of the body on the motor cortex illustrates the sequence of representation as well as the disproportionate representation given to the various muscles involved in skilled movements (Penfield, 1954).

back. In mice the vibrissae are most heavily innervated, and in raccoons it is their hands.

Central representations of the somatosensory system are flexible and may depend on sensory stimulation, especially during early life. In the mouse, single cortical areas, called barrels, are devoted to each individual vibrissa (whisker). The barrel fields of the cortex are almost equal in size to the somatosensory cortex devoted to the rest of the body (Woolsey and Van der Loos, 1970). There are five rows of barrels that correspond to the five rows of vibrissae. When a bristle is destroyed by cauterization in early life, the cortical barrel that represents it shrinks, while the neighboring barrels expand into the territory of the cortex originally devoted to the cauterized whisker (Dietrich *et al.*, 1981; Simons *et al.*, 1984) (Fig. 6.13). When two whiskers are glued together, their cortical barrels fuse. Perhaps the most surprising finding is the case of a mouse that was born with an extra whisker, as sometimes happens. This mouse had an extra barrel in its cortex (Van der Loos *et al.*, 1984).

From these results, it is clear that the neural representation of the body surface has flexibility in its structure. The sensory fields themselves and their activity guide this flexibility. In a later chapter we examine the mechanisms by which the activity of inputs influences their targets fields. Here, we only mention that a particular class of glutamate receptor, the NMDA receptor, has been implicated in the refinement of topographic maps in this and many other systems (Jablonska *et al.*, 1999). A study using mutant mice in which the NMDA receptor has been knocked out by homologous recombination shows that this system may be involved in establishing the boundaries of the barrel fields (Iwasato *et al.*, 1997). Mutant mice showed normal pathfinding of trigeminal axons in the brain stem, and even a normal somatosensory projection to the cortex. But mutant mice failed to develop whisker-specific patches or barrels, which demonstrates involvement of the NMDA in the segregation of these fields (Chapter 9).

The representation of vibrissae in discrete units of neural tissue is also seen in the hindbrain, where the trigeminal axons from each whisker make their first synapses. By applying fluorescent dyes to label the axons of single trigeminal neurons, it has been shown that these axons form an orderly topographic projection in the brain stem (Killackey *et al.*, 1995). The brain stem barrelettes are also sensitive to damaging parts of the whisker pad, but the sensitivity extends to an earlier prenatal stage of development. From the brain stem, there is a topographic projection preserving the body representation to the thalamus. To a certain extent, the thalamic map is also flexible in neonatal animals as indicated from the responses to injuries that damage sensory neurons (Florence *et al.*, 1998; Jones and Pons, 1998; Merzenich, 1998) (Fig. 6.14). The cortical somatotopic map, as we see below, can transform throughout life and changes in activity patterns are sufficient for such reorganizations.

When an adult, through accident or medical intervention loses sensation in one area of the body as happens when a peripheral nerve is cut, the cortical representation of that area may be invaded by representation from neighboring parts. This is thought to be one reason why people who have lost a limb may report sensations in the phantom limb, especially when a part of the body is touched whose cortical representation is adjacent to the missing limb. A touch to the face in such a person can be experienced as a touch on the missing hand. The explanation is that nerve fibers that carry information about touch on the face invade the neighboring cortical area that used to receive such information from the lost limb. The rest of the brain, however, has not yet "learned" the change in the meaning of the input to this part of the cortex and still interprets it as a touch to the hand. Experiments with monkeys, in which a single finger is temporarily paralyzed by a cuff of TTX on the nerve, have shown that there is a rapid reorganization of the somatosensory map in the cortex. Within days, the representation of the insensitive finger shrinks and the representation of the neighboring fingers expands (Merzenich and Jenkins, 1993). These cortical changes in the representation of somatotopy can be extremely large even in normal animals, as was revealed by an unusual experiment at the National Institutes of

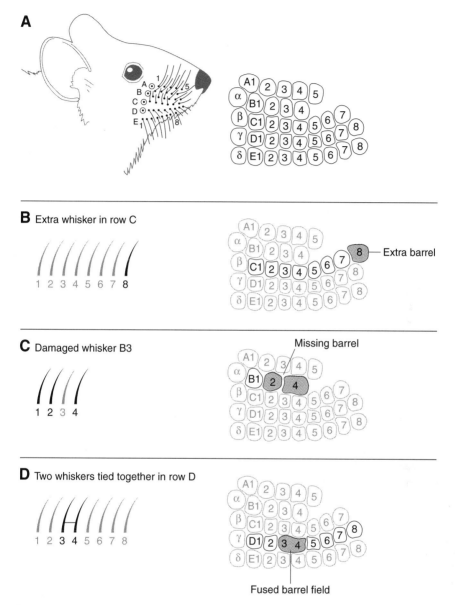

Figure 6.13 Plasticity of the mouse barrel field in the somatosensory cortex. (A) The correspondence between bristles and barrel field in the cortex of a normal mouse. (B) An extra whisker in row C leads to the formation of an extra barrel in the appropriate location in the cortex. (C) Neonatal damage to the B3 whisker causes the shrinkage of this barrel and the expansion of neighboring ones. (D) Tying two whiskers together causes their barrel field to coalesce (Woolsey and Van der Loos, 1970).

Health. Anti-vivisectionists stole a set of experimental monkeys after their somatosensory cortex was first mapped, and the monkeys were not recovered until about 10 years later. When the scientists remapped their somatosensory cortices, they found that the extent of the rearrangement was dramatic, a matter of tens of millimeters (Palca, 1991; Pons *et al.*, 1991). Thus, minor

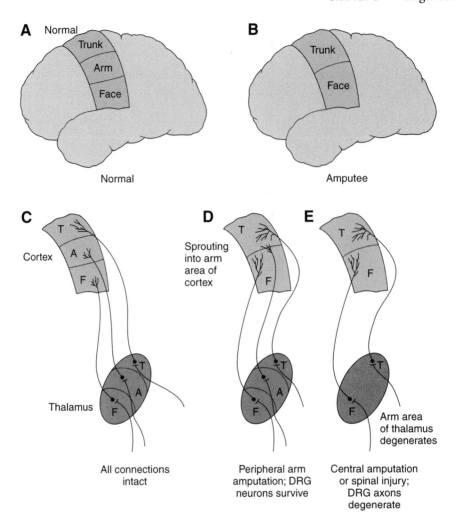

Figure 6.14 Large-scale plasticity in the somatosensory cortex. (A) The normal organization of the cortical topography in the somatosensory system. (B) Damage to the arm may result in large-scale reorganization of the cortical map. (C) There is an isomorphic mapping of the somatosensory thalamus onto the primary cortex. (D) When the arm is damaged peripherally and the sensory neurons in the DRG survive, the reorganization is cortical rather than thalamic. (E) When the damage is more central causing the DRG cells to degenerate, both the thalamus and the cortex get reorganized (Adapted from Merzenich, *Science* **282,** 1062–1063. Copyright 1998 American Association for the Advancement of Science. Credit: K. Sutliff).

reorganization of the cortical somatosensory map is happening throughout life, and is presumably influenced by experience and activity. Even normal use can change topographic representations in an impressive way. Monkeys were trained to use just one fingertip to feel textural differences for a few hours a day over a period of months. The result was a hugely expanded cortical representation of that fingertip with respect to its neighbors (Recanzone *et al.,* 1992). We examine

the cellular mechanisms underlying these changes in a later chapter.

Visual Maps and the Theory of Chemospecificity

In the early 1940s, Roger Sperry cut the optic nerve of a newt, rotated the detached eye 180° in its orbit, and assayed the visuomotor behavior of the animal after its nerve had regenerated. The newts, and in subsequent studies, frogs, behaved as if their visual world were back-to-front and upside-down: when a lure was presented in front of them "they wheeled rapidly to the rear instead of striking forward..." and when the lure was presented above "the animals struck downward in front of them and got a mouthful of mud and moss," (Sperry, 1943) (Fig. 6.15). This led him to propose that topographic nerve connections between the retina and its main central target, the optic tectum, were the result of anatomical rather than experiential features of the nervous system. These experiments invalidated the then prevailing notion that the brain could learn to sort out jumbled connections into appropriate pathways by behavioral feedback. Sperry's unlucky frogs never did learn to snap in the correct direction. Sperry reasoned that the retinal fibers mapped onto the tectum according to original anatomical coordinates of the eye. The explanation he gave was the possible existence of biochemical tags across the retina and the tectum. He envisaged that cells in the retina and their postsynaptic partners in the tectum acquire a matching set of affinities, or cytochemical tags, during development and that retinal ganglion cell fibers are guided to the appropriate tectal areas according to these complementary affinities. He postulated the existence of two or more cytochemical gradients "that spread across and through each other with their axes roughly perpendicular. These separate gradients successively superimposed on the retinal and tectal fields and surroundings would stamp each cell with its appropriate latitude and longitude expressed in a kind of chemical code with matching values between retinal and tectal maps" (Sperry, 1963).

Various alternative ideas were put forward to challenge Sperry's chemospecificity hypothesis. One simple mechanism for creating an ordered map is to merely preserve the organization of the axons from the retina to the tectum. In the optic nerves of certain fish, retinal fibers are precisely ordered according to retinal position, so that the map is already formed in the nerve. *In vitro* studies have shown that axons from the temporal retina tend to stick together and to avoid nasal fibers (Bonhoeffer and Huf, 1985). These studies support the idea that fiber order is an important mapping mechanism. However, in many vertebrates the optic nerve appears to be topographically disordered, suggesting that the preservation of specific neighbors in the axons developing optic projection can not be the key to map formation. In all vertebrates examined there is a dramatic reorganization of fibers as they leave the optic nerve and enter the brain. In *Xenopus,* it is possible to transplant half eyes and thus make animals, that have duplicated retinas such as dorsal–dorsal retinas or ventral–ventral retinas. Normally, the optic tract bifurcates into medial and lateral branches (or brachia) close to the tectum with axons from ventral retina traveling in the medial brachium and those from dorsal retina in the lateral brachium. Fibers from double ventral eyes all enter the medial brachium and the lateral brachium fails to form (Fawcett and Gaze, 1982) (Fig. 6.16). Thus it seems that the tips of retinal axons make step-by-step decisions about their position as they extend through the neuroepithelium and map onto the tectum. Axon tracing techniques have shown that regenerating retinal axons, despite being completely disorganized as they enter the target, take quite circuitous and abnormal routes to arrive at the appropriate tectal position (Fujisawa, 1981). Therefore, although fiber ordering may help, it certainly does not explain topographic mapping in this system.

Another mechanism that could create order in the projection is to keep the axons sorted by their time of arrival at the tectum. In many vertebrates, there is a temporal gradient of differentiation in the retina, often central to peripheral. In goldfish, this order is striking as their eyes grow throughout life, adding new rings of cells at the margins. Axons of ganglion cells of the same age tend to fasciculate and grow together to the tectum, which is also growing at its caudal peripheral edges. Thus arriving axons map onto the perimeter of the tectum in orderly age-related fascicles, making it possible to imagine that the time of axon ingrowth is an important cue for the origins of the map (Stuermer and Easter, 1984).

This idea has been tested in Xenopus retinae (Holt, 1984). Here, dorsal axons grow out first,

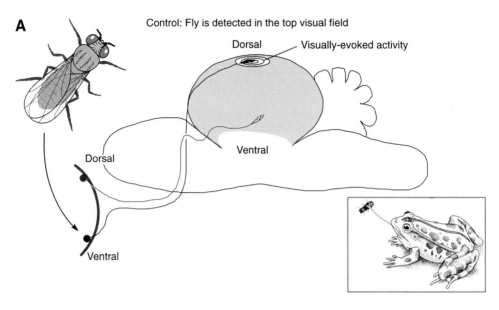

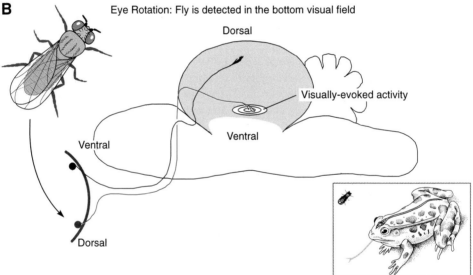

Figure 6.15 The preservation of maladaptive topography. (A) A normal frog sees a fly above its head because the image falls on the ventral retina. The image is relayed to the dorsal tectum by retinal axons. Thus, a hungry frog will jump in the appropriate upward direction. (B) A frog with a rotated eye receives the same fly image on what used to be the dorsal retina. Retinal axons from this part of the eye project to the ventral tectum. Thus, the frog leaps in the wrong downward direction away from the actual position of the fly (Sperry, 1943).

pioneering the way to the tectum and innervating the lateral neuropil which happens to be closest. Ventral axons start out later, arrive later, and, perhaps finding the lateral sites already occupied, travel further to synapse with the next closest available sites in the medial regions of the tectum. Experiments, however, show that the consequences of this temporal gradient from

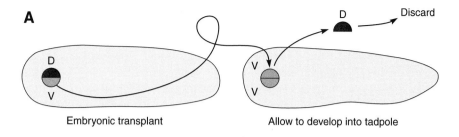

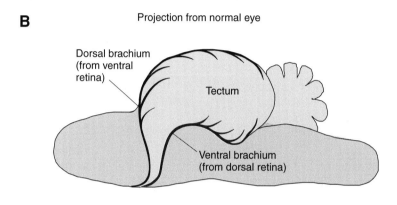

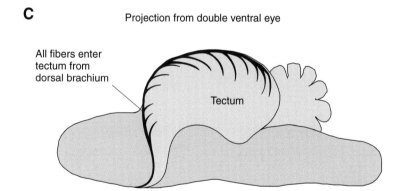

Figure 6.16 Topography in the pathway. (A) Transplantation of a ventral half eye bud from a donor embryo in place of a dorsal half eye bud in a host embryo leads to a double ventral eye. (B) In the normal frog, fibers from the ventral retina enter the tectum via the dorsal brachium whereas fibers from the dorsal retina enter the tectum from the ventral brachium. (C) In the brains of double ventral eyed animals all retinal fibers enter the tectum via the dorsal brachium (Fawcett and Gaze, 1982).

dorsal to ventral are insignificant to axonal navigation and targeting. Specifically, when a dorsal half retina is transplanted from a younger to an older embryo, the dorsal axons are relatively delayed so that they follow rather than precede ventral axons. Therefore, the axons from both dorsal retina and ventral retina innervate the tectum in accordance with their position in the retina rather than their time of arrival in the tectum (Fig. 6.17).

Thus, spatial and chronological ordering of axons on route to the tectum does not appear to be critical to map formation in the target. Instead, there are several pieces of evidence that demonstrate that the tectum is intrinsically labeled as Sperry suggested. First, when a small piece of tectum is rotated, regenerating retinal fibers recognize this piece as rotated and map onto it according to its original orientation, showing that labels of some sort do exist on tectal cells (Yoon, 1975). Second, regenerating and developing retinal axons map correctly when forced to grow onto a previously uninnervated tectum, showing that retinal axons do not just brand tectal cells with their own label, and when regenerating find their own marking (Feldman *et al.,* 1971; Harris, 1982). Third, rostral and caudal membrane stripes from uninnervated tectum can serve as differential substrates for the growth of temporal and nasal axons (Walter *et al.,* 1987). Fourth, as we see below, the orientation of the tectum can be reversed by embryological or genetic manipulation long before innervation. From these various studies, the picture emerges that the formation of the retinotectal map depends on the intrinsic initial polarity of both the retina and the tectum. The crucial determinants are the original position of a retinal ganglion cell in the eye field and the original position of a target cell within the tectal field.

To establish when the topographic map first arises, neuroanatomical fiber tracing and physiological recordings have been performed on younger and younger embryos. In frogs and zebrafish, such studies show that there is order in the very earliest projection to the tectum (Holt and Harris, 1983; Stuermer, 1988). Early terminal arbors of individual RGCs stretch over a large extent of the tectum in *Xenopus,* but as the tectum grows the overlap of retina terminals decreases and the map becomes increasingly refined (Sakaguchi and Murphey, 1985). Interestingly, this is not done by pruning down the terminal arbors of the original innervating RGCs. In fact,

terminal arbors continue to expand with development. They do not, however, grow as fast as the tectum itself. The result is that individual terminal arbors occupy a decreasing fraction of the tectal neuropil and make contact with a small ratio of possible target cells as development proceeds. Thus, tectal polarity and positional identity are present from the earliest stages of normal retinotectal projection, but become refined with development. The next questions that arise are: How do these structures get this positional information? What is the molecular nature of this information?

Determination of Retinotopic Identity

To understand when pre- and postsynaptic populations establish their positional identity, the effects of rotating the retina or the tectum at early stages of development have been explored. When similar experiments were done with limb buds, it was found that rotations at a very early stage were followed by complete regulation, and the limb developed normally. A similar rotation slightly later produced a limb with just one axis inverted and the other regulated, while a still later rotation, after both axes had been fixed, produced a totally inverted limb.

At first, it appeared that something similar was going on with the eye bud (Hunt and Jacobson, 1974). But these experiments could not be replicated and a consensus of results from rotations of the eye in several species of lower vertebrates showed that the eye is polarized with respect to its dorsoventral and nasotemporal axes at very early stages (Sharma and Hollyfield, 1980). In fact, eye rotations in *Xenopus* show that the retinal axes are specified as early as anyone has been able to rotate the eye bud, which is soon after closure of the neural tube and long before the cells in the retina are even born. It has even been reported that single retinal precursors transplanted to different retinal locations retain their original retinotectal specificity, suggesting that they have inherited positional values in a

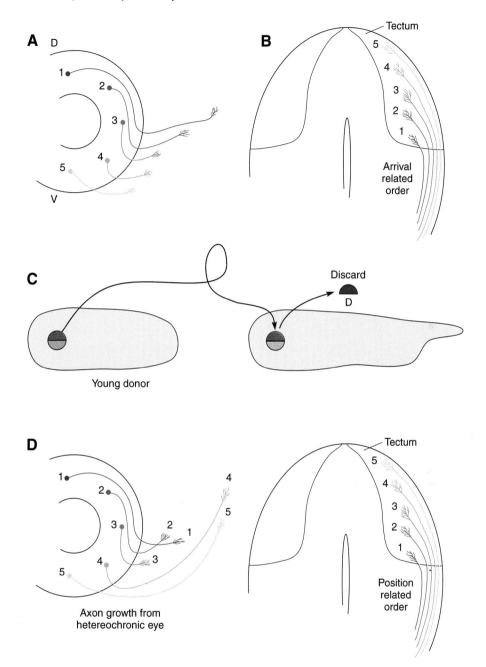

Figure 6.17 Topographic connections with heterochronic innervation. (A) In a normal *Xenopus* embryo retinal ganglion cells from the dorsal retina grow out of the eye first and innervate the lateral tectum. Axons from the ventral retina grow later and behind the dorsal axons, and when they reach the tectum they innervate the medial part. (B) An experimental heterochronic embryo in which a young dorsal half eye has been transplanted to an older ventral half. (C and D) The result is that now ventral axons lead dorsal axons to the tectum. When they arrive, however, normal topographic mapping is immediately established (Holt, 1984).

rather stable way. What about the tectum? Here the story is different. Tectal transplants done at Embryonic Day 2 in chicks generally reverse their rostrocaudal axis as assessed by the patterns of tectal histogenesis and the orientation of the retinotectal map, but those that are done at Embryonic Day 3 retain their original polarity (Itasaki and Nakamura, 1992) (Fig. 6.18). It may be that the retinal axes are specified earlier than it has been possible to rotate the eye primordium. Perhaps we would do better to examine the mechanism rather than the timing of positional specification.

What is the nature of the polarizing signals? Current thinking is that retinal and tectal positional information may originate with the positional information genes that are turned on during gastrulation and neurulation or even earlier, when the dorsoventral and anteroposterior axes of the embryo are first set up (see Chapter 2). Retinoic acid (RA) has been implicated in helping to set up the retinal axis (McCaffery and Drager, 1993). Duplicated eyes with two ventral but no dorsal halves result from treatment of the late gastrula or early neural plate in *Xenopus* and zebrafish with retinoic acid (RA) suggesting that the dorsal–ventral axis may be set up by this type of signaling pathway (Manns and Fritzsch, 1991; Hyatt *et al.,* 1996) (Chapter 2). In the developing retina, there is a strong dorsal to ventral gradient of one form of aldehyde dehydrogenase, a key enzyme in the manufacture of RA. Dorsal retinal cells have been shown to be a much richer source of RA than ventral cells. When zebrafish embryos are exposed to pharmacological agents that interfere with this enzyme they exhibit defects in the genesis of the dorsal retina (Marsh-Armstrong *et al.,* 1994).

Several genes are expressed differentially along the nasotemporal (anterior–posterior) axis in the embryonic chicken retina. Among these are two molecules called BF-1 and BF-2 that belong to a particular family of homeobox-containing transcription factors called the *winged–helix* factors because of their proposed structure (Hatini *et al.,* 1994). They are expressed in nonoverlapping regions of the eye: BF-1 in the anterior or

nasal half and BF-2 in the posterior or temporal half. Misexpression of either factor causes RGCs to project to incorrect locations along the rostrocaudal axis of the tectum (Yuasa *et al.,* 1996). Thus, topographical expression of these transcription factors appears to control formation of the retinotectal map by giving nasal or temporal identity to the retinal cells. Similarly, other transcription factors are found in dorsal to ventral gradients and these may have roles in setting the positional information in this axis.

Polarity in the tectum appears to come about as a result of another homeobox transcription factor, *engrailed* (En), which is normally expressed at highest levels in the posterior tectum and anterior cerebellum (Itasaki *et al.,* 1991). In optic tecta that are grafted to an anterior location in the diencephalon of chick embryos, the gradient of En expression is reversed, and the strength of expression depends on the distance from the mesencephalic–diencephalic junction (Martinez and Alvarado-Mallart, 1990; Itasaki and Nakamura, 1992) (Fig. 6.19). In these animals, retinal axons projecting to the ectopic tectum follow the gradient of En expression. That is, axons from temporal retina project to the tectal region exhibiting the least *engrailed* staining, while axons from nasal retina project to tectal regions expressing more En (Itasaki and Nakamura, 1992). To establish a direct link between *engrailed* expression and retinotopy, a retroviral vector encoding the *engrailed* gene was used to infect the tectum and produce animals that had high levels of ectopic En expression throughout the tectum. In these brains, the nasal fibers that normally terminate in the posterior tectum instead arborize at ectopic sites in the anterior tectum (Itasaki and Nakamura, 1996). Temporal fibers that normally synapse on anterior neurons failed to innervate the tectum and often degenerated. This series of experiments shows that En expression level is tightly linked to retinotopy and strongly suggests a causal relationship between En and retinotectal topography.

Tectal transplants reveal that *engrailed* expression is regulated in part by an activating influence emanating from the hindbrain. The region of the brain with the strongest En-inducing ca-

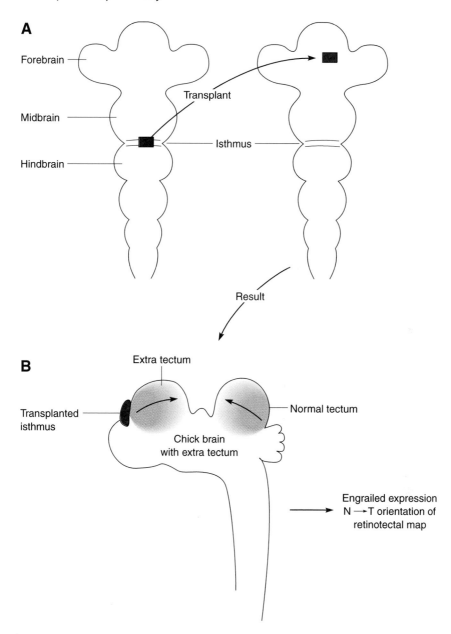

Figure 6.18 Induction of an ectopic midbrain in a chick embryo. (A) Part of the isthmus at the mid-hindbrain junction is transplanted into the forebrain of a host embryo. (B) As a result of the transplant an ectopic extra tectum is formed with reversed AP polarity, both in terms of *engrailed* expression and retinotectal mapping (Martinez and Alvarado-Mallart, 1990; Itasaki *et al.,* 1991).

pacity is the junction between the midbrain and the hindbrain, called the isthmus (Martinez *et al.,* 1991). When this region is transplanted by itself it induces En expression in nearby tissue and can even induce an entire ectopic tectum out of forebrain tissue, acting as a sort of organizer. A

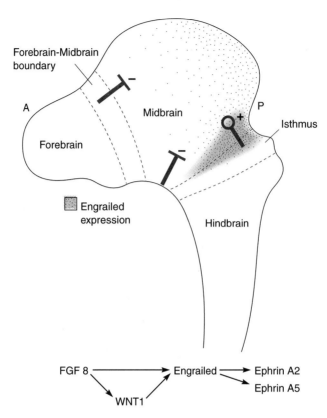

Figure 6.19 Influences on tectal AP polarity. The isthmus by means of FGF8 and Wnt1 expression turns on *engrailed* in the posterior tectum. The forebrain–midbrain boundary and the floor plate by means of unknown factors repress *engrailed* expression rostrally and ventrally. The resulting *engrailed* gradient in the dorsal midbrain positively regulates the ephrin ligands that are critical for retinotectal mapping (Retaux and Harris, 1996).

molecule that is expressed first in the mesoderm and then in the overlying isthmus, FGF8, has midbrain inducing and polarizing effects. Beads soaked in FGF8 and implanted into the forebrain induce ectopic En expression in the caudal diencephalon and cause a mirror image duplication of the mesencephalon (Crossley *et al.*, 1996). The fact that FGF8 is sufficient to induce En expression, together with the observation that FGF8 is expressed in mesoderm underlying the neural plate at a stage before En induction, suggests that mesodermal FGF8 could be the inducer of isthmic En expression. The isthmus also expresses the secreted molecule Wnt1, the vertebrate homolog of *Drosophila wingless* and the best-known regulator of En expression in flies.

Wnt1 knockout mice progressively lose En expression which suggests that Wnt-1 is involved in En maintenance (Danielian and McMahon, 1996). The forebrain–midbrain junction has a negative influence on En expression (Itasaki *et al.*, 1991). This was demonstrated in experiments in which En expression in posterior midbrain was downregulated when it was transplanted next to this junction. The floor plate and notochord also suppress En expression, as seen when En-expressing midbrain is transplanted near this tissue (Darnell and Schoenwolf, 1995). Clearly, the pattern of *engrailed* expression is highly regulated by extrinsic factors that we are beginning to understand and trace the origins of in the developing embryo (Fig. 6.19).

Engrailed is a transcription factor that by itself cannot steer axons within the tectum, but must somehow regulate the graded expression of effector chemospecificity molecules that Sperry first hypothesized were on cell surfaces. Many molecules have been discovered that may play such a role, but few have been proven to be involved. For instance, monoclonal antibodies were used to find an antigen called TOP_{DV}, a membrane protein that is 40-fold more concentrated in the dorsal than in the ventral retina and 10-fold higher in the lateral than in the medial tectum. TOP_{AP} is another such molecule with higher expression in the temporal retina and anterior tectum (Trisler, 1990). Such reciprocal gradients of potentially homophilic molecules could well support the formation of a topographic map from the retina to the tectum, but no studies with these molecules have yet revealed such a function.

A more successful functional approach to identifying the relevant molecules used membranes from anterior and posterior parts of the tectum to make a striped carpet. When retinal tissue is grown on such a carpet, nasal retinal axons grow preferentially on posterior tectal membranes, and temporal retinal axons grow preferentially on anterior tectal membranes (Walter *et al.*, 1987b) (Fig. 6.20). Surprisingly, when the posterior membrane fragment is heated, or exposed to an enzyme (PI–PLC) that removes phosphotidyl-inosotol (PI)-linked membrane molecules, temporal axons no longer avoid caudal membranes (Walter *et al.*, 1987a, 1990). This suggests that the relevant activity is proteinaceous, membrane-linked, and repulsive to temporal axons. Nasal axons are rather insensitive to this inhibitory factor. By examining the choices that temporal axons make between membranes extracted from successive rostrocaudal sixths of the tectum, it became clear that this inhibitory activity is graded. Temporal axons challenged with a gradient of the posterior membranes, steered away, slowed down, and stopped when they encountered increasing concentrations (Baier and Bonhoeffer, 1992). These experiments suggest that this graded activity, by itself, is capable of guiding temporal axons to the posterior tectum and thus contributing to topographic map formation. Using this assay, a 33-kDa GPI-linked repulsive guiding molecule (RGM) was partially purified. The role of this 33-kDa protein was examined with chromophore assisted laser inactivation (CALI) studies (Stahl *et al.*, 1990; Muller *et al.*, 1996). In this technique, malachite green-labeled antibodies are allowed to bind to RGM and were then blasted with a laser to produce intense fluorescence in the malachite green. The fluorescence produces a very localized concentration of oxygen radicals that is thought to destroy neighboring molecules. When RGM is inactivated in this manner, temporal axons grow onto posterior stripes.

Two other repulsive factors RAGS and ELF1 (now called ephrin A5 and ephrin A2) have also been implicated in the rostrocaudal mapping in the retinotectal system (Cheng *et al.*, 1995; Drescher *et al.*, 1995). The Eph family of tyrosine kinase receptors is the largest known family of such receptors and is expressed in complex patterns throughout the nervous system. Ligands come in two subfamilies, GPI-linked or A type and transmembrane or B type, as do their receptors. All the members of A-type ligands are able to activate all the members of A-type receptors, while each of the B-type ligands can activate all of the B-type receptors (Flanagan and Vanderhaeghen, 1998). Throughout the nervous system, one finds reciprocal arrangements of A-type ligands with A-type receptors and B-type ligands with B-type receptors. Besides the tectum, these ligand–receptor interactions have been implicated in axon growth and targeting in various other systems such as the hippocampus. The promiscuity between various receptors and ligands does not necessarily indicate a lack of specificity because of the differential affinities of the receptors for the ligands within a subfamily. That the CNS is painted with rich patterns of these ligands and receptors suggests that these molecules are involved in axonal targeting and topography in many parts of the nervous system.

Both ephrin A5 and ephrin A2 are ligands for EphA tyrosine kinases and are expressed in a posterior (high) to anterior (low) gradient in the tectum or superior colliculus (Fig. 6.21). The

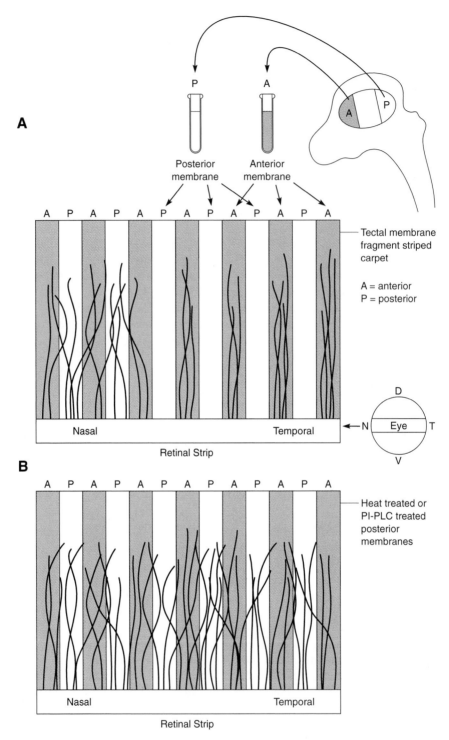

Figure 6.20 The striped carpet assay. (A) An equatorial strip of retina spanning the nasal (N)–temporal (T) extent is positioned on a striped carpet of alternating anterior, (A) and posterior (P) tectal membranes. The nasal fibers from the retinal explant grow on both A and P tectal membranes but the temporal fibers grow only on the A membranes. (B) If the tectal membranes are denatured or treated with PI–PLC, which releases PI-linked membrane proteins, the temporal axons also grow on both types of membranes, suggesting that the P membranes normally have a PI-linked repulsive guidance molecule (Walter *et al.,* 1987a,b,1990).

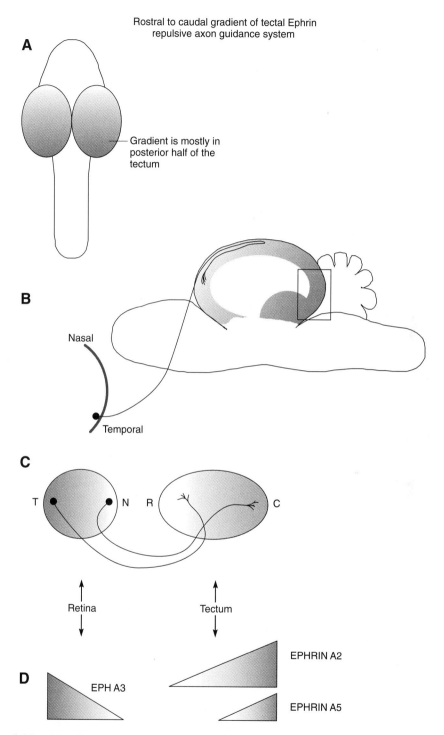

Figure 6.21 AP retinotopic guidance system. (A) There is a gradient of ephrins in the tectum, high in the posterior pole and low in the anterior pole. (B) A retinal ganglion cell in the temporal retina expresses active receptors for these tectal ephrins and avoids the posterior tectum. (C, D) Opposing gradients of active EphA receptor expressed in the retina and the gradients of A-type ephrins in the tectum. This system can at least partially account for topographic mapping in this axis (Cheng *et al.,* 1995; Drescher *et al.,* 1995).

ephrin A5 (RAGS), expressed primarily on tectal glia, was found in a search for PI-linked membrane proteins expressed more on posterior than on anterior membranes (Drescher *et al.,* 1995), while ephrin A2 (ELF1), expressed primarily on posterior tectal neurons, was found in a search for ligands of Mek4 (EphA3) which is expressed in many places in the brain, including the retina (Cheng *et al.,* 1995). EphA3 is a receptor for both ligands but has 10-fold higher affinity for ephrin A5 than for ephrin A2 (Monschau *et al.,* 1997). Temporal axons that have high levels of EphA3 avoid the posterior pole of the tectum that has the highest level of the ephrin ligands to this receptor. When viruses carrying genes for these ligands are used to overexpress ephrin A2 across the entire tectum in chick embryos, temporal axons fail to make terminal arbors in the tectum. When membrane stripes are made from the anterior tectal cells transfected with ephrin A2, temporal axons will not grow on them. When ephrin A5 is knocked out, temporal axons invade posterior tectum and some retinal axons leave the posterior border of the tectum altogether, showing that this molecule also has a role as an exit barrier from the target (Frisen *et al.,* 1998). Thus there appear to be at least three repulsive molecules, RGM, ephrin A2, and ephrin A5, involved in the proper mapping of temporal axons. Now that we have identified some of the tectal factors involved, we can ask if they are regulated by *engrailed* in the expected way. Misexpression studies with *engrailed* show that high levels of *engrailed* across the tectum lead to matching high levels of ephrin A5 and ephrin A2, and, as expected, topographical defects in the retinotectal projection occur, with temporal retinal axons avoiding anterior tectum (Friedman and O'Leary, 1996; Logan *et al.,* 1996).

We might imagine that there are similar graded repulsive activities for nasal axons and, although ephrins and their receptors have not been shown to be involved in the formation of the dorsoventral axis of the retinotectal map, at least one ephrin receptor, EphB2, has been found in a ventral (high) to dorsal (low) gradient in the retina, while its ligand ephrin b1 is found in a medial (high) to lateral (low) gradient in the tectum, suggesting that such molecules might be involved in this axis of the map as well (Braisted *et al.,* 1997; Holash *et al.,* 1997). In addition to repulsive factors, evidence suggests that there are also attractive or adhesive factors that help stick nasal retinal fibers to posterior tectal membranes, temporal to anterior tectal membranes, and so on. So, although we are beginning to understand the molecular basis of retinotopy in the tectum, there are lots of molecules involved in this process that we have yet to identify and understand.

Recently, a genetic approach has been taken to the study of topography in the visual system using zebrafish. Zebrafish males were treated with a chemical mutagen and then mated with nonmutant females. Separate lines were founded from individual offspring that could be tested in the F3 generation with one quarter of the fish having the possibility of uncovering a recessive phenotype. A rapid method of displaying retinotectal topography was employed in which DiI was injected into the dorsonasal retina and DiA was injected into the ventrotemporal retina. By screening about eight fish per family from several thousand families, dozens of mutants with affected retinotectal projection were recovered (Baier *et al.,* 1996). The mutations define genetically distinct steps in this process. Some affect pathfinding between the eye and the tectum, while others affect map formation in the tectum (Karlstrom *et al.,* 1996; Trowe *et al.,* 1996). Interestingly, mutations that disturb axon pathfinding to the tectum do not disrupt retinotopic mapping, and vice versa, suggesting that the process of targeting is molecularly distinct from that of pathfinding.

Mutations in two genes, *nevermind* and *who-cares,* affect the dorsoventral patterning of the projection. In embryos homozygous for either of these mutations, axons from dorsal retinal ganglion cells terminate both ventrally and dorsally in the tectum. In *nevermind,* the retinotopic order of axons along the optic nerve and tract is changed as well, suggesting, perhaps, that the axons themselves are totally confused about their topographic identities. Mutants in two other genes, *gnarled* and *macho,* affect the anteroposterior patterning of the projection. In these mutants, dorsonasal axons branch and ter-minate too soon in the anterior tectum (Fig. 6.22). Mutations of six other genes lead retinal axons to form abnormal terminal fields in the

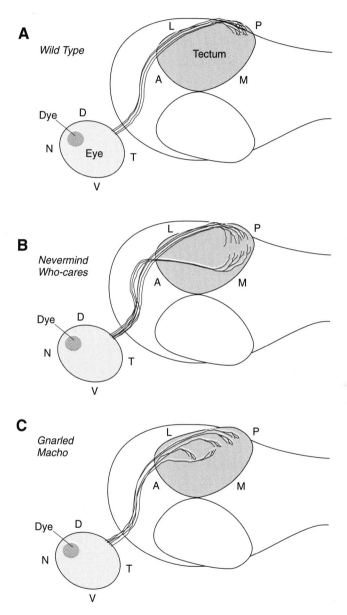

Figure 6.22 Fish mutants with retinotectal mapping problems. (A) In wild-type fish axons labeled in the nasal dorsal retina project to the lateral posterior tectum. (B) In *nevermind* and *who-cares* mutants, there is a problem with the DV axis and the same axons terminate both laterally and medially. (C) In *gnarled* and *macho* mutants, there is more of an AP problem, and the same axons terminate in both the anterior and the posterior tectum (Trowe *et al.,* 1996).

tectum. The molecular defects that these mutants encode is not yet known and awaits the cloning of the associated genes. Because this particular screen was part of a larger screen for embryonic defects, most of the retinotectal mutants have other defects in body or brain formation. This suggests that genes used in topographic map formation in the visual pathway are pleiotropic and essential for other aspects of development. It also leaves open the possibility, however, that there are other genes that are essential for and primarily involved in map formation that have not been identified and still others which when mutant show no phenotype because of functional molecular redundancy in the system. In the later case, the lack of some component of the topography system is covered for by another molecule that can do a similar job. If this were the case, then a single mutant screen would clearly not uncover these genes.

Shifting Connections, Fine Tuning, and Registration

While correct in the broad sense, Sperry's idea that the topography of the retina and the tectum is specified by stable chemical differences on the surfaces of the cells, has some shortcomings. Consider the case of a goldfish. It hatches as a tiny 1-mg animal and over the course of its life, if it is nurtured in flowing water, may attain a weight of 1 kg. It has increased in mass a millionfold. As the animal grows, the retina grows in proportion, by adding cells circumferentially at the rim or margin. The tectum grows as well, but mostly at the caudal end. In order for the retinotectal map to remain evenly distributed, the retinal axons must continually break their connections from one set of postsynaptic cells and move posteriorly across the tectum (Gaze *et al.,* 1979). For example, axons from the center of a large adult retina were born first when the fish was just a small larva (Fig. 6.23). These axons initially project to target neurons at the center of the larval tectum. However, these tectal neurons become limited to the ante-

rior pole of the tectum as new tectal cells are added caudally. Thus, these central retinal axons have continued to switch their preferred targets to more posterior tectal cells throughout the animal's lifetime (Easter and Stuermer, 1984). This fact is not easily reconciled with stable chemical cues.

A similar type of shifting reorganization of connections is evident when half of the retina or half of the tectum of a fish is ablated. When half the retina is ablated the remaining half retina's projection expands to cover the entire tectum. When half the tectum is removed, the retina's projection compresses to cover the remaining half (Schmidt, 1978; Schmidt and Coen, 1995). This sort of regulation is also observed in neonatal hamsters with a partially deleted superior colliculus (Fig. 6.23). This form of topographic expansion or compression, like the natural shift that is a consequence of the asymmetric growth of the tectum, does not depend on the activity patterns in retinal fibers. The regulation can occur in the dark or even in the continuous presence of TTX (Meyer and Wolcott, 1987). The distribution of ephrins has not been checked in these cases, so it is possible that the chemospecificity cues do change as a result of such operations. Another possible explanation is that retinal fibers tend to spread out evenly over the tectal surface using some form of fiber–fiber repulsion. Thus, even if the position cue is not an ideal match, as occurs following ablation, the ingrowing fibers will, nevertheless, tend to occupy all available tectal space by repelling each other.

These shifting connections are part of a larger developmental phenomenon whereby once a topographic map is established it is adjusted, modified, and fine-tuned. The projections from eye to midbrain in the chick and the rat are well ordered from the outset, yet some nasal and temporal axons overshoot their topographic targets. Subsequently, these connections are refined as the retinal fibers elaborate sidebranches in the vicinity of their appropriate targets and withdraw the inappropriate projections. Temporal retinal fibers in culture prefer to branch on anterior tectal membranes, suggesting that the appropriate tectal area may induce terminal field branches

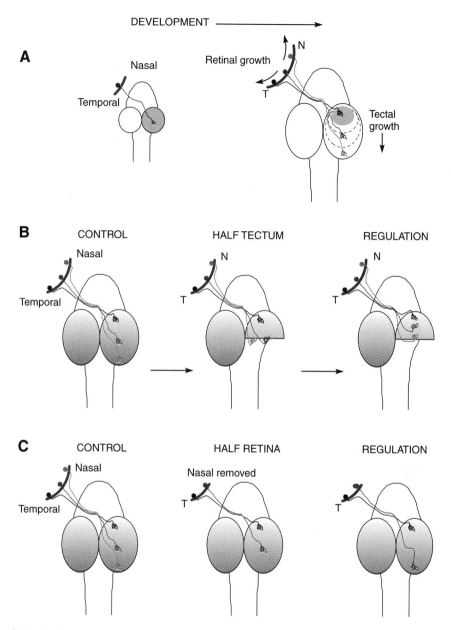

Figure 6.23 Shifting connections. (A) During the lifetime of a frog or fish, its eye and brain continues to grow. The retina grows circumferentially like a tree, but the tectum grows in expanding posterior crescents. As a result new retina that is added temporally must send axons to the anterior primordial tectum, while fibers from the central primordial retina must shift posteriorly, and new nasal fibers map to the new posterior tectum in order to keep the map in topographic order. (B) If half the tectum is removed from a fish, after about a month the retinotopic map will regulate and compress, mapping out evenly over the remaining half tectum. (C) Similar regulation occurs when half the retina is removed. The remaining projection eventually expands over the whole tectum (Schmidt, 1978; Gaze *et al.*, 1979; Schmidt and Coen, 1995).

(Roskies and O'Leary, 1994). A similar phenomenon has been observed along the mediolateral axis. Such corrections were first observed in the regenerating optic nerve fibers of fish and amphibians. Unlike the shifting described connections above, this type of refinement in the topography of the map, especially during regeneration, is dependent on activity. Without impulse activity, the map may be roughly topographic, but the size of the receptive fields recorded at a single site become larger and less precise than normal. Analysis of individual retinal axonal arbors shows that they are up to four times as large as normal ones (Schmidt and Buzzard, 1990). Similar effects arise when regenerating fish are kept in a stroboscopic environment, which shows that it is not activity per se but the pattern of firing that is responsible for fine tuning and arbor restriction (Schmidt and Eisele, 1985; Cook and Rankin, 1986) (Chapter 9).

The mapping of retinal projections onto the tectum is often in spatial register with the afferents from other sensory modalities that also project onto the midbrain, including, for example, the auditory and somatosensory systems (Drager and Hubel, 1975). This registration of inputs may be crucial to the animal's ability to form a coherent map of the world that can be transmitted to the motor system for orientation movements. Predictable orientation movements are evoked by electrical stimulation to a specific area of the superior colliculus. When the auditory and somatosensory fields were mapped on the tectum of eyeless mice and salamanders, the orientation of each sensory field was organized correctly, even though there was no retinal input (Drager and Hubel, 1978; Harris, 1982). This suggests that each set of afferents respond to the intrinsic polarity of the tectum. Thus, if the eye of a ferret is deflected during development, there is an immediate misregistration of the visual and auditory maps, but over the course of weeks the auditory map realigned with the visual one (King *et al.,* 1988). These studies show that the visual map is somehow dominant and can influence the auditory map. The visual map also seems to dominate or instruct the development of the auditory map in barn owls. A shift in the auditory map accomplished by the use of earplugs, or a shift in the visual map by the use of prisms, knocks the two maps out of alignment (Knudsen, 1991; Knudsen, 1985). If either of these manipulations is performed early in life, the auditory map slowly shifts to come into register with the visual map. Moreover, in owls blinded from birth, the auditory map of space on the tectum is poorly organized (Chapter 9).

To summarize, the establishment of the appropriate topographic axes arises as a result of molecular gradients, such as the ephrins and their receptors. However, these cues are not absolute positional markers. Rather, a second mechanism tends to spread the afferents across the available target population. All this happens in the absence of synaptic activity. Thus, when lower vertebrates are raised in the continuous presence of TTX, the development of retinotectal projections proceeds normally, and the precision of the topography does not appear to be appreciably compromised. However, during the final stage of map formation, retinal arborizations are refined and this process requires synaptic activity.

Olfactory Maps

The map of olfactory receptors onto the brain has proven to be an elusive subject. In the vertebrate nervous system, olfactory receptors in the sensory epithelium send axons into the olfactory bulb where they make connections with second-order mitral and tufted cells in synaptic complexes called glomeruli. Activity measurements from the main olfactory bulb of vertebrates reveal that distinct odorants cause activity in distinct glomeruli, as if somehow information about a particular odor came to be processed in particular regions of the bulb. In the zebrafish, a careful anatomical study of the olfactory bulb has shown that, as in insects, there is an invariant pattern of about 80 glomeruli that have the same position and size from individual to individual (Baier and Korsching, 1994). This suggests that odorant coding may already be spatially segregated at the bulb. Indeed, glomeruli in certain positions are consistently activated by the application of specific odorants (Friedrich and Korsching, 1997). Thus, each odor causes a specific spatial constellation of activity in the bulb. In contrast, retrograde labeling studies show that the receptors projecting to a single glomerulus are scattered over the olfactory epithelium and there is no clear regionalization of odorant receptors on the sensory epithelium. Thus, point-to-point mapping does not occur as it does in the visual or somatosensory systems. Distributed spacing is seen by *in situ* hybridization for olfac-

tory neurons expressing the same odorant receptor mRNA (Buck and Axel, 1991). These two pieces of data indicate that olfactory neurons which respond to the same odor are scattered over the peripheral sensory epithelium and yet project to the same glomerulus (Fig. 6.24). In the mouse or rat there are about 1000 subtypes of sensory neurons, each expressing one specific odorant receptor.

Despite the fact that olfactory receptors of a particular type are spread out over the olfactory epithelium, there is, nevertheless, a rough

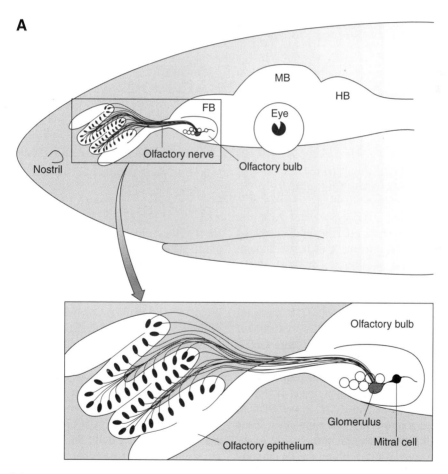

Figure 6.24 Olfactory mapping in a fish. (A) Olfactory receptors of the same type are spread out over the olfactory epithelium, but their axons all converge on a single glomerulus. (B) Comparison of topographic mapping in the visual system, where neighboring cells project to neighboring targets creating a central representation of visual space; and the olfactory system where cells of the same type are intermingled and yet their axons sort out and converge forming an odor representation map (Baier and Korsching, 1994).

B

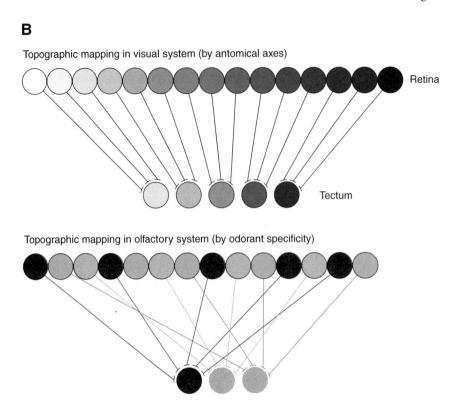

Figure 6.24 *(Continued)*

topography between the olfactory epithelium and the olfactory bulb in the rat. This has to do with zone-to-zone representation (Ressler *et al.*, 1993). Particular receptors that are expressed in specific zones of the epithelium project to a set of glomeruli within subregions of the bulb (Vassar *et al.*, 1994). Recent evidence suggests that several carbohydrates influence this zone-to-zone targeting. Subpopulations of olfactory sensory neurons express two carbohydrates present on NCAM, called NOC-3 and NOC-4 (Dowsing *et al.*, 1997). Some axons express both NOC-3 and NOC-4, while others express just one or neither. Thus NOC-3 and NOC-4 may be part of a combinatorial code used in establishing the topography of connections between the olfactory neuroepithelium and bulb. In fact removing the core protein has a significant effect on olfactory targeting. In mice lacking NCAM, many axons fail to exit the olfactory nerve fiber layer and stop

short of their glomerular targets. Another homophilic adhesion glycoprotein, OCAM, is also expressed on subsets of olfactory axons in a zone-specific manner (Yoshihara and Mori, 1997). The axons of sensory neurons expressing OCAM project to glomeruli in OCAM-expressing zones of the olfactory bulb, suggesting a role in zone-to-zone projection of the primary olfactory axons. Galectin-1 is a galactose-binding vertebrate lectin that is also expressed on subsets of cells in the olfactory system (Puche *et al.*, 1996). Mutants for Galectin-1 show topographical errors in the projection of sensory neurons to specific areas of the olfactory bulb. So, we might be able to account for zone-to-zone mapping through these homophilic adhesion systems, but what about the precise mapping?

Some of the mRNA for the olfactory receptor subtypes is found in the axons of these cells, so it is possible to use *in situ* analysis to study the spatial arrangement of the axons of a single class of receptor though the cells are scattered cells throughout the nasal epithelium. These studies confirm that scattered axons from a given receptor type converge onto topographically fixed glomeruli so that a consistent olfactory map is created in the brain (Vassar et al., 1994). Moreover, when one compares the two sides of the brain or the brains of two different animals, the position of the glomerulus that receives input from a particular subtype of olfactory receptors is preserved. So, although we can't name all the glomeruli in a mammal, we believe that, just as in fish, there is a conserved map and the glomeruli that serve the distinct odorant receptors create an olfactory map with fixed and highly specific topography. It is not known how this odor topography is further processed in the brain, but it appears that each glomerulus projects to several locations in the olfactory cortex and that each region of the olfactory cortex receives input from multiple glomeruli. Each region of the olfactory cortex may then receive convergent input from a unique combination of glomeruli to form a higher order map of odor quality (Axel, 1995).

To explain how receptors of a given class all find the right glomerulus, one might imagine that the expression of a receptor gene is be linked to the expression of particular guidance molecules. Another possibility, however, is that the odorant receptor molecules themselves are expressed on axonal growth cones and are involved in selecting the correct postsynaptic target area (Mombaerts et al., 1996). One can test this by following axons in which the odorant receptors are altered in transgenic animals and knockouts. First, what happens when a receptor is knocked out? Are the axons unable to find their targets? In these knockouts, the olfactory neurons express a bacterial marker enzyme (lacZ) that has been inserted into a specific receptor, (the lacZ gene has disrupted its function) but the cells do express lacZ and so can be identified anatomically. By examining the distribution of lacZ one can see how axons behave when they can no longer express the correct receptor. In such cases, the axons expressing lacZ appear

disoriented and do not converge on their target glomerulus or indeed on any glomerulus (Wang et al., 1998). This suggests that the olfactory receptors are indeed critical for accurate targeting in the bulb. Swapping receptors is the best way to test this (Mombaerts et al., 1996). So, in another set of experiments, a specific odorant receptor gene was replaced by a fusion gene driving not only lacZ but also the cDNA for a different receptor so that the axons misexpressing this receptor were easy to visualize (Fig. 6.25). Surprisingly, when olfactory neurons that target to distinct regions of the bulb have their receptors swapped, they target neither to their normal glomeruli (P2 in this case) nor to the glomeruli typical of their new odorant receptor. Instead, they map to a new specific glomerulus somewhere in between, suggesting that while odorant receptors do have some role in targeting there must be other factors that guide these axons to their particular targets. However, when receptors are swapped between sensory neurons that have nearby targets in the same region such as when the P3 receptor is expressed under the P2 promoter, the axons do target to a glomerulus in the exact vicinity of P3, proving that the odorant receptor is important for targeting to the right place (Wang et al., 1998). Just as their dendrites sniff the air, it seems that the growth cones of olfactory neurons use the same receptors to sniff their way inside the brain and home in on the appropriate glomerulus once they get close enough.

A similar situation exists in insects where the pattern of glomeruli may be very reproducible from individual to individual within a single species. This is particularly obvious in the male moth who has a specific set of olfactory receptors on the antenna that are involved in smelling the female pheromone bombykol. In the male moth's brain there is a distinct glomerulus, called the macroglomerular complex, that contains the synaptic terminals of all the bombykol-sensitive receptors. When tobacco hornworm moths (Manduca sexta) are tested in a wind tunnel with a source of female pheromones upwind, the males show pheromone-modulated anemotaxis. This is a characteristic mate-seeking

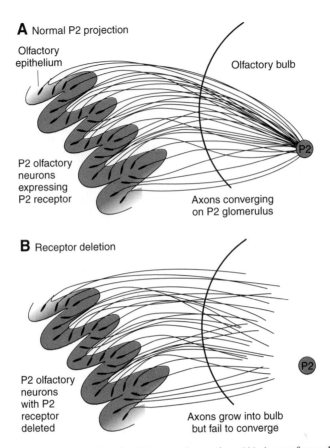

A Normal P2 projection

Olfactory
epithelium

Olfactory bulb

P2 olfactory
neurons
expressing
P2 receptor

Axons converging
on P2 glomerulus

P2

B Receptor deletion

P2 olfactory
neurons
with P2
receptor
deleted

Axons grow into bulb
but fail to converge

P2

Figure 6.25 Olfactory receptors are involved in central targeting. (A) Axons from olfactory neurons expressing the P2 receptor converge on the P2 glomerulus. (B) If the P2 receptor is deleted, these axons do not converge on any glomerulus. (C) If these neurons are made to express the M71 receptor instead of the P2 receptor, they converge on a glomerulus somewhere in between P2 and M71. (D) If they are forced to express the P3 receptor and the P3 glomerulus is in the same zone as the P2 glomerulus, they converge on a glomerulus right next to P3 (Mombaerts *et al.,* 1996; Wang *et al.,* 1998).

behavioral sequence initiated by stimulation of thesensory neurons found only in male antennae. To test the developmental relationship between specific sensory receptors and specific glomeruli, antennae were transplanted from male to female moths during pupal stages (Schneiderman *et al.,* 1986). In these cases, the female moths end up with antennal lobe interneurons that respond postsynaptically to stimulation with bombykol at the transplanted antennae. These interneurons branch into a region resembling the male-specific macroglomerular complex that is induced by the male receptors. Females with male antennae even respond to pheromonal stimulation with anemotaxis.

Computational Maps

The cochlea of the mammalian inner ear performs a spectral analysis of incoming sound. High sound frequencies activate hair cells at one end of the cochlea (the base), while low sound frequencies activate hair cells at the other end (the apex). Thus, instead of stimulus location in space, as is seen with the visual and somatosen-

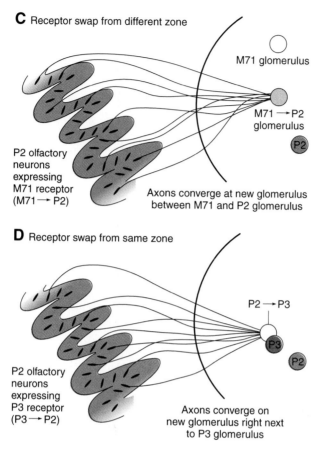

C Receptor swap from different zone

M71 glomerulus

M71 →P2 glomerulus

P2

P2 olfactory neurons expressing M71 receptor (M71 → P2)

Axons converge at new glomerulus between M71 and P2 glomerulus

D Receptor swap from same zone

P2 → P3

P3

P2

P2 olfactory neurons expressing P3 receptor (P3 → P2)

Axons converge on new glomerulus right next to P3 glomerulus

Figure 6.25 *(Continued)*

sory systems, it is the pitch of the stimulus that is mapped systematically across the receptor surface. This tonotopic organization maps onto higher order nuclei along the central auditory pathway up to and including the auditory cortex (Knudsen *et al.*, 1987).

In addition to this isomorphic cochleotopic map, which is a simple reflection of the spatial arrangement of cells on a sensory surface, the brain is capable of creating central maps that have no bearing to the spatial arrangement of receptors. Rather, these maps reflect some higher order processing of sensory information. A stunning example of these computational maps is found in the auditory cortex of mustached bats (Suga, 1989) (Fig. 6.26). Here, there are several maps based on echolocation, where neurons are

sensitive to two distinct signals one from an emitted sound and one from the echo of that sound. There is a map coding for the distance of a target, with neurons sensitive to short delays between the emitted sound and the echo (close objects) at one end of the cortical area and neurons sensitive to long delays (distant objects) at the other end. There is also a map of the relative speeds of the target based on the change in frequency that relative movement imparts to a sound by means of the Doppler effect. Neurons tuned to echoes that are higher in frequency than the emitted cry encode for approaching objects, while neurons that respond to frequencies lower than the emitted cry code for objects moving away. This speed axis is also mapped in the auditory cortex.

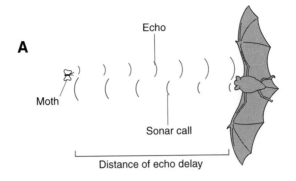

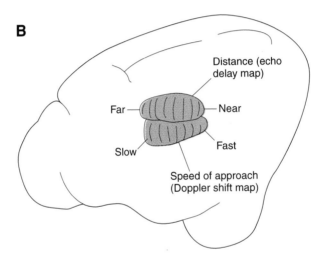

Figure 6.26 A computational map. (A) A bat detects a moth by processing echoes in its auditory cortex. (B) The distance of the moth is detected by the time delay between the call and the echo and mapped onto a near–far map in the auditory cortex. The speed that the bat is approaching the moth is detected by a Doppler shift in the echo and mapped onto a slow–fast map in the cortex (Suga, 1989).

In the barn owl, single neurons in the auditory midbrain receive afferent projections from brain stem neurons that are sensitive to interaural time and intensity differences. These neurons respond best to a particular azimuth due to their interaural time sensitivity and a particular elevation due to their interaural intensity sensitivity. These "space-sensitive" neurons are arranged systematically in the auditory midbrain, forming a map of auditory space. Many animals can locate objects in space with one ear because of the shape and sound-absorbing properties of the pinna which filters the sound in different ways depending on the direction from which it arrives. It is not understood how monaural maps of space are computed. Nor is it well understood how these maps, or the binaural maps, originally develop. However, it is clear that these maps are modifiable during the course of development, if for no other reason than the size of the animals head usually grows in early life, thus changing the distance between the two ears.

The auditory space map found in the guinea pig superior colliculus does not mature until 32 days postnatal. Moreover, it appears that auditory experience plays an important role in the formation of the map. If interaural cues are disrupted by plugging one ear early in postnatal life, then the auditory map of space compensates for this reduced unilateral input and remains aligned with the visual space map. Removing the pinnae from both ears of a guinea pig before the onset of hearing causes both the monaural and binaural cues to be disrupted, and these animals never achieve normal topography of the auditory map in the superior colliculus.

Experience dependent map formation or large-scale refinement is probably common to computational maps, which appear to need functioning circuitry to calculate the topographic coordinates. Where maps can be made on the basis of the anatomical placement of receptors, experience-dependent refinement appears to play a more minor role. One imagines then that maps in the brain come in all intermediate levels, based partly on computation and partly on anatomy. Understanding how maps are made and preserved through projections and how topography is refined is critical for understanding the making of a mature brain.

Summary

Pathfinding to the vicinity of a correct target is only the first step in the process of selecting appropriate postsynaptic cells on which to synapse. Having come to the doorstep of the target population, axons use a variety of signals, such as relative changes in growth factors, to slow down, enter the target and begin to arborize. Growing axons are often encouraged to enter the target at one site and discouraged from exiting the target at another site through repulsive barriers. There are a variety of molecules within the target zone, including gradients of ephrins and CAMs that conspire, often in combination, to encode different possible target cells along various axes and layers. The incoming afferents are distinguished from each other by the presence of different amounts of various receptors on their surfaces so that they respond differentially to the different target cells. These gradients of ligands and receptors are often the result of very early patterning events in the embryo, such as those that lay down rostrocaudal and dorsoventral patterns. Transcription factors expressed in such patterns control the expression of these molecules and so one can imagine a nervous system that wires up to a fairly high degree of precision, even in the absence of function. But, as we have seen here, the fine-tuning of neural connections, and the formation of computational maps, is heavily dependent on synaptic activity. In Chapter 9, we learn much more about the role of neural activity in synapse formation.

CHAPTER 7

Survival and Growth

Introduction

Neuron birth and migration is often followed not by a celebration, but by a requiem. Even as they differentiate and become interconnected, most neurons face a life-or-death challenge that leaves 20 to 80% of them dead from "natural causes" (Oppenheim, 1991). During embryonic or fetal development, neuron survival often depends upon molecular signals that are supplied by the postsynaptic target, the presynaptic afferents, or by neighboring cells (Fig. 7.1). If a sufficient amount of these survival factors can not be obtained, then death may result. Many neurons also depend upon the synaptic contacts that they receive, and denervation can lead to atrophy or death. This diverse group of mechanisms is referred to as *trophic* interactions because one cell is "nourished" by another. The first part of this chapter describes the characteristics of normal cell death in the developing nervous system. We then discuss the molecular mechanisms that are thought to regulate this process. Finally, we learn that electrical activity and synaptic transmission can have an important influence on neuron survival.

What Does Neuron Death Look Like?

Once naturally occurring cell death begins, the nerve cell participates actively in its own demise through gene transcription and protein synthesis. This process is often termed *apoptosis* or programmed cell death (PCD). To the trained eye, a dying neuron looks quite different from a healthy one (Fig. 7.2). In fact, naturally occurring neuron death was discovered over a century ago by John Beard (1896), who followed the fate of a very large, easily recognized neuron found at the surface of the skate spinal cord. He found that these Rohon–Beard cells were born in the neural crest and differentiated in the spinal cord, sending out processes to the ectoderm before degenerating. At first, it was difficult to accept the concept that neurons were born only to die a

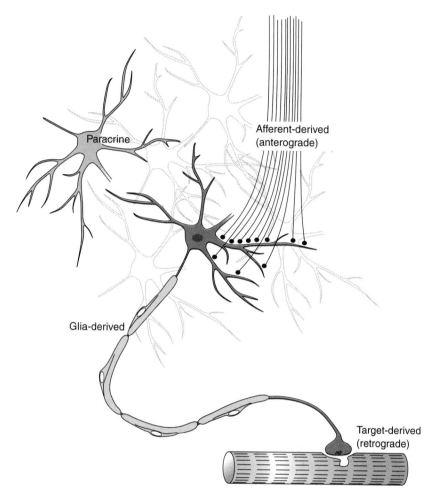

Paracrine

Afferent-derived (anterograde)

Glia-derived

Target-derived (retrograde)

Figure 7.1 Four sources that influence neuron survival. Neurons receive signals that influence their survival from the cells that they innervate (target-derived), from their synaptic inputs (afferent-derived), from neighboring neuron cell bodies (paracrine), and from nonneuronal cells (glia-derived).

short time later. Although there were many reports of neuron death following the removal of their target (see below), it was not clear that postmitotic neurons were lost in any significant number during normal development.

The appearance of apoptotic cells is characterized by a condensation of nuclear material (pyknosis) and a blebbing of the plasma membrane (Fig. 7.3). The protuberances eventually separate from the cell body and are phagocytosed by macrophages. As the large, crescent-shaped aggregates of nuclear material form, enzymes are activated that cleave the DNA, producing fragments of about 200 base pairs. Although this process is too small to see directly, it is now possible to stain the broken ends of DNA strands with molecular markers. The TUNEL technique (for **T**erminal transferase **U**TP **N**ick **E**nd Labeling) employs an enzyme that attaches labeled nucleotides to the exposed 3'-hydroxyl ends of the DNA fragments. This approach is useful when studying cell death in a large population of cells that has no clear boundaries, such as an area of cerebral cortex.

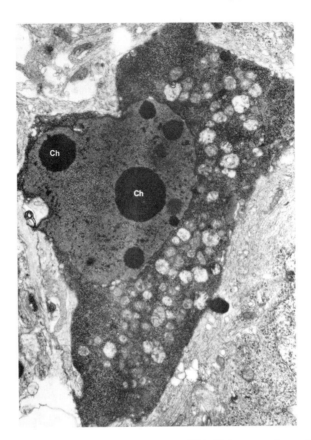

Figure 7.2 Electron micrograph of a dying motor neuron. This high-power photomicrograph shows a late phase of motor neuron degeneration in the Embryonic Day 6 chick spinal cord. The cytoplasm is darkly stained, and the nucleus contains large condensed chromatin (Ch) masses. (Reprinted from Chu-Wang and Oppenheim, Cell death of motoneurons in the chick embryo, *J. Comp. Neurol.,* Copyright © 1978, by permission of Wiley–Liss, Inc., a subsidiary of John Wiley & Sons, Inc.)

The changes that typically follow a traumatic injury, called *necrosis,* are quite distinct from apoptosis. Mitochondria stop producing energy and, as the cell becomes unable to regulate ionic content, its organelles swell up. The cell's lysosomal enzymes become activated, which breaks down cytoplasmic components, and the cell finally bursts open (Fig. 7.3). There is an important difference between a cell that dies gracefully by budding off neat little packages of membrane (apoptosis), compared to one that dies violently by retching catabolic enzymes on its neighbors (necrosis). Clearly, a graceful death is unlikely to injure healthy neurons, and serves as an efficient means to eliminate these cells.

How Many Neurons Die?

It might seem a rather straightforward matter to determine whether neurons are being added or removed from a population: Simply count the neurons in a young animal and subtract this number from an identical count obtained in an adult. If the number is positive, then neurons must have been born. If the number is negative, then neurons must have died. However, it is more difficult to obtain an accurate neuron count than one might suppose. For example, cell counts can remain relatively stable when neurogenesis and cell death overlap in time. A second problem revolves around the counting strategy, since it is often too laborious to count all of the neurons

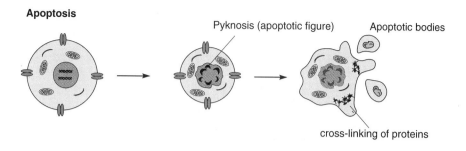

Apoptosis

Pyknosis (apoptotic figure)   Apoptotic bodies

cross-linking of proteins

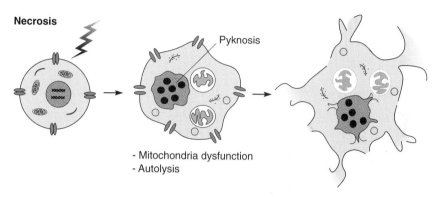

Necrosis

Pyknosis

- Mitochondria dysfunction
- Autolysis

Figure 7.3   A comparison between apoptosis and necrosis. Naturally occurring cell death is usually accomplished through a process called apoptosis. During apoptosis, the neuron begins to shrink and the nuclear matter becomes condensed (pyknosis), forming crescent-shaped figures. As proteins become cross-linked at the membrane, small apoptotic bodies break off and are phagocytized. In contrast, injured neurons tend to die through a process of necrosis. During necrosis, neurons can not maintain osmotic balance and swell up, finally bursting open.

in a structure. Estimates of neuron number are made from stained tissue sections, and the total neuron counts can be affected by the size and density of the cell bodies, each of which changes during development. Finally, neurons are not the only type of cell to die during development. For example, about 50% of oligodendrocytes in the rat optic nerve die during development, and their survival depends upon the presence of retinal axons (Barres *et al.,* 1992).

The overproliferation of neurons in most areas of the CNS suggests that it is a valuable mechanism. For example, cell death may ensure that the number of afferents is well-matched to the size of the target population. This theory makes the rational assumption, known to every woodworker, that it is much easier to trim off the

excess than to paste on a little bit extra later. Thus, we expect an elephant to have a far greater number of motor neurons innervating its bulky leg muscles as compared to the mouse with its short, skinny legs. There are many interesting examples of this principle, such as the limbless lizard, *Anguis fragilis,* which produces a set of motor neurons in the limb region that then proceed to die (Raynaud *et al.,* 1977). Therefore, neurogenesis provides a primary point of regulation for setting neuron number (see Chapter 3) and cell death provides a second. This concept is raised again when we discuss the overproliferation and elimination of synaptic contacts (see Chapter 9).

If cell death is a developmental mechanism for matching the size of a presynaptic population

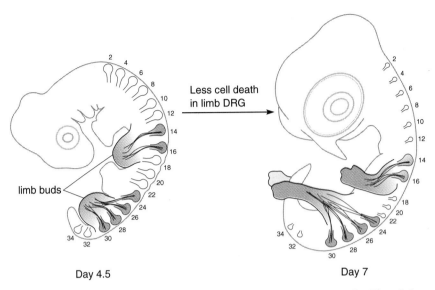

Day 4.5   **Day 7**

Figure 7.4 The pattern of naturally occurring cell death in chick dorsal root ganglia. There is less cell death amongst neurons in the DRGs that innervate limbs (red filled) than in those that innervate the axial musculature (white filled). Since there is a relatively greater amount of muscle mass in the limbs, survival is correlated with the amount of target tissue. (Adapted from Hamburger and Levi-Montalcini, 1949)

to its target, then it should occur at a discrete time and place. This was explored in dorsal root ganglia (DRG), where about 30% of neurons die during normal development (Fig. 7.4). The first observation was that neurons die during a specific time interval. In the chick, DRG neurons begin to degenerate at Embryonic Day 4.5, and the degeneration lasts for 2½ days. The second observation is that natural cell death occurs most predominantly in those DRGs that innervate axial musculature. The DRGs that innervate wings and legs have more tissue to innervate, and cell death is much reduced in these ganglia. Furthermore, the central and peripheral projections of DRG neurons make contact with their target before cell death occurs. Therefore, naturally occurring cell death does appear to be an important mechanism for selective elimination of those neurons with less target to innervate (Ernst, 1926; Hamburger and Levi-Montalcini, 1949).

Once it became clear that cell death was a general feature of the developing nervous system, its magnitude became the subject of rigorous cell counting studies. One of the most convincing ways to demonstrate that neurons are dying is to count both the healthy cells and the pyknotic cells in the same tissue section (Hughes, 1961). For example, counts of spinal motor neuron (MN) cell bodies in the chick and frog demonstrate that the decrease in the number of healthy looking MNs is perfectly correlated with the appearance of pyknotic cells (Fig. 7.5). Again, the period of cell death occurs when MN axons are synapsing onto muscles and their cell bodies are receiving afferent contacts.

The only case where cell death has been quantified in both pre- and postsynaptic neuronal populations is for two nuclei in the chick auditory brain stem (Fig. 7.6). The presynaptic population of cells, called nucleus magnocellularis (NM), is the first region of the chick brain to receive input from the ear, and these cells project to a second-order auditory nucleus, called nucleus laminaris (NL). Both groups of cells undergo their final mitosis, migrate to their final positions, and begin a period of normal cell death that occurs primarily from Embryonic Day 11 to 13. The percentages of cells that die in the two nuclei are quite similar. About 18% of the presynaptic NM neurons die during this inter-

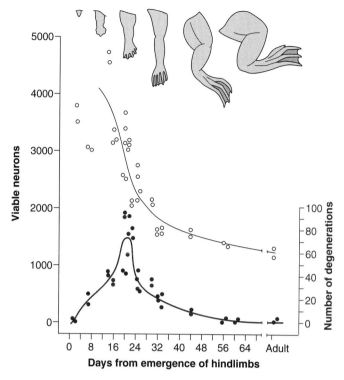

Figure 7.5 The period of cell death in frog motor neurons. The graph shows the total number of healthy (black) and pyknotic (red) motor neurons that innervate the frog hind limb during each of several developmental stages. At the top is a picture of leg size during this period. The number of pyknotic (degenerating) neurons reaches a peak at precisely the time when the loss of healthy (viable) neurons is most rapid. (Adapted from Hughes, 1961, with permission, Company of Biologists Ltd.)

val, while 19% of the postsynaptic NL neurons are wiped out (Rubel *et al.,* 1976; Solum *et al.,* 1997). Thus, the magnitude of cell death is well-correlated in these two interconnected cell groups.

Cell death has now been detected at all levels of the nervous system, including the cortex. Of course, it is virtually impossible to count the neurons in any one area of cortex because the number of cells is great and the borders are poorly defined. Therefore, the TUNEL technique (described above) has been used to show that DNA fragmentation is present during early development. Surprisingly, this technique suggests that about 70% of cortical cells are dying at Embryonic Day 14, but the majority of apoptotic cells are found within the proliferative zone (Blaschke *et al.,* 1996).

Survival Depends on the Synaptic Target

Even before normal cell death was a well-accepted event, it was known that developing nerve cells died when their target was removed. A common manipulation was to remove a limb bud around the time of innervation and then examine the motor neurons or DRG cells that would have made synapses there. These studies were performed on amphibian or chick embryos because it was relatively easy to carry out the surgeries. The removal of an appendage was usually devastating to the pool of presynaptic neurons (Fig. 7.7). In the salamander, *Amblystoma,* the sensory ganglia that normally innervate a limb are much smaller when the limb is excised. In contrast, sensory ganglia that normally

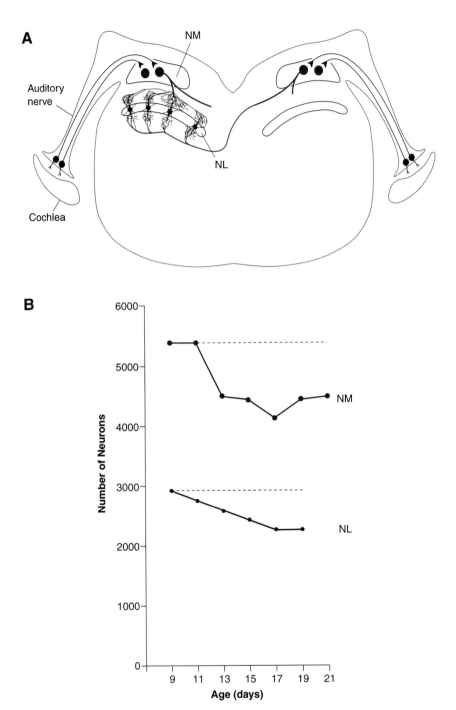

Figure 7.6 The period of cell death in pre- and postsynaptic nuclei in the chick. (A) A transverse section through the chick auditory brain stem. The nucleus magnocellularis (NM) is a central auditory nucleus that is innervated by auditory nerve terminals. It projects to a second-order nucleus, called nucleus laminaris (NL), on both sides of the brain. (B) The graph shows the total number of cell bodies in NM and NL during the latter period of embryonic development. In both nuclei, about 20% of the neurons are lost between Embryonic Days 9 and 17. (Adapted from Rubel *et al.*, 1976, and Solum *et al.*, 1997)

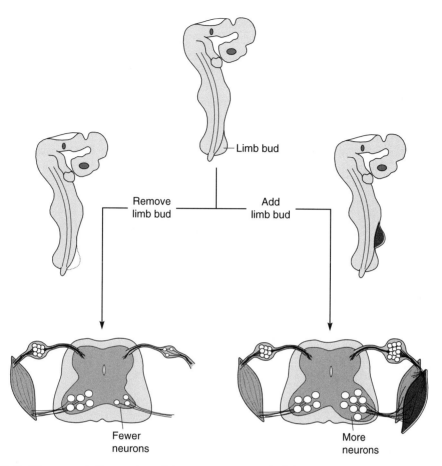

Figure 7.7 The amount of target tissue influences neuron survival. Two experimental strategies have been used to test whether target tissue provides neurons with a survival factor. In the embryonic chick, a limb bud can be surgically removed or an extra limb bud can be grafted nearby. (Left) When a limb bud is removed, the process of cell death is enhanced, and there are fewer motor neurons and DRG cells. (Right) When an extra limb bud (red) is grafted on, the process of cell death is decreased, and there are a greater number of motor neurons and DRG cells. (Adapted from Hamburger, 1943; Hollyday and Hamburger, 1976)

innervate axial musculature are much larger than normal if provided with a transplanted limb (Detwiler, 1936).

The relationship between motor neuron number and target size is remarkably linear in the chick. As greater and greater amounts of muscle are removed from a developing chick embryo, the ventral horn of the spinal cord becomes smaller (Fig. 7.7). When an extra limb bud is transplanted next to the original one, providing a larger than normal target region, developing processes grow into the added target, and the population of motor and DRG neurons are found

to be much larger than normal. The addition of an extra limb bud saved up to 25% of the motor neurons that would otherwise have died. Experimental alteration in the size of the periphery led to the hypothesis that the target provides a survival factor. When it was eliminated there were fewer neurons to be found in the adult, and when it was enlarged neurons were found in greater than normal numbers (Hamburger, 1943; Hollyday and Hamburger, 1976).

A complementary experiment can be performed by reducing the number of neurons projecting to a target and determining whether the remaining cells die off anyway. In one such experiment, about two-thirds of the ciliary ganglion neurons innervating one eye were killed off by cutting their axons. After the normal period of cell death had ended, the number of ganglion cells remaining was almost 40% greater than expected. Furthermore, several of the surviving axons sprouted into the peripheral territory that was vacated by the death of axotomized ciliary neurons. Therefore, particular neurons are not preordained to die, but appear to do so through some sort of competition for an attribute of the target (Pilar *et al.,* 1980).

A basic question that arises from these studies is whether the target influences neuron proliferation or cell death. By carefully studying the pattern of degeneration of DRG neurons following wing bud removal in the chick, Viktor Hamburger and Rita Levi-Montalcini (1949) demonstrated that target removal leads to an increase in the number of dying neurons. One wing bud was removed at about 3 days of incubation, and the dorsal root ganglia were examined ipsilateral and contralateral to the ablation. Within 2 to 3 days, the ganglia ipsilateral to the extirpated wing buds were much smaller than normal and contained a large number of darkly stained pyknotic cells (Fig. 7.8). Although the number of mitotic cells was also reported to vary with target size, subsequent studies show that target removal has little or no effect on the amount of tritiated-thymidine that is incorporated into DRG neurons (Carr and Simpson, 1978).

NGF: A Target-Derived Survival Factor

Neuron survival clearly depends on the presence of target tissue, but what is being procured? One simple hypothesis is that the target cells secrete a chemical that presynaptic neurons require for their survival. In fact, an extraordinary series of experiments, coupled with a few strokes of serendipity, led to the first endogenous neuro-

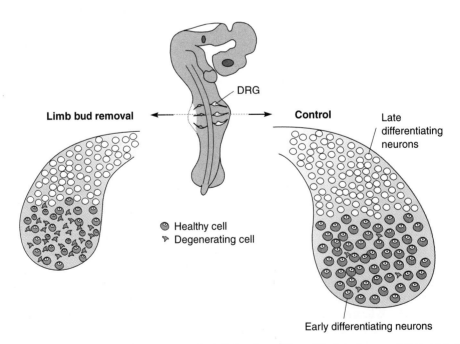

Figure 7.8   The target influences neuron survival. Following unilateral limb bud removal (left side), there is an increase in the number of degenerating cells in the DRG ipsilateral to the ablated limb, compared to the control side (right). (Adapted from Hamburger and Levi-Montalcini, 1949)

trophic substance to be discovered, the nerve growth factor (NGF). NGF has since been shown to largely control the survival of sympathetic neurons and contribute to the survival of sensory DRG neurons during development. Although NGF turns out to be the tip of an enormous iceberg of growth and survival factors (below), we examine its discovery in some detail because it remains the best understood system.

How did scientists arrive at the neurotrophic theory of cell survival? Viktor Hamburger (1934) first suggested that the target produces a factor that is retrogradely transported by the innervating neurons and influences their development. Initially, it was not clear whether this hypothetical substance upregulated neurogenesis, recruited cells to differentiate as neurons, or prevented differentiated neurons from dying. As described above, two sets of careful observations strongly suggested that the hypothetical substance worked by maintaining the survival of differentiating neurons (Levi-Montalcini and Levi, 1942; Hamburger and Levi-Montalcini, 1949).

By modern standards, the next step would be to harvest the target tissue (e.g., muscle) and try to isolated a soluble substance that enhances survival. However, most of the necessary biochemical tools did not yet exist in the 1950s. The isolation of a neurotrophic factor took a few decades to achieve, and it began with a surprising set of observations. In an effort to provide neurons with an "unlimited" amount of target tissue, various mouse tumors were implanted into the chick hindlimb (Bueker, 1948; Levi-Montalcini and Hamburger, 1951; Levi-Montalcini and Hamburger, 1953). One tumor, a connective tissue cell line called sarcoma, grew rapidly and was invaded by nerve fibers. Within 5 days of the transplant, there was a dramatic increase in the survival of sensory and sympathetic neurons, while motor neurons were unaffected (Fig. 7.9). When the tissue was examined in a little more detail, a key observation was made: ganglia with no apparent physical connection to the tumor were also greatly enlarged. This provided the first indication that cell survival was mediated by a diffusible chemical.

A more direct demonstration came from experiments in which tumor cells were placed on a vascularized respiratory membrane in the chick egg called the chorioallantois. In this case, the tumor was not in contact with sympathetic and sensory ganglia, but it did share the same blood supply. Even though the tumor was physically isolated from the nervous system, it was able to elicit a strong growth-promoting effect (Fig. 7.9). Thus, sarcoma tumor cells must release a soluble factor that can be transported to the neurons through the circulatory system.

As a first step toward isolating the putative survival factor found in mouse sarcoma, an *in vitro* assay system was developed. Sympathetic ganglia were obtained from chick embryos and placed in a tissue culture dish, either by themselves or next to mouse sarcoma tumor cells. When grown next to tumor, the neurons survived and grew a dense halo of axons within hours, providing a simple and convenient assay system. Although biochemical isolation was a slow process, it was possible to obtain a tumor cell fraction that had only proteins and nucleic acids. To determine whether either of these components contained the growth factor, a biochemical trick was employed. Snake venom was known to contain high levels of an enzyme that breaks down nucleic acids and it was, therefore, added to the extract (Cohen and Levi-Montalcini, 1956; Levi-Montalcini and Cohen, 1956). If the biological activity were lost, then one could conclude that growth factor contained nucleic acids. Surprisingly, the tumor fraction containing the snake venom was even more potent than the origin protein–nucleic acid fraction. Even more curious, the snake venom, itself, was found to support nerve growth (Fig. 7.10).

As it turned out, the discovery of a growth-promoting effect in snake venom was extremely fortunate. It suggested that growth-promoting activity would also be found in a mammalian analog, the salivary gland. In fact, the mouse submaxillary gland proved to be a wonderful source for the nerve growth factor, and this eventually led to its complete isolation and sequencing.

Once the NGF was purified, it was possible to perform two critical experiments *in vivo* to determine whether this protein is both necessary and sufficient to keep sensory and sympathetic neurons alive during development. First, the NGF

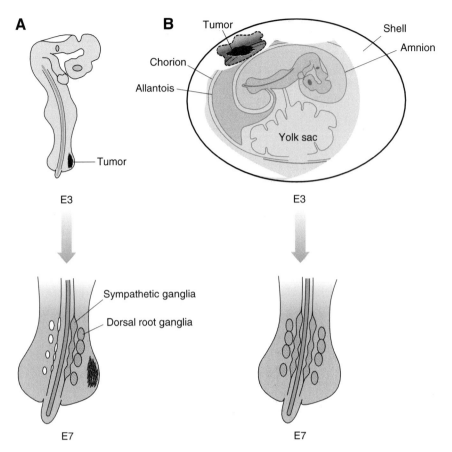

Figure 7.9 A target-derived soluble factor can support neuron survival. (A) When a tumor cell line (red) is placed in the chick embryo at E3, the size of sympathetic ganglia and DRGs is much larger ipsilateral to the tumor by E7. (B) When the same tumor cell line (red) is placed on the chorioallantoic membrane at E3, such that nerve fibers have no direct access, all of the sympathetic and dorsal root ganglia are much increased in size by E7. Thus, the tumor must have secreted a soluble factor that enhanced neuron survival. (Adapted from Bueker, 1948; Levi-Montalcini and Hamburger, 1951, 1953)

protein that was purified from snake venom was injected directly into neonatal rodents, and it did produce a dramatic increase in the size of sensory and sympathetic ganglia (Levi-Montalcini and Cohen, 1956). In addition to keeping neurons alive, it is also clear that NGF promotes process outgrowth. For example, when NGF is injected into neonatal rodents, sympathetic nerve fibers are no longer restricted to their normal synaptic target, but grow widely in the peripheral field and can even invade blood vessels or the central nervous system (see Chapter 4).

In a second experiment to determine whether endogenous NGF is necessary for survival, an antibody directed against the NGF protein was injected into neonatal rodents. This leads to the loss of almost all sympathetic neurons (Levi-Montalcini and Booker, 1960). It was later found that DRG cells are no longer dependent on NGF at the age when antibody was administered, but they can be destroyed by prenatal exposure to NGF antibody (Johnson *et al.,* 1978). In fact, not all sensory neurons are dependent on NGF for survival. Those sensory neurons that derive from sensory placodes (e.g., nodose ganglion), rather than the neural crest, are unresponsive to NGF treatment. In the DRG, only small peptidergic neurons that carry nociceptive signals to

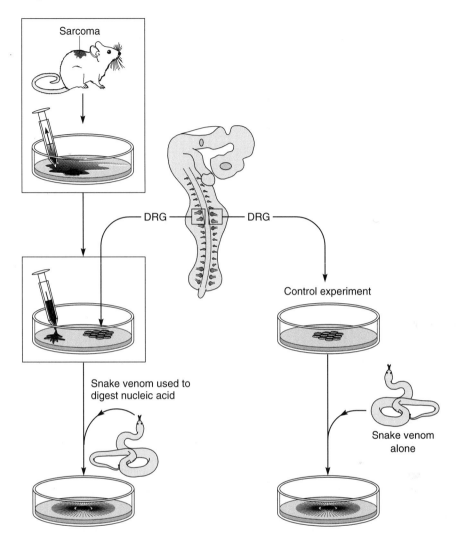

Figure 7.10 A soluble factor that supports the survival and growth of DRG neurons is discovered in a mouse sarcoma and, later, in snake venom. (Left) DRG neurons obtained from chick embryos were placed in a tissue culture dish and conditioned medium from a mouse sarcoma was added. The venom of a snake was added to the culture to determine whether nucleic acids mediate the trophic effects. The DRG neurons survived and grew processes under these conditions. (Right) When the control experiment was performed, in which only snake venom was added to the DRG neuron cultures, a surprising discovery was made. The DRG neurons survived and grew, indicating that the snake venom must also have contained a soluble survival factor. (Adapted from Cohen and Levi-Montalcini, 1956; Levi-Montalcini and Cohen, 1956)

the spinal cord are killed following loss of the NGF signal. More recently, it has been possible to reproduce the effects of antibody treatment in genetically engineered mice. When a deletion is made in the coding sequence of the NGF gene, homozygous animals display profound cell loss in both sympathetic and sensory ganglia (Crowley *et al.,* 1994).

If NGF is the endogenous survival factor, then it should be present at the sympathetic and sensory ganglion target regions during an appropriate period of development. Although NGF levels are extremely low (except in the fortuitous case of the male mouse salivary gland, from which it was purified), it has been possible to localize the protein with immunohistochemical staining and the NGF mRNA with *in situ* hybridization. For example, trigeminal axons arrive at their cutaneous target just before the NGF mRNA and protein are manufactured, and the initial outgrowth of trigeminal axons is NGF independent (Davies *et al.,* 1987), suggesting that the maintenance of trigeminal neurons depends on NGF derived from their target. Taken together, the experiments performed *in vivo* and *in vitro* provide the clearest example of a neuron survival signal. As this great success was achieved by 1960, it was reasonable to assume that there were many other neurotrophic substances in the brain and that these would be found with somewhat less effort. While several growth and survival factors were discovered in nonneuronal systems, the search for another bona fide neurotrophic substance was, at first, somewhat frustrating.

NGF Is a Member of the Neurotrophin Family

The full amino acid sequence of NGF was obtained by 1971, yet a full decade elapsed before a second neurotrophic factor was identified. The search began with the innocent observation that, in contrast to its effect on the retinae from lower vertebrates, NGF does not stimulate neurite outgrowth from cultured rat retina. Working under the assumption that there must be a growth factor or factors for the mammalian retina, a soluble extract was prepared from pig brain tissue. This extract did, in fact, stimulate retinal process outgrowth in a dose-dependent manner. When the active substance, named brain-derived growth factor (BDNF), was purified and its amino acid sequence determined, its structure displayed a striking similarity to that of NGF (Turner *et al.,* 1982; Leibrock *et al.,* 1989).

Several members of the neurotrophin family have now been isolated, and they are found in both the peripheral and the central nervous system. The more recent additions to the family have been given the less colorful names: neurotrophin-3 (NT-3), NT-4, NT-5, and NT-6 (Fig. 7.11). In each case, a precursor protein of about 250 amino acids is processed posttranslationally to produce the active peptide which forms a dimer. The family members share about 50% sequence homology with one another, particularly within six hydrophobic regions that are responsible for linking the two protomers together. Each neurotrophin also contains a unique amino acid sequence, and it is this variable region that is responsible for binding to a specific receptor (Ibanez, 1994).

Individual members of the neurotrophin family play a role in the survival of specific peripheral neuron populations. As with NGF, two general classes of experiments have been performed: Either excess neurotrophin was provided (*in vivo* or *in vitro*) or the amount of endogenous neurotrophin was decreased, commonly by single gene knockout experiments (Chapter 2). Experiments of this sort indicate that BDNF is a necessary endogenous signal for the survival of vestibular ganglia, while NT-3 is an endogenous survival signal for cochlear ganglia. A comparison between the two experimental approaches shows that positive results must be treated cautiously. While BDNF is able to save chick motor neurons when administered during the period of naturally occurring cell death, there is no effect on motor neuron survival in BDNF knockout mice (Oppenheim *et al.,* 1992; Ernfors *et al.,* 1994, 1995). Both BDNF and NT-3 also contribute to the survival of neurons in the sensory, trigeminal, and nodose ganglia. Unlike NGF, they may not serve only as a target-derived survival factor because each is expressed within the ganglia, suggesting a paracrine mechanism (Fig. 7.1).

There Is a Family of Neurotrophin Receptors

Even before a receptor for NGF was discovered, it was known that NGF binds with high affinity to axon terminals. The protein can also

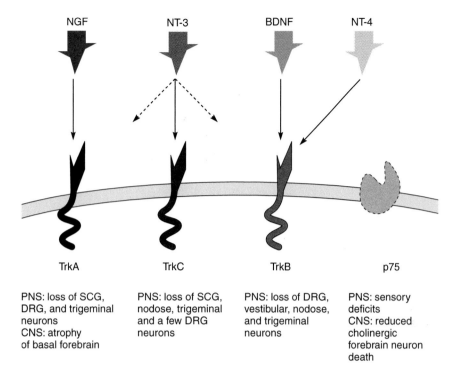

Figure 7.11 Neurotrophins and their receptors. Following the discovery of NGF, several homologous proteins were discovered, including NT-3, BDNF, and NT-4. Each of these proteins binds selectively to a member of the Trk receptor tyrosine kinase family (solid arrows). NT-3 binds with somewhat lower affinity to TrkA and TrkB (dashed arrows). In addition, there is a low-affinity receptor, called p75. The effect of eliminating the neurotrophin or its receptor in mice is shown beneath each pair.

be taken up into membrane vesicles and transported back to the cell body where it is broken down eventually (Hendry *et al.,* 1974; Johnson *et al.,* 1978). However, it is the interaction of NGF with its receptor at the cell membrane that appears to be critical for neuron survival. For example, when NGF is placed directly into the cytoplasm of NGF-responsive PC12 cells, it fails to induce the production of the enzyme choline acetyltransferase, even though externally applied NGF is quite able of doing so. Moreover, injecting antibodies to NGF into the cytoplasm does not prevent external NGF from inducing the enzyme (Heuman *et al.,* 1984). Although the presence of NGF in the cell body does not appear to be critical for cell survival, the retrograde transport of some signal is important. Sympathetic neurons die when vinblas-

tine is used to disrupt their retrograde transport, and the cells can be saved with NGF treatment (Johnson, 1978).

Exposure of the growing tips of axons to NGF is sufficient to prevent cell death. This was demonstrated in an elegant tissue culture study where sympathetic neuron cell bodies were placed in a central chamber that was physically isolated from the growth media that bathed the neuritic processes (Fig. 7.12). When NGF is provided only to neurites that grow out and reach one of the isolated side chambers, the neurons survive. This result suggests that the signal for survival is somehow relayed back to the cell body, perhaps via a second messenger system (see below). NGF also has a local effect on the neurites receiving the treatment. They grow rapidly when exposed to the peptide, but neurites

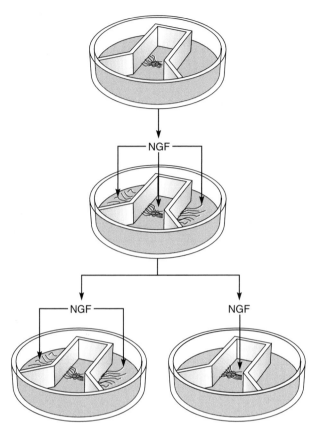

Figure 7.12 The NGF signal can be transduced at the tips of growing neuronal processes. Sympathetic neurons were placed in a special tissue culture system that permitted the cell bodies and neurites to be bathed in different media. Neurons could be kept alive by adding NGF to each compartment (center), to the neurites only (bottom left), or to the cell bodies only (bottom right). (Adapted from Campenot, 1977, 1982)

that are not directly exposed to NGF are found to retract (Campenot, 1977, 1982).

When ^{125}I-labeled βNGF binding studies are performed on freshly dissociated chick sensory neurons, there are two types of binding site (Sutter *et al.,* 1979). The first type displays a lower affinity for NGF (e.g., nanomolar concentrations saturate the binding sites), while the second type displays a higher affinity for NGF (e.g., picomolar concentrations saturate the binding sites). In fact, there are two different types of NGF receptor proteins that are associated with these binding kinetics, and each one has now been isolated.

The high-affinity receptor was discovered following the observation that a NGF-dependent cell line exhibited protein phosphorylation on the tyrosine amino acids when treated with NGF (Fig. 7.13; Maher, 1988). Soon after, an oncogene was discovered in human colon carcinoma cells, and this turned out to be a transmembrane protein containing a tyrosine kinase on its cytoplasmic tail (Martin-Zanca *et al.,* 1986). The oncogene apparently results from a genetic rearrangement that fuses a tyrosine kinase with part of a nonmuscle tropomyosin sequence, leading to its name: tropomyosin receptor kinase or Trk (later called TrkA). The *trk* proto-oncogene was cloned and the distribution of its mRNA was examined *in vivo.* The highest levels of expression are confined to the cranial sensory, dorsal root, and sympathetic ganglia (Martin-Zanca

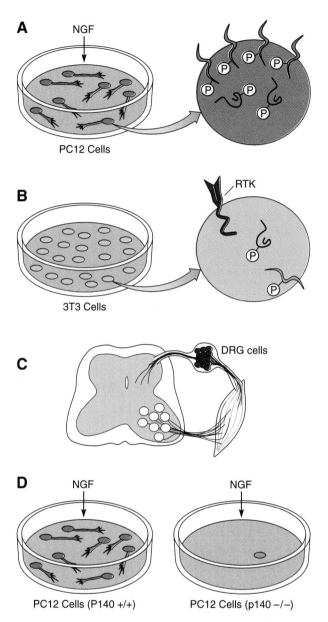

Figure 7.13 The high-affinity NGF receptor was discovered through a series of disparate observations. (A) NGF was found to elicit protein phosphorylation in PC12 cells. (B) The oncogene in a cancer cell line was found to be a transmembrane receptor tyrosine kinase (RTK). (C) The messenger RNA for this RTK (red) was found in extremely high levels in DRG neurons. (D) When this RTK, called p140, was eliminated from PC12 cells, they became unresponsive to NGF. (Adapted from Maher, 1988; Martin-Zanca *et al.,* 1986, 1990; Loeb *et al.,* 1991)

et al., 1990). Most importantly, the TrkA protein (also called p140) is a high-affinity binding site for NGF, and the binding event induces tyrosine kinase activity (Kaplan *et al.,* 1991a).

Several lines of evidence indicate that TrkA does transduce the NGF survival signal. A mutant line of PC12 cells that lack Trk protein are unresponsive to NGF, although they can be rescued if they are transfected with expression vectors encoding the full-length rat *trk* cDNA (Loeb *et al.,* 1991). Perhaps the most compelling evidence is that transgenic mice lacking TrkA receptors exhibit extensive neuron cell death in sympathetic and dorsal root ganglia (Smeyne *et al.,* 1994). It is worth noting that a population of NGF-sensitive neurons, cholinergic cells of the basal forebrain, have been identified in the central nervous system (Gage *et al.,* 1988). When their axons are cut in adult rats, infusion of NGF into the CNS is able to keep them alive. While NGF does not appear to play a role in their survival during development, it is found that *trkA* -/- mice have fewer axonal projections from cholinergic basal forebrain neurons to the hippocampus and cortex, suggesting a role in process outgrowth (see Chapter 4).

Three high-affinity neurotrophin receptors have now been isolated: TrkA, TrkB, and TrkC. The latter two were discovered by taking the *trk* sequence and performing low-stringency binding screens with cDNA libraries. In this manner, two sequences were isolated that encoded for 145-kDa receptor tyrosine kinases, named TrkB and TrkC (Barbacid, 1994). Each Trk receptor has two immunoglobulin-like repeats in the extracellular domain and a tyrosine kinase with autophosphorylation sites in the cytoplasmic domain. The extracellular domains are about 50% homologous, but each Trk displays a specific affinity for one or two of the neurotrophins: TrkA is specifically activated by NGF, TrkB is specifically activated by BDNF or NT-4, and TrkC is specifically activated by NT-3. There are a number of truncated Trk receptors (those missing the tyrosine kinase domain) that are able to bind to their cognate ligand, and these are generally expressed only by glial cells during development.

In fact, the *trkC* genes may encode for up to eight different TrkC receptor proteins.

Expression of TrkB and TrkC is widely distributed in the CNS and levels remain quite high into adulthood (Barbacid, 1994). When mice lacking either the TrkB or the TrkC receptor are analyzed, the effects on cell survival are in general agreement with those found in BDNF -/- and NT-3 -/- mice, respectively (Klein *et al.,* 1993, 1994). However, the effects of TrkB disruption may be quantitatively greater than the effects of BDNF disruption because TrkB also serves as a receptor for NT-4. Targeted disruption of the *trkB* gene is particularly devastating in that all mice die within 2 days of birth and several peripheral populations are effected, such as the trigeminal, nodose, and dorsal root ganglia. Primary vestibular neurons are almost completely eliminated. In contrast, targeted disruption of the *trkC* gene results in the loss of a small number of DRG neurons and a larger loss of nodose ganglion neurons.

The Low-Affinity Neurotrophin Receptor

The low-affinity NGF receptor was isolated by expression cloning. It is a 75-kDa transmembrane glycoprotein (hence, its name, p75) that shares homology with members of the tumor necrosis factor (TNF) family of receptors (Johnson *et al.,* 1986). Although its functional role in cell death remains a subject of debate, there is evidence that p75 collaborates with the Trk receptors to enhance ligand binding and phosphorylation (Chao, 1994). For example, cutaneous sensory trigeminal neurons cultured from p75 knockout mice require a fourfold greater concentration of NGF in order to survive (Davies *et al.,* 1993). That is, in the absence of p75, TrkA is able to transduce the survival signal, but less efficiently. However p75 knockout mice display only minor cell loss among sensory neurons, being nowhere near the level found in *trkA* -/- animals (Lee *et al.,* 1992).

Recent studies indicate that p75 may play a dual role in cell survival. For example, rat brain oligodendrocytes grown in culture express the p75 receptor, but not TrkA, and NGF treatment kills the majority of these cells (Casaccia-Bonnefil *et al.*, 1996). In the developing retina, the depletion of endogenous NGF with antibody results in better survival of retinal neurons (Fig. 7.14). The ability of NGF to kill retinal neurons is apparently mediated by p75 because antibodies against this receptor prevent the cell death (Frade *et al.*, 1996). The survival of TrkA-negative brain stem cholinergic neurons is actually enhanced in p75 -/- mice, or normal animals injected with a p75-inhibiting peptide, again supporting the notion that this receptor promotes cell death during development (Van Der Zee *et al.*, 1996). In cultured sympathetic neurons, BDNF is also able to kill cells through activation of the p75 receptor (Bamji *et al.*, 1998).

In another scenario, the presence of p75 can lead to cell death if NGF is absent. When the level of p75 receptor is decreased in cultured E12–15 mouse DRG neurons by transfecting them with an antisense oligonucleotide, NGF is unable to promote cell survival. A much different effect is obtained for older sensory neurons, from E19 to P2. These older p75-negative cells survive better *without* NGF, suggesting that p75 is providing a constitutive death signal (Barrett and Bartlett, 1994). Similarly, the expression of p75 induces cell death in an immortalized neural cell line when no ligand is present, but the addition of NGF inhibits cell death (Rabizadeh *et al.*, 1993).

Whether p75 kills neurons due to ligand binding or in its absence, there is still little understanding about the molecular signal. Unlike the Trk receptors, p75 does not have an intracellular catalytic domain. TNF receptor family members have been shown to activate two intracellular signaling pathways: a transcription activator called nuclear factor κB (NF-κB) is recruited to enter the nucleus, and the sphingomyelinase activity is raised to create a lipid second messenger molecule called ceramide. One intriguing clue about the function of p75 comes from its homology to other members of the TNF receptor family. Each

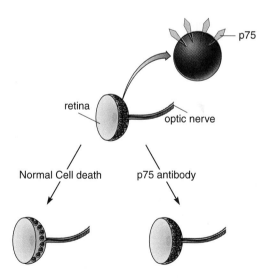

Figure 7.14 The low-affinity NGF receptor p75 may facilitate cell death. Retinal ganglion cells undergo a period of naturally occurring cell death during development (left). However, when antibodies directed against p75 are injected into the retina (right), they effectively block NGF binding, and the cell death is much reduced. (Adapted from Frade *et al.*, 1996)

of these proteins has a "death domain" on the cytoplasmic tail that is similar to the *reaper* gene product in *Drosophila*. The deletion of *reaper* blocks most cell death in the embryonic fly nervous system, and its over-expression in the retina leads to the complete loss of cells (White *et al.,* 1996).

The Expanding World of Survival Factors

The old razor about taking care not to wish for something else it may come true has some validity in the world of survival factors. Whereas neuroscientists were vigorously searching for even a single new survival factor in 1980, there are now several families of factors and receptors. Unfortunately, the trophic influence of most factors has been tested in few brain regions during development. Of the neurons that have been investigated, most are influenced by several trophic factors, and the array of factors (or receptors) can vary during the course of development.

The cytokines form a diverse family of secreted proteins that were originally discovered as growth factors in lymphocyte cultures, and many of these have turned out to have a primary role in neuron survival as well. The names of individual cytokines derive from the first biological activity that they were discovered to have, such as killing tumors (tumor necrosis factor) or promoting mitosis of hematopoietic stem cells (colony-stimulating factor).

In recent years, several cytokines have been found to keep neurons alive in dissociated primary culture. For example, ciliary neurotrophic factor (CNTF) supports the survival of autonomic, DRG, hippocampal, and motor neurons. CNTF binds to an intrinsic membrane protein, called CNTFRα, and this binding event recruits two other transmembrane proteins (gp130 and LIFRb) that form the β subunit of the receptor complex (Fig. 7.15). The α subunit provides specificity to the trimeric receptor, while the β subunits are responsible for signal transduction (Stahl and Yancopolous, 1994). When the recep-

tor complex forms, a tyrosine kinase (member of the Jak family) that is associated with the cytoplasmic tail of each β subunit becomes activated and phosphorylates a DNA-binding protein (p91) that translocates to the nucleus and apparently activates transcription (Bonni *et al.,* 1993).

Of particular interest is the effect on motor neurons because cell death in this population has been well characterized and closely linked to the target, yet no survival factor has been identified. When chick embryos are treated with human recombinant CNTF, half of the naturally occurring motor neuron death is prevented (Oppenheim *et al.,* 1991). Surprisingly, parasympathetic, sympathetic, and sensory neuron cell death are unaffected. Although CNTF knockout mice display little effect on cell survival during development, including motor neurons, a null mutation of CNTFRα does increase normal motor neuron cell death by about a third (DeChiara *et al.,* 1995). This result implies that at least one cytokine signaling pathway, utilizing CNTFRα, plays an important role in motor neuron survival, although the endogenous ligand is yet to be identified. Furthermore, since most motor neurons survive without the CNTFR, there must be other target-derived survival signals.

Two other factors have been identified as preventing naturally occurring motor neuron death *in vivo*. As its name implies, glial-derived neurotrophic factor (GDNF) was isolated from a glial cell line, and it was initially characterized by its ability to keep midbrain dopaminergic cells alive *in vitro*. This assay was chosen because Parkinson's disease involves the death of these dopaminergic neurons, and a survival factor may have important therapeutic value (Lin *et al.,* 1993). Like CNTF and other cytokines, the GDNF receptor is composed of a ligand recognition α subunit (GDNFRα) and a transmembrane tyrosine kinase β subunit. Although GDNF treatment prevents naturally occurring motor neuron death in chick embryos, null mutations of GDNF in mice have very little effect on MN cell death (Oppenheim *et al.,* 1995; Sánchez *et al.,* 1996). It may be that manipulations of the GDNF receptor will clarify its role in motor neuron development. A more recent entry to the field of motor

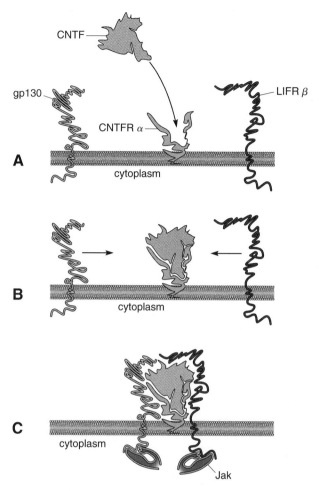

Figure 7.15 Cytokine signaling. (A) CNTF binds first to an intrinsic membrane protein called CNTFRα. (B) This event causes two other transmembrane proteins (gp130 and LIFR) to form the β subunit of the receptor complex. (C) The activated receptor complex signals via a tyrosine kinase (Jak) that is associated with the cytoplasmic tail of each β subunit.

neuron trophic factors is a cytokine called hepatocyte growth factor/scatter factor (HGF/SF), which is known to act as both a chemoattractant and a muscle-derived survival factor (Ebens *et al.*, 1996).

Despite the expansion of candidate growth factors, few of them seem to have an effect on the survival of CNS neurons when they are eliminated from the developing system. One hypothesis is that central neurons, unlike peripheral ganglion cells, have multiple targets and afferents, perhaps giving them access to many different growth factors during development. The prediction from this hypothesis is that one must eliminate two or more growth factors or receptors in order to disrupt survival. It is also likely that many survival factors have yet to be identified. For example, the survival of embryonic retinal ganglion cells is enhanced by tectal cell-conditioned medium in a manner that cannot be duplicated by CNTF or the neurotrophins (Meyer-Franke *et al.*, 1995). A final consideration is that many trophic factors also promote certain aspects of differentiation (see Chapters 2–4) and progress along these pathways may be necessary for survival.

Endocrine Control of Cell Survival

Hormonal signaling controls many aspects of development, including cell survival. There are now several examples of brain structure that are quantitatively different in males and females of the same species, often referred to as a sexual dimorphism (Chapter 10). These sexual dimorphisms are thought to arise from regional differences in the amount of steroid hormones or their receptors. Steroid hormones (e.g., estrogens and androgens) are lipid-soluble molecules that bind to cytoplasmic receptors, and these receptors can translocate to the nucleus where they regulate gene transcription. For example, normal cell death amongst developing superior cervical ganglion (SCG) neurons is greater in female rats than in male rats. Furthermore, castration of neonatal male rats significantly increases the number of dying neurons, suggesting that a gonadal hormone may be responsible for better neuron survival in the male SCG. In fact, treatment of neonatal animals with a sex hormone (estradiol or testosterone) improves SCG neurons survival, even in female animals (Wright and Smolen, 1987). While such discoveries have sparked much interest and theorizing about the neural substrates of male- and female-specific behavior, there remain few solid examples that correlate structure to function. These are considered in more detail below (see Chapter 10).

The survival of some motor neurons are also dependent on the presence of specific sex hormones. In the lumbar spinal cord of male rats, there are two motor nuclei that innervate striated muscle of the penis: the spinal nucleus of the bulbocavernosus (SNB) and the dorsolateral nucleus. As one might expect, these nuclei and the muscles that they innervate are present in males, but are nearly absent in female rats. This sexual dimorphism arises from the selec-

tive loss of motor neurons in female rats. During the first 10 postnatal days, the total number of SNB neurons decreases by nearly 70% in females, although the number only decreases by about 30% in males (Fig. 7.16). However, when females are treated with the androgen steroid hormone testosterone, the amount of cell death is decreased and resembles the pattern seen in males (Nordeen et al., 1985). When males are castrated and reared with an androgen antagonist, flutamide, their SNB neurons are as scarce as in female rats (Breedlove and Arnold, 1983). Thus, an endogenous androgen signal is probably necessary to keep more male SNB neurons alive during development.

Endocrine signals can lead to extensive remodeling throughout the nervous system. In the moth, there are a great many neurons that are necessary in larvae or required for the process of metamorphosis from caterpillar to pupa to moth. However, when the adult moth emerges from its pupa, nearly 40% of its abdominal neurons are lost over a few days. This period of normal cell death is initiated when a steroid hormone, 20-hydroxecdysone (20-HE), is eliminated from the circulation (Truman, 1983; Truman and Schwartz, 1984). In fruit flies, there are about 300 neurons in the ventral cord that express much higher levels of the 20-HE receptor, and these are precisely the cells that die at metamorphosis (Robinow et al., 1993). Apparently, the cells that are to be eliminated become extremely dependent on 20-HE and this period of cell death can be delayed by treatment with 20-HE in both the moth and the fruit fly. Endocrine signaling is also responsible for neuron death during vertebrate metamorphosis (Decker, 1976, 1977). The surge of thyroxine that initiates metamorphosis from tadpole to frog causes lysosomal activity to increase in motor neurons. The motor neurons that innervate regressing tail musculature of tadpoles are eliminated directly by a thyroid hormone signal.

Endocrine signals have also been implicated in cell survival amongst the sexually dimorphic telencephalic nuclei of songbirds: those species where males learn to produce mating calls, while females vocalize little, if at all. In

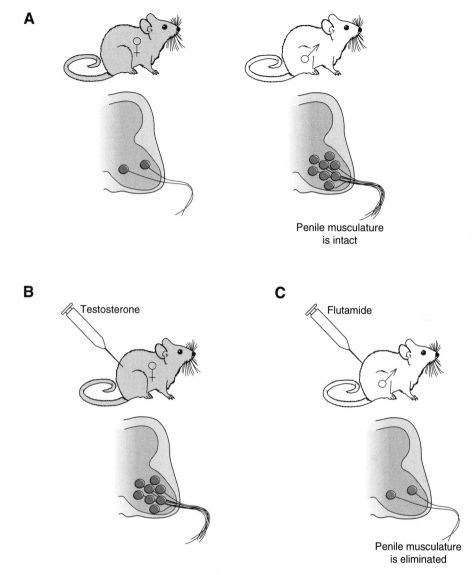

A

Penile musculature
is intact

B Testosterone

C Flutamide

Penile musculature
is eliminated

Figure 7.16 Hormonal influence on motor neuron survival. (A) Areas of the lumbar spinal cord that inner-vate penile muscles in male rats are nearly absent in female rats, due to motor neuron death during development. (B) When females are treated with the androgen steroid hormone testosterone, lumbar motor neuron death is decreased. (C) In contrast, when males are castrated and reared with an androgen antagonist, flutamide, lumber motor neurons display enhanced cell death. (Adapted from Nordeen *et al.,* 1985; Breedlove and Arnold, 1983)

canaries and zebra finches, at least three areas of the brain that support song production are much larger in males than in females (Nottebohm and Arnold, 1976). In some nuclei such as the robustus nucleus of the archistriatum (RA), which shares some features with motor cortex, the differences in neuron number arise from a selective loss of neurons in the female (Nordeen and Nordeen, 1988; Kirn and DeVoogd, 1989). What is the evidence that steroid hormones influence cell survival in males? If developing females are treated with testosterone, then the number of neurons in RA becomes masculinized, and the birds can acquire male-like vocalizations (Gurney, 1981). More recently, the idea that steroid hormones can account for sexual dimorphism of songbird vocal nuclei has been challenged. For example, it has not been possible to feminize the song nuclei of male birds by castration or with pharmacological treatments that decrease the active metabolite of testosterone, estrogen. Furthermore, when genetic females are "engineered" to grow testicular tissue that secretes androgens, their vocal nuclei do not become masculinized (Wade and Arnold, 1996). Therefore, there are strong reasons to think that steroid hormones play a role in control of cell number in male and female songbirds, but the precise mechanisms remain elusive.

Cell Death Requires Protein Synthesis

One might suppose that when a neuron is deprived of a trophic factor, it fails to maintain normal levels of protein synthesis and metabolism and simply "passes away." In fact, neurons collaborate in their own death by activating genes and synthesizing proteins that injure the cell. That is, they "commit suicide." The first indication that an active process could account for cell death came from studies of nonneuronal cells. For example, cultured tadpole tail cells die when exposed to thyroxine, but this can be prevented by blockers of RNA and protein synthesis (Tata, 1966). A major breakthrough came from genetic studies of cell death in the nematode *Caenorhabditis elegans* (Driscoll and Chalfie, 1992). About 10% of cells die during development in *C. elegans,* most of them being neurons, but inactivation of two specific genes (called *ced-3* and *ced-4*) rescues all of these cells, including neurons (discussed in more detail below). Is it possible that neuron cell death can actually be prevented by blocking protein or RNA synthesis?

This hypothesis was tested by asking whether neurons could be rescued by blocking their protein synthesis. As described above, embryonic sympathetic neurons are able to survive *in vitro* when grown in the presence of NGF. When NGF is removed from the culture medium, few neurons remain after 2 days. Therefore, the first experiment determined whether inhibitors of RNA or protein synthesis could save NGF-deprived neurons (Fig. 7.17). Actinomycin D blocks transcription by binding to DNA and preventing the movement of RNA polymerase, while cycloheximide prevents translation by blocking the peptidyl transferase reaction on ribosomes. Each of these treatments rescued sympathetic neurons following NGF deprivation, demonstrating that new RNA and proteins must be manufactured to bring about cell death. To determine when the harmful phase of translation occurs, cycloheximide was delivered at several times after NGF deprivation, and it was found that the cell death-promoting proteins are produced at about 18 h (Martin *et al.,* 1988). If all the molecular machinery for cell death was present in the cytoplasm, one would expect that neurons would be committed to die within a few hours.

To determine whether mRNA and protein synthesis are general features of cell death *in vivo,* animals were treated with synthesis inhibitors at the age when neurons are normally lost (Fig. 7.18). When chick embryos are treated with either cycloheximide or actinomycin D on Embryonic Day 8, the time of maximum motor neuron and DRG cell death, they exhibit a striking reduction in the number of dying neurons (Oppenheim *et al.,* 1990). Similarly, the cell death that occurs in response to declining levels of 20-HE in moths can be reduced by RNA or protein synthesis inhibitors (Fahrbach *et al.,* 1994). These studies suggest that trophic signals may stimulate the production of proteins that protect the neuron from death, and in the absence of a trophic signal harmful proteins may be synthesized. The search for such proteins is discussed below.

Much of the cell death machinery seems to be present at all times in a neuron's cytoplasm. In fact, recent studies have shown that, under

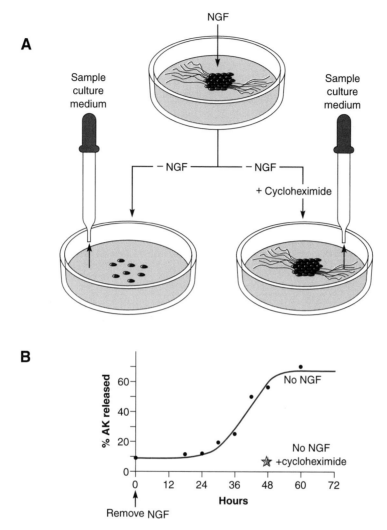

Figure 7.17 Neuron cell death can be delayed by blocking protein synthesis. (A) Sympathetic neurons die within 2 days when NGF is removed from the culture medium (left). When the translation blocker cyclohex-amide was added to NGF-deprived cultures sympathetic neurons were rescued (right) (B) Significant levels of a cytoplasmic enzyme, adenylate kinase (AK), could be measured in the tissue culture medium when neuronal membranes became leaky as the cells began to die. As shown in the graph, AK levels rose to about 65% in NGF-deprived neurons (black dots), but remained unchanged when cyclohexamide was added (star). (Adapted from Martin *et al., The Journal of Cell Biology,* 1988, **106,** 829–844, by copyright permission of the Rocke-feller University Press.)

certain conditions, cells can undergo apoptosis even if their nucleus is removed. Therefore, it will be important to study naturally occurring cell death in many areas of the nervous system in order to determine whether protein synthesis is an obligate part of the death pathway.

Intracellular Signaling

The fact that most identified survival factor receptors are kinases suggests that protein phos-phorylation plays a prominent role in the cell death pathway. NGF signal transduction, the best

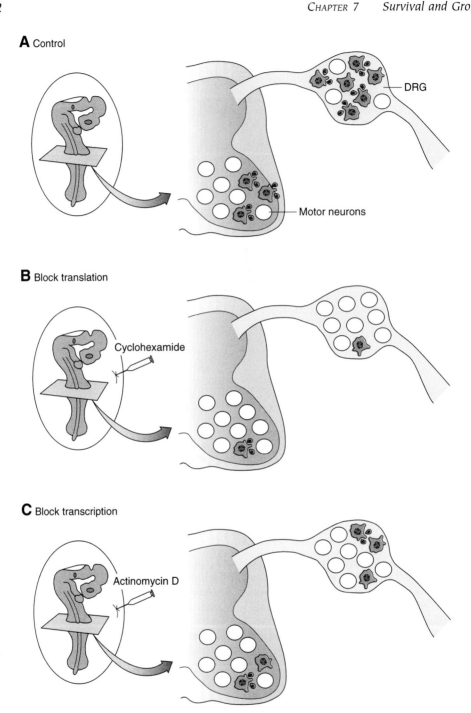

Figure 7.18 The synthesis of mRNA and protein is required for naturally occurring cell death *in vivo*. (A) Pyknotic (light red) motor neurons and DRG neurons were counted during normal development in the chick. (B) Chick embryos were treated with a protein synthesis antagonist, cyclohexamide, when motor neuron and DRG cell death was greatest, and the number of pyknotic neurons was decreased. (C) Similarly, when chick embryos were treated with a transcription inhibitor, actinomycin D, there was a reduction in the number of pyknotic neurons. (Adapted from Oppenheim *et al.,* 1990)

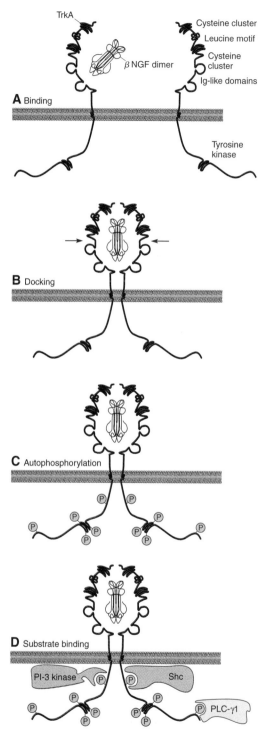

Figure 7.19 NGF–receptor interaction. (A) The biologically active form of NGF is a dimer of identical 13-kDa peptide chains called the β subunit. The NGF dimer binds to the TrkA protein (Binding). (B) The binding induces two receptors to form a dimer (Docking). (C) The bound receptor complex leads to phosphorylation of neighboring Trk receptors (Autophosphorylation). (D) Cytoplasmic molecules (PI-3 kinase, Shc, PLC-γ1) then dock at the cytoplasmic tail (Substrate binding).

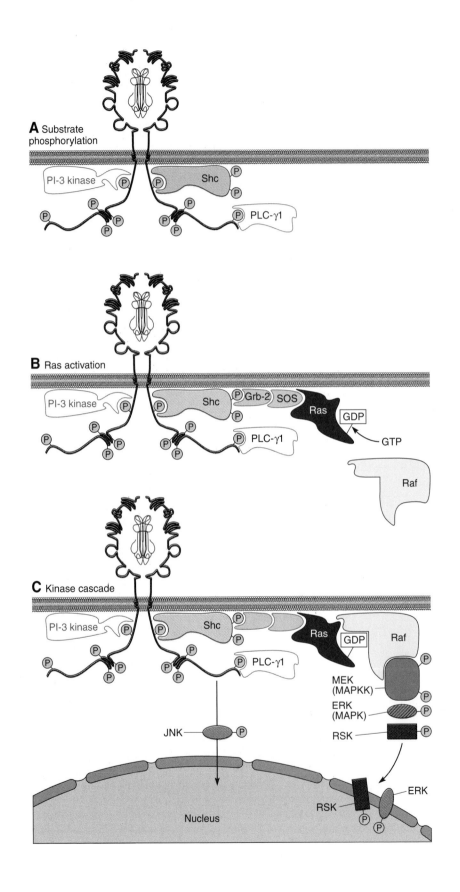

A Substrate phosphorylation

PI-3 kinase

Shc

PLC-γ1

B Ras activation

PI-3 kinase

Shc Grb-2 SOS Ras GDP

GTP

PLC-γ1

Raf

C Kinase cascade

PI-3 kinase

Shc Ras GDP Raf

PLC-γ1

MEK (MAPKK)

ERK (MAPK)

RSK

JNK

RSK

ERK

Nucleus

characterized pathway, involves the sequential activation of cytoplasmic molecules. Some of these molecules modify existing cytoplasmic or membrane proteins, while others enter the nucleus and regulate gene transcription. Since NGF can influence many developmental events besides cell survival (e.g., process outgrowth), this discussion is restricted to cytoplasmic signals that are most relevant to survival.

The binding of NGF to the TrkA receptor is thought to induce dimerization, followed by the rapid phosphorylation of five tyrosine residues on the cytoplasmic tail by neighboring Trk receptors (Kaplan *et al.,* 1991b). The phosphorylation sites on the Trk receptor apparently serve as docking sites for the cytoplasmic molecules that will propagate the signal toward the nucleus (Fig. 7.19). For example, Trk can activate a phospholipase (PLC-γ1) and phosphatidylinositol 3-kinase (PI-3) resulting in the production of several second messengers. One of the proteins that binds to, and is phosphorylated by, the Trk receptor, called Shc, initiates a series of events that leads to activation of a protooncogene, called Ras (Fig. 7.20). Shc first recruits two proteins, Grb-2 and SOS, to the membrane. The SOS protein is able to activate Ras by enhancing the exchange of GDP for GTP.

The potential importance of Ras signaling to neuron survival is demonstrated in experiments where the Ras protein is injected directly into cultured chick DRG neurons. Although DRG neurons depend on NGF for their survival, the Ras protein is sufficient to prevent cell death (Borasio *et al.,* 1989). Furthermore, the same treatment promotes the survival of BDNF-dependent nodose ganglion neurons and CNTF-dependent ciliary ganglion neurons. Because activated Ras is able to phosphorylate many substrates, the intracellular signal can diverge along different molecular pathways. However, a major substrate for activated Ras is a serine/threonine kinase, called Raf. Once Raf is activated, there occurs a sequential activation of mitogen-activated protein kinases (MAPKs), termed the kinase cascade, eventually resulting in translocation into the nucleus (Fig. 7.20). One group of proteins that enters the nucleus and regulates gene transcription is called the extracellular receptor-activated kinases (ERK).

Which MAPKs are responsible for the positive effects of NGF binding, and which ones produce the negative effects following its withdrawal? In PC12 cells, there is evidence for both types of signal (Xia *et al.,* 1995). NGF promotes the survival of PC12 cells, and this is accompanied by activation of several MAPKs. Within 6 h of NGF withdrawal, PC12 cells begin to die in great numbers, and there is a prominent decrease in ERK activity. To test whether ERK is responsible for the positive effect of NGF, PC12 cells were engineered to produce constitutively high levels of ERK activity (Fig. 7.21). These cells survived much better following NGF withdrawal. There is also a MAPK signal, called JNK, that appears to turn on following NGF withdrawal. In fact, PC12 cell death will occur in the presence of NGF if JNK is constitutively activated. Thus, NGF may upregulate proteins needed for cell survival through ERK, while proteins needed for suicide are upregulated by JNK.

Experiments in primary neuron cultures also suggest that JNK and its target (c-Jun) are involved in the cell death pathway. In cultures of NGF-dependent sympathetic neurons, expression of c-Jun is induced immediately after withdrawal of the neurotrophin. Experimental reduction of c-Jun is sufficient to rescue NGF-deprived neu-

---

Figure 7.20 Trk signaling pathway. (A) The Trk receptor activates several intracellular proteins, including Shc (substrate phosphorylation). (B) Two proteins, Grb-2 and SOS, are then recruited to the membrane, resulting in the activation of a protooncogene called Ras (Ras activation). (C) The activated Ras phosphorylates several substrates, including a serine/threonine kinase, called Raf. A sequence of mitogen-activated protein kinases are then activated (kinase cascade). This intracellular signaling system concludes with the translocation of proteins into the nucleus (ERK, JNK, RSK).

rons, and constitutive overexpression of c-Jun is sufficient to kill neurons in the presence of NGF (Ham *et al.,* 1995). Similarly, rat spinal motor neurons can be kept alive *in vitro* by blocking JNK activity (Maroney *et al.,* 1998).

Although we have tried to present a unified picture of cell survival signaling, it is likely that different neurons will employ specific cytoplasmic mechanisms. For example, Ras appears to be a principal cytoplasmic signal for NGF signaling in DRG neurons However, it has also been found that NGF-dependent sympathetic neurons from caudal regions of nervous system are *not* saved by Ras injection, while sympathetic neurons from the rostral SCG are saved (Markus *et al.,* 1997). Furthermore, the many molecular pathways between receptor and nucleus interact with one another, producing another level complexity. This is demonstrated by experiments in which the binding of an intracellular protein to TrkA is disrupted. For example, activation of ERK requires binding and activation of both Shc and PLC-γ1 (Stephans *et al.,* 1994). A complete intracellular pathway mediating survival and death is yet to be described, but we now have the likely candidates that pass

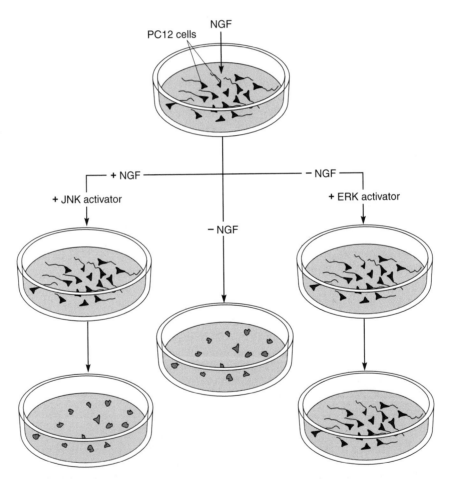

Figure 7.21 ERK and JNK mediate the effects of NGF. When NGF is withdrawn from the culture medium, PC12 cells die (center). NGF in not able to support PC12 cell survival when the MAP kinase JNK is constitutively activated (left). In contrast, when ERK is constitutively activated in PC12 cells, they are able to survive even in the absence of NGF (right). (Adapted from Xia *et al.,* 1995)

the signal from membrane to nucleus. Fortunately, this part of the mystery need not be complete for us to consider the cytoplasmic weapons that neurons use to kill themselves.

Caspases: Agents of Death

The discovery of specific genes that are directly involved in apoptosis was made in genetic experiments on the nematode *C. elegans*. Since death appears to involve a series of discreet genetic steps, it came to be known as programmed cell death. Two genes, *ced-3* and *ced-4, must* be expressed by each *C. elegans* cell if it is to die during development (*ced* stands for cell death abnormal). When either of these genes is mutated, almost all of the PCD is prevented (Yuan and Horvitz, 1990). Analysis of mosaic animals (i.e., animal in which the *ced* gene is expressed in only a few identified cells) indicates that the gene product acts within the cell that produces it, showing that PCD proceeds by suicide rather than a violent neighbor. What are these gene products and how do they control the life or death decision?

Proteases appear to be the weapon of choice for cell death. While it has been known for some time that one can rescue injured cells by blocking proteolytic enzymes, the evidence for protease involvement in normally occurring cell death only came recently. In fact, one of the gene products that kills *C. elegans* neurons, CED-3, turns out to be a cysteine protease, an enzyme that specifically cuts up proteins after an aspartate residue. In mammals, there is a CED-3-like protease called interleukin-1β-converting enzyme (ICE). While ICE plays a life-affirming role in processing pro-interleukin-1β for the purpose of blood cell production, it also serves as an angel of death in the developing nervous system. New cysteine proteases have been identified in many species, and they are now generally referred to as **C**ysteine requiring **ASP**artate prote**ASE**s, or caspases (Fig. 7.22). Thus, ICE is now called caspase-1.

Several caspases have now been implicated in neuron cell death. When a caspase inhibitor (a cytokine response modifier, crmA) is microin-

jected into chick DRG neurons *in vitro,* they can survive the withdrawal of NGF (Gagliardini *et al.,* 1994). Caspases may also mediate the death-promoting effect of "death domain" containing proteins, such as the low-affinity neurotrophin receptor p75 and the *Drosophila* protein caller Reaper (discussed above). For example, Reaper overexpression in the *Drosophila* eye causes all the cells to die, but a caspase inhibitor is able to block this effect (White *et al.,* 1996).

To determine whether caspases are involved in the normal period of cell death, chick embryos were treated with a synthetic peptide inhibitor of caspase on Embryonic Day 8, the peak of motor neuron death. After 24 h, the number of pyknotic cell bodies was cut in half compared to animals treated with a less selective protease inhibitor (Milligan *et al.,* 1995). However, it remains possible that the synthetic peptide inhibitor blocked more than one member of the caspase family. To examine the effect of a single protease, transgenic mice were produced lacking caspase-3, the closest mammalian homolog of CED-3 (Kuida *et al.,* 1996). The brains of these animals were disorganized, and there were few signs of the pyknotic cell clusters that accompany nervous system morphogenesis, suggesting a decrease in normal cell death.

Caspase-3 activity may be selectively expressed in cells that die by apoptosis, but not necrosis (described above). Cultured cerebellar granule cells become apoptotic when deprived of serum containing high potassium, and these cells are rescued with a selective inhibitor of caspase-3. The same treatment has no effect on neurons that become necrotic when exposed to high concentrations of glutamate (Armstrong *et al.,* 1997).

It is not too surprising to learn that nerve cells commit suicide by destroying their own proteins, but it is not yet clear whether a critical substrate must be catalyzed by caspase for cell death to proceed. At this point there are a few interesting candidates (Lazebnik *et al.,* 1994; Loetscher *et al.,* 1997). The first target is a DNA repair enzyme called poly(ADP-ribose) polymerase (PARP), suggesting that cell death is achieved by compromising the neuron's tran-

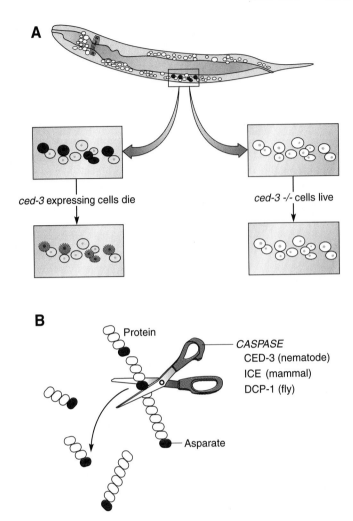

Figure 7.22   The role of caspases in cell death. (A) In *C. elegans*, CED-3-expressing cells (red) die during development, but almost all cell death is prevented when the *ced-3* gene is mutated. (B) CED-3 is a member of the caspase family, enzymes that specifically cut up proteins after an aspartate residue. There are homologs of CED-3 in mammlas (ICE) and fruit flies (DCP-1). (Panel A adapted from Yuan and Horvitz, 1990)

scription machinery. A second target, of some interest to those studying Alzheimer's disease, is the transmembrane proteins called presenilins that are apparently involved in the *Notch signaling* pathway (see Chapter 2). Although NGF-deprived PC12 cells normally die, they can be rescued by transfection with presenilin 2 anti-sense mRNA.

While no final arrests have been made, caspases appear to be a primary agent of death in the developing nervous system. However, smoking guns abound, and it is still too soon to rule out other mechanisms of normal cell death. For example, cells must constantly decrease the amount of superoxide (O_2^-) that accumulates as a result of oxygen usage in the mitochondrial respiratory chain. Free radicals such as O_2^- have unpaired electrons, making them an extremely reactive species. Excess O_2^- can disrupt membrane integrity, inhibit pumps, and break DNA.

Superoxide dismutase (SOD) is the housekeeping enzyme that eliminates O_2^- by catalyzing a reaction to O_2 and H_2O_2. Interestingly, sympathetic neurons can survive for a longer period of time after NGF deprivation if injected with SOD. However, a caspase has been identified that carries out the cell death process initiated by trophic factor deprivation, but *not* that due to increases in free radicals (Troy *et al.,* 1997). Thus, a single neuron type can die in very different ways, even though the process looks identical by visual inspection.

Regulating Death Proteins

There are a number of important checks and balances to ensure that only the right neurons die. The first two regulators of cell death were discovered in genetic studies of *C. elegans.* The *ced-4* gene product, discussed above as a necessary constituent of the death pathway, appears to be a protease-activating factor. CED-4 binds to the inactive form of CED-3 (a homolog of caspase-3) and leads to its activation. The activation of another gene, *ced-9,* can prevent apoptosis in all cells. Mutations that inactive *ced-9* lead to death amongst cells that would normally survive through development (Hengartner *et al.,* 1992). CED-9 apparently blocks death by complexing with CED-4 and interfering with its ability to activate the caspase.

A number of death promoters and death inhibitors have now been identified in mammals, some of which are homologous to CED-4 and CED-9 (Fig. 7.23). The mammalian homologs of CED-4 are called apoptosis protease-activating factors (Apaf). In one scenario, a heterodimer forms between two Apafs, and one of them cleaves caspase-3 to form the active enzyme. Mutations of this Apaf lead to a decrease in cell death *in vivo* (Li *et al.,* 1997), similar to the effects of CED inactivation. The mammalian homolog of CED-9 is a membrane-associated protein called Bcl-2 (named for its discovery in B cell lymphoma cells). Transgenic mice that overexpress Bcl-2 in their neurons have much bigger brains than normal animals, and cell counts in the facial nucleus and retina reveal that there are over 40% more neurons (Martinou *et al.,* 1994).

The family of Bcl-2-like protein has grown tremendously. While some of them turn out to be cell death inhibitors (like CED-9), others are found to promote cell death. Genetic studies suggest that there is some redundancy amongst survival-promoting *bcl-2*-like genes: Targeted disruption of the *bcl-2* gene does not appear to have any effect on neuron survival, but disruption of another family member, *bcl-x,* produces distinct signs of apoptosis (Motoyama *et al.,* 1995). BAX is a death-promoting member of the BCL-2 family, and it can apparently inactivate BCL-2 by dimerizing with it. Thus, cell death in ganglia and motor neurons is virtually eliminated in *bax* knockout mice, and it is significantly reduced in many areas of the CNS (White *et al.,* 1998).

Despite the striking phenotypes that are observed when *bcl-2* family members are manipulated genetically, their mechanism of action is far from clear. In fact, the interaction of cell death regulators with one another and with caspases is certain to become a tangled web. Recently discovered proteins that interact with BCL-2 family members include BAD (*bcl-2*-associated death promotor), BAK (*bcl-2* homologous antagonist killer), and BAG (*bcl-2*-associated gene). Furthermore, BCL-2 itself is a caspase substrate, and its protective influence can be obliterated by cleavage (Cheng *et al.,* 1997). Finally, an entirely new families of regulators has recently emerged, the inhibitors of apoptosis (IAP). These proteins appear to directly inhibit caspases, and one member of the IAP family has been found to be deleted in humans with a disorder called spinal muscular atrophy in which spinal cord motor neurons become depleted (Roy *et al.,* 1995).

Synaptic Transmission at the Target

Some of the earliest experimental manipulations of target size suggested that functional

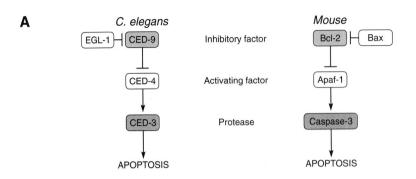

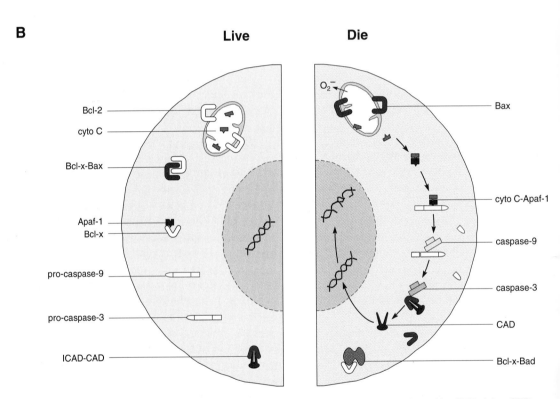

Figure 7.23 Regulation of cell death machinery. (A) In *C. elegans,* CED-3 is activated by CED-4, but CED-9 can complex with CED-4 and interfere with activation. EGL-1 can bind to CED-9 and facilitate the processing of CED-3. A similar regulatory pathway is found in the mouse. Caspase-3 is activated by Apaf-1, but BCL-2 family members can block Apaf activity. Bax family members can promote cell death by interfering with specific Bcl-2 proteins. (B) The hypothetical events that permit a cell to live or cause it to die. Living cells (left) express BCL-2, which is associated with mitochondria. Bcl-x can complex with Apaf-1 and prevent caspase activation. In dying neurons (right) Bax enters the mitochondrial membrane, perhaps permitting cytochrome C (cyto C) to leak out. Bad can complex with bcl-x and prevent it from interacting with Apaf-1. When cyto C is released from the mitochondira, it complexes with Apaf-1 and activates caspase-9, which goes on to activate caspase-3. One target of caspase-3 is ICAD, an inhibitor of a nuclease that is responsible for DNA fragmentation, caspase-activated deoxyribonuclease (CAD).

synaptic contacts were correlated with survival. Removal of the nasal placodes in salamander embryos did not, at first, decrease the size of the innervating forebrain region. However, after the system became functional, loss of the target did produce a hypoplasia (Burr, 1916). Observations from the NMJ also suggest that functional synapses are involved in motor neuron survival. There is a very tight correlation between the onset of neuromuscular activity in chicks and the onset of normal motor neuron cell death.

If synapse activity is necessary for survival, then one would predict that more neurons would die in its absence. To test this hypothesis, chick embryos were treated with an acetylcholine receptor antagonist (curare or bungarotoxin) during a 4-day period that overlapped the normal period of motor neuron death. Curare was quite effective at blocking neuromuscular transmission, as spontaneous movements were virtually eliminated for much of the treatment period. Rather than increasing cell death, the surprising result was that synapse blockade saved motor neurons (Fig. 7.24). Over 40% of the motor neurons that would have died were still alive after the period of normal cell death ended and the curare had been removed (Pittman and Oppenheim, 1979). Furthermore, curare produced a three-fold increase in the number of motor axon branches and synapses during the period when normal cell death occurs (Dahm and Landmesser, 1991). A similar decrease in normal cell death is found in the isthmo-optic nucleus when activity is blocked in its target, the eye, by injecting TTX during development (Péquignot and Clarke, 1992).

Since TTX-poisoned neurons sprouted new terminals, neuron survival may depend on proper access to the target-derived survival factor, rather than on the total amount of factor produced by the target (Oppenheim, 1989). Access could be provided by a greater number of synapses. In fact, several observations suggest a correlation between synapse formation and survival factor expression. Embryonic hippocampal neurons grown in dissociated culture for 7 days make numerous synaptic contacts with one another, and the expression of NGF and BDNF mRNA gradually increases over this period. However, NMDA re-

ceptor blockade decreases neurotrophin expression and GABAA receptor blockade increases it (Zafra *et al.,* 1991). Neurotrophin expression is also regulated by neuronal activity in embryonic cortex cultures, and this mechanism enhances survival (Fig. 7.25). Depolarization-evoked calcium entry increases both BDNF expression and cell survival *in vitro*. When function-blocking antibodies directed against BDNF are added to the cultures, however, the trophic effect of depolarization is eliminated (Ghosh *et al.,* 1994). Therefore, neurons may have some influence over the survival factors that they seek from a target: increased branching may provide better access and synaptic transmission can regulate the amount of factor produced.

Afferent Regulation of Cell Survival

Neuron growth and differentiation occurs without synaptic contacts at first, but maturation and survival quickly become dependent on neurotransmission and electrical activity. If the amount of synaptic transmission is too low during development, then postsynaptic neurons can cease protein synthesis and become atrophic; they may even die. Paradoxically, too much excitatory activation has been shown to kill neurons by loading their cytoplasm with calcium. In this section, we discuss the relationship between innervation, synaptic activity, and neuron survival and ask what trophic signal is being provided by afferent terminals.

Many of the original studies involved removing centrally projecting axons to see whether the central target developed properly in their absence. For example, Larsell (1931) removed an eye in tree frog larvae and found that its target, the contralateral optic tectum, had many fewer cells than expected. However, these studies were not able to discriminate between effects on neurogenesis or migration versus effects on neuron survival.

One of the best studied cases of afferent regulated survival is the nucleus magnocellularis (NM) in the chick central auditory system (Fig.

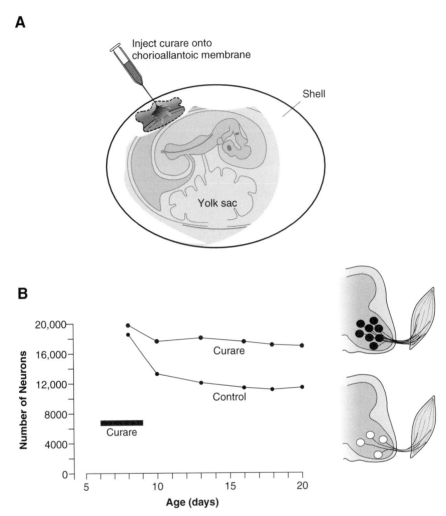

Figure 7.24 Blocking synaptic transmission prevents normal motor neuron cell death. (A) Neuromuscular transmission can be blocked by applying curare onto the chorioallantoic membrane of chick embryos. (B) In control animals, over 30% of motor neurons die after Embryonic Day 5. When animals are treated with curare from E6 to E9, the magnitude of normal cell death is greatly diminished. (Adapted from Pittman and Oppenheim, Cell death of motoneurons in the chick embryo spinal cord, *J. Comp. Neurol.*, Copyright © 1979 by permission of Wiley–Liss Inc., a subsidiary of John Wiley & Sons, Inc.)

7.26). Just before taking up her studies of NGF (above), Rita Levi-Montalcini had been studying the effect of cochlear nerve fibers on the survival of NM neurons and other brain stem nuclei. These studies have fascinated students of biology because they were performed with very little equipment in the countryside of Italy while World War II raged around her. Despite these privations, Levi-Montalcini (1949) was able to show that the period of normal cell death is elevated when the cochlea is removed. Although there was little sign of degeneration at E11, the age at which auditory nerve fibers first activate NM neurons, there was a dramatic loss of cells by E21. Subsequent studies showed that about 30% of NM neurons are lost following cochlear ablation, and the effect of denervation is much reduced in adult animals (Parks, 1979; Born and Rubel, 1985).

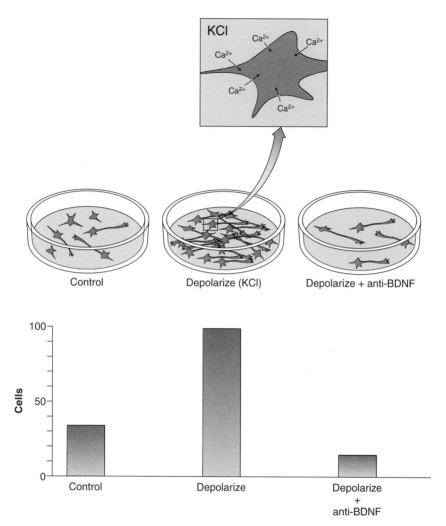

Figure 7.25 Electrical activity enhances the survival of embryonic cortex neurons by way of a neurotrophic signal. When the cultures are depolarized by adding KCl to the culture medium, calcium enters the neurons and the level of BDNF expression increases, leading to greater neuron survival compared to control medium. The trophic influence of depolarization is eliminated by adding a function-blocking anti-BDNF antibody to the growth medium. (Panel B adapted from Ghosh *et al.,* 1994)

Survival in other peripheral and central neurons also depends, in part, on afferent connections during development (Linden, 1994). However, surgical removal of the afferent population does not really address what the trophic signal is. Does the synapse provide a survival factor such as NGF? Does the neurotransmitter itself enhance survival? To address this question, intact afferent pathways were treated with agents that block neuronal activity (Maderdrut *et al.,* 1988; Born and Rubel, 1988). In the chick ciliary ganglion, cell death is increased when transmission is blocked, although neurogenesis and migration proceed normally. Similarly, action potential blockade in the cochlea for 48 h is also sufficient to increase normal cell death in the chick NM. Therefore, synaptic activity seems to play a critical role in postsynaptic neuron survival.

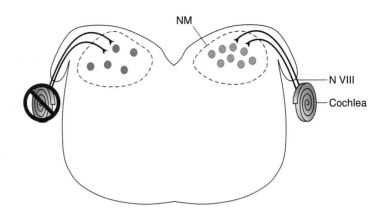

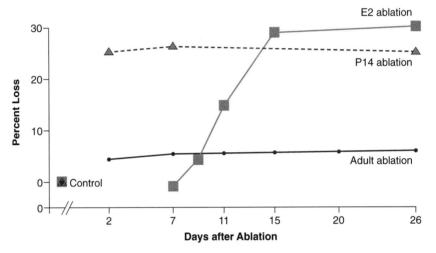

Figure 7.26   Afferent innervation regulates neuron survival in a chick central auditory nucleus. (A) Auditory neurons (NVIII) from the cochlea innervate the nucleus magnocellularis (NM) in the chick auditory brain stem. The removal of a cochlea (left) completely denervates NM neurons on the ipsilateral side. (B) When a cochlea is removed at Embryonic Day 2 (E2), about 30% of NM neurons are lost during the ensuing 2 weeks, although cell death does not begin until E10. When the cochlea is removed at Posthatch Day 14, about 25% of neurons die within 2 days. In adults, cochlear ablation results in the loss of only about 5% of NM neurons. (Adapted from Parks, 1979; Born and Rubel, 1985)

What is it about synaptic activity that promotes neuron survival? One possibility is that synaptic transmission provides a positive survival signal. Alternatively, synaptic transmission may evoke action potentials, and the associated voltage-gated currents may affect survival. To distinguish between these two possibilities, brain slices containing the chick NM and its auditory nerve afferents were placed *in vitro* and provided with two different stimulation protocols (Fig. 7.27). Although the experimental period was too brief to observe dying neurons, denervation of NM neurons leads to a rapid decrease in protein synthesis that is thought to be a condition preceding cell death in this and many other neural systems. When the auditory nerve is stimulated, NM neurons receive synaptically evoked activity, and protein synthesis is main-

Anterograde stimulation (synaptic)

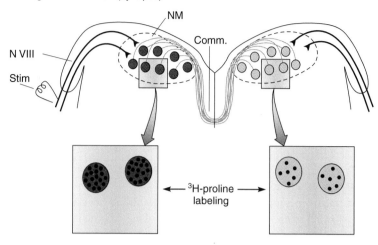

Retrograde stimulation (action potentials only)

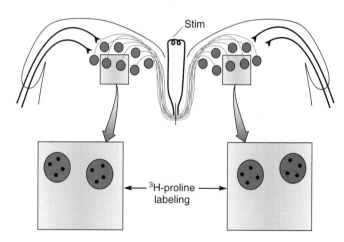

Figure 7.27 Synaptic activity regulates postsynaptic protein synthesis in chick auditory brain stem. (Top) Brain slices containing the chick nucleus magnocellularis (NM) and its auditory nerve afferents (NVIII) were incubated in an oxygenated solution containing [³H]-proline. Synaptic transmission in one NM was elicited by electrically stimulating NVIII afferents (left). When the tissue was processed for autoradiography, it was found that synaptically stimulated NM neurons incorporated far more proline (black dots) into newly synthesized proteins compared to the control side (right). (Bottom) When the axons of NM neurons were stimulated at the commissure, evoking a retrograde action potential in the cell body, protein synthesis was not maintained. (Adapted from Hyson and Rubel, 1989)

tained. In contrast, when NM axons are stimulated to produce antidromic action potentials in their cell body, protein synthesis is not maintained (Hyson and Rubel, 1989). Thus, the preservation of postsynaptic neuron metabolism, and presumably its survival, depends on the release of something from the synaptic terminal.

Although we do not yet know what the trophic substance might be, there is some indication that the neurotransmitter itself may play a role. Auditory nerve fibers release glutamate at their synapse on NM neurons, and this transmitter produces large excitatory postsynaptic potentials. However, glutamate also acts to limit the amount of calcium that enters NM neurons by activating a metabotropic glutamate receptor (mGluR). When auditory nerve fibers are stimulated in the brain slice preparation, NM cytoplasmic calcium levels remain low, but the addition of an mGluR antagonist during continued orthodromic stimulation results in a rapid increase in calcium (Zirpel and Rubel, 1996). It is interesting that blockade of ionotropic glutamate receptors *in vivo* can decrease normal cell death in NM and block it entirely in nucleus laminaris (Solum *et al.*, 1997). Thus, excitatory afferents may jeopardize survival through ionotropic glutamate receptor activation, but promote survival through activation of mGluRs.

It is possible that afferents also release trophic factors during development. Neurotrophins, such as NT-3, are produced in the developing retina, and they are transported anterogradely down retinal ganglion cell axons to the optic tectum (von Bartheld *et al.*, 1996). Since the survival of optic tectum neurons depends on both axonal transport and electrical activity by retinal axons, it seems possible that NT-3 mediates this afferent regulation (Catsicas *et al.*, 1992). Of course, if neurotrophins provided an anterograde signal, then the target neurons would be expected to have Trk receptors at the synapse. In fact, an electron microscopic study of TrkB and TrkC receptors showed that they are located at postsynaptic profiles in the developing (and adult) central nervous system (Hafidi *et al.*, 1996).

It is also interesting to consider that membrane depolarization, which is often found to enhance the survival of cultured neurons, actually promotes the expression of survival factor receptors. In a sympathetic neuron cell line, membrane depolarization causes the cells to produce TrkA receptor, and this allows NGF to become an effective survival factor (Birren *et al.*, 1992).

In fact, some neurons depend on sufficient levels of cytoplasmic calcium even before they become dependent on neurotrophins (Larmet *et al.*, 1992). Thus, synapses may be employing more than one mechanism in keeping neurons alive, and these may include postsynaptic depolarization (and calcium homeostasis), activation of metabotropic receptors, and stimulation of neurotrophin receptors.

Summary

Naturally occurring cell death claims up to 80% of the differentiating neurons in the developing brain. Depending on the particular group of neurons, survival may depend on target-derived trophic substances, afferent synaptic activity, blood-born hormonal signals, and other cues that have yet to be confirmed *in vivo*. The diversity in survival signals is mirrored by a diversity of cytoplasmic mechanisms for dying. However, most forms of normal cell death require either the production or the activation of proteins that can do damage to the neuron, such as caspases. Given the danger of keeping death machinery in place, neurons also have a broad range of regulatory proteins that presumably ensure that the correct number of neurons are killed off.

Despite the wealth of candidate molecular mechanisms that have been identified as contributing to cell death, the process is little understood in the central nervous system. Perhaps there are CNS trophic factors that have yet to be discovered. Alternatively, CNS neurons tend to receive a broad array of afferents and often project to more than one target, suggesting that their survival is "well-distributed." As we search for additional factors, we must be cautious of evidence supporting a role for each individual factor in supporting neuron survival. There are innumerable ways to save neurons that are removed from the body and placed in culture, but many of these methods do *not* duplicate *in vivo* mechanisms, just as our need to wear a life vest in the ocean does not mean that we need one while eating supper. In contrast, the survival of many central neurons may include multiple factors, and the failure to observe an effect in genetically altered animals does not remove a factor from the list of candidates.

The role of electrical activity in cell survival points out the tremendous plasticity of the developing nervous system. Small perturbations of synaptic activity can have a profound impact on the number of cells and the amount of postsynaptic membrane on which the synapses form (see Chapter 9). It is not too difficult to imagine that these mechanisms are necessary to optimize the diverse kinds of neural circuitry found within each animal.

CHAPTER 8 · · · · · · · · · · · ·

Synapse Formation and Electric Function

· · · · ·

The average mammalian cortical neuron receives over 10,000 synapses along its soma and dendrites. Some of these synapses release glutamate which excites the postsynaptic neuron, while others release GABA which acts to inhibit the cell. At a single glutamatergic synapse there are several receptors that may open ion channels or activate second messenger systems. The change in membrane potential brought about by synaptic transmission can activate ion channels and, in the case of voltage-gated sodium channels, lead to an action potential. While this description is a sanitized version of synaptic organization in the CNS, it highlights some of the challenges for the study of neural development. For example, the excitatory and inhibitory contacts are not formed at random on the surface of cortical neurons. Having located a prefectly fine postsynaptic cell on which to synapse, each axonal process must identify the correct patch of membrane on which to set up shop. Most glutamatergic synapses are located on postsynaptic specializations, called spines, while GABAergic synapses tend to form on the cell body and proximal dendrite. There must also be a mechanism to control the total number of synapses that can form on any one neuron, with plenty of leftover membrane that is covered by glial endfeet.

Meanwhile, the cortical neuron is busy determining the appropriate type of transmitter receptors to place in the membrane. A tight little cluster of $GABA_A$ receptors on a dendritic spine head would be of little use to the glutamate-releasing terminals that are located there. At the same time that synapses are being constructed, each cortical neuron is producing and positioning many types of voltage-gated channels across its membrane. The correct type of calcium channel seems to be critical to the formation of synapses, as well as their subsequent function. However, if too many sodium channels are placed right next to an excitatory synapse it might lead to a full blown action potential before synaptic integration can occur. Alternatively, sodium channels may need to be localized right in some synapses, such as the neuromuscular junction, to ensure that neurotransmission produces an action potential reliably.

To begin to understand this complexity we first consider separately how presynaptic terminals and postsynaptic specializations arise. There seem to be two general truths that emerge from this section. First, neurons manufacture many of the synaptic building blocks even before making contact with one another. Second, a great deal of intercellular communication accompanies the maturation of these emerging contacts. Once we have understood something about how synapses are fabricated, we can begin to discuss how they work (or fail to work) at birth. Of course, the function of a neuron depends on more than just its synapses, so we conclude by learning about the development a neuron's electrical properties.

Synaptogenesis

The formation of synaptic connections distinguishes nervous system development from that of all other tissues in the body. We have already seen that axon terminals follow a set of extracellular cues to reach the correct target and then selectively arborize in one part of the target based upon positional cues (see Chapters 5 and 6). Synaptogenesis begins when a growth cone comes in contact with an appropriate postsynaptic cell and continues as the growth cone differentiates into a presynaptic terminal. The decision to stop growing and differentiate is made in concert with the postsynaptic cell. However, both the growth cone and the postsynaptic cell begin to generate essential components for neurotransmission even before the initial contact. Therefore, the pace of synaptogenesis is rather explosive, and little mistakes in connectivity are corrected during a later period of development (see Chapter 9).

One general problem in studying synapses at any age is that they are extremely small, often having a contact length of about 1 μm. This makes them nearly impossible to see with a light microscope, and one might wonder how they were discovered in the first place. In fact, at the turn of the century, one group of biologists believed that neuronal processes fused with one another to produce long fibers with a continuous protoplasm, called a syncytium (Fig. 8.1). Another group of scientists felt that neurons were separate cells, as had been shown for other cell types, and these neurons must be in contact with one another at the tips of their processes (Ramon y Cajal, 1905). The great interest that was then focused on the tips of neuronal processes led both to the discovery of growth cones in very young tissue (see Chapter 4), and to the first descriptions of presynaptic terminals in older animals (Held, 1897). Charles Sherrington, winner of the 1932 Nobel Prize in Medicine, realized that a separation between nerve cells would allow for a new form of intercellular communication (cf. chemical transmission), and he popularized the term synapse (Sherrington, 1906).

The fundamental questions of synaptogenesis concern how a growth cone becomes transformed into a presynaptic terminal and how a uniform postsynaptic membrane becomes specialized at discrete loci along its surface. Moreover, we would like to understand the mechanisms that control pre- and postsynaptic differentiation. While some synaptic features arise intrinsically, there is now a great deal of evidence to suggest that signals emanating from glia, ECM, or other neurons participate in synaptogenesis.

What Does Synapse Formation Look Like?

Studies of the synapse began in earnest during the early 1950s. With the arrival of two new techniques, electron microscopy and intracellular recordings, one finally had the ability to see the complex structure of synaptic contacts and to observe their behavior (Palade and Palay, 1954; Fatt and Katz, 1951). Together, these techniques established the yardstick by which we determine whether two nerve cells are, in fact, connected to one another. At the functional level, a brief change in postsynaptic membrane potential in response to afferent stimulation is the key identifying feature of a synapse. At the structural level, an accumulation of presynaptic vesicles, a

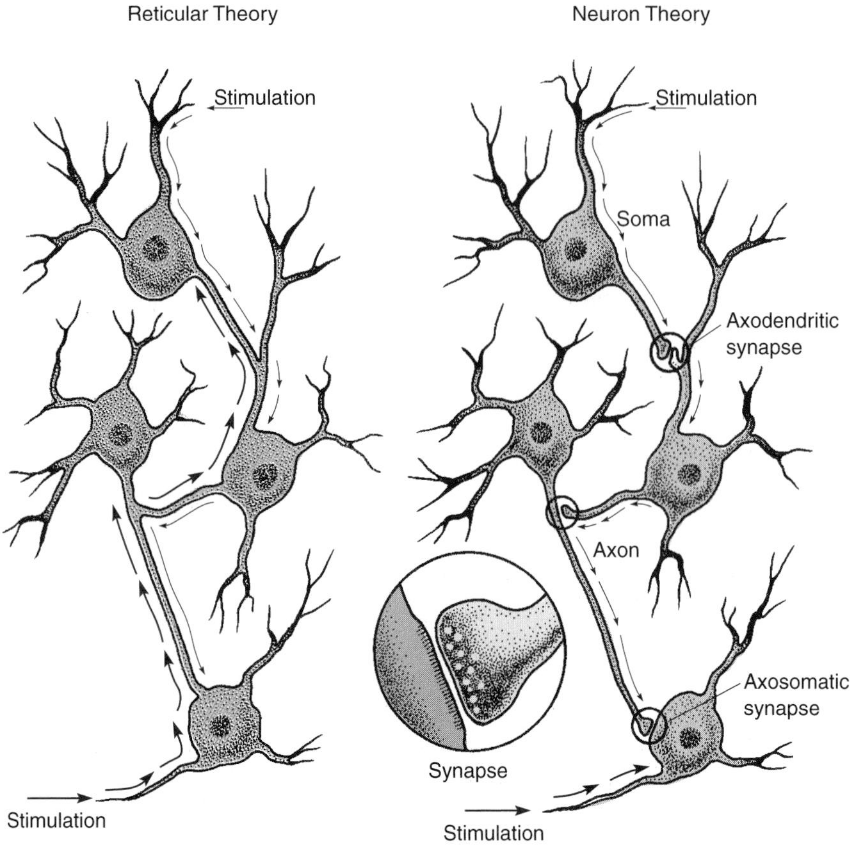

Figure 8.1 Reticular versus neuron theory. Over a century ago, the nervous sytem was thought to be a syncytium (left) of cells that were joined together by their processes. This arrangement would permit electrical activity to travel through the syncytium in either direction (thin and thick arrows) upon stimulation. As evidence mounted that neurons were separate cells (right), it was recognized that a chemical synapse (inset) would permit electrical activity to travel in only one direction (thin arrows).

narrow cleft between membranes, and a post-synaptic membrane thickening are all clear signs of synapse formation. One of the most common observations at newly formed synapses is that the number of synaptic vesicles in the presynaptic terminal profile is extremely low (Fig. 8.2). In the rodent cortex, the average number of vesicles found in a synaptic profile increases almost three-fold during the first postnatal month (Dyson and Jones, 1980).

Neither anatomy nor physiology alone is sufficient to identify a developing synapse. Purely anatomical measures of synapse formation can

be misleading because some functional contacts are known to develop rapidly, with little evidence of specialized morphology. On the other hand, an exclusively functional assay of synapse formation may create problems because there is evidence that "silent" synapses exist in the CNS that nonethless display normal structure. For the sake of simplicity, we begin with an anatomical description of synaptogenesis, and the molecular and physiological transformations that accompany them are considered below.

Ultrastructural studies provide the strongest evidence for the time period when synapses are

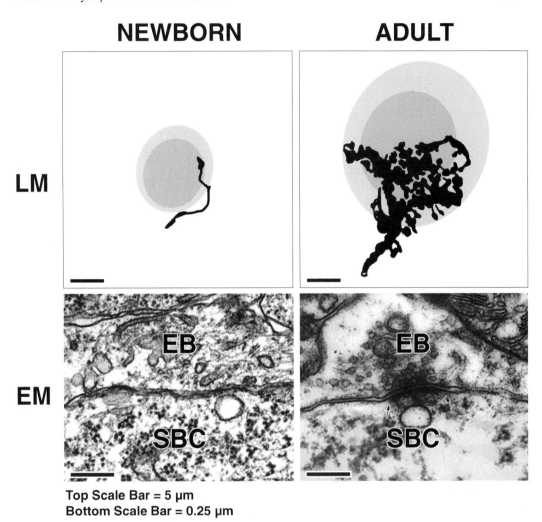

NEWBORN   **ADULT**

LM

EM

EB

SBC

EB

SBC

Top Scale Bar = 5 μm
Bottom Scale Bar = 0.25 μm

Figure 8.2 Development of synapse morphology. The contact of an auditory nerve endbulb (EB) onto its postsynaptic target, the spherical bushy cell (SBC), in the newborn and adult mouse. (Left) As shown in the drawing of a light microscopic (LM) view, the endbulb initially forms a small contact on the spherical bushy cell in newborn mice. When these contacts are examined at the ultrastructural level, there is little evidence of synapse differentiation. (Right) In adults, the endbulb forms an extremely large ending on the spherical busy cell. At the ultrastructural level, these contacts display many signs of mature synapses, including presynaptic vesicles and a postsynaptic membrane density. (C. J. Limb, T. Pongstaporn, and D. K. Ryugo, presented at the 1999 Assoc. Res. in Otolaryngol. Meeting)

added in the peripheral and central nervous systems. Bursts of synapse formation are found throughout the nervous system, but the timing and duration vary greatly (Vaughn, 1989). In the mouse olfactory bulb, synaptic profiles can first be recognized in electron micrographs at Embryonic Day 14 (E14). The total number of synaptic profiles increases exponentially through

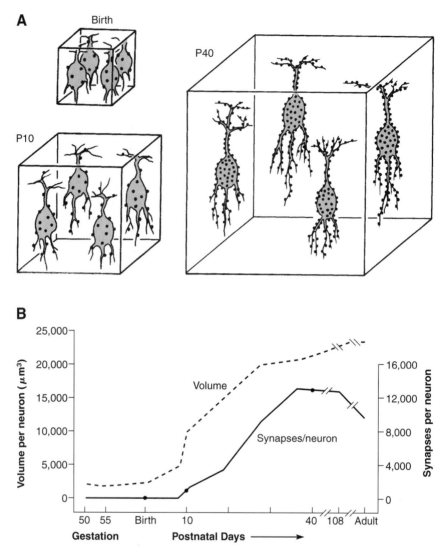

Figure 8.3 Growth of neuronal elements during cat visual cortex development. (A) From birth until Post-natal Day 40 (P40), the density of neuronal cell bodies decreases as gliogenesis and angiogenesis occur. During this same period, dendritic arbors are expanding, and synaptic terminals (black dots) are accumulating on the postsynaptic membrane. (B) The total volume of visual cortex occupied by each neuron increases by almost 10-fold during the first postnatal month. When neuron packing density is taken into consideration, the accumulation of synapses can be expressed as synapses per neuron. As shown in the graph, there is a dramatic increase in synapses from P10 to P30 and a significant decline after P108. (Adapted from Cragg, 1975)

the first postnatal week and then continues to increase at a lower rate over the next several weeks (Fig. 8.3). Therefore, new synaptic contacts continue to be manufactured over a long time period after axons invade their target. One reason for this extended period of synaptogenesis is that dendrites are still growing and the addition of postsynaptic membrane may attract new contacts. It is also likely that certain afferent projections may arborize at different times. In the rat visual cortex, where the synaptic profiles of excitatory and inhibitory synapses can be recognized, their increase in number occurs at different times. Other areas display a steady increase in synapse number, such as the the rat superior cervical ganglion, where the process occurs gradually from innervation at E14 to over 1 month after birth (Smolen, 1981).

Where Do Synaptic Specializations Form?

The location of synapse formation is extremely important to the operation of the nervous system. Even at the nerve–muscle junction, motor synapses form at distinct central locations on the myofibers. On the typical central neuron there are many more options. Synapses that form near the soma are thought to have a greater voice in deciding whether the neuron will fire an action potential or not. Thus, inhibitory synapses are often found nestled up around the cell body so that they can halt activity efficiently. In contrast, many synapses form on dendritic spines where their activity provides tiny potentials that must be summed together to produce a significant change in the neuron's activity. When many different types of afferents synapse on a postsynaptic neuron, each with a distinct functional role, then the problem becomes quite difficult indeed. Does synaptogenesis proceed in any particular sequence, and how does each synapse know where to form on the postsynaptic cell?

There is some reason to believe that dendrites initially provide a more suitable contact site than the soma. Again, the electron microscopist has been able to show where synapses are added because both the presynaptic terminal and the postsynaptic location (e.g., soma, dendrite, spine) are identifiable at high magnification. In many systems, including the spinal cord, the hippocampus, and the cortex, synapses seem to form initially on the dendritic processes. For example, nearly 75% of axodendritic synapses are found on dendritic growth cones in the embryonic mouse spinal cord (Vaughn *et al.*, 1974).

Even in the cortex and hippocampus, axodendritic synapses are present in newborn tissue, while few axosomatic synapses are found until 2–3 weeks later (Pappas and Purpura, 1964; Schwartz *et al.*, 1968).

Early observations from Golgi-stained spinal cord material showed axonal growth cones and dendritic growth cones seemingly reaching for one another, suggesting that axodendritic synapses result from an early trophic interaction. In fact, dendrite growth is quite dependent on the presence of afferent connections and possibly the transmitters that they release. More recently, it has been suggested that synapses may actually be prevented from forming at some locations by the presence of glial cell processes that wrap around parts of the postsynaptic neuron. For example, excitatory connections to an auditory brain stem nucleus called the medial superior olive (MSO) are at first restricted to the dendritic regions of the cell. At this stage, MSO cell bodies are completely surrounded by glial membrane. As the glial membrane regresses, synapses are formed on the MSO cell bodies (Brunso-Bechtold *et al.*, 1992). In this regard, it is interesting that elimination of a putative cell adhesion molecule at the neuromuscular junction (cf. s-laminin) permits glial processes to invade the synaptic region and impede synapse maturation (Noakes *et al.*, 1995). Therefore, glial cells may serve as a bodyguard, determining when and where synapses can be formed, and the postsynaptic cell can dismiss the bodyguard by expressing specific cell surface proteins.

During the time when synapses are forming between nerve cells, it is quite common to see pre- and postsynaptic structures all by themselves, essentially, synapses to nowhere (Fig. 8.4). From the amphibian spinal cord to the rodent olfactory cortex, presynaptic-like structures with an accumulation of vesicles apparently develop in the absence of a postsynaptic cell. Similarly, postsynaptic densities that are not in contact with a presynaptic terminal have been found in the olfactory bulb and cortex. These lonesome structures indicate that growth cones and dendrites are poised on the brink of differentiating into synaptic specializations (Hayes

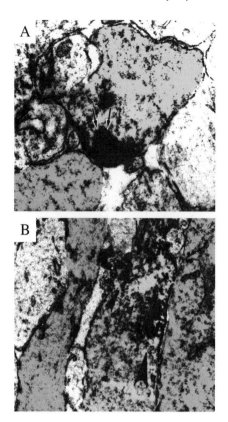

Figure 8.4 Postsynaptic differentiation without a presynaptic contact. (A) An electron micrograph showing clustering of $\alpha2$-adrenergic receptor (arrows) in a Postnatal Day 4 rat visual cortex neuron. Both of the tinted structures are dendrites. (B) An electron micrograph showing clustering of the AMPA-type receptor subunit GluR2 (arrowheads) in a Postnatal Day 4 rat visual cortex neuron. All three of the tinted structures are dendrites. (From C. Aoki, unpublished observations)

and Roberts, 1973; Newman-Gage *et al.,* 1987; Westrum, 1975; Hinds and Hinds, 1976b).

Presynaptic terminal differentiation has even been found to occur on nonneuronal cells. Transient presynaptic-like terminals have been identified on glial cells during axon ingrowth, particularly in areas without dendritic processes (Hendrikson and Vaughn, 1974). In a *Drosophila* mutant that has no mesoderm, and therefore no muscle, motor axons continue to form presynaptic-like profiles on glia and other cells (Prokop *et al.,* 1996). However, some cells appear to be crucial for synapse differentiation. Ablation of selected embryonic muscle precursors in *Caenorhabditis*

results in gaps in a set of dorsal muscles and prevents presynaptic varicosity formation (Plunkett *et al.,* 1996).

The general significance of these observations are threefold. First, synaptogenesis does not take place over a uniform time frame throughout the nervous system, even within a single species. Second, synapse formation proceeds for days to months after the ingrowth of afferents and may even occur at low levels in adult animals. Third, growing neuronal processes may express a synaptic phenotype with little or no encouragement from its appropriate partner. Nevertheless, we will see that the normal maturation of stable synapses does involve a substantial number of interactions.

Initial Signs of Synaptogenesis in Vitro

Even the highest power electron microscope can not detect the onset of synaptogenesis between a growth cone and a postsynaptic cell (Vaughn, 1989). There is simply not much to be seen. More importantly, the morphology can not tell us how the synapse is working. To get around these problems, many scientists have turned to the tissue culture technique where it is possible to watch cells come into contact with one another and monitor synapse morphology and function from moment to moment (see Chapter 5, Box: Tissue Culture Advantage). The earliest tissue culture studies demonstrated that mature synapses could form in isolated pieces of neural tissue, but the temporal resolution was comparable to the best *in vivo* studies. When it became possible to observe the growth cone approaching a postsynaptic target neuron, then observations were first made close to the onset of synaptogenesis.

One of the first *in vitro* systems consisted of a piece of fetal rat spinal cord plated next to dissociated neurons from the superior cervical ganglion, a target of autonomic motor neurons (Rees *et al.,* 1976). Within the first several hours of contact, there are only subtle changes in morphology to indicate that synapse formation is underway (Fig. 8.5). Of course, this is precisely why *in vivo* observations could not detect the very onset of synapse formation. At first, the growth cone loses its filopodia and forms a punctate contact that is unusually close to the postsynaptic cell membrane (about 7 nm, less than the diameter of a hemoglobin molecule). This suggests that an adhesive interaction may be involved in the initial stages of synaptogenesis (Rees *et al.,* 1976; Buchanan *et al.,* 1989). There are also many examples of presynaptic protrusions being engulfed by muscle membrane, termed coated pits. These observations show an intense interaction at the initial site of contact. The first sign of differentiation is found below the postsynaptic membrane, where the Golgi apparatus accumulates and coated vesicles proliferate, both of which probably contribute to the construction of the postsynaptic density. As for the presynaptic terminal, it is only after about 24 h of contact that vesicles begin to accumulate at the site of contact. Thus, the *structure* of a synapse appears to mature over a relatively long period, and the postsynaptic cell is the first to display any signs of differentiation.

At the moment a growth cone comes in contact with its postsynaptic target it begins a metamorphosis, transforming from a homely pathfinding organelle to a radiant presynaptic terminal. One surprise is that the growth cone already has a rudimentary transmitter-releasing mechanism. This was shown in tissue culture preparations where the postsynaptic neuron could be recorded from while the growth cone approached and made contact. (Young and Poo, 1983; Hume *et al.,* 1983). During the first 2 days of a *Xenopus* spinal neuron and myocyte culture, neurons produce growth cones, extend neurites, and form functional contacts with neighboring muscle cells. A special electrode was constructed having an excised piece of muscle cell membrane at its tip, and this membrane contained ACh receptors (see Box: Biophysics: Nuts and Bolts of Functional Maturation). When a patch of AChR-containing membrane is brought close to the growth cone, the AChR-coupled channels open and current flows, indicating that the growth cone is releasing ACh spontaneously (Fig. 8.6). Growth cones are also able to release transmitter in response to electrical stimulation of their cell bodies. Therefore, some of the presynaptic neurotransmission machinery is present even before synaptogenesis, albeit in an immature form.

Role of Calcium during Presynaptic Differentiation

The adult-like morphology of a synapse usually emerges only after nerve cells have been

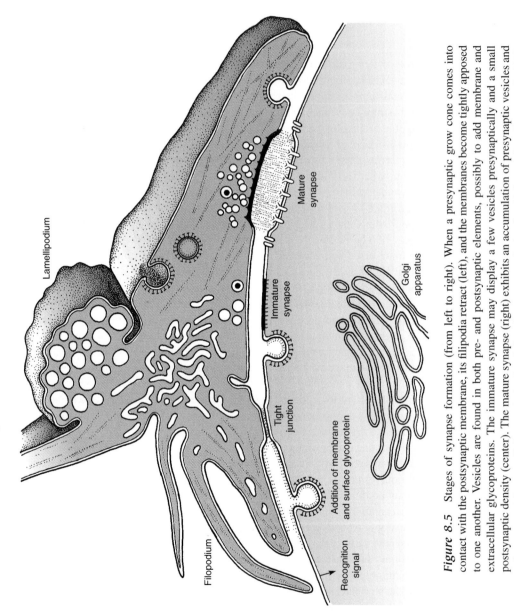

Figure 8.5 Stages of synapse formation (from left to right). When a presynaptic grow cone comes into contact with the postsynaptic membrane, its filipodia retract (left), and the membranes become tightly apposed to one another. Vesicles are found in both pre- and postsynaptic elements, possibly to add membrane and extracellular glycoproteins. The immature synapse may display a few vesicles presynaptically and a small postsynaptic density (center). The mature synapse (right) exhibits an accumulation of presynaptic vesicles and a dense material extracellular matrix in the cleft and a postsynaptic density. (Adapted from Rees *et al.*, 1978, with permission)

Biophysics: Nuts and Bolts of Functional Maturation

The study of neural tissue development is unique because the cells possess diverse electrical properties. These properties result from two essential components. First, the neuron must produce batteries by selectively pumping ions from one side of the membrane to the other. Second, the neuron must produce switches, commonly referred to as voltage- and ligand-gated channels, that allow the batteries to discharge (i.e., ionic currents flow due to an electrochemical gradient) across the membrane. To determine how pumps and channels operate, one must be able to record from a single neuron (or a portion of it) and to control the neuron's environment. The most important parameters that must be controlled include ionic composition, voltage across the membrane, and the presence of ligands. The technical challenges presented by these requirements have largely been overcome in the past 4 decades, providing some fundamental discoveries about developing neurons.

To study the voltage-gated channels, one must be able to move the membrane potential to different holding voltages (voltage-clamp) and then observe whether current flows across the membrane. Thus, if one depolarizes an axon, voltage-gated sodium channels will open at some criterion voltage, termed threshold, and Na^+ will enter the cell (i.e., inward current). A novel set of recording techniques, call patch-clamping, was introduced to fully characterize different types of channels. Patch-clamp electrodes can form high resistance seals ("giga-seals") with small areas of membrane, and these patches of membrane can then be excised from the cell (Hamill *et al.,* 1981). There are several advantage of this approach. Small patches of membrane often contain single channels; they are relatively easy to voltage-clamp, and either side of the membrane may be exposed to the defined media. These techniques allow one to determine a channel's signature properties: the voltage at which activation and inactivation occur, the mean channel open time, the mean current amplitude, the relative permeability to different ions, and the pharmacological profile. Finally, when the excised patches of tissue contain a known class of neurotransmitter receptors, then the recording pipet may be used to detect the release of neurotransmitter ("sniffer pipets"). This approach has led to the discovery that growth cones release transmitter (Young and Poo, 1983; Hume *et al.,* 1983).

It is also possible to form a giga-seal with the neuron of interest and then rupture the membrane, forming a whole-cell recording configuration. Although this technique is qualitatively similar to a standard sharp electrode intracellular recording, there are added benefits. The tip of the recording electrode is much larger than that of the sharp electrode, both improving the signal-to-noise ratio and allowing for relatively large current injections. The large tip diameter translates into a large hole in the membrane through which the patch pipet solution travels quite easily, allowing the intracellular composition to be controlled within a matter of minutes. In a more elegant form of this technique, a perfusion system is added to the recording pipet such that intracellular composition can be altered during a recording session (Chen *et al.,* 1990).

While the patch-clamp techniques offer rigid biophysical measures, they seldom allow one to evaluate the movement of a single type of ion. One common strategy requires the use of several antagonists to block the contribution of contaminating ions (e.g., magnesium ions block the flow of calcium). A second approach makes use of a novel group of electrodes, each of which is responsive to changes in the concentration of a specific ion, such

(continued)

Biophysics: Nuts and Bolts of Functional Maturation *continued*

as potassium (Syková, 1992). The tips of these electrodes are filled with a liquid membrane that is selectively permeable to one species of ion, such that local changes in concentration result in the net movement of that ion across the membrane, resulting in a detectable potential difference. When employed in the central nervous system, these electrodes reveal substantial developmental changes in the regulation of extracellular potassium and pH (Connors *et al.,* 1982; Davis *et al.,* 1987; Jendelová and Syková, 1991)

The fields of electrophysiology and image processing have found a productive relationship in the area of membrane channels. The introduction of ion-sensitive fluorescent dyes has provided a noninvasive means of assessing functional properties while providing a high degree of spacial resolution. Each of these dyes emit light at a specific wavelength when activated with an exciting beam of light at a different wavelength. The amount of emitted light is proportional to the free concentration of a specific species of ion. That is because a dye's absorption or emission properties are altered when it binds to the ion. Selective indicator dyes now exist for a wide range of ions including Na^+, Ca^{2+}, C^-, and H^+. The indicator dye fluo-3 has been used to demonstrate an elevation of Ca^{2+} immediately following contact between growth cone and target cell (Dai and Peng, 1993). A novel variation of this technology makes use of compounds that exist in a "caged" configuration and which only become activated when exposed to light of a specific wavelength. In this manner, one may elevate the concentration of a specific substance with great temporal and spatial resolution.

in contact with one another for some time, a time during which intercellular communication exerts a strong influence. In fact, growth cones usually slow down when they enter their target, and this may involve a signal to halt growth cone motility and encourage synapse formation. Evidence for a target stop signal was found in a system where newborn mouse basilar pontine nuclei were cocultured with their target neurons, the granule cells of the cerebellum (Baird *et al.,* 1992). Pontine neurites grow slowly (>50 μm/h) on polylysine or laminin, but grow rapidly (>100 μm/h) on cerebellar glial cells. When pontine nuclei were cultured on a bed of glia along with dissociated granule cells, the outgrowth of neurites was depressed. By closely examining individual neurites it was found that the decreased growth was due to contact with granule cells. Neurites that did not come upon a granule cell during their outgrowth continued to grow for a normal distance. Moreover, when granule cells

were suspended above the pontine explants, the neurites grew at a normal rate. Thus, neurite outgrowth can be terminated at the appropriate target by a contact-dependent mechanism.

The dialogue between pre- and postsynaptic cells begins as soon as the growth cone filopodia make contact. Calcium levels suddenly increase in the growth cone (Dai and Peng, 1993; Zoran *et al.,* 1993). This was determined for both frog and snail motor neurons that were grown in dissociated tissue culture and filled with a Ca^{2+}-sensitive indicator dye. When a muscle cell is manipulated into contact with a growth cone, the Ca^{2+} increases locally within seconds (Fig. 8.7). This response exhibits some target specificity. The Ca^{2+} rise only occurs when appropriate postsynaptic cells are manipulated into contact with the motor neuron. This mechanism is similar to the collapse of growth cones as they contact specific pathfinding cues, which is often accompanied by an elevation of intracellular

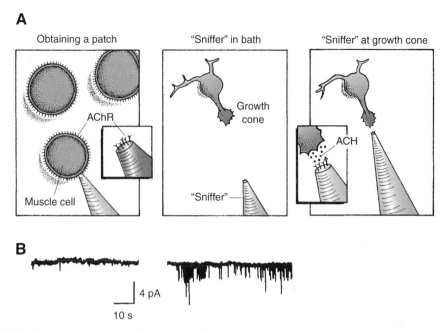

A

Obtaining a patch

AChR

Muscle cell

"Sniffer" in bath

Growth cone

"Sniffer"

"Sniffer" at growth cone

ACH

B

4 pA

10 s

Figure 8.6 Spontaneous release of neurotransmitter from growth cones. (A) A biological sensor for ACh (a "sniffer") was created by excising a patch of membrane from a muscle cell with a recording pipet. The membrane contained AChRs that were facing outward. Thus, when the pipet was advanced near a growth cone, a current could be recorded when ACh bound to the receptors. (B) Recording of ACh-evoked currents (downward deflections) when the sniffer pipet was distant from the growth cone (left) and when it was within a few micrometers of the growth cone (right). The increased activity indicates that the growth cone was releasing ACh. (Traces from Young and Poo, adapted with permission from *Nature* **305:** 634–637, Copyright 1983 Macmillan Magazines Limited)

Ca^{2+} (see Chapter 4). It is not yet clear how calcium levels increase, but one possibility is that calcium is released from internal stores. In the rat central nervous system, IP_3 receptors, which transduce calcium release from endoplasmic reticulum, are upregulated during the period of intense synaptogenesis (Dent *et al.,* 1996).

What is the evidence that a contact-evoked rise in Ca^{2+} provides a signal for growth cone differentiation? Intracellular Ca^{2+} can be manipulated in growth cones by exposing them to ionophores such as A23187, a molecule that spontaneously inserts into a neuron's membrane allowing Ca^{2+} to pass freely into the cell (Mattson and Kater, 1987). As calcium rises, growth cones are often found to slow down and to assume a rounded appearance (Fig. 8.8A). The effect of increased calcium can even be detected on growth cones that have been isolated from their cell

body, indicating that calcium acts locally. When the Ca^{2+} concentration within the growth cone is adjusted to differerent levels by setting extracellular Ca^{2+} concentration, cultured chick DRG growth cones became stationary in all but a limited range of Ca^{2+} concentrations: from 200 to 300 nM (Lankford and Letourneau, 1991).

Second Messengers Mediate Presynaptic Differentiation

Because changes in free Ca^{2+} are relatively easy to observe with fluorescent dyes, we tend to emphasize the importance of these events. The activity of other second messenger systems can not be observed directly, but we can find out whether they play a role by using pharmacological agents

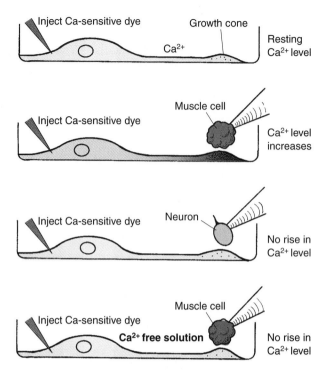

Figure 8.7   Contact with target increases free calcium in the growth cone. Dissociated neurons were filled with a Ca^{2+}-sensitive dye (top), and the growth cone was imaged while either a muscle cell or a neuron was brought into contact (middle). Intracellular free calcium increased only during contact with the muscle (red). The muscle-evoked rise in Ca^{2+} did not occur when the cells were bathed in a Ca^{2+}-free medium (bottom), indicating the involvement of calcium channels. (Adapted from Dai and Peng, 1993)

that activate or block the substance. For example, cAMP levels can be artificially increased by introducing membrane-permeable analogs, by activating synthesis with adenylate cyclase, or by inhibiting cAMP breakdown with phosphodiesterases. In fact, each of these manipulations can decrease neurite extension in certain neuronal populations (Mattson *et al.,* 1988; Lankford and Letourneau, 1991).

To study this mechanism in more detail, a giant growth cone preparation was made from cultured *Aplysia* bag cells (Forscher *et al.,* 1987). When these growth cones come into contact with a target, microtubules extend toward the site of contact and filamentous actin begins to accumulate. A similar transformation can be produced by raising cAMP levels within the growth cone. The cytoskeleton reorganizes and neurosecretory granules invade the growth cone's lamellapodia,

resulting in a presynaptic-like morphology (Fig. 8.8B). Interestingly, cAMP signaling continues to play a role in the formation and stability of synaptic connections (see Chapter 9). Another signaling pathway may also contribute to the transformation of bag cell growth cones into presynaptic-like structures. Activation of protein kinase C (PKC), an enzyme that is normally regulated by calcium and a phospholipid (diacylglycerol, DAG), results in the rapid appearance of new calcium channels at the edge of the grow cone (Knox *et al.,* 1992).

Calcium, PKC, and cAMP probably work together to produce a terminal that has secretory vesicles at the sight of contact as well as the appropriate ion channels for excitation–secretion coupling. In fact, the contact-evoked increase in calcium may actually be a result of cAMP signaling. When an identified snail motor neuron is

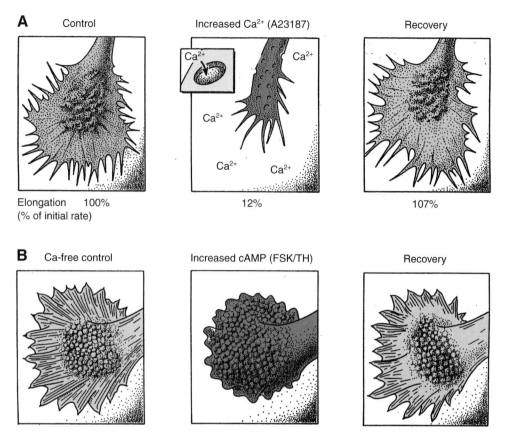

Figure 8.8 Calcium and cAMP may initiate presynaptic differentiation. (A) Intracellular free calcium is increased in cultured snail buccal neurons using the Ca^{2+} ionophore A23187. As calcium enters the growth cone (dark red), it slows down and retracts its lamellipodia and most of its filopodia. When the ionophore is removed, the growth cone is once again elaborated. (B) Intracellular cAMP levels are increased in cultured *Aplysia* bag cell neurons by exposing them to an adenylate cyclase activator, forskolin (FSK), and a phosphodiesterase inhibitor, theophylline (TH). When cAMP levels rise (dark grey), growth cone motility ceases and organelles fill the lamellipodia. When the drugs are removed, the growth cone morphology is restored. (Adapted from Mattson and Kater, 1987; Forscher *et al.*, 1987)

manipulated into contact with its normal target *in vitro*, it exhibits an increase in calcium (Funte and Haydon, 1993). This calcium increase can be mimicked by a membrane permeable analog of cAMP, and it can be prevented when an inhibitor of cAMP-dependent protein kinase (PKA) is injected into the motor neuron.

How are these intracellular signals activated during growth cone differentiation? Certain neurotransmitter receptors can evoke a Ca^{2+} influx, and some of these receptors have been shown to inhibit growth cone motility (Mattson and Kater, 1989). Cell adhesion molecules are also capable

of transducing cell surface signals to produce an elevation of internal Ca^{2+} (Doherty *et al.*, 1991). However, the receptor–ligand interactions that activate PKA or PKC have yet to be identified.

Molecular Signals and Presynaptic Differentiation

Adhesion between growth cones and target cells increases rapidly upon contact (Evers *et al.*, 1989). To demonstrate this sort of adhesion *in vitro*, round muscle cells, known as myoballs, were lifted off the culture dish with a pipet and placed in contact with the growing tip of a *Xenopus* spinal neuron (Fig. 8.9). At either 1.5 or 15 min after a contact was initiated, the intercellular adhesion was evaluated by observing how much the neurite was deformed as the myoball was pulled away. While a low level of adhesion is evident after 1.5 min, the percentage of tightly adherent contacts doubles during the first 15 min of contact.

What kinds of adhesion molecules are involved in the formation of early contacts? At the nerve–muscle junction, NCAM is gradually lost during innervation, but reappears at the endplate following denervation. This suggests that NCAM facilitates synapse formation, but nerve–muscle contacts appear to develop normally in NCAM knockout mice (Covault and Sanes, 1985; Moscoso *et al.*, 1998). The initial development of motor synapses in fruit flies is also normal in the absence of FasII, a homolog of NCAM (Schuster *et al.*, 1996a). However, the synapses retract from the muscle in slightly older fasII -/- animals, suggesting that this cell adhesion molecule is required for the stabilization of connections. Another family of cell adhesion molecules, called cadherins, are located at many different central synapses, including the cerebellum and the hippocampus. In the hippocampus, two members of the family, N-cadherin and E-cadherin, are restricted to separate synapses along the dendrite, suggesting a role in specific innervation patterns (Fannon and Colman, 1996). However, we still do not know how they contribute to the initial formation of hippocampal synapses.

Another set of adhesion molecules that could facilitate synapse differentiation is found in the extracellular matrix (see Chapter 5). One ECM molecule that is synthesized by muscle and deposited in the synaptic cleft, called s-laminin, can inhibit neurite outgrowth. Thus, s-laminin may slow the growth cone and promote its transformation into a presynaptic terminal (Porter *et al.*, 1995). Furthermore, s-laminin may directly influence the presynaptic differentiation. In s-laminin knockout mice, there is a dramatic decrease of vesicle-associated phosphoproteins, called synapsins, in presynaptic motor terminals (Noakes *et al.*, 1995).

Synapsins, themselves, appear to play an important role in synapse development. For example, overexpression of synapsin IIb in a neuroblastoma × glioma hybrid cell line leads to an increase in the number of synapse-like contacts (Han *et al.*, 1991). In order to decrease synapsin expression, hippocampal cultures were exposed to synapsin II antisense oligonucleotides (Fig. 8.10). When the number of synapses was assessed by staining for other presynaptic proteins, synapse formation was found to be prevented, or even reversed (Ferreira *et al.*, 1995).

Endogenous signals can also actively prevent synapse formation. For example, when semaphorin II is misexpressed in a set of identified fly muscle fibers, their motor axons do not make synaptic contacts (Fig. 8.11). As the semaphorin II misexpression gradually declines with age, the motor axons eventually begin to innervate the muscle fibers (Matthes *et al.*, 1995). Thus, both permissive and restrictive signaling systems regulate the differentiation of growth cones into presynaptic terminals.

Receptor Clustering Signifies Postsynaptic Differentiation at NMJ

Many neurotransmitter receptors are produced before innervation occurs. However, the aggregation of these proteins is the most important hallmark of synapse formation. Is receptor clustering a cell-autonomous process or is it induced by the presynaptic terminal? At first inspection, the postsynaptic site appears to be produced in an autonomous fashion. Acetylcholine receptors (AChRs) form small clusters on the muscle cell membrane even before the motor axon terminals arrive (Fischbach and Cohen, 1973). Structures that resemble postsynaptic densities, but which do not appear to contact a presynaptic element, have also been found in the developing olfactory bulb and visual cortex during early development (Hinds and Hinds, 1976b; Bahr and Wolff, 1985).

The process of receptor clustering has been explored most thoroughly at the NMJ, and many

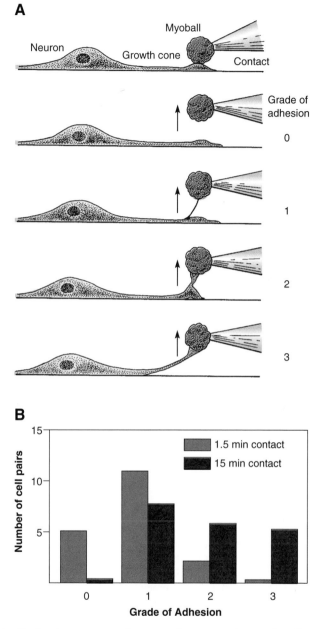

Figure 8.9 Rapid adhesion between growth cone and postsynaptic muscle cell. (A) A muscle cell was manipulated into contact with a growth cone in dissociated cultures of *Xenopus* spinal cord. After 1.5 or 15 min, the muscle cell was withdrawn, and the degree of adhesion was graded: 0, no attachment; 1, filamentous attachment; 2, deformation of growth cone; and 3, detachment of growth cone from substrate. (B) After 1.5 min of contact, most pairs exhibited only grade 0–1 adhesion. However, after 15 min of contact, the level of adhesion shifted to grade 1–3. (Adapted from Evers *et al.,* 1989, with permission)

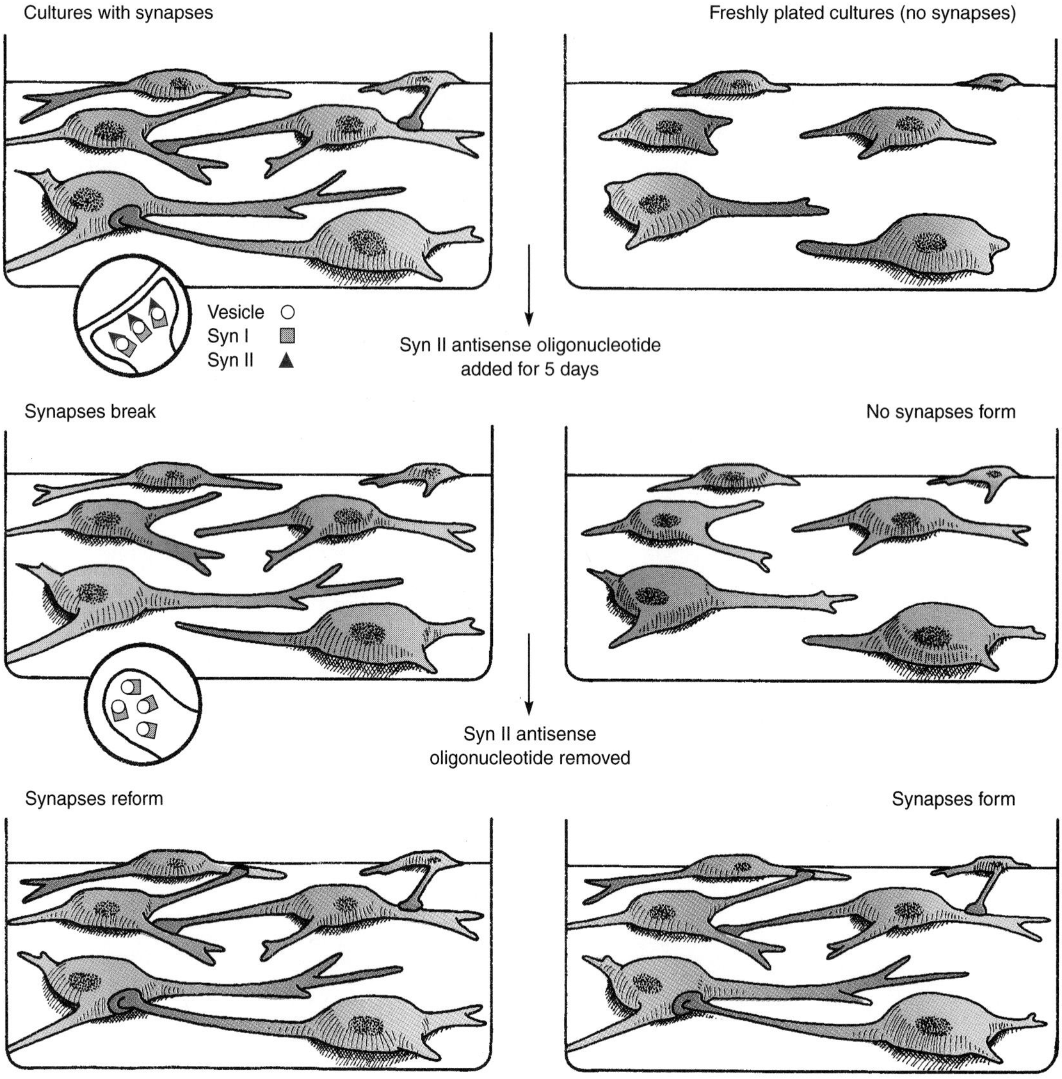

Cultures with synapses

Freshly plated cultures (no synapses)

Vesicle ○
Syn I ▪
Syn II ▲

Syn II antisense oligonucleotide
added for 5 days

Synapses break

No synapses form

Syn II antisense
oligonucleotide removed

Synapses reform

Synapses form

Figure 8.10 The vesicle-associated proteins synapsin II is necessary for synapse formation. In dissociated hippocampal cultures, the addition of a synapsin II antisense oligonucleotide will cause existing synapses to be broken (left column), or prevent new synapses from forming (right column). When the antisense oligonucleotide is removed, synapses can form once again. (Adapted from Ferreira *et al.,* 1995)

of the mechanisms are now well understood. At the time of innervation, muscle cell membrane contains a relatively even distribution of AChRs (Fig. 8.12). This was originally demonstrated by recording the response from rat muscle cells *in vivo* as ACh was applied at different places along the myofiber surface (Diamond and Miledi, 1962). Early in development, ACh application at each site evokes a similar shift in membrane potential. As the muscle became innervated, the ACh-evoked response becomes much larger at the site of innervation, and the response at extrasynaptic regions declines. It then became possible to visualize the distribution

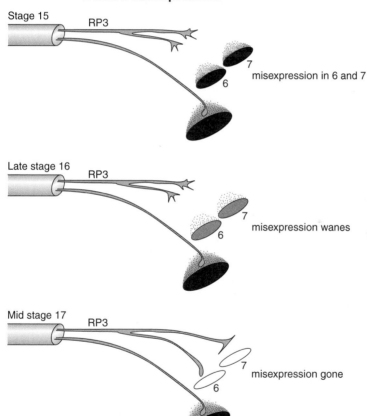

Figure 8.11 Postsynaptic expression of semaphorin II can block synapse formation. In normal *Drosophila* embryos (+/+), different motor axons innervate semaII-expressing muscle cells (33) and semaII-negative muscle cells (6 and 7). When semaII is misexpressed in muscles 6 and 7 during development, the RP3 motor axons do not make contact (stage 15). As the level of misexpressed semaII declines (stage 16 and 17), the RP3 axons gradually come to innervate muscles 6 and 7. (Adapted from Matthes *et al.,* 1995)

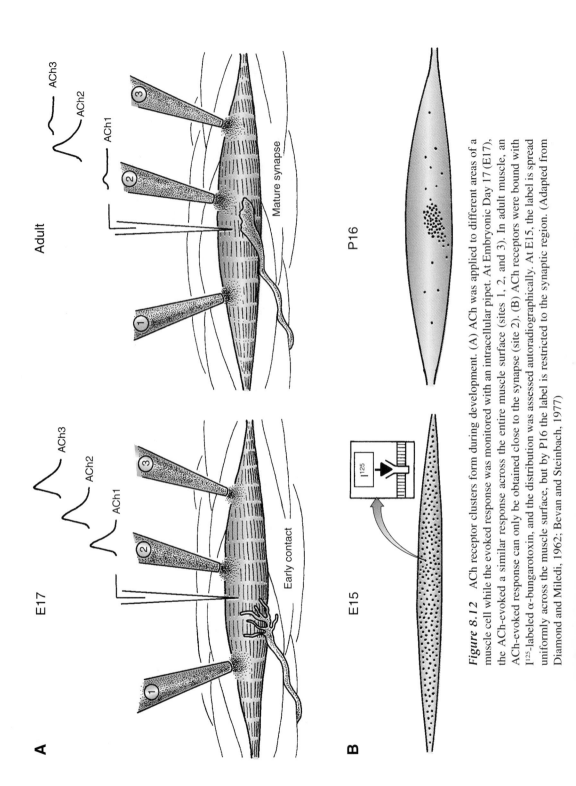

Figure 8.12 ACh receptor clusters form during development. (A) ACh was applied to different areas of a muscle cell while the evoked response was monitored with an intracellular pipet. At Embryonic Day 17 (E17), the ACh-evoked a similar response across the entire muscle surface (sites 1, 2, and 3). In adult muscle, an ACh-evoked response can only be obtained close to the synapse (site 2). (B) ACh receptors were bound with I^{125}-labeled α-bungarotoxin, and the distribution was assessed autoradiographically. At E15, the label is spread uniformly across the muscle surface, but by P16 the label is restricted to the synaptic region. (Adapted from Diamond and Miledi, 1962; Bevan and Steinbach, 1977)

of AChRs by labeling them with radioactive α-bungarotoxin (α-Btx), a high-affinity peptide from the venom of the Taiwanese cobra (Bevan and Steinbach, 1977; Burden, 1977a). Consistent with the electrophysiological measures, α-Btx labeling is evenly distributed at first and then becomes highly localized to the synapse (Fig. 8.12). The process of clustering leads to a dramatic disparity in receptor concentration: there are >10,000 AChRs/μm^2 at the synaptic region, but <10/μm^2 in the extrasynaptic regions (Fertuck and Salpeter, 1976; Burden, 1977a; Salpeter and Harris, 1983).

Presynaptic Terminals Induce Receptor Aggregation

The appearance of spontaneous AChR clusters on muscle cells, or "free" postsynaptic densities in the CNS, raises the possibility that "mature" regions of the postsynaptic cell might serve as preferred sites of innervation. Do these early postsynaptic sites induce the growth cone to terminate and form synapses? If one carefully watches a growth cone in tissue culture, it is seen to induce new postsynaptic sites at its initial site of contact. When dissociated cultures are made of cholinergic spinal cord neurons and myocytes, it is possible to follow the clustering of AChRs during the period of innervation by labeling the muscles with a fluorescent α-Btx (Anderson and Cohen, 1977; Cohen et al., 1979). Although small AChR clusters are seen prior to innervation, they do not serve as preferred sites of innervation. Rather, the growing neurites induce the rapid accumulation of AChRs as they extend across the muscle (Fig. 8.13A). When the temporal relationship between innervation and AChR cluster formation is estimated in the *Xenopus* embryo, nerve terminals precede the appearance of AChR clusters by about 3 h (Chow and Cohen, 1983). Indeed, the clustering of GABA$_A$ and AMPA receptors also appears to correlate with the presence of presynaptic contacts in hippocampal cultures, although precise measures have not yet been made (Killisch et al., 1991; Craig et al., 1993).

The ability to induce AChR clusters is specific to certain types of presynaptic neurons (Fig. 8.13B). In *Xenopus* dissociated cultures, dorsal root and sympathetic ganglion neurites can contact muscle cells, but they are associated with few AChR clusters. In contrast, neurites from spinal cord neurons, which presumably include motor neurons, are associated with AChR clusters at 70% of contact sites (Cohen and Weldon, 1980; Kidokoro et al., 1980). When spinal motor neurons are selectively prelabeled *in vivo*, and then dissociated in the presence of myocytes, their ability to induce AChR clusters can be compared to the unlabeled spinal interneurons (Role et al., 1985). Motor neurons and ciliary ganglion cells, both of which secrete ACh, are able to induce AChR clusters on all contacted myocytes, whereas the interneurons do not induce significant AChR clustering.

Studies at the NMJ suggest that appropriate nerve terminals (i.e., cholinergic) support the induction of AChR clusters. Does the neurotransmitter receptor have to be activated in order to cluster? When myocytes and spinal cord are cultured in the presence of an AChR antagonist, D-tubocurarine, they develop an identical number of functional contacts compared to control cultures (Cohen, 1972). To directly assess AChR clustering during the blockade of neurotransmission, fluorescently labeled α-Btx was first applied to visualize the AChRs that were present on muscle cell membrane, and excess unlabeled α-Btx was then added to prevent visualization of newly inserted AChRs (Anderson and Cohen, 1977). In these experiments, the clustering of AChRs occurs normally at the site of neurite contact in the absence of cholinergic transmission.

The clustering of AChRs is a result of both migration within the muscle membrane and, after several hours, insertion of newly synthesized protein. The speed with which AChRs can migrate along the muscle cell membrane was demonstrated by recording the amplitude of ACh-evoked depolarizations before and after the local iontophoresis of α-Btx onto a small area of the muscle cell surface (Poo, 1982). When the α-Btx is first applied, the ACh-evoked potential

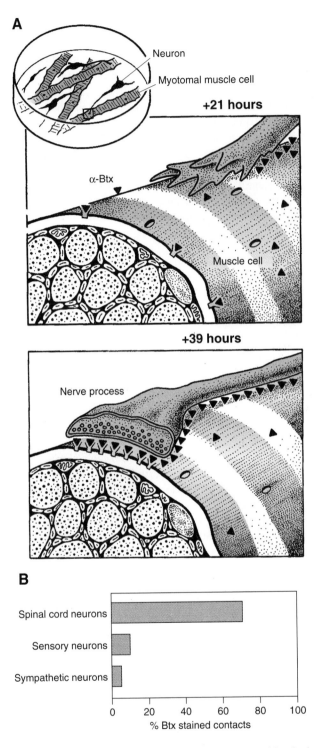

Figure 8.13 ACh receptor clustering on muscle fibers is induced by contact with spinal neurites. (A) A culture of spinal neurons and muscle cells was labeled with a fluorescent α-Btx at 21 and 39 h after plating. Soon after the spinal neurite grew across the muscle surface, fluorescent α-Btx (black triangles) appeared at the contact site, indicating that cluster formation was inducted. (B) The ability to induce AChR clusters is neuron-specific. When muscle cells were cultured with spinal neurons, DRG neurons, and sympathetic neurons, only the spinal neurons induced significant α-Btx labeling. (Adapted from Anderson and Cohen, 1977; Cohen and Weldon, 1980)

decreases in size as a local region of receptors is blocked (Fig. 8.14). However, the size of the potential gradually recovers over several minutes as neighboring AChRs, which were not exposed to α-Btx, migrate into the "silenced" area (Fig. 8.14). At the onset of synaptogenesis, the AChR clusters are labile and will disperse if the muscle is denervated. When α-Btx-labeled muscles from embryonic mice are denervated and placed in calcium-depleted culture media, the AChR clusters are lost (Bloch and Steinbach, 1981). By birth, the labeled AChR clusters have become resistant to this treatment.

Agrin, a Transynaptic Clustering Signal

The studies discussed above strongly suggest that nerve terminals produce a signal that initiates receptor clustering at the postsynaptic cell. Interestingly, AChR clustering can also be produced by the basal lamina, an extracellular matrix that ensheathes each muscle cell. When muscle cells are damaged in adult frogs, they degenerate, leaving behind the basal lamina (Fig. 8.15). New myofibers then regenerate beneath this basal lamina, and AChR clusters form at the original synaptic sites along the basal lamina, even if motor nerve terminals are absent (Burden *et al.*, 1979). These results motivated a search for a "clustering" signal within the extracellular matrix. A protein that is able to mimic the clustering ability of nerve terminals or the basal lamina, named agrin, was subsequently isolated from the electric organ of the marine ray *Torpedo californica*, a site rich in cholinergic synapses (Godfrey *et al.*, 1984; Nitkin *et al.*, 1987). Monoclonal antibodies directed against agrin have been used to localize this protein to motor neuron cell bodies, the synaptic basal lamina, and muscle cells (Reist *et al.*, 1987; Magill-Solc and McMahon, 1988; Fallon and Gelfman, 1989). To test whether release of neuronal agrin is responsible for AChR cluster formation, polyclonal antibodies were used to block its function *in vitro* (Reist *et al.*, 1992). Polyclonal antibodies that were raised against *Torpedo* agrin, were

found to bind selectively to chick agrin, and blocked cluster formation in chick nerve–muscle cultures. However, muscle cells also produce agrin, and it was important to determine whether muscle agrin could induce clustering. Since the polyclonal antiserum does not block rat agrin, a coculture experiment was designed that made use of tissue from chicks and rats (Fig. 8.16). The antiserum does prevent clustering on rat muscle cells that are innervated by chick neurons (Fig. 8.16). However, it does not block AChR cluster formation on chick muscle cells that are innervated by *rat* neurons. Thus, rat neurons must be releasing the agrin that elicits cluster formation. A neuron-specific isoform of agrin, generated by alternative splicing of the mRNA, has since been shown to have greater cluster-inducing activity than that found in muscles (Ruegg *et al.*, 1992; Ferns *et al.*, 1993).

The results suggest that neuron-derived agrin is necessary for AChR cluster formation *in vitro*, but its contribution to neuromuscular formation *in situ* was only recently addressed with homologous recombination (Chapter 2). Mice with decreased agrin expression have smaller AChR clusters. Furthermore, postsynaptic sites appear to be less mature than normal, suggesting that this signaling pathway regulates more than just receptor clustering (Gautam *et al.*, 1996).

Agrin-like molecules probably serve a similar role throughout the nervous system. Agrin mRNA has been detected in the brains of embryonic rats and chicks (Rupp *et al.*, 1991; Tsim *et al.*, 1992). Four different forms of agrin, each deriving from the alternative splicing of agrin RNA (Ferns *et al.*, 1992), are distributed throughout the adult rat brain, and these are not restricted to areas of the brain with cholinergic synapses (O'Connor *et al.*, 1994). Furthermore, the centrally expressed agrins are functionally different from those at the NMJ. Thus, cerebellar granule cell-specific agrin is not able to induce AChR clusters in chick myotybes (So *et al.*, 1996).

Postsynaptic Response to Agrin

While there is strong evidence that neural agrin initiates AChR clustering at the developing

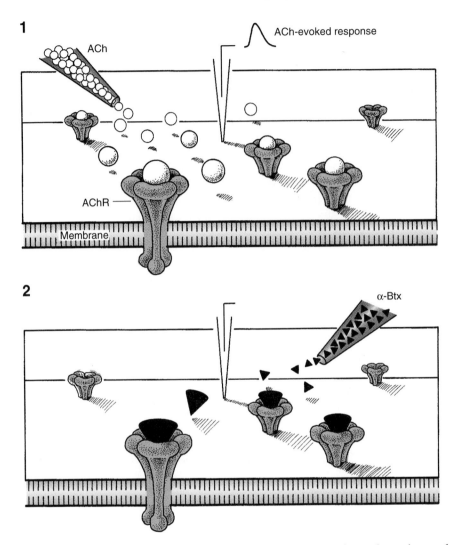

Figure 8.14 ACh receptor mobility in the muscle membrane. (1) ACh is ionophoresed onto the muscle cell, and the evoked response is recorded with an intracellular pipet. (2) A small patch of muscle membrane is then exposed to α-bungarotoxin (α-Btx), blocking the AChRs in the immediate region. (3) Immediately after α-Btx is applied, the ACh-evoked response is diminished. (4) The ACh-evoked response gradually recovers as AChRs that had not been bound by α-Btx move into the exposed region (arrows). The electrophysiological trace shows ACh-evoked responses (positive deflections) throughout each stage (indicated by the numbers 1 to 4) of the manipulation. (Adapted from Poo, with permission from *Nature* **295**: 332–334, Copyright 1982, Macmillan Magazines Limited)

NMJ, the signal transduction mechanism is not fully resolved. It is known that agrin induces postsynaptic tyrosine phosphorylation and that the AChR β subunit is one site of action in chick and mouse muscle cells (Wallace *et al.,* 1991; Qu and Huganir, 1994). In fact, an inhibitor of tyrosine kinase can prevent AChR clustering in response to agrin (Wallace, 1994; Ferns *et al.,* 1996). The temporal relationship between β subunit phosphorylation and receptor clustering is quite close. Receptor phosphorylation reaches a peak within 1 h, and receptor clustering then

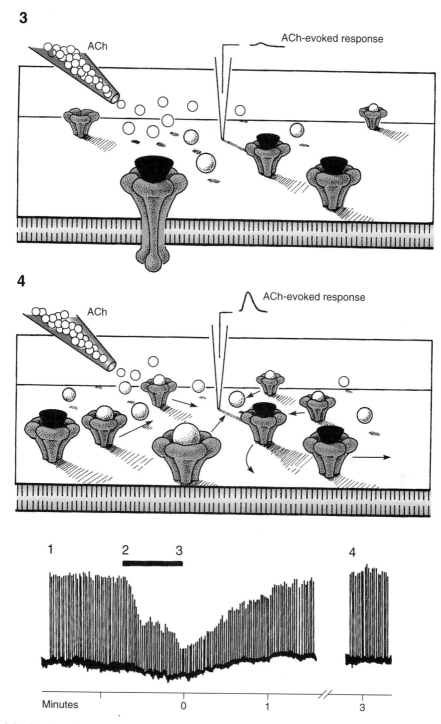

Figure 8.14 (Continued)

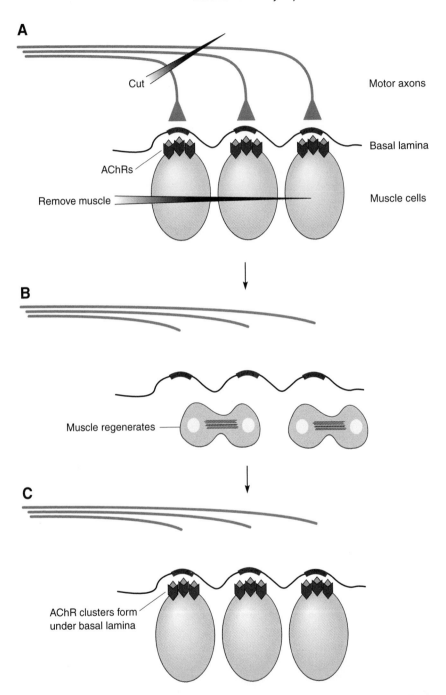

A

Cut

Motor axons

AChRs

Basal lamina

Remove muscle

Muscle cells

B

Muscle regenerates

C

AChR clusters form
under basal lamina

Figure 8.15   The extracellular matrix contains a factor that induces AChR clustering. (A) In the adult frog cutaneous pectoris muscle, the motor axons were cut and the muscle cells were destroyed, leaving only the basal lamina which contains extracellular matrix molecules. (B) New myofibers are generated as a result of cell division. (C) AChR clusters form on the regenerated muscle fibers, directly beneath the synaptic portion of the basal lamina. (Adapted from Burden *et al.,* 1979)

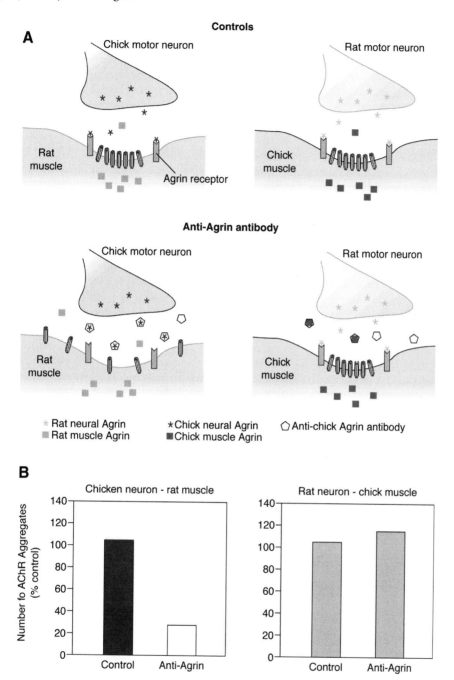

Figure 8.16 Neural agrin induces ACh receptor clusters. (A) To test whether neural agrin (dark red stars) or muscle agrin (light red stars) induced AChR clusters, mixed chick–rat cultures were produced. The reason for this strategy was that a function blocking antibody existed for chick agrin. The antibody blocked receptor clustering when the motor neurons were from chick (left), but not when the muscle cells were from chick (right). (B) These results were quantified for each type of culture. The anti-agrin antibody decreased the number of AChR aggregates to 25% of controls in chick motor neuron cultures (left). (Adapted from Reist *et al.,* © 1992 Cell Press, with permission)

occurs over the next 6 h. By the time that receptor clustering has reached a maximum, phosphorylation is in steep decline (Fig. 8.17). The amount or location of receptor subunit phosphorylation may also interfere with cluster formation. For example, a phosphatase inhibitor that leads to increased β subunit phosphorylation can actually prevent agrin-induced receptor clustering (Wallace, 1995). Although a number of cytoplasmic enzymes, such as PKA or PKC, have been implicated in phosphorylating AChR subunits, the key events are not yet known (Huganir and Greengard, 1983; Huganir *et al.*, 1984).

During a widespread search for the postsynaptic agrin receptor, two candidates have emerged, one of which appears to transduce the clustering activity. The first, muscle-specific kinase (MuSK), was identified in a search for a novel receptor tyrosine kinase in denervated muscle and was found to be restricted to the synaptic junction (Valenzuela *et al.*, 1995). The functional importance of MuSK was verified in a targeted disruption of the gene in mice (Fig. 8.18). These animals display a dramatic loss of postsynaptic maturation, including the loss of AChR clustering (DeChiara *et al.*, 1996). While agrin and MuSK display strong binding kinetics, this is only apparent for MuSK that is expressed in muscle cells, suggesting that the protein must form a complex with accessory proteins (Glass *et al.*, 1996).

The dystrophin-associated glycoprotein α-dystroglycan also appears to be a postsynaptic agrin binding protein (Gee *et al.*, 1994; Campanelli *et al.*, 1994; Bowe *et al.*, 1994; Sugiyama *et al.*, 1994). However, agrin mutants that have poor affinity for α-dystroglycan are nonetheless able to induce AChR clusters (Meier *et al.*, 1996; Hopf and Hoch, 1996). Therefore, α-dystroglycan is probably not directly involved in this part of synaptogenesis. The absence of dystrophin in Duchenne's muscular dystrophy leads to reduced expression of associated proteins in the sarcolemma, resulting in damage during contraction, poor calcium homeostasis, and eventual necrosis (Davies *et al.*, 1995).

A muscle cell peripheral membrane protein, called rapsyn (aka, 43-kDa protein), is involved

in transducing the clustering signal (Sealock *et al.*, 1984). Messenger RNA for rapsyn is present in muscle cells prior to AChR cluster formation, and the protein colocalizes with newly formed clusters *in vivo* (Noakes *et al.*, 1993). When AChR subunits were introduced into cells that do not ordinarily express this molecule, no clusters formed. However, the coexpression of rapsyn is sufficient to promote AChR clustering (Frohner *et al.*, 1990; Phillips *et al.*, 1991). The phenotype of rapsyn-deficient mice is fully consistent with a primary role in cluster formation (Gautam *et al.*, 1995). AChR mRNA and protein are restricted to the central region of muscle fibers, but do not aggregate at the site of neural contact. Rapsyn probably acts as more than just an intermediate signal for MuSK. The presence of rapsyn is able to induce MuSK clusters in a fibroblast expression system, and it is also able to activate the tyrosine kinase activity (Gillespie *et al.*, 1996). There are other molecules that also accumulate at the nerve-muscle synaptic cleft, including acetylcholinesterase and s-laminin. Therefore, it is possible that other signaling pathways that regulate postsynaptic maturation have not yet been identified.

Receptor Clustering Mechanisms in the CNS

Several clustering proteins, located at the cytoplasmic surface, have now been identified in the central nervous system. One of these proteins, called gephyrin, was originally discovered during the purification of glycine receptor subunits (Kirsh *et al.*, 1993a,b). Spinal neurons grown in dissociated culture normally display clusters of glycine receptor. However, when the cells are grown in the presence of a gephyrin antisense nucleotide, which presumably prevents the translation of gephyrin mRNA, then the clusters do not form (Fig. 8.19).

A family of molecules, called membrane-associated guanylate kinases (MAGUK), have also been implicated in synapse formation (Cho *et al.*, 1992; Kistner *et al.*, 1993). One of these

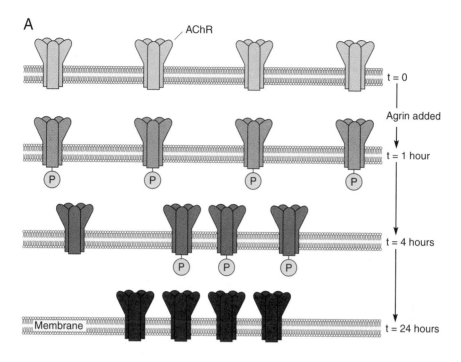

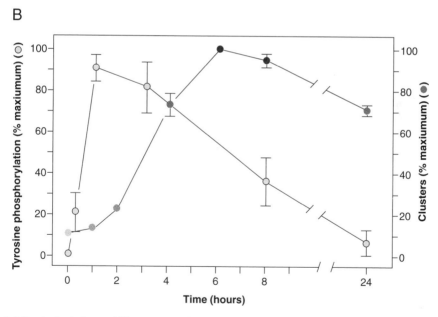

Figure 8.17 Agrin induces ACh receptor phosphorylation prior to clustering. (A) When cultures were exposed to agrin, AChRs were maximally phosphorylated within an hour. Receptor aggregation occurs over the next few hours as the level of phosphorylation begins to decline. (B) The results of these experiments are plotted and show a gradual decline in phosphorylation over 24 h. In contrast, AChR clustering is maximal by 6 h after agrin exposure and declines slightly by 24 h. (Adapted from Ferns *et al.,* from *The Journal of Cell Biology,* 1996, **132:** 937–944, by copyright permission of the Rockefeller University Press)

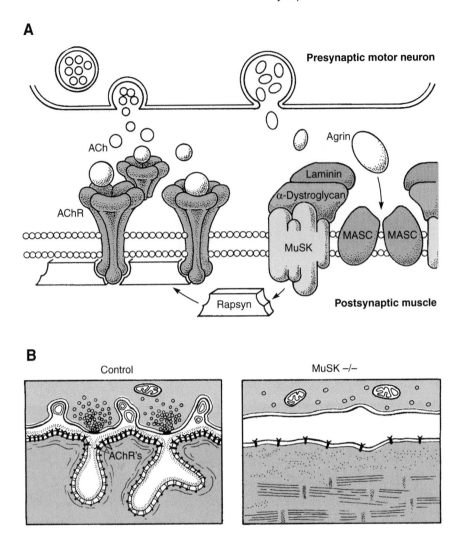

Figure 8.18 Agrin binds to a receptor complex, and MuSK is required for clustering. (A) This schematic shows that agrin is released from the presynaptic terminal and activates a receptor complex that includes muscle-specific kinase (MuSK) and an unidentified accesory protein (MASC). There are many other agrin binding sites, including laminin and α-dystroglycan. The intracellular peripheral membrane protein rapsyn is required for the agrin-mediated MuSK activation to produce AChR phosphorylation, and it participates in receptor clustering. (B) In normal mice, AChRs aggregate at the nerve–muscle junction (left), but in MuSK-deficient mice (right) there is no clustering and the postsynaptic site does not differentiate. (Panel B adapted from DeChiara *et al.,* 1996)

proteins, PSD-95 (aka, SAP-90), is located in the postsynaptic density of hippocampal neurons, and it participates in the clustering of both NMDA receptors and potassium channels at the postsynaptic membrane (Kim *et al.,* 1995; Kor-nau *et al.,* 1995; Kim and Sheng, 1996; Nie-thammer *et al.,* 1996). Synaptic channels and receptors apparently bind to a similar amino acid sequence, called the PDZ domain, on each of the clustering proteins. Furthermore, cluster forma-

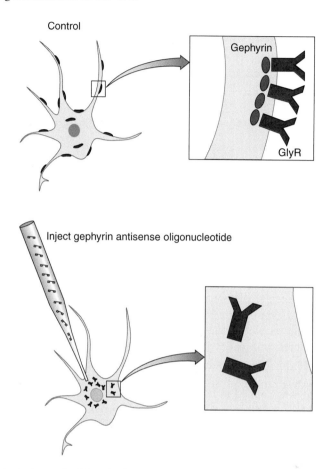

Figure 8.19 Gephyrin is required for glycine receptor clustering. When spinal neurons are grown in culture, the peripheral membrane protein gephyrin colocalizes with glycine receptor clusters (top). When translation of the gephyrin protein is blocked with an antisense oligonucleotide (bottom), the glycine receptors do not form clusters in the neuronal membrane. Rather, they remain within the cytoplasm. (Adapted from Kirsh *et al.,* 1993b)

tion is regulated by protein phosphorylation. In fact, there is a specific four amino acid sequence on the C-terminal tail of receptors and channels, called ET/SXV, that serves as an important phosphorylation site (Niethammer *et al.,* 1996; Cohen *et al.,* 1996).

Clustering proteins are conserved across species. A MAGUK family member, called discs-large (DLG), colocalizes with glutamate receptors at the *Drosophila* nerve–muscle junction. When the *dlg* gene is inactivated, synaptic structure and function are profoundly altered (Woods

and Bryant, 1991; Lahey *et al.,* 1994; Budnick *et al.,* 1996). In fact, DLG is necessary for the localization of FasII, a cell adhesion molecule that regulates synapse formation (see Chapter 9). As with the mammalian family members, the DLG protein has a PDZ binding domain, and the membrane proteins that it anchors have the conserved C-terminal motif. The precise role that MAGUKs and channel C-terminal domains play during synaptogenesis remains to be determined. If receptor clustering in the CNS is initiated by the nerve terminal, as it is at the NMJ, then the transynaptic signaling will likely be a focus of future research.

Regulation of Receptor Expression and Synthesis

Even while receptor clustering is underway, the synthesis of new synaptic proteins is dramatically increased. In fact, the majority of AChRs within a cluster are newly inserted a short time after innervation (Salpeter and Harris, 1983; Ziskind-Conhaim et al., 1984; Role et al., 1985; Dubinsky et al., 1989). The contribution of existing and newly inserted AChRs was examined at newly formed synapses in chick nerve–muscle cultures by labeling the receptors before and after innervation (Fig. 8.20). Before innervation, all of the AChRs present on the muscle membrane surface were labeled with α-Btx ("old" AChRs). Following the addition of neurons, a monoclonal antibody directed against an extracellular AChR epitope was applied to label all AChRs ("old" and "new" AChRs). In this way, it was possible to determine the contribution of both old receptors (i.e., α-Btx labeled) and new receptors (i.e., antibody-labeled minus α-Btx labeled). Within 8 h of neuron addition, more than 60% of the AChRs are newly inserted into the muscle membrane, indicating that synthesis is rapidly upregulated (Role et al., 1985). These results suggest that synthesis is regulated by the presynaptic terminal. In fact, when innervation of the Drosophila neuromuscular junction is delayed or prevented in prospero mutants, the normal increase in functional glutamate receptors fails to occur (Broadie and Bate, 1993b).

Further evidence that motoneuron terminals regulate AChR synthesis comes from the localized expression of the specific mRNAs. Muscle cells are polynuclear, and the nuclei that lay directly below the synaptic cleft are distinctive from those found extrasynaptically in that they specifically transcribe AChR mRNA, and this is controlled by the presence of motoneuron terminals (Klarsfeld et al., 1991; Sanes et al., 1991; Simon et al., 1992; Merlie and Sanes, 1985). To

date, there is no evidence that receptor mRNAs are localized subsynaptically in CNS. In situ hybridization with glutamate receptor probes does not indicate the presence of mRNA in hippocampal neuron dendrites, either in situ or in vitro (Steward, 1994; Craig et al., 1993), although it is possible the levels are below the level of detection.

Innervation can also regulate the expression of receptors at neuron–neuron contacts. In cocultures of chick spinal cord and dissociated sympathetic neurons, the ACh-evoked response recorded in sympathetic neurons increases almost 10-fold after innervation (Role, 1985). This effect can also be produced with spinal cord-conditioned media, suggesting that the signal is a soluble factor (Gardette et al., 1991). The influence of innervation on receptor synthesis can be quite specific, as revealed by culturing chick motoneurons in the presence or absence of spinal cord interneurons. Motoneurons were first selectively labeled with fluorescent dye in vivo, such that they could be identified in a dissociated cell culture (O'Brien and Fischbach, 1986a, b). In some preparations, the motoneurons were isolated with a fluorescence-activated cell sorter and plated with only myotubes. When cultured in the absence of spinal interneurons, dissociated chick motoneurons exhibit much smaller glutamate-evoked currents, although their sensitivity to GABA and glycine is unaffected, at least over the 6 day culture period examined (Fig. 8.21). The presence of interneurons also serves to localize glutamate sensitivity to the motoneuron processes, whereas the somata were maximally sensitive to glutamate in sorted cultures.

As new receptors are added, they also become more stable. This has been shown by measuring how long the receptors remain in the membrane before being replaced. In the chick, the rate of AChR turnover gradually increases from from a half-life of ≈30 h at the time of synaptogenesis to ≥50 days at 3 weeks posthatch (Burden, 1977a,b). In the rat diaphragm muscle, the AChRs that appear during synaptogenesis at E15 also have a half-life of ≈30 h, and this increases to a mature half-life of 6–11 days by E21 (Reiness and Weinberg, 1981). The

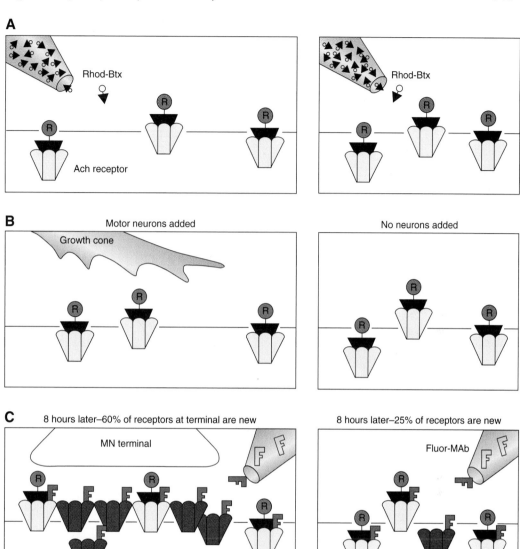

Figure 8.20 Insertion of new ACh receptors occurs within hours of innervation. (A) Cultures of muscle cells were labeled with rhodamine-conjugated bungarotoxin (Rhod-Btx). (B) In one set of cultures, motor neurons were added (left), while a second set of remained within neurons (right). (C) After 8 h, both cultures were labeled with a fluorescein-conjugated antibody against AChRs (Fluor-MAb). The cultures with motor neurons contained many AChRs (red) that were labeled only with antibody, indicating that they had been inserted after the Rhod-Btx labeling. The muscle cell cultures had AChRs (gray) that were primarily labeled by both Rhod-Btx and Fluor-MAb, indicating that the receptors had been in the membrane when the experiment began. (Adapted from Role *et al.*, 1985)

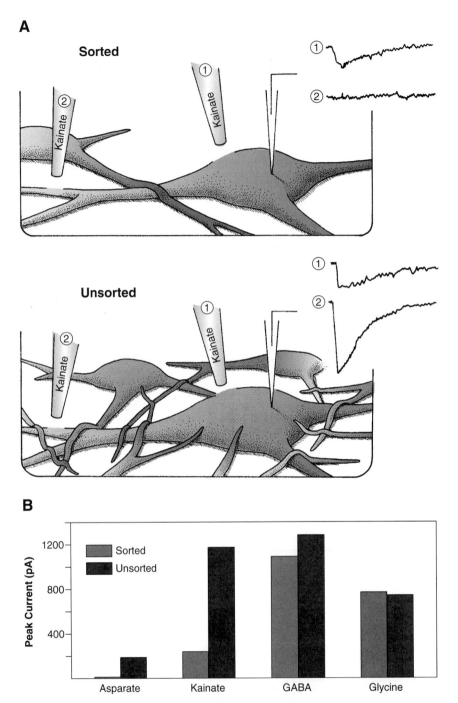

Figure 8.21 Neuronal contacts induce kainate receptors in dissociated spinal cultures. (A) Cultures contained either motor neurons only (Sorted) or a mixture of motor neurons and interneurons (Unsorted). Intracellular recordings were obtained while kainate was applied to the neuron. Sorted neurons (gray) exhibited relatively small kainate-evoked currents, particularly on their dendrites (electrode 2). Unsorted neurons (red) exhibited very large kainate-evoked currents on their dendrites. (B) The extra contacts in unsorted cultures specifically induced kainate and aspartate receptors, but not GABA or glycine receptors. (Adapted from O'Brien and Fischbach, 1986b)

signal that leads to increased receptor stability is not yet known, but it may involve common second messenger systems. Receptor half-life is prolonged either by the influx of postsynaptic calcium or a rise in cAMP (Rotzler *et al.,* 1991; Shyng *et al.,* 1991).

Neuronal Activity Limits Receptor Expression

The increase in receptor synthesis that accompanies synapse formation suggests that the presynaptic terminal is providing a signal of some sort. One simple possibility is that the transmitter itself is able to regulate the transcription of synaptic proteins. However, synaptic activity actually inhibits AChR synthesis in adult muscle, particularly in the extrasynaptic region. When adult cat muscle is denervated, the muscle cells become highly responsive to ACh applied at any position along the surface (Axelsson and Thesleff, 1959). This denervation supersensitivity is due to new receptor synthesis (Merlie *et al.,* 1984).

What is it about the nerve terminal that limits receptor production? In fact, denervation supersensitivity can be produced by decreasing the transmission of an intact terminal (Fig. 8.22). When presynaptic action potentials are blocked or cholinergic transmission is eliminated, there is a dramatic increase in AChRs (Lømo and Rosenthal, 1972; Berg and Hall, 1975). The opposite manipulation, direct electrical stimulation of muscle cells *in vitro,* produces a decrease in AChR synthesis (Shainberg and Burstein, 1976). At least in muscle cells, synaptic activity appears to contain receptor synthesis through increasing postsynaptic calcium and activating a PKC (Klarsfeld *et al.,* 1989; Laufer *et al.,* 1991; Huang *et al.,* 1992).

A similar sort of regulation probably occurs in neurons. Unlike in the NMJ, supersensitivity can not be observed as directly in the central nervous system because neurons are embedded in a web of glia, matrix, and blood vessels. However, many areas of the nervous system express high levels of the NMDA receptor during development, and this expression seems to be regulated by innervation. For example, the functional expression of NMDA receptors decreases with age in the visual cortex of normal kittens, but when animals are reared in complete darkness to decrease visually driven activity, NMDAR-mediated transmission remains at an unusually high level (Fox *et al.,* 1992). Similar sorts of observations have been made for AMPA receptors and GABA$_A$ receptors.

ARIA, a Transynaptic Regulator of Transcription

If synaptic activity represses receptor synthesis, how does the presence of motor nerve terminals cause an increase of AChR synthesis by the postsynaptic muscle cells? An initial screen of soluble factors present in the chick brain revealed a substance that could stimulate AChR synthesis in isolated myotubes (Jessell *et al.,* 1979). Subsequently, a 42-kDa glycoprotein with Acetylcholine Receptor Inducing Activity (hence its name, ARIA) was isolated from the chick central nervous system (Usdin and Fischbach, 1986). The increase in AChR synthesis apparently results from an accumulation of mRNAs for specific AChR subunits, particularly the ε-subunit (Harris *et al.,* 1988; Martinou *et al.,* 1991). Thus ARIA appears to regulate transcription (Fig. 8.23).

An ARIA knockout mouse has now been generated, and although the homozygotes die before the NMJ can form, the heterozygotes express less ARIA protein and display a significant reduction of AChRs (Sandrock *et al.,* 1997). This was studied by measuring the size of individual synaptic events, called quanta, which are probably due to the release of ACh from a single synaptic vesicle. These quantal events are smaller in heterozygote mice, presumably because there is less AChR to transduce the signal (Fig. 8.23). Interestingly, the size of nerve-evoked potentials, consisting of many quanta, is actually larger in heterozygotes. Apparently, the heterozygote nerve terminal releases more

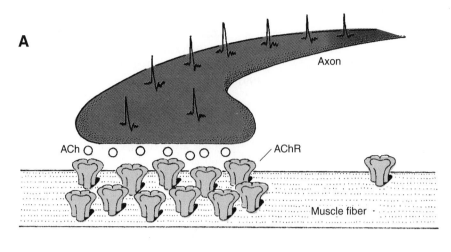

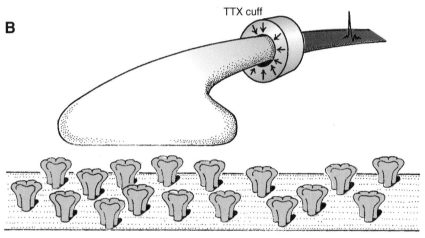

Figure 8.22 Extrasynaptic ACh receptors accumulate when the nerve is inactive. (A) At the control nerve–muscle junctions, the electrically active terminal (red, action potentials) releases ACh and the receptors are clustered at the postsynaptic membrane. (B) When motor axon activity is blocked (white, no action potentials) with the sodium channel blocker tetrodotoxin (TTX), extrajunctional ACh receptors are distributed over the entire muscle surface. (Adapted from Lømo and Rosenthal, 1972)

quanta, suggesting that the presynaptic nerve terminal compensates for the loss of postsynaptic receptors by releasing more transmitter than normal.

ARIA message is localized to motor neurons, and the protein is transported to the synaptic junction, as assessed with immunohistochemical staining (Falls *et al.,* 1993; Sandrock *et al.,* 1995). Furthermore, electron microscopic analysis indicates that once ARIA is released at the neuromuscular junction, it then becomes concentrated on the presynaptic side of the basal lamina (Goodearl *et al.,* 1995). In fact, the basal lamina has previously been shown to also contain a signal that activates AChR transcription in the absence of motor nerve terminals (Goldman *et al.,* 1991).

Sequence analysis of the ARIA cDNA indicates that it is a member of the Neu protooncogene ligand family (Falls *et al.,* 1993). In the

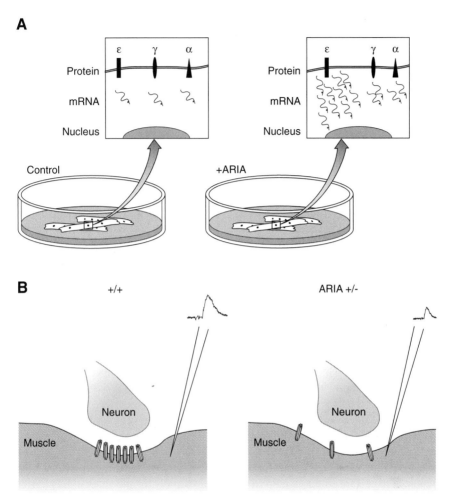

Figure 8.23 ARIA selectively upregulates the ε subunit mRNA. (A) In control muscle cell cultures, approximately equal amounts mRNA for the ε, γ, and α AChR subunits are produced. The addition of ARIA increases mRNA for all subunits, but the ε subunit is selectively enhanced. (B) When intracellular recording are obtained from control (+/+) and heterozygous ARIA-deficient mice (+/-), the latter exhibit smaller quantal events and decreased accumulation of receptor. (Adapted from Sandrock *et al.,* 1997)

nervous system, members of this protein family are now referred to as the neuregulins (NRGs), and they play a broad role in neural development. The receptors for neuregulins are actually members of another large family: the EGF receptor tyrosine kinase family (erbBs). At the neuromuscular junction, ARIA colocalizes with at least three of these erbB receptors. ARIA signaling may involve a common kinase pathway. In one cell line, ARIA stimulates tyrosine phos-

phorylation of erbBs and mitogen-activated protein kinase (MAPK). Furthermore, a specific inhibitor of MAPK abolishes ARIA-induced AChR subunit expression (Si *et al.,* 1996).

ARIA immunostaining has been found in the chick and rat CNS, and other NRGs are also found in the mammalian CNS. Similarly, erbB2, erbB3, and erbB4 are expressed by neurons and glia in the chick CNS during development. Thus, NRG signaling is likely to be involved in the development of central synapses, although specific evidence for this has yet to emerge.

Synaptic Transmission

There appears to be more than one "time constant" for the maturation of synaptic transmission. A rapid phase of maturation, occurring over minutes, can occur because the growth cone is able to release transmitter and postsynaptic cell expression neurotransmitter receptors. There is a slower phase of development, occurring over several hours, during which an array of synapse-specific proteins accumulate (e.g., receptor clustering). During the longest phase of maturation, lasting days to weeks, the adult forms of synapse-specific proteins are synthesized and incorporated into the membrane, and the functional properties of excitatory and inhibitory synapses become adult-like.

In some systems, particularly in the peripheral nervous system or the NMJ, the timing of axon ingrowth and synaptic transmission has been followed with great precision *in vivo.* In the rat superior cervical ganglion, axons first enter the target between E12 and E13, and afferent-evoked postsynaptic potential is recorded by E13. Similarly, motor axons grow out of the *Xenopus* spinal cord and form functional synapses on the developing myotubes over a period of hours (Kullberg *et al.,* 1977). In the fruit fly, it takes only 8 h for neuromuscular transmission to reach a mature level of function (Broadie and Bate, 1993a). However, it is nearly impossible to record from a cell at the exact moment that it is first contacted by a growth cone *in vivo.*

Fortunately, the appearance of synaptic transmission can be explored with great accuracy in dissociated cultures. When intracellular recordings were obtained from isolated *Xenopus* muscle cells, and the formation of a neurite contact was visually monitored on a microscope, it was found that synaptic potentials could be elicited within minutes of lamellopodial contact (Kidokoro and Yeh, 1982). To provide even better temporal resolution, muscle cells were manipulated into contact with growing neurites while they were being recorded from (Fig. 8.24A). The tight seal between the large tip of a whole-cell recording electrode and the muscle membrane (see Box: Biophysics: Nuts and Bolts of Functional Maturation) permits the recordings to continue while a small round muscle cell, called a myoball, is detached from the substrate and repositioned in the culture dish. Using this technique, it is possible to observe nerve-evoked synaptic transmission that is great enough to elicit an action potential within 15 s of nerve–muscle contact (Fig. 8.24C). In most cases, the synaptically evoked response increases during the first 15 min of contact (Sun and Poo, 1987; Evers *et al.,* 1989). Certain adult-like characteristics of synaptic transmission, such as depression and facilitation, are also present immediately after contact. While spontaneous synaptic events appear within seconds of contact (Fig. 8.24B), they continue to increase in both rate and amplitude over the first 10–20 min (Xie and Poo, 1986). Clearly, functional maturation proceeds briskly at the NMJ *in vitro.* However, most analyses of the mammalian CNS, both *in vitro* and *in vivo,* indicate that synaptic properties take days or weeks to reach maturity (see below).

In comparing the development of synaptic structure and function, it is interesting that the maturation of transmission seems to evolve far more rapidly. In the chick ciliary ganglion, synaptic potentials can be recorded before synapses are detected with an electron microscope (Landmesser and Pilar, 1972). Similarly, when a muscle is manipulated into contact with a growth cone in a *Xenopus* culture, the recorded synaptic currents can be quite large at contacts that show no differentiation at the ultrastructural level (Buchanan *et al.,* 1989).

Rapid Modulation of Release and Receptor Function

The membrane from muscle cells probably induces an increase in transmitter release from cholinergic neurons with a specific signal. When an outside-out patch of AChR-containing membrane (see Box: Biophysics: Nuts and Bolts of

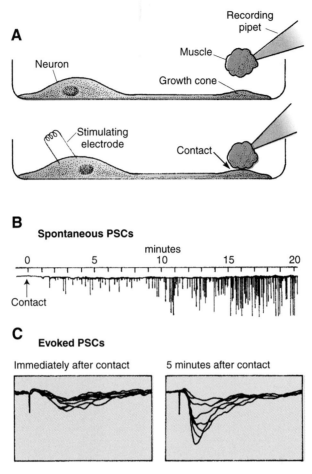

Figure 8.24 Muscle cell contact enhances spontaneous and evoked transmission. (A) Cultures of *Xenopus* spinal neurons were grown in culture and whole cell pipets were used to record from round muscle cells and to manipulate them into contact with the neuron. (B) A continuous recording from a muscle cell shows spontaneous transmission (downward deflections) during the first 20 min after contact. (C) Nerve-evoked postsynaptic currents (downward deflections) increased in amplitude from the moment of contact to 5 min later. (Adapted from Evers *et al.,* 1989, with permission; Xie and Poo, 1986)

Functional Maturation) is used to monitor transmitter release from a neurite, direct contact with a muscle cell, or the muscle cell membrane patch itself, is able to induce transmitter release (Fig. 8.25). When the growth cone is contacted by other neurons or with a glass probe, sustained release is not induced (Xie and Poo, 1986). The contact-mediated signal has not yet been found, but there are several secreted proteins that might serve as retrograde signals, from muscle to presynaptic terminal.

When added to the media in *Xenopus* nerve–muscle cultures, two members of the neurotrophin family of growth factors, BDNF and NT-3, are able to potentiate the release of ACh by presynaptic terminals, as assessed by an increase in the rate of spontaneous synaptic events (Lohoff *et al.,* 1992). These neurotrophins also potentiate stimulus-induced synaptic transmission and increase the levels of two synaptic vesicle proteins, synaptophysin and synapsin 1, in the cultured spinal neurons (Wang *et al.,* 1995). Ciliary

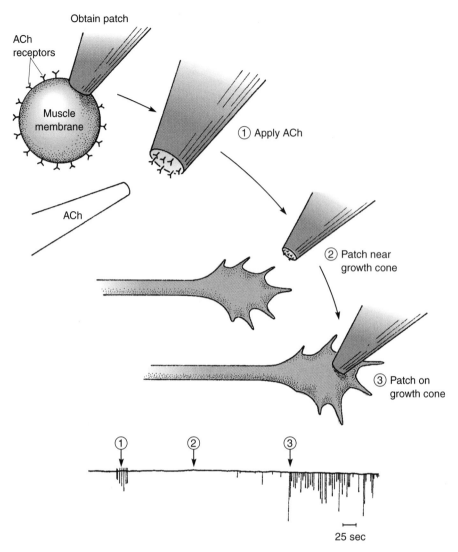

Figure 8.25 Muscle membrane induces transmitter release from growth cone. (1) A sniffer pipet is generated as described in Fig. 8.6. (2) ACh is applied to the sniffer to evoke a response. (3) The sniffer is moved near the growth cone and records little ACh release. (4) The patch of membrane is brought into contact with the growth cone and induces a long-lasting burst of transmitter release. (Adapted from Xie and Poo, 1986)

neurotrophic factor (CNTF) has also been shown to potentiate spontaneous and evoked transmitter release (Fig. 8.26A), but the cellular mechanism appears to differ from that of BDNF (Stoop and Poo, 1996). BDNF exerts its effect at the synaptic terminal through a calcium-dependent process, whereas CNTF seems to act at the soma. It take approximately 10 min for BDNF

or CNTF to effect transmission, and neurotransmission remains altered for hours after these compounds are removed (Fig. 8.26B).

Retrograde signaling may also involve metabolites of arachidonic acid (AA), a membrane-soluble polyunsaturated fatty acid (Harish and Poo, 1992). Injection of AA into muscle cells dramatically increases the frequency of sponta-

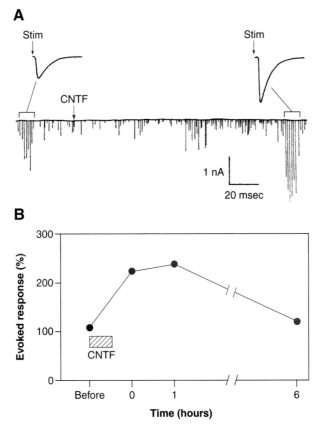

Figure 8.26 CNTF enhances evoked synaptic responses. (A) A series of nerve-evoked synaptic currents (downward deflections) were recorded from *Xenopus* muscle cells *in vitro*. Following exposure to ciliary neurotrophic factor (CNTF), the size of nerve-evoked currents increased dramatically. (B) As shown in the graph, exposure to CNTF causes the size of evoked synatic responses to double (red points) and this effect lasts for several hours. (Adapted from Stoop and Poo, 1996, with permission)

neous transmitter release from the presynaptic terminals. Apparently, the injected compound diffuses across membrane to reach the terminal. This effect is blocked with inhibitors of AA metabolism.

The enhancement of synaptic transmission that is observed soon after innervation could also occur if existing receptors on the postsynaptic membrane were modulated. For example, when embryonic rat medullary neurons are placed in dissociated culture, there is no sign of glycine-evoked currents during the first 6 days *in vitro*. However, glycine-evoked currents can be observed in excised patches of membrane within a day of plating. This result suggests that the glycine receptors are converted from an inactive to an active state during development (Lewis *et al.,* 1990). It seems likely that intercellular signaling affects receptor function. Calcitonin gene-related peptide (CGRP) is released from motor terminals and is able to rapidly increase the mean open time of AChR channels in *Xenopus* nerve–muscle cultures (Lu *et al.,* 1993). This effect appears to be mediated through an elevation of cAMP in the muscle cell and is blocked by inhibitors of cAMP-dependent protein kinase (PKA). A second protein kinase, PKC, is also able to modulate the kinetics of low-conductance AChRs (Fu and Lin,

1993). Therefore, phosphorylation of "immature" AChRs may prolong their open state, thereby increasing the size of transmitter-evoked postsynaptic potentials at the time of innervation.

Maturation of Transmission and Receptor Isoform Transitions

Although synaptic connections can form rapidly, their functional properties are gradually adjusted during development. One of the most common observations is that the duration of excitatory or inhibitory synaptic potentials declines over the course of days. For example, in the rat neocortex, the duration of excitatory postsynaptic potentials (EPSPs) decreases from approximately 400 to 100 ms during the first 2 postnatal weeks of development (Burgard and Hablitz, 1993), and synaptic potentials in the rat hippocampus display a similar schedule of maturation. Even synapses in the brain stem display marked alterations during postnatal development (Fig. 8.27). In the lateral superior olive, the maximum duration of both glutamatergic EPSPs and glycinergic inhibitory postsynaptic potentials (IPSPs) declines approximately 10-fold during the first 3 postnatal weeks (Sanes, 1993). The declines in IPSP and EPSP durations have similar rates of development, suggesting that some of the underlying mechanisms are the same. These long-lasting synaptic potentials probably limit the perceptual capabilities of young animals (see Chapter 10).

Why are synaptic potentials of such long duration in developing neurons? One common difference is that young synapses usually express a unique form of the neurotransmitter receptor, called a neonatal isoform. These transiently expressed receptors tend to have functional properties different than those of the receptor that is expressed by adult neurons. In particular, the receptor-coupled ion channels in young cells remain open for a longer period of time, compared to those in mature cells. In mammalian muscle cells, recordings were made from single channels with the patch-clamp recording technique

(see Box: Biophysics: Nuts and Bolts of Functional Maturation), and the mean channel open times were found to decline from about 6 to 1 ms during development (Siegelbaum *et al.,* 1984; Vicini and Schuetze, 1985).

The relationship between the function and molecular composition of AChRs was first revealed by a set of studies that utilized the serum from patients with myasthenia gravis, an autoimmune disease that result in weakness of the voluntary muscles. Antibodies from myasthenia serum were found to bind to specific AChR epitopes, and when these antibodies were used to label the rodent NMJ, the pattern of staining was found to change during development. This suggested that there must be a transition in the molecular properties of the AChR (Weinberg and Hall, 1979; Reiness and Hall, 1981). In fact, the basis for both the functional and immunological changes is a transcriptional switch (Fig. 8.28). The AChR is initially composed of four subunits, $\alpha_2\beta\gamma\zeta$, but during the first 2 postnatal weeks in rat, the many nuclei beneath each synapse stop expressing the γ subunit and increase expression of the ϵ subunit transcripts, resulting in a new heteromeric receptor, $\alpha_2\beta\epsilon\zeta$ (Gu and Hall, 1988). This transition occurs even when muscle is denervated, indicating that the nerve terminal may deposit a signal in the basal lamina.

Even though nerve cells limp along on one nucleus in the soma, it appears that they are able to respond to innervation by altering the receptor isoform expression. When chick sympathetic ganglion neurons are innervated, their sensitivity to ACh is enhanced, and this is correlated with increased expression of five AChR transcripts (Moss and Role, 1993; Corriveau and Berg, 1993). At E11, only 30% of neurons have significant AChR activity, and each individual patch of membrane contains a mixture of AChRs. At E17, the great majority of patches have a single functional type of receptor. Similar changes in specific AChR subunits have been observed in rat brain stem, spinal cord, and dorsal root ganglia during prenatal development.

A developmental switch in receptor subunits has now been demonstrated in nearly every transmitter system in the central nervous system.

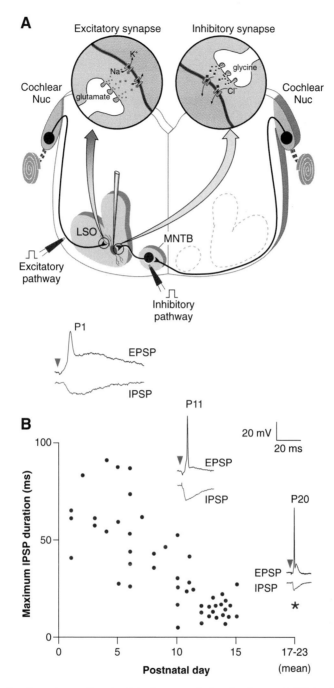

Figure 8.27 The duration of synaptic potentials decreases during development. (A) A schematic of a central auditory nucleus, the lateral superior olive (LSO), which receives excitatory synapses from the ipsilateral cochlear nucleus, and inhibitory synapses from the medial nucleus of the trapezoid body (MNTB). The inset at left shows that excitatory terminals release glutamate and open receptors that are permeable to Na^+ and K^+ (postsynaptic neuron is light red). The inset at right shows that inhibitory terminals release glycine and open receptors that are permeable to Cl^-. (B) When intracellular recordings are made from LSO neurons during the first 3 postnatal weeks, the afferent-evoked action potential/EPSP and IPSP durations decline by about 10-fold. Examples for Postnatal Days 1, 11, and 20 are shown at the top, and a summary of all recordings is plotted in the graph (red asterisk represents mean value). (Adapted from Sanes, 1993, with permission)

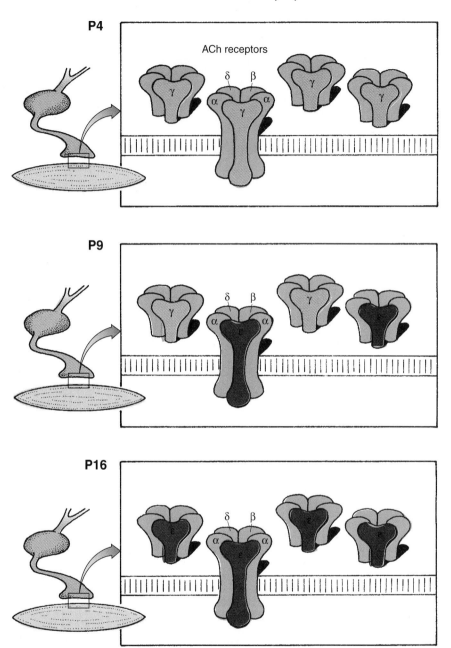

Figure 8.28 Substitution of ACh receptors' subunits during development. In rat muscle, AChRs are composed of α, β, δ, and γ subunits at Postnatal Day 4 (P4). By P9, there is a mix of receptors: some have the initial complement of subunits, and others have substituted the ε subunit (dark red) in place of the γ subunit (light red). At P16, all receptors contain the ε subunit. (Adapted from Gu and Hall, 1988)

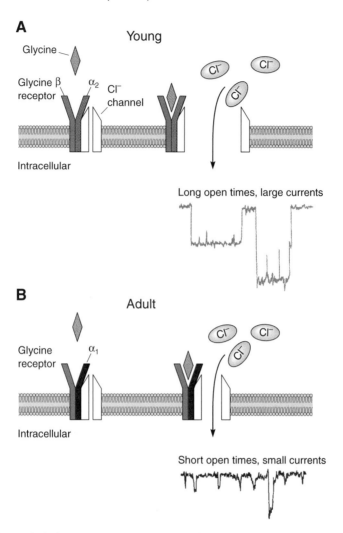

A Young

Glycine

Glycine β receptor α_2

Cl^- channel

Intracellular

Long open times, large currents

B Adult

Glycine receptor α_1

Intracellular

Short open times, small currents

Figure 8.29 Neonatal glycine receptors have immature functional properties. (A) In neontal mammalian neurons, the glycine receptor is composed of β and α_2 subunits. When bound by glycine, the receptors remain open for a relatively long time and pass a relatively large current. (B) In adult neurons, the glycine receptor contains a β subunit, but the neonatal isoform α_2 is replaced by the α_1 subunit. These receptors open briefly and pass less current than the neonatal form. (Adapted from Takahashi *et al.*, Copyright 1992 Cell Press, with permission)

For example, the adult form of the glycine receptor heteromer involves the substitution of a 48-kDa ligand-binding subunit for a neonatal isoform (Becker *et al.*, 1988). Recordings from outside-out from rat dorsal spinal cord neurons during development show that there is a complementary change in function (Takahashi *et al.*, 1992). The glycine-gated channels from young animals (<P5) open for a much longer period of time and pass a greater amount of current, compared to older postnatal animals (Fig. 8.29). By examining the properties of two different glycine receptor subunits in a *Xenopus* expression system, it was determined that a transition from the α_2 to the α_1 subunit could explain the functional change.

When a receptor family has many subunits, the type of receptor that is produced becomes a combinatorial problem. The temporal and regional expression of 13 different $GABA_A$ receptor subunits in the developing rat brain provides an interesting example (Laurie *et al.,* 1992). The expression patterns are determined by *in situ* hybridization, a technique in which radiolabeled antisense oligonucleotides are used as probes for each species of mRNA (Fig. 8.30). The onset of expression and the adult level of expression can vary greatly for a single subunit, depending on location. Moreover, there are a large number of subunits that are transiently expressed within a given structure. As one of many examples, the onset of γ_2 subunit expression occurs throughout the brain at E17. Whereas the level of γ_2 expression gradually increases in the hippocampus and cerebellum, it ceases to be expressed in the cortex and thalamus.

The long duration of excitatory synaptic events in many regions of the CNS is at least partly due to a neonatal form of the NMDA-gated glutamate receptor (Fig. 8.31). The duration of afferent-evoked excitatory postsynaptic currents (EPSCs) in the rat superior colliculus that are mediated by NMDA receptors declines severalfold during the first 3 postnatal weeks (Hestrin, 1992). Similar observations have been made in the ferret lateral geniculate nucleus and rat cortex. NMDAR subunit composition probably affects other functional properties of the receptor. For example, NMDARs are sensitive to the presence of both ligand (glutamate) and membrane depolarization in adults, but voltage sensitivity may be absent in the neonatal hippocampus (Ben-Ari *et al.,* 1988). Apparently, the neontal receptors are less sensitive to Mg^{2+}, the ion that must be expelled from the channel pore during depolarization, thus permitting Na^+ and Ca^{2+} to pass through (Bowe and Nadler, 1990). Together, these observation suggest that there are fewer limitations on excitatory transmission through the NMDAR early in development.

The signals that are responsible for receptor switches may come from neurotransmission itself. For example, the waning of NMDAR-mediated responses in many areas of the brain (see above) is often accompanied by increased transmission through a second class of glutamate receptors, called AMPA receptors. In fact, functional AMPARs can be rapidly recruited by NMDAR activity. In the neonatal rat, glutamatergic synaptic transmission appears to be absent because most synapses have only functional NMDARs, and NMDA receptors tend to remain closed at the resting membrane potential. These are sometimes refered to as "silent synapses." When NMDARs are permitted to be active by stimulating the synapse during depolarizing current pulses, the synapses are soon found to have functional AMPARs (Durand *et al.,* 1996). A similar pattern of maturation occurs in the optic tectum of *Xenopus* tadpoles. Whe calcium–calmodulin-dependent protein kinase II (CaMKII) is constitutively expressed in the tectal neurons, the appearance of AMPAergic transmission can be facilitated. This suggests that calcium entry through NMDARs may activate CaMKII which mediates the recruitment of functional AMPARs (Wu *et al.,* 1996). Activation of silent synapses has also been observed at slightly later periods of development and may, in fact, underlay certain forms of learning or memory (see Chapter 9).

Maturation of Transmitter Reuptake

The time that neurotransmitter remains in the synaptic cleft will also affect the duration of synaptic potentials, and the development of transmitter uptake systems is critical for the appearance of mature function. Neurotransmitter transporter protein development has been studied by expressing polyadenylated brain RNA (polyadenylation, or the addition of about 200 adenylate residues, is a common modification to transcripts in eukaryotic cells) in *Xenopus* oocytes (Blakely *et al.,* 1991). Messenger RNA was obtained from animals of different ages and placed in a *Xenopus* oocyte expression system. The amount of transport was quantified by incubating the oocyte in a radiolabeled amino acid neurotransmitter, such as [³H]-glycine, and the

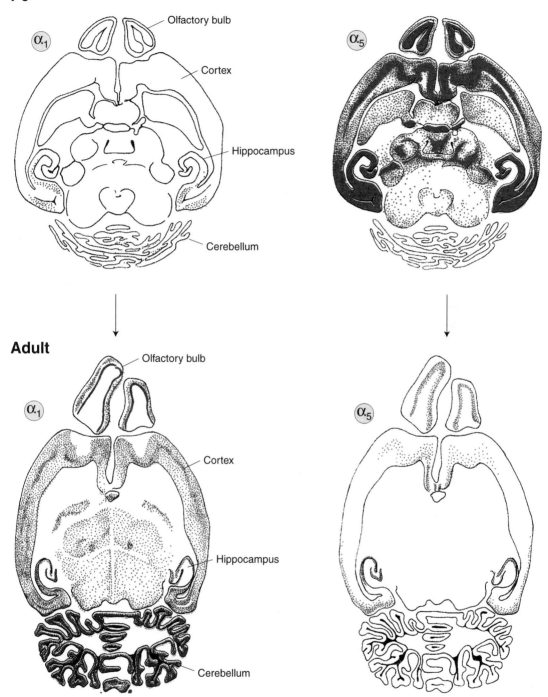

P6

Olfactory bulb

α_1

Cortex

Hippocampus

Cerebellum

α_5

Adult

Olfactory bulb

α_1

Cortex

Hippocampus

Cerebellum

α_5

Figure 8.30 Anatomical distribution of GABA$_A$ receptor subunits (red) changes dramatically during development. Each panel displays the staining pattern of an antibody directed against either the α_1 or the α_5 GABA$_A$R subunits. (Top) At P6, there is little α_1 in the brain, whereas α_5 is heavily expressed in the hippocampus and cortex. (Bottom) In adult, α_1 is heavily expressed, and α_5 is nearly absent. (Adapted from Laurie *et al.,* 1992, with permission)

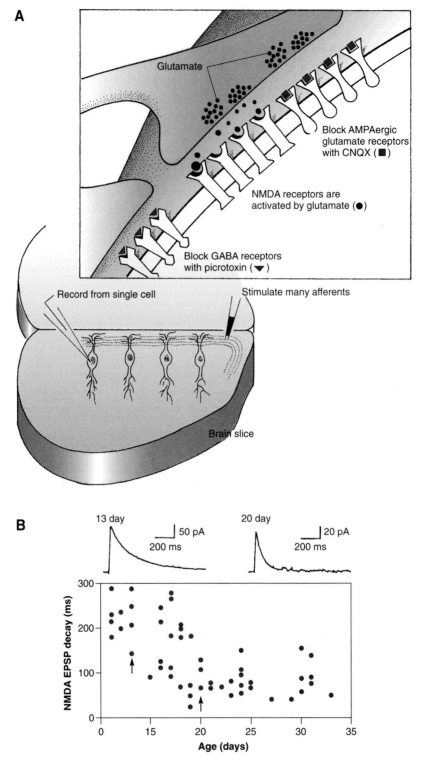

Figure 8.31 The NMDA-type glutamate receptors close more rapidly with age. (A) Intracellular recordings were obtained from rat hippocampal neurons in a brain slice preparation, and AMPA-type glutamate receptors and GABA receptors were blocked (black triangles and squares). Thus, stimulation of afferents evoked glutamate release, and only postsynaptic NMDA-type receptors were activated. (B) The afferent-evoked EPSPs were longer lasting in neurons from young rats due to the slow decay time. (Adapted from Hestrin, 1992, with permission from *Nature* **357:** 686–689, Copyright 1992 Macmillan Magazines Limited)

amount of ³H was quantified with a liquid scintillation counter. Using this assay, it was found that glutamate and GABA transporters first appear in the cortex at Postnatal Day 3 and increase to adult levels over the next 2 weeks. In the brain stem, the expression of a glycine transporter gradually increases to adult levels over the first 3 postnatal weeks.

A number of amino acid transporters have now been identified at the molecular level, and a few studies have traced their developmental appearance using *in situ* hybridization. The excitatory amino acid transporters mEAAT1 and mEAAT2 are first found in the proliferative zone of mouse forebrain and midbrain during gliogenesis (E15–E19). However, mEAAT2 mRNA continues to increase in many areas of the CNS during the first 2–3 postnatal weeks (Sutherland *et al.,* 1996). Transcripts for the Na^+/Cl^--dependent glycine transporter (GlyT1), found almost exclusively in glial cells, achieve maximal levels in E13 mice, quite early in neural development (Adams *et al.,* 1995). Although the presence of transporter mRNA suggests that neurotransmitter could be efficiently cleared at the onset of synaptogenesis, studies of amino acid transporter function suggest that their physiology remains immature for some time (Blakely *et al.,* 1991). Therefore, the maturation of transporter proteins probably limits the kinetics of synaptic transmission.

Appearance of Synaptic Inhibition

Up to this point, our discussion has focused on excitatory synapses, and these connections have provided the great majority of information on synaptogenesis (and most of that from the cholinergic NMJ). Initially, it was thought that inhibitory synapses, those releasing GABA or glycine, matured after excitatory synapses. This is because IPSPs are often not observed in neonatal animals. For example, intracellular recordings from the kitten visual cortex demonstrate that afferent-evoked IPSPs are absent from over half the neurons during the first postnatal week, whereas all neurons display IPSPs by adulthood (Komatsu and Iwakiri, 1991). Similar observations have been made on the developing rat neocortex (Luhman and Prince, 1991).

However, synaptic inhibition appears with a similar time course as synaptic excitation in diverse areas such as the spinal cord, cerebellar nuclei, olfactory bulb, lateral superior olive, and somatosensory cortex (Oppenheim and Reitzel, 1975; Sanes, 1993). Inhibitory events are probably more difficult to detect in young animals, because they are concealed by excitatory events (Agmon *et al.,* 1996), and because their equilibrium potential is close to the resting membrane potential (Zhang *et al.,* 1991). Therefore, it is likely that inhibitory synapses are present from the outset but that their functional properties are immature.

Is Inhibition Really Inhibitory during Development?

In adult animals, synaptic inhibitory potentials are generally hyperpolarizing because the receptor is coupled to a Cl^- channel, and the Cl^- equilibrium potential is more negative than the cell's resting potential. However, inhibitory synaptic transmission usually produce *depolarizing* potentials during the initial phase of development (Obata *et al.,* 1978; Bixby and Spitzer, 1982; Mueller *et al.,* 1983, 1984; Ben-Ari *et al.,* 1989). For example, during the first postnatal week, rat hippocampal neurons display large spontaneous and evoked depolarizations that are blocked by the $GABA_A$ receptor antagonist bicuculline (Fig. 8.32A).

These depolarizing IPSPs are apparently large enough to open voltage-gated calcium channels. In dissociated cultures obtained from embryonic rat hypothalamus, intracellular free calcium is decreased by bicuculline during the first 10 days *in vitro* (Obrietan and van den Pol, 1995). As the cultures mature, bicuculline increases calcium, presumably by allowing excitatory synaptic acitivity to have a greater

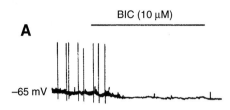

A

−65 mV

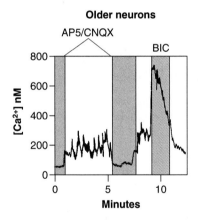

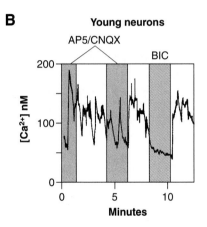

Figure 8.32 GABAergic inhibition initially evokes membrane depolization and calcium entry. (A) Intracellular recording from a neonatal rat hippocampal neuron shows that the $GABA_A$ receptor antagonist bicuculline (BIC) blocks the spontaneous action potential and causes the cell to hyperpolarize. (B) Intracellular free calcium was monitored in hypothalamic cultures during exposure either to glutamate receptor antagonists (AP5/CNQX) or to a $GABA_A$ receptor antagonist (BIC). After 8 days *in vitro* (young neurons), only BIC produced a decrease in calcium. At 33 days *in vitro* (older neurons), AP5/CNQX produced a decrease in calcium, and BIC increased calcium. (Adapted from Ben-Ari *et al.,* 1989, Obrietan and van den Pol, 1995, with permission)

depolarizing influence (Fig. 8.32B). Therefore, inhibitory synapses may provide a qualitatively different input to postsynaptic neurons during development.

Inhibitory postsynaptic potentials gradually become hyperpolarizing during development, as has been demonstrated in the spinal cord, brain stem, hippocampus, and cortex (Kandler and Friauf, 1995; Agmon *et al.*, 1996; Zhang *et al.*, 1991). The depolarizing inhibitory potentials seen in young animals are probably due to the outward flow of Cl- through $GABA_A$ or glycine receptor-coupled channels (Reichling *et al.*, 1994; Owens *et al.*, 1996). Therefore, intracellular chloride must be elevated in young neurons, and it is important to understand how chloride is distrubuted across the membrane. The ability of cortical neurons to regulate intracellular Cl^- was tested by loading them with Cl^- (i.e., making the Cl^- equilibrium potential more positive) and observing the IPSP size (Luhmann and Prince, 1991). Loading the neurons with Cl^- resulted in depolarizing IPSPs at all ages, but the youngest neurons did *not* recover (Fig. 8.33). Thus, the Cl^- pump is probably not operating at a mature level.

In some cases, the depolarizing nature of inhibitory synaptic potentials are maintained by an active process. For example, even when recordings are made with a whole-cell electrode that presumably sets the intracellular chloride concentration of a neuron, the IPSC reversal potential becomes more negative as development progresses (Agmon *et al.*, 1996). Surprisingly, it seems that some developing neurons maintain high intracellular Cl^- levels by pumping the ion in. For example, Na^+ and Cl^- are cotransported into Rohon–Beard cells in the developing *Xenopus* spinal cord, producing GABA-evoked depolarizations in these cells (Rohrbough and Spitzer, 1996). Recently, it has been shown that the expression of two chloride transporters is developmentally regulated. A transporter that extrudes chloride (KCC2) increases during maturation, and a transporter that moves chloride into the neuron (NKCC) declines with age (Plotkin *et al.*, 1997; Rivera *et al.*, 1999; Lu *et al.*, 1999; Williams *et al.*, 1999).

Electrical Properties

Action potentials are the unit of currency in the nervous system. The membrane spanning proteins that permit sodium, potassium, and calcium to permeate neuron membranes are critical to action potential generation. When a neuron becomes slightly depolarized, perhaps due to a synaptic potential, the opening of voltage-gated sodium channels permits a large depolarizing current due to the high sodium concentration extracellularly and the low sodium concentration of the cytoplasm. As the sodium influx depolarizes the neuron, a second set of voltage-gated channels is activated that permits potassium to leave the cell, thus returning the membrane potential to rest. In many cases, the initial depolarization recruits a third type of voltage-gated channel that permits calcium to enter the neuron. From a developmental perspective, calcium channels are of greatest importance because intracellular calcium serves as a second messenger throughout neuronal differentiation.

Resting Potential and Membrane Properties

The resting membrane potential of most neurons becomes more negative during the course of development (Kullberg *et al.*, 1977; Burgard and Hablitz, 1993; Tepper and Trent, 1993; Sanes, 1993; Ramoa and McCormick, 1994; Warren and Jones, 1997). This is due, in part, to the appearance of energy-dependent ionic transporters whose expression may itself depend on ionic composition (Wolitzky and Fambrough, 1986; Schmidt *et al.*, 1992; Brandt and Neve, 1992; Fukuda and Prince, 1992). The membrane potential is actually due to the precise type of channels that are open at rest and, surprisingly, this is poorly understood even for adult neurons.

There are a few fundamental changes in the nervous system environment that affect all functional properties. For example, extracellular space decreases by more than half, and extracellular

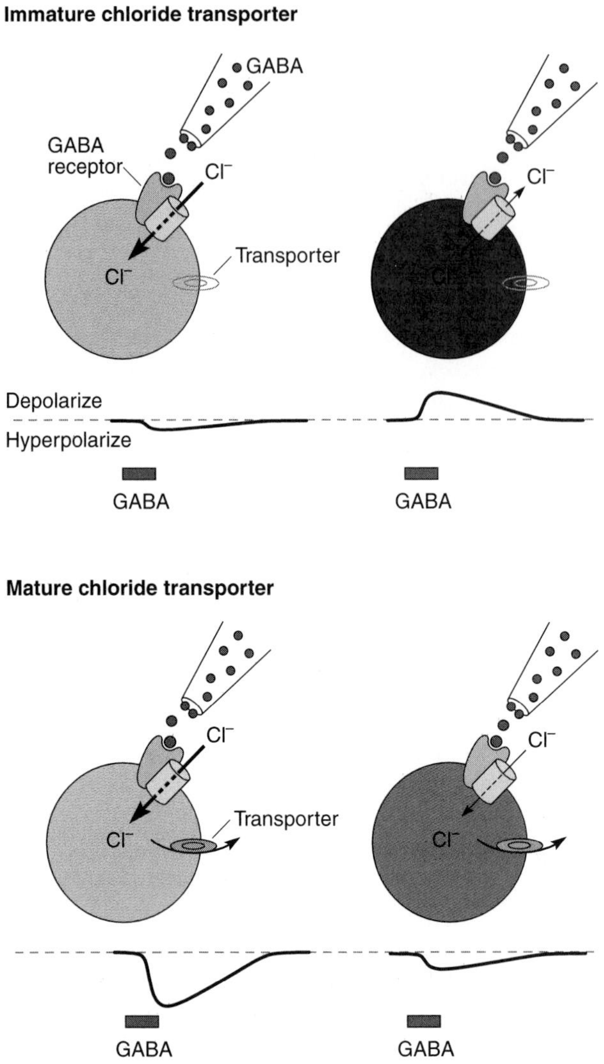

Immature chloride transporter

Mature chloride transporter

Figure 8.33 An immature chloride pumping mechanism allows inhibitory synapses to evoke membrane depolarizations. Intracellular recordings are obtained with low (light red) and high (dark red) chloride concentrations in the pipet, indicated by the shade of red. (Top) In young neurons, GABA evokes a membrane hyperpolarization when chloride concentration is low. However, it can not recover when the intracelluar chloride concentration is raised, and GABA depolarizes the cell. (Bottom) In older neurons, the chloride transport mechanism is mature. Thus, when the intracelluar chloride concentration is raised, the cell can recover, and GABA continues to evoke a membrane hyperpolarization. (Adapted from Luhmann and Prince, 1991)

K^+ becomes well-regulated, dropping from as much as 35 mM in the cortex of newborn rabbits to about 3 mM in adults (Mutani *et al.,* 1974). Since extracellular K^+ largely determines the resting membrane potential, this difference would translate into a shift of almost 35 mV. The regulation of extracellular space matures during the same time period when glial cells proliferate

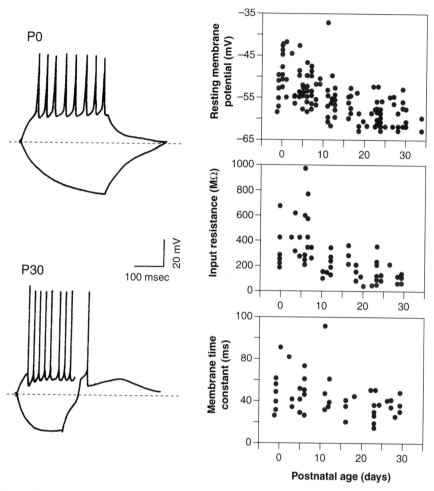

Figure 8.34 Development of passive membrane properties. (Left) The intracellularly recorded voltage response to positive and negative current pulses in a P0 and a P30 neuron from ferret lateral geniculate nucleus (LGN) brain slices. The P0 neuron displayed a longer time constant and larger voltage deflection. (Right) Plots of membrane potential, input resistance, and time constant from LGN neurons during postnatal development. Membrane potential becomes about 10 mV more negative, input resistance decreases by about 200 MΩ, and the time constant decreases by about 10 ms (Adapted from Ramoa and McCormick, 1994, with permission).

and differentiate (Connors *et al.*, 1982; Skoff *et al.*, 1976). Thus, when glial precursor cells in the neonatal rat spinal cord are killed with X-irradiation, extracellular K$^+$ remains poorly regulated (Syková *et al.*, 1992).

A few simple properties determine the size and speed of electrical events. These membrane properties depend on the total amount of membrane and its permeability to ions. For instance,

membrane input resistance determines how much the membrane voltage will change for a given current pulse. The membrane time constant determines how rapidly the membrane will reach a new voltage when current is injected. Both of these properties tend to decrease with age (Fig. 8.34), probably reflecting an increase in cell size (i.e., total membrane). Thus, input resistance would decrease because the number of resistors (i.e., channels) tends to increase as membrane is added to a cell.

The Action Potential

Neurons are in possession of some ionic channels from birth. However, the initial density of channels in the neuronal membrane is quite low, and they display immature properties. As with neurotransmitter receptors, this is due partly to the transient expression of neonatal isoforms. To determine how much current flows through a given membrane area, whole-cell voltage-clamp recordings are obtained from the neuron of interest (see Box: Biophysics: Nuts and Bolts of Functional Maturation), and pharmacological agents are employed to block all but a single type of channel. For example, to measure the density of sodium channels, one places the neuron in potassium and calcium channel blockers. A series of voltage command pulses are then delivered through the electrode while observing the current amplitude produced by the opening of voltage-sensitive channels in the neuronal membrane. In this way, it is also possible to characterize the potential at which channels are maximally activated.

In some developing systems, the action potential duration is first carried by calcium ions, and the calcium channels tend to remain open for a longer time. Thus, *Xenoupus* neurons begin life with 60 to 90 ms action potentials, although they quickly decrease to about 1 ms in duration (Fig. 8.35). There are two basic changes that explain this decreased duration. First, sodium channels become the major path for ionic current (Spitzer and Lamborghini, 1976; Baccaglini and Spitzer, 1977). Second, there is a 3.5-fold increase in the current through a potassium channel, called the delayed rectifier, that is activated during membrane depolarization (Barish, 1986). The maturation of this large outward current is also expected to limit the amount of calcium that enters a neuron during action potentials.

When ion channel composition does change, the transition can be explosinve (Fig. 8.36). The sodium and potassium currents, as measured in dissociated *Xenopus* spinal neurons, increase dramatically within about 24 h of their terminal mitosis (O'Dowd *et al.,* 1988). Similar observations have been made in explants of chick cortex (Mori-Okamoto *et al.,* 1983). The accumulation of sodium channels is of special interest because the amount of information that the nervous system can process, in terms of action potentials, is directly dependent on this protein. In acutely dissociated rat cortical neurons, the sodium current density increases six-fold during the first 2 postnatal weeks (Huguenard *et al.,* 1988). The density of a second sodium current, called persistent because it inactivates slowly at depolarized membrane potentials, also doubles in cortical pyramidal cells during the first 3 postnatal weeks (Alzheimer *et al.,* 1993).

Channel Diversity

It is important to recognize that there is no uniform order of channel appearance in the nervous system. For example, chick motor neurons have significant sodium and delayed rectifying potassium currents from the outset. There is a relatively late appearance of at least one type of potassium channel and two types of calcium channels (McCobb *et al.,* 1989, 1990). As with neurotransmitter receptors, there are switches in isoform that effect channel function. For example, when single voltage-gated potassium channels are examined by patch-clamp analysis during the maturation of cerebellar Purkinje cells *in vitro,* it is found that channels with larger conductances (i.e., the amount of current for a given change in potential) develop later (Yool *et al.,* 1988). In the majority of patches recorded at 5 days *in vitro,* 27 pS channels are observed but channels of 100 pS began to appear in patches at 8–14 days (Fig. 8.37). A larger conductance potassium channel also appears later in *Xenopus* spinal neurons.

There are many other types of potassium channels in addition to the delayed rectifier, and they generally appear later in development. For example, there is a fast transient potassium current, termed the A current, that becomes activated only *after* a period of hyperpolarization

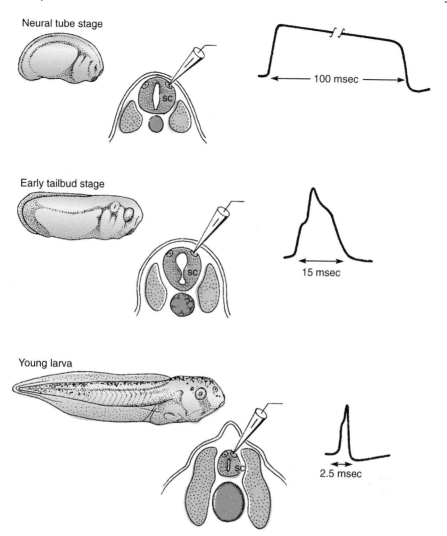

Figure 8.35   Action potentials are initally calcium-dependent. (Top) When intracellular recordings were made from spinal cord (sc) Rohon–Beard neurons in neural tube stage *Xenopus* embryos, depolarizing current injection produced long-lasting calcium action potentials. (Middle) In early tailbud embryos, current injection evoked a mixed sodium/calcium response. (Bottom) In the young larva, current evoked a brief sodium-dependent action potential. (Adapted from *TINS* **4** Spitzer, Development of membrane properties in vertebrates, pp. 169–172, Copyright 1981, with permission from Elsevier Science)

and contributes to oscillatory neuronal discharge. The appearance of A channels can be demonstrated by measuring potassium currents evoked with depolarizing voltage pulses from two different holding potentials. Since the A channel is maximally activated at −80 mV, a depolarizing command from this level will recruit both the delayed rectifier current (I_{KV}) and the A current (I_A). However, when the depolarizing command is initiated from −40 mV, *only* I_{KV} is activated. Therefore, one can subtract the current obtained at −40 mV from that obtained at −80 mV to obtain an isolated I_A record (Fig. 8.38). In chick motor neurons, the density of I_A increases 10-fold during a one week period, while I_{KV} remains at a relatively constant value (McCobb *et al.*, 1990).

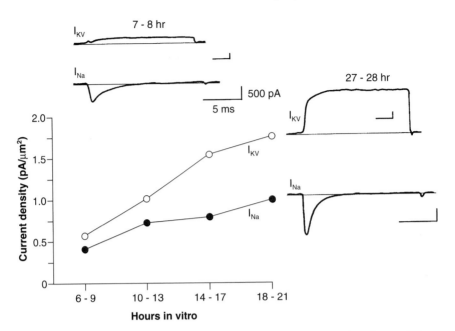

Figure 8.36 The densities of sodium and potassium currents increase rapidly in cultures of *Xenopus* spinal neurons. The graph shows that both potassium (open circles) and sodium currents (red circles) increase during the first 24 h *in vitro*. Currents were normalized based on the size of the cell body (pA/μm²). Examples of these currents are shown for 7–8 h and 27–28 h. (Adapted from O'Dowd *et al.,* 1988, with permission)

A third potassium channel depends upon both membrane potential *and* the intracellular calcium concentration to open (Fig. 8.38). These calcium-sensitive potassium channels also tend to be expressed after the delayed rectifier (O'Dowd *et al.,* 1988; Duorado and Dryer, 1992). Likewise, an inward potassium current that is activated by hyperpolarization, called the anomalous rectifier (I_h), increases about 10-fold in rat hypoglossal motoneurons from P8 to P21 (Bayliss *et al.,* 1994).

Significance of Calcium Channel Expression

Calcium currents that are activated by small depolarizations, called low-voltage-activated (LVA) or T currents, are broadly expressed in developing tissue. As the nervous system matures, there is an increasing prominence of calcium channels that activate only when the cell is greatly depolarized (Fig. 8.39). These are referred to as high-voltage-activated (HVA) or N and L currents. When hippocampal neurons from E19 rats are placed in a dissociated culture, only LVA currents are recorded at first. However, HVA currents appear over the next few days and become a major contributor (Yaari *et al.,* 1987). Similarly, it is the LVA calcium currents that are primarily observed when neurons from chick dorsal root ganglia, ciliary ganglia, or ventral horn are first recorded from (Gottmann *et al.,* 1988; McCobb *et al.,* 1989). These are overtaken by HVA currents within about 24–48 h.

The initial appearance of LVA calcium channels can contribute greatly to a neuron's differentiation. For example, spontaneous calcium transients in developing *Xenopus* spinal neurons, largely carried by LVA calcium channels, have been implicated in the acquisition of GABAergic phenotype and process outgrowth (Spitzer, 1994). In fact, these calcium transients regulate the maturation of electrical properties, including a switch

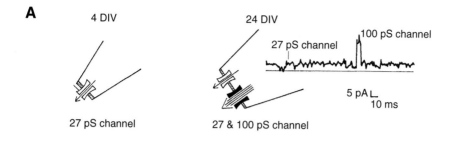

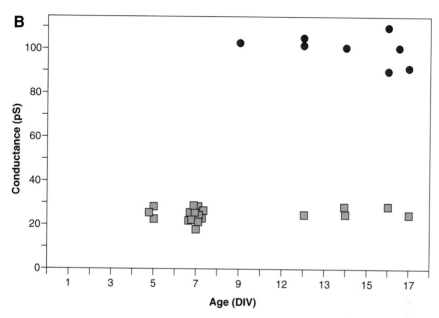

Figure 8.37 A high-conductance potassium channel appears later in development. (A) When a small patch of membrane is obtained from cultured rat cerebellar Purkinje neurons, one can record only small conductance channels at 5 days *in vitro* (DIV). In older cultures, one observes both small- and large-conductance channel openings. (B) The graph shows that channels with a small conductance (gray squares) are present by 5 DIV, while large-conductance channels (red circles) are not observed until 9 DIV. (Adapted from Yool *et al.,* 1988, with permission)

in potassium channel isoforms. The rate of activation for single potassium channels also increases by 2–3 times as *Xenopus* spinal neurons mature *in vitro* (Fig. 8.40). This transition in channel kinetics is dependent upon calcium influx and can be induced by activation of a protein kinase C (Desarmenien and Spitzer, 1991). The new potassium channel might appear either as a result of post-translational modification, activation of "silent" channels, or protein synthesis.

Regulation of Ionic Channel Expression

The addition of new channels to the membrane is necessary for most increases in current density. For example, when *Xenopus* neurons are grown in the presence of RNA or protein synthesis inhibitors, the transition from calcium- to sodium-dependent action potentials is prevented (Blair, 1983; O'Dowd, 1983). In a like manner, transcription blockers prevent the normal

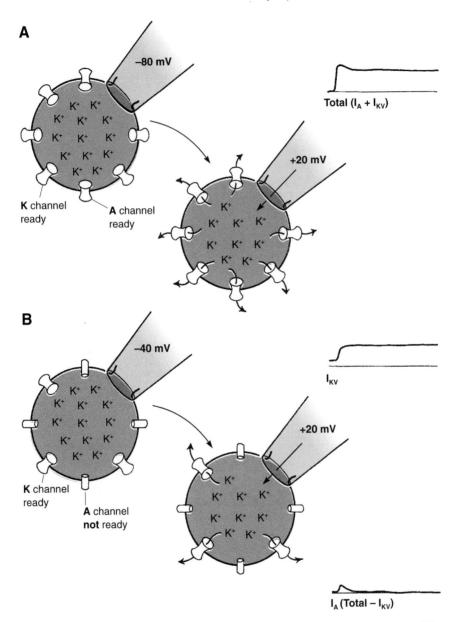

Figure 8.38 The developmental increase in two potassium currents has the same time course. The current flowing through the A-type potassium channel (I_A) is determined with a two-step process. (A) First, total potassium current is recorded by holding the neuron at -80 mV and then moving to $+20$ mV. (B) Next the potassium current flowing through the delayed rectifier (IK_V) is recorded by holding the neuron at -40 mV and then moving to $+20$ mV. I_A is then obtained by subtracting IK_V from Total current. (C) Graph showing that I_A and the calcium-dependent potassium current $I_{K(Ca)}$ increase with the same time course in chick ciliary ganglion neurons. (Adapted from Duorado and Dryer, 1992)

C

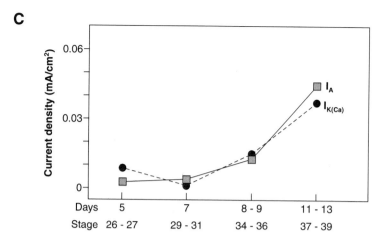

Figure 8.38 (*Continued*)

increase in potassium current density (Ribera and Spitzer, 1989). The signal to increase production of potassium channels is present for only a brief period of time. A 9-h exposure to an RNA synthesis inhibitor prevents the normal increase in potassium current density, even though RNA synthesis resumes upon withdrawal of the inhibitor. However, the appearance of A currents is not permanently blocked by transcription inhibitors.

If transsynaptic signals regulate ion channel maturation, they remain largely unknown. However, the glycoprotein that stimulates AChR synthesis in muscle cells, ARIA, can induce a two-fold increase in sodium channels (Corfas and Fischbach, 1993). Other well-described growth factors, such as FGF, can upregulate the density of calcium channels in dissociated cultures of hippocampal neurons, and the effect requires protein synthesis (Shitaka *et al.*, 1996). Electrical activity itself may affect the expression level of certain channels. Action potential blockade delays or prevents the normal increase in sodium and potassium current density in *Xenopus* myocytes *in vitro* (Linsdell and Moody, 1995).

The extrinsic signals that regulate ion channel expression are beginning to be understood in parasympathetic neurons of the chick ciliary ganglion. The expression of an A type (I_A) and a calcium-activated current ($I_{K[Ca]}$) is reduced when ciliary neurons are grown in dissociated culture,

in the absence of their target or preganglionic afferents (Duorado and Dryer, 1992). To determine whether synaptic connectivity influences potassium channel expression, *in vivo* manipulations were performed in which either the optic vesicle containing the target tissue was removed or a portion of the midbrain primordium containing the preganglionic nucleus was removed (Duorado *et al.*, 1994). The neurons were then acutely dissociated so that whole-cell voltage-clamp recordings could be obtained easily. The density of I_A was unaffected by either manipulation, although the channels did appear to open and close more rapidly than normal. In contrast, $I_{K[Ca]}$ was reduced by 90–100% following either target removal or deafferentation.

A factor has now been isolated from a target of the ciliary ganglion, the iris, that is able to upregulate the density of $I_{K[Ca]}$ (Subramony *et al.*, 1996). When neurons are cultured in the presence of iris extract, the density of $I_{K[Ca]}$ reaches reach normal levels within 7 h (Fig. 8.41). This factor turns out to be a TGFβ. When an antibody directed against the TGFβ family is added to iris extract or injected into the eye, the expression of $I_{K[Ca]}$ is inhibited (Cameron *et al.*, 1998). Interestingly, transcripts of the calcium-activated potassium channel are present in cultured ganglia before the current can be recorded, and the effect of iris extract does not require protein synthesis. These results suggest that

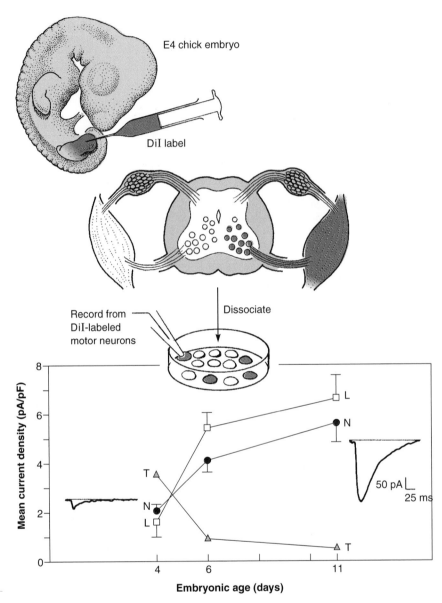

Figure 8.39 Two calcium currents increase while a third declines in developing spinal motor neurons. (Top) To obtain identified motorneurons, a dye (DiI, red) was injected into the leg bud, and this dye was retrogradely transported by motor neurons. Thus, when the tissue was dissociated, it was possible to identify motor neurons because they carried the DiI label. (Bottom) When calcium currents were recorded from the dissociated motor neurons, it was found that T-type calcium channels declined with age, while N- and L-type channels increased. (Adapted from McCobb *et al.,* © 1989 Cell Press, with permission)

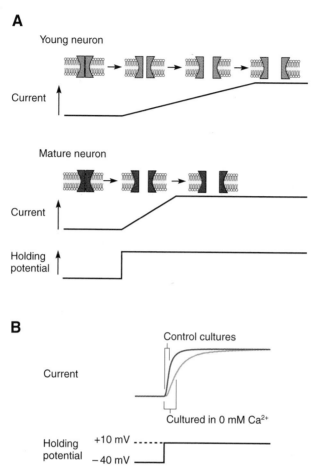

Figure 8.40 Calcium-dependent maturation of potassium channel activation. (A) When voltage-dependent potassium currents are recorded during a depolarizing voltage command in *Xenopus* spinal neurons, the currents activate more rapidly with time *in vitro*. This is schematized by showing the individual channels opening more rapidly in mature neurons. (B) IK$_V$ was recorded in *Xenopus* spinal neurons *in vitro*. When cultures were grown in normal medium the current activated rapidly (dark red), but when grown in the absence of calcium for about 1 day, the current activated more slowly (light red). (Adapted from O'Dowd *et al.*, 1988; Desarmenien and Spitzer, 1991)

retrograde signals can affect the translation, insertion, or modification of this potassium channel with a very short latency.

Summary

The generic cortical neuron that we began the chapter with somehow manages to express just the right complement of receptors and chan-nels and place them at the correct part of the cell. The differentiation of these properties depends upon an ongoing discussion between neuronal connections. Fortunately, we now have a basic understanding of synapse formation, including a few of the transynaptic signaling pathways. As extraordinary as these accomplishments are, it is important to recognize that we know very little about most of the modulatory afferents, many of the neurotransmitter receptors, and several of the

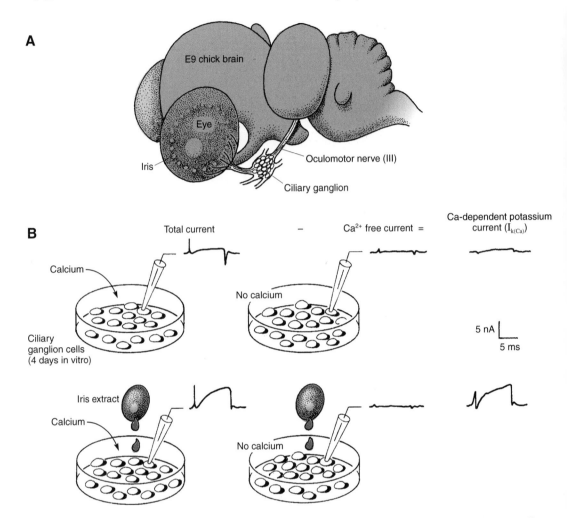

Figure 8.41   An extract from iris induces calcium-dependent potassium currents. (A) Ciliary ganglion neurons, which innervate the iris, were isolated from E9 chicks and placed in dissociated culture. (B) When the cultures were grown in control culture medium, one could record very little calcium-dependent potassium current ($I_{K(Ca)}$). This is shown by recording total current and subtracting the current in Ca^{2+}-free media. When an extract from the iris (red) was added to the cultured neurons, a much larger $I_{K(Ca)}$ was subsequently recorded. (Adapted from Subramony *et al.*, 1996)

cytoplasmic signaling pathways. Furthermore, we have begun to understand how the most basic attributes of transmission and electrogenesis develop, yet we have little understanding of how these functional building blocks shape the computational properties of a developing neuron. After all, that is a major goal of neural development. Why is 50,000 synapses the correct number of inputs for a cortical neuron? How would the neuron work with half that number? How

does the number or glutamatergic synapses influence the number of GABAergic or serotonergic synapses? How would a neuron operate if inhibitory synapses formed on dendritic spines and glutamatergic synapses were restricted to the soma? As we start to understand how individual synapses are constructed, it will be fascinating to explore the mechanisms that regulate their placement on a neuron and their relationship to specific ion channels.

Refinement of Synaptic Connections

· · · · ·

Most axons grow to the correct location, begin to arborize, and make functional contacts on the appropriate type of postsynaptic cell. The precision of innervation is accomplished with a host of signals that supervise the axon's direction of growth as well as the site of arborization. Yet even as the number of synapses is increasing in a target region (see Chapter 8), another mechanism is often set in motion, one that leads to a *loss* of synapses. For example, in the kitten visual cortex there is a burst of synaptogenesis during the first 40 postnatal days, and the number of synapses per neuron soars from a few hundred to 12,000. As synapse proliferation reaches a peak rate, afferent projections from the thalamus begin to retract from neighboring regions of the cortex, leading to a "striped" pattern of innervation (Cragg, 1975; LeVay *et al.,* 1978). There are also examples of connections that are eliminated entirely during development. Turning again to the kitten visual cortex, it has been shown that commissural afferents from the opposite side of the brain are lost in great numbers during first 3 postnatal months.

Why are synapses being assembled and destroyed at the same time, particularly when the pathfinding and mapping mechanisms produce such accurate results? A traditional answer to this question states that there is not enough genetic information to specify the adult pattern of innervation. It is also true that the brain is a piece of tissue designed for continuous modification, even into adulthood (cf. learning and memory). The addition and loss of synapses may reflect a major goal of nervous system function: to optimize behavioral performance in a given environment. One might argue that there is no better time for learning and optimizing performance than during early development. Therefore, the consequence of synapse elimination would appear to be greater specificity of neural connections, and the correct complement of afferents may optimize the computational properties of a neuron.

Rearranging Synaptic Connections

During the period of synapse formation, there are two types of inappropriate connections that are generated. First, individual axons that arborize in the correct topographic position (see Chapter 6) may spread out a little bit too far, perhaps a few tens of micrometers past their proper boundary (Fig. 9.1A). While this may seem to be a trivial distance, if millions of neurons make errors of this magnitude, then neural computations could be adversely affected. A second way in which innervation may be immature

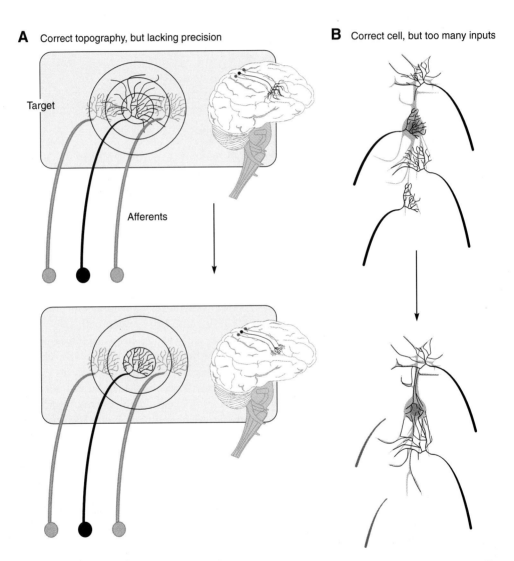

A Correct topography, but lacking precision

Target

Afferents

B Correct cell, but too many inputs

Figure 9.1 Two kinds of afferent projection errors during development. (A) The projection of three afferents to the cortex is shown, and each one centers its arborization at the topographically correct position in the target. However, one of the arbors initally extends too far (top) and these local branches are eliminated (bottom) during development. (B) A single neuron is shown to receive input from four afferents initially (top), and two of these inputs are eliminated (bottom) during development. Note that the remaining afferent arbors may spread out on the postsynaptic neuron.

occurs when a postsynaptic neuron receives synapses from the wrong number of afferents. The ratio of innervating afferent axons per postsynaptic neuron, referred to as convergence, varies greatly in the nervous system. At the mammalian nerve–muscle junction there is one motor axon synapse per muscle cell. In the cerebellum each Purkinje cell receives innervation from a single climbing fiber axon (cf. climbing fiber convergence is 1) but is contacted by thousands of parallel fiber synapses on its dendritic tree (parallel fiber convergence is ≈200,000). As we shall see, many postsynaptic neurons receive the adult number of afferents only after a fraction of their functional contacts are eliminated (Fig. 9.1B).

The addition or elimination of synapses during development is certainly the most extreme way to modify synaptic function during development. However, it is likely that the postsynaptic response magnitude that is produced by an individual synapse (cf. synaptic strength) is also regulated, perhaps without any structural changes. In the adult nervous system, the strength of synaptic transmission has been shown to change with use, and these alterations are thought to underlie the storage of memories (see Box: Remaining Flexible: Adult Mechanisms of Learning and Memory). Sensory deprivation studies conducted on developing animals provided some of the earliest evidence that the strength of neural connection is also dependent upon their continued activation. In the early 1960s, Torsten Wiesel and David Hubel began a remarkable series of experiments on visual experience and the maturation of cortical function. They found that if one eye is deprived of visual stimulation during development, then it largely loses the ability to activate cortical neurons, indicating that the synapses driven by the closed eye were either eliminated or weakened. These experiments suggest that the initial connectivity of the visual pathway is not stable. It can be permanently altered by a developmental mechanism that utilizes nervous system activity.

What is the evidence for synapse elimination in the developing nervous system? How widespread is this mechanism? Three experimental approaches have been taken to determine whether a loss of synapses occurs during development. First, intracellular recordings have been used to show changes in the number of functional afferents per postsynaptic neuron. Second, anatomical studies have revealed that single axonal arborizations become spatially restricted within the target population. But how do these detailed synaptic decisions impact on nervous system performance? To answer this, we shift our attention from the molecular level to experiments that explore nervous system function and behavioral performance. Third, it is possible to examine whether all of the synapses are working together correctly by studying the response of single neurons to sensory stimuli, such as light or sound. Many auditory neurons respond with great accuracy to the location of a sound source in space, and this reflects both the number and the strength of their synaptic inputs. If there are errors in synaptogenesis, then one might expect that auditory neurons will respond to an unusually broad range of spatial stimuli. Therefore, a neuron's computational abilities are a fairly sensitive assay of synaptic refinement. We will consider the results from each of these three approaches in the following sections.

Functional Synapses Are Eliminated

The developmental loss of synaptic contacts has been observed in systems as diverse as the nerve–muscle junction of invertebrates to the cerebral cortex of primates. In the majority of cases these changes are not apparent by casually observing neonatal and adult tissue sections under the microscope. Instead quantitative comparisons must be made using measurements from many neurons. How is it possible to count the number of afferents per postsynaptic neuron? An imaginative approach to this problem, first employed in the early 1970s, used intracellular recordings and electrical stimulation of the afferent pathway (Fig. 9.2). The basic assumptions are that each axon will evoke a postsynaptic potential (PSP) when stimulated and that the

Remaining Flexible: Adult Mechanisms of Learning and Memory

The cellular mechanisms responsible for changes in synaptic strength have been explored most thoroughly in adult animals because of their importance in learning and memory. Synaptic plasticity has been studied in a wide variety of neuronal systems, from molluscan ganglia to mammalian cerebral cortices, yet the catalog of cellular, molecular, and genetic mechanisms seems to expand daily. This is probably good news for those interested in developmental plasticity because many of the ideas and techniques have been imported successfully.

The very first inquiries into synaptic mechanisms of plasticity demonstrated that synaptic transmission could be enhanced for about 1 min following a period of intense stimulation. Recording from muscle cells revealed that post-tetanic facilitation occurred because more neurotransmitter was released from the presynaptic terminal (Larrabee and Bronk, 1947; Lloyd, 1949). For the most part, contemporary studies continue to rely on intracellular recordings, usually in conjunction with a drove of "magic bullets" that are designed to block the function of a specific molecule. A relatively new approach makes use of genetic manipulations in the fruit fly and the mouse (Chapter 2) to provide an important experimental link between gene products, synaptic function, and behavior.

The modern era of cellular research began in the 1960s when the classical conditioning paradigm of paired stimuli was applied directly to a molluscan nervous system. In an intact sea slug, *Aplysia,* it is possible to enhance a touch-evoked withdrawal of the siphon when the tactile stimulus is paired with an electric shock during a training period. To study the neural basis of this sensitization, afferent-evoked EPSPs were recorded intracellularly from an identified neuron in the abdominal ganglion and stimuli were delivered to both afferent pathways simultaneously. Following paired stimulation, one of the synapses produced much larger EPSPs and this effect lasted for up to 40 min (Kandel and Tauc, 1965). The increase was termed heterosynaptic facilitation because synaptic transmission at one set of synapses modified the functional status of a second, independent set.

One of the most compelling examples of synaptic plasticity, called long-term potentiation (LTP), was first identified in the early 1970s. By recording extracellularly from the

PSPs will summate in discrete steps as the additional fibers are recruited by increasing the electric stimulus (Fig. 9.2). Therefore, the increments in PSP size serve to estimate the number of axons making functional contacts on a single postsynaptic neuron or muscle fiber.

When this experiment is performed at the mature neuromuscular junction, a single large PSP is recorded, indicating that the muscle fiber is innervated by a single motor nerve terminal. However, when the same experiment is performed in neonatal animals, the PSP size first doubles and then triples in amplitude as the stimulus activates two and then three motor axons (Fig. 9.3). Similar observations have been made in developing chick, rat, and kitten muscles (Redfern, 1970; Bagust *et al.,* 1973; Bennett and Pettigrew, 1974). The elimination of convergent motor axons at the rat soleus muscle results in a decrease from three axons per muscle fiber to only one during the second postnatal week.

The precise time course over which synapse elimination occurs and the proportion of afferents lost vary greatly between areas of the nervous system, even within a single species. In the rat cerebellum, for example, the elimination of

hippocampus of anesthetized rabbits, it was found that a brief, high-frequency stimulus to the afferent pathway resulted in an enhancement of the evoked potential that lasted for hours to days (Bliss and Lmo, 1973). Over the next few years, intracellular recordings from mammalian brain slice preparations demonstrated that the size of EPSPs also increases following tetanic afferent stimulation. LTP is now thought to be one mechanism by which synapses store information because humans with hippocampal lesions display memory deficits, and a drug that blocks LTP *in vitro* is also able to impair spacial learning in rodents.

The discovery of a cellular analog of learning has raised many questions about the cellular mechanisms and the molecular pathways involved. Recent studies have indicated that two types of changes can occur at a potentiated synapse: increased transmitter release and enhanced postsynaptic response. One likely scenario for LTP in the hippocampus has glutamatergic transmission and postsynaptic depolarization combining to activate NMDARs, allowing calcium to flood the postsynaptic cell. The calcium then activates one or more kinases which, in turn, phosphorylate proteins at the synapse. Although it is still not clear which proteins are modified, there is evidence that functional glutamate receptors are added to the membrane, thus enhancing the postsynaptic response. A very simple form of learning in the *Aplysia,* long-term facilitation of transmitter release, illustrates another important molecular pathway. An increase in presynaptic cAMP leads to the activation of a cAMP-dependent protein kinase (PKA). Once activated, the PKA subunit travels to the nucleus where it phosphorylates a transcription factor. The facilitated transmitter release involves new gene expression and protein synthesis, although these products have yet to be identified (Kaang *et al.,* 1993).

The cAMP signaling pathway seems to be a primary bridge to the formation of long-term memories in fruit flies and mice. There are two cAMP-dependent transcription factors, one that activates gene expression and a second that represses it. Thus, when transgenic flies are bred to express the activator, they remember an odor with much less training. However, flies that express the repressor are unable to store long-term olfactory memories (Yin *et al.,* 1994, 1995). The genetic approach to learning and memory clearly holds the promise of uniting cellular and behavioral findings, and it is likely that studies of developmental plasticity will profit as well.

climbing fiber synapses onto Purkinje cells occurs during the second postnatal week, about the same time course as observed at the neuromuscular junction (Mariani and Changeux, 1981). In contrast, the elimination of preganglionic synapses onto neurons of the rat submandibular ganglion occurs over at least 5 postnatal weeks (Lichtman, 1977), far longer than is required for elimination at the neuromuscular junction (Fig. 9.3). The number of cochlear nerve synapses on neurons of the chick cochlear nucleus declines rapidly, from about four to two afferents (Fig. 9.3) and reaches a mature state even before

hatching (Jackson and Parks, 1982). Therefore, synapse elimination appears to be a widespread phenomenon, although there are no general rules about the percentage of afferents that is lost or the duration of time required.

As the number of presynaptic afferents increases, it becomes difficult to resolve small differences in PSP size. However, functional estimates of synaptic convergence suggest that elimination occurs even in systems that remain multiply innervated as adults (Lichtman and Purves, 1980; Sanes, 1993). This physiological method is not sensitive to certain forms of synapse

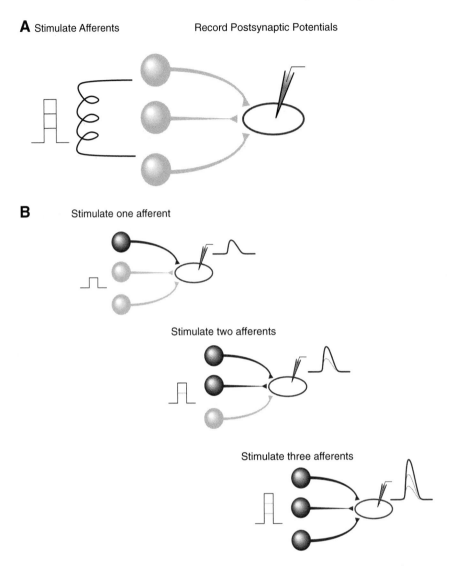

A Stimulate Afferents   Record Postsynaptic Potentials

B   Stimulate one afferent

                              Stimulate two afferents

                                        Stimulate three afferents

Figure 9.2 An electrophysiological method for determining the number of inputs converging onto a neuron. (A) A stimulating electrode is placed on the afferent population while an intracellular recording is obtained from the postsynaptic cell. (B) As the stimulation current is increased, the afferent inputs are recruited to become active (red). When a single afferent is active, the postsynaptic potential (PSP) is small. When two and then three afferents are activated, the PSP become quantally larger. One can estimate the number of inputs by counting the number of quantal increases in PSP amplitude, in this case three.

elimination. For example, climbing fiber axons innervate the soma and dendrite of cerebellar Purkinje cells in neonates, but the somatic synapses are eliminated during the course of development (Altman, 1972).

Axonal Arbors Are Refined or Eliminated

How is it possible to know whether synapse elimination occurs at central neurons that re-

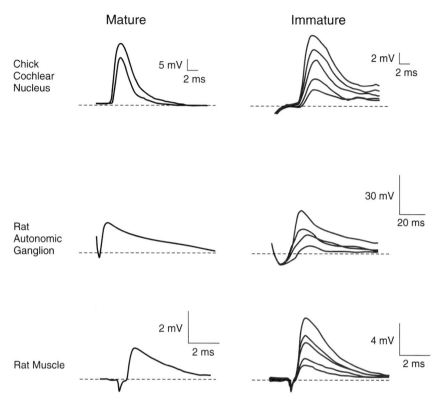

Mature   **Immature**

Chick Cochlear Nucleus

5 mV | 2 ms   2 mV | 2 ms

Rat Autonomic Ganglion

30 mV | 20 ms

Rat Muscle

2 mV | 2 ms   4 mV | 2 ms

Figure 9.3   Three examples of decreased convergence, as measured electrophysiologically (see Fig 9.2). On the right are shown the increases in afferent evoked PSP recorded in immature neurons (red) of the chick cochlear nucleus, rat autonomic ganglion, and rat NMJ. There are 3–5 quantal increases in PSP amplitude. On the left are shown the increases in afferent evoked PSP amplitude in mature neurons (black). There are 1–2 quantal increases in PSP amplitude, indicating the functional elimination of inputs. (Adapted from Jackson and Parks, 1982, Lichtman, 1977, O'Brien *et al.*, 1978, with permission.)

ceive contacts from hundreds or thousands of afferents? The simple answer is that it is not yet possible to demonstrate elimination directly in such systems. The size of individual PSPs is too small and their amplitude is too variable, leaving one with a cloud of potentials that do not increase in crisp steps. One approach is to count all the synaptic contacts on a neuron at several postnatal ages. For example, measures of synapse number and contact length taken from motor neurons provide an estimate that 50% of synaptic contacts are lost during development, and comparable changes are found in the human cortex (Conradi and Ronnevi, 1975; Huttenlocher and de Courten, 1987). In addition, a rat

raised with many objects in its cage (cf. enriched environment) has almost 25% more synapses per neuron in the visual cortex (Turner and Greenough, 1985).

Impressive as these numbers are, there are two potential problems. First, they do not tell us whether the actual number of axons making synapses onto postsynaptic neurons changes during development. For example, a single afferent could initially make 100 weak synapses that gradually transform into 50 strong ones. Second, *total* synapse number may increase in some systems during the time when *some* synapses are being eliminated, and this would go unnoticed.

If we assume for a moment that axons make synapses wherever they arborize, then it should be possible to study synapse elimination indirectly by looking at the amount of territory occupied by the axon. The most obvious case occurs when a projection is eliminated due to the death of nerve cell bodies. In chicks, there is a projection from a brain stem nucleus, the isthmooptic nucleus, to the retina in which nearly 60% of the projecting cells die, particularly those projecting to the wrong place in the retina (Casticas *et al.*, 1987).

However, elimination of commissural axons' projections from one side of the cerebral cortex to the other occurs even in the absence of cell death (Innocenti *et al.*, 1977). This was demonstrated in rats by labeling commissural neurons twice, once early in development and then once again after certain axons retracted. Neurons that projected to the other hemisphere are retrogradely labeled with a yellow dye at birth by injecting the dye on one side of the brain and allowing commissural axons to transport it back (Fig. 9.4). Two weeks later, a second dye, this time blue, is injected in the same spot, and the remaining commissural axons retrogradely transport it to their cell bodies. When the tissue is examined, many cells are stained yellow, but only a fraction of these labeled cells also contain the blue dye (O'Leary *et al.*, 1981). The yellow cells send axons through the commissure at birth, but some of the cells retract their axons before the blue dye is injected. Therefore, many cortical neurons generate transient projections through the cerebral commissure (corpus callosum), and some of these axons are eliminated during development.

The wholesale withdrawal of axons provides a wonderful example of developmental refinement, but unfortunately for the anatomist it is not the norm. In fact, changes in terminal arbor morphology are usually quite subtle. An axon will tend to innervate the correct target region (see Chapter 6), extend a bit beyond the correct topographic position, and then pull back to the adult boundary. Perhaps the best-characterized examples of axon terminal elimination come from the developing visual pathway. In cats and primates, retinal ganglion cells from each eye

project to separate layers in the lateral geniculate nucleus (LGN). The LGN neurons then project to layer IV of the visual cortex, forming segregated eye-specific termination zones, called ocular dominance columns or "stripes" (Fig. 9.5A).

It is possible to visualize the projection pattern of an entire eye by injecting [³H]-proline into the eye cup. This label is taken up by retinal ganglion cells and transported down their axons to the LGN where is crosses the synapse, enters the postsynaptic LGN neuron, and is carried by the axons to their terminals in the cortex. When the cortex tissue sections are exposed to film, an autoradiographic image of the LGN axon terminals from one eye is observed (Fig. 9.5B). By applying this technique to the cat visual pathway during postnatal development, it is found that the LGN afferents from one eye are at first widespread in cortical layer IV. Over the next several weeks, this diffuse label breaks up into discrete patches that represent eye-specific termination zones (LeVay *et al.*, 1978). The light-evoked responses of layer IV visual cortex neurons are perfectly consistent with the anatomy. At first, most layer IV cortical neurons respond to stimulation of either eye, while many are only driven by a single eye in adult animals. Therefore, individual LGN arbors from one eye must retract a portion of their terminals during development or there is a selective elimination of the entire geniculate axon. More recently, the morphologies of single LGN axon terminals have been examined in the primate visual cortex, and the area occupied by one type of terminal decreases by 50%, consistent with the autoradiographic studies (Florence and Casagrande, 1990).

The development of retinal arbors in the LGN illustrates how targeting errors are widespread, yet subtle in appearance. In mammals, retinal axons grow to the correct area of the LGN from the outset, but they also make two kinds of inappropriate contacts. First, nearly all of them produce a few small collaterals, about 10–20 μm in length, in a part of the LGN that will eventually be innervated by the other eye only. In the cat, the formation of eye-specific layers occurs *in utero* when these side branches are selectively eliminated (Fig. 9.6). A second phase

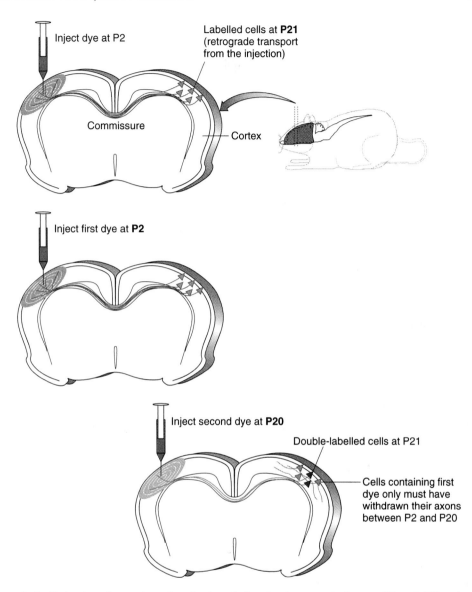

Figure 9.4 limination of commissural projections during development. At Postnatal Day 2 (P2), a dye was injected into the cortex (gray), and it was retrogradely transported by commissural neurons. At P21, the animal was sacrificed and the tissue was processed to reveal the labeled neurons. In a second experiment, the first dye (gray) was injected at P2, and a second dye (red) was injected at P20. When the tissue was processed, some commissural neurons were double labeled (gray/red), whereas others contained only the first dye (gray). Thus, the first-labeled cells projected to the contralateral cortex at P2, but retracted their axons during postnatal development and maintained local connections. (Adapted from O'Leary *et al.,* 1981.)

of refinement occurs postnatally when retinal terminals become more focused in the LGN (Fig. 9.6). Retinal ganglion cells that have small visual receptive fields (cf. X cells) decrease the width of LGN tissue that they innervate by a distance of only about 60 μm, yet this amounts

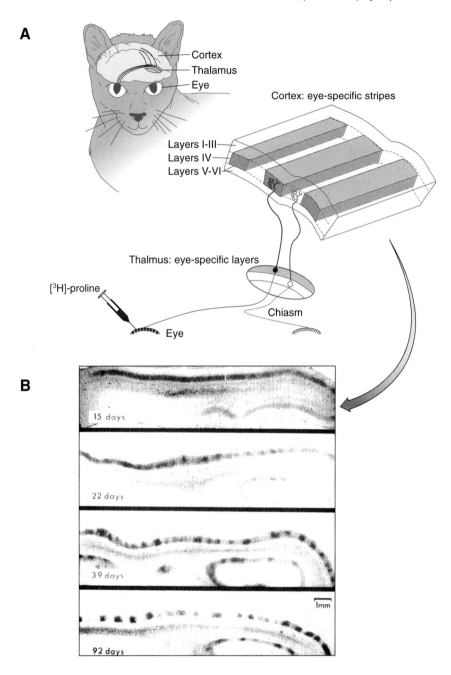

Figure 9.5 Thalamic afferents form eye-specific terminal zones in cat primary visual cortex. (A) When [³H]-proline is injected into one eye, it is transported transynaptically to the cortex. A schematic shows the visual pathway from eye to cortex. Retinal ganglion cells project to an eye-specific layer in the thalamus, and thalamic neurons project to eye-specific stripes in cortex layer IV. (B) Autoradiograms of [³H]-proline in postnatal cat visual cortex show that the terminal field from one eye initially spreads across the whole of layer IV (15 days), but gradually becomes restricted to stripes. (Adapted from LeVay *et al., J. Comp. Neurol.* **191:** 1–51, Copyright © 1978. By permission of Wiley–Liss, Inc., a subsidiary of John Wiley & Sons, Inc.)

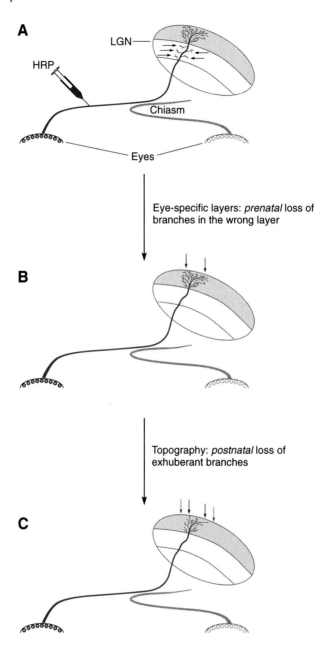

Figure 9.6 Development of retinal ganglion cell terminals in the cat lateral geniculate nucleus (LGN). (A) When individual retinal fibers are labeled with horseradish peroxidase (HRP) on Embryonic Days 43–55, they have many sidebranches in the inappropriate layer of LGN (arrows). (B) By birth, most of the side branches have been eliminated and terminal arborizations are restricted to the correct layer. However, the terminal zone remained wider in the eye-specific lamina at 3–4 weeks postnatal (arrows) (C) When fibers of retinal X-cells were filled in adult cats, they were found to have retracted (black arrows). (Adapted from Sur *et al.,* 1984; Sretavan and Shatz, 1986.)

to a highly significant reduction (Sur *et al.,* 1984; Sretavan and Shatz, 1986). Thus, errors are numerous but modest in size.

Are synapses actually being formed by these transient projections? The answer can be found by first filling entire axons with a tracer, such as horseradish peroxidase, and then examining the terminals with an electron microscope. In fact, labeled presynaptic terminals have been found in parts of the target where they never remain in the adult, indicating that these structurally mature synapses will eventually have to be broken (Reh and Constantine-Paton, 1984; Campbell and Shatz, 1992).

Just how commonplace is axonal refinement and the loss of synaptic connections? It is found in a great variety of species and neural structures, although there are exceptions. There is significant remodeling of retinal axons during topographic map formation in the visual midbrain (Reh and Constantine-Paton, 1984; Simon and O'Leary, 1992). In frogs, single retinal afferents innervate successively posterior locations within the tectum as development proceeds. In mammals, retinal axons innervate topographically incorrect positions at birth, and these terminals are gradually withdrawn over 2 weeks.

Synapse elimination is also found in invertebrates. In the cricket, single sensory neurons are functionally connected with two different interneurons during an early stage of development. Gradually, the strength of one connection doubles while the other connection is completely eliminated (Chiba *et al.,* 1988). As we see below, excitatory synaptic transmission has been implicated in the rearrangement of connections. However, inhibitory afferents can also become more refined during development. The arbor size of single glycinergic afferents decreases by about 25% along the tonotopic axis in a mammalian auditory brain stem nucleus during postnatal development (Sanes and Siverls, 1991).

Some Terminals Expand or Remain Stable

Although many axons make a few inappropriate connections, there are some afferent path-

ways where synapse elimination is either scarce or absent. In contrast to the axonal arbors described above (see Figs. 9.5 and 9.6), there are retinal ganglion cells with large visual receptive fields (Y cells) whose arbors expand during development (Sur *et al.,* 1984; Florence and Casagrande, 1990). While the functional implications of terminal expansion are not clear, some neural circuits probably require broad connectivity with the sensory world. Many systems may employ a mixed strategy: some axons expanding in territory while others retract. In the chick auditory system, two sets of axons converge on the nucleus laminaris, one innervating the dorsal dendrites and the other the ventral dendrites. Both sets of afferents spread out along the tonotopic axis during the embryonic period, suggesting that synapses are being added (Young and Rubel, 1986). However, the ventral terminal arbors form directly above their parent axon at first, but nearly half of them are found at a significant distance later in development. Since it is unlikely that the entire axon shifts its position, individual synaptic contacts are probably eliminated from one region of the terminal and new synapses are added at a different position. The connections from sensory axons to motor neurons appear to be accurate from the outset. Inappropriate monosynaptic connections from sensory axons to spinal motor neurons are not found with intracellular recordings, although there may be significant errors through polysynaptic pathways (Seebach and Ziskind-Conhaim, 1994; Mears and Frank, 1997).

Neural Activity Regulates Synaptic Connections

Each of us experiences use-dependent changes is our nervous system on a regular basis. Visual and auditory information is processed by our nervous system and stored as memories (see Box: Remaining Flexible). Our hands gradually become more adept at working with a newly purchased tool or paintbrush. When the level of noise or illumination changes abruptly, our ears, eyes, and nervous system adjust to maintain the fidelity of the signal. Similarly, we accept the notion that our rearing environment influences many aspects of our adult behavior (see Chapter 10). To take an obvious example, we produce the language to which we were exposed as infants, whether it was Hindi, American Sign Language, or Spanish. But how much is the developing nervous system really altered by the environment? Is synaptogenesis and synapse elimination influenced directly by a use-dependent process?

An early approach to this problem, one that is still in regular use, involved the elimination of sensory structures. Denervation studies of this sort indicated that neuron growth and survival depend on intact connections during development (see Chapter 7). However, it was not known whether improperly used synapses would become weak or lost entirely. The next experimental step was to leave the nervous system intact, but to change its activity in some known manner. With this goal in mind, Wiesel and Hubel (1963a, 1965) began to explore the effects of monocular and binocular deprivation on the development of visual coding properties in the CNS. Their results clearly show that synaptic activity is necessary for the maintenance or elimination of neural connections during development.

Before we can understand the functional changes brought about by visual deprivation, it is necessary to review some basic properties of the visual cortex. As described above, each neuron in layer IV of the visual cortex receives projections that are largely driven by one eye or the other (see Fig. 9.5). Thus, when visual stimuli are delivered to the appropriate eye, layer IV neurons respond with a burst of action potentials. Cortical neurons that respond to only one eye are referred to as monocular neurons. The majority of cortical neurons, particularly those laying outside of layer IV, are activated by both eyes and are referred to as binocular neurons. When an extracellular electrode passes through the visual cortex, recording from many neurons in succession, most cells are found to be activated by either eye. That is, most binocular neurons are recorded outside of layer IV. Hubel and Wiesel (1962) divided the cortex neurons into seven groups, based upon the relative ability of each eye to evoke a response. For example, if a neuron was driven solely by the contralateral eye, then it was assigned to group one. If it was driven equivalently by each eye, then it was assigned to group four, and so forth. These data can be conveniently represented as a histogram of ocular dominance (Fig. 9.7). Judged by their continued use during the past 35 years, ocular dominance histograms provide a sensitive measure of binocularity in the visual pathway.

A series of experiments was performed in which light-evoked activity was decreased by keeping the eyelid closed, referred to as visual deprivation (Wiesel and Hubel, 1963a,b, 1965). This manipulation does no damage to the retina, and LGN neurons remain responsive to visual stimulation after the eyelid is reopened. At first, a single eyelid was kept closed for a few months, and recordings were made from the visual cortex after the eye was reopened. The effect was unmistakable: Most cortical neurons no longer responded to stimulation of the deprived eye (Fig. 9.8), although they continued to respond to the unmanipulated eye.

Reasoning that disuse must have weakened the synapses from the deprived eye, Wiesel and Hubel recorded from binocularly deprived kittens, expecting to see a total absence of visually evoked activity. It came as a great surprise, then, that most cortical neurons remained responsive to stimuli through either eye. That is, the ocular dominance histogram obtained from binocularly deprived animals resemble that of normal animals (Fig. 9.9). "It was as if the expected ill effects from closing one eye had been averted by closing the other" (Wiesel and Hubel, 1965). However, many neurons display abnormal responses, and a large fraction of neurons are unresponsive to light, as originally predicted (Sherman and Spear, 1982).

The total amount of evoked activity does not necessarily predict whether a synapse will be strong or weak. Rather, differences in the amount of synaptic activity seem to determine the strength of a connection. This idea came to be known as the *competition hypothesis*. Under this scheme, retinal synapses in the LGN should not be affected by deprivation because LGN neurons are monocular and receive afferents that are either uniformly active or uniformly deprived

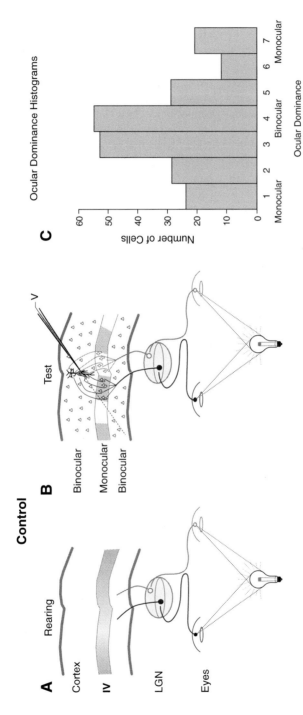

Figure 9.7 Response properties of visual cortex neurons in normally reared cats. (A) The visual system received normal stimulation until the time of recording. (B) Single neuron recordings were made with an extracellular electrode passed tangentially through the cortex. Neurons respond to only one eye in layer IV (monocular). In layers I–III and V–VI, neurons respond to both eyes (binocular) due to convergent connections. In normal cats, the terminal stripes from each eye-specific layer of the LGN occupy a similar amount of space. (C) Each neuron was characterized as responding to a single eye (monocular) or as responding to both eyes (binocular). In normal animals, most visual cortical neurons are binocular. (Adapted from Wiesel and Hubel, 1962.)

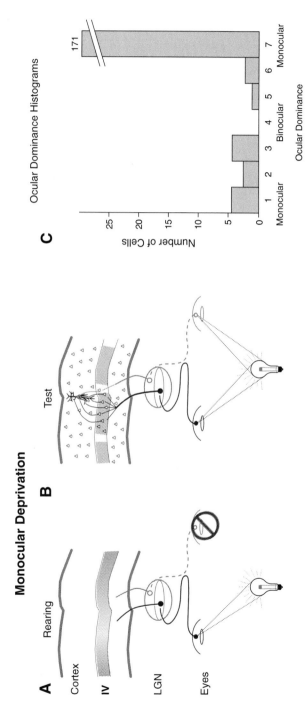

Figure 9.8 Response properties of visual cortex neurons in monocularly deprived cats. (A) The visual system received normal stimulation through one eye (red), and the other eye (gray) was kept closed until the time of recording. (B) The terminal stripes from the deprived eye became much narrower, and the visual responses of neurons outside of layer IV were more responsive to the open eye. (C) In monocularly deprived cats, the vast majority of cortical neurons responded to the open eye only. (Adapted from Wiesel and Hubel, 1963a.)

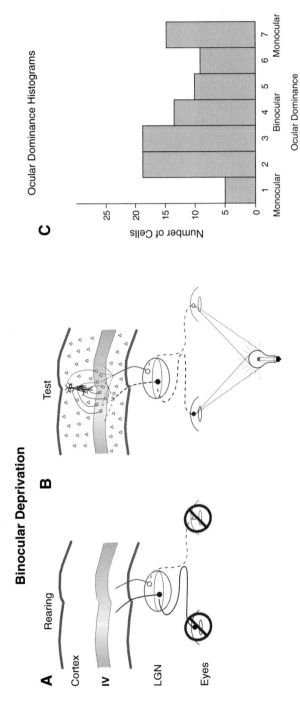

Figure 9.9 Response properties of visual cortex neurons in binocularly deprived cats. (A) Both eyes were kept closed until the time of recording. (B) The terminal stripes from each eye occupied a similar amount of space. (C) The majority of visually responsive neurons was driven by both eyes. (Adapted from Wiesel and Hubel, 1965 with permission.)

of light. Similarly, binocular deprivation evens the playing field, as none of the afferents to the cortex should be more active than any other. Monocular deprivation creates a situation in which cortical neurons receive a set of active afferents from the open eye and a group of afferents with lowered activity from the closed eye, placing the latter at a disadvantage.

In a pivotal test of the competition hypothesis, kittens were raised with an artificial strabismus (cf. misalignment of the eyes), produced by surgically manipulating one of the extraocular muscles (Hubel and Wiesel, 1965). This manipulation mimics a clinical condition in humans, called amblyopia, that commonly results in the suppression of vision through one of the eyes, presumably to avoid double vision. In strabismic kittens, visual stimuli activate different positions on the two retinas, meaning that cortical neurons are rarely activated by both eyes at the same time (Fig. 9.10). Following several months of strabismus, recordings were once again made from the visual cortex. In strabismic cats, both eyes effectively activate neurons in the cortex, but most cortical neurons respond to stimulation of one eye or the other. Few binocular neurons are observed. Therefore, an equivalent amount of activity in the two pathways is not sufficient to explain the results. Instead, it seems that the *timing* of synaptic activity must somehow be involved in allowing inputs to remain active on cortical neurons. These experiments suggest that synapses from each eye must be active at nearly the same instant if both are to keep strong functional contacts with the same postsynaptic neuron (Fig. 9.10). Small disparities in the timing of synaptic activity may determine the strength of a synapse, an idea that has since been tested in tissue culture (below).

Does synapse elimination actually underlie the activity-dependent modulation of synapse strength? It is possible that changes in ocular dominance may be explained by the elimination or expansion of LGN synapses in layer IV of the cortex. In fact, the ocular dominance columns (stripes) formed by geniculate terminals provide a particularly good model for studies of synapse elimination. In normal animals, when [³H]-proline is injected into one eye, there is a periodic variation in silver grain density in layer IV of the cortex. Labeled and nonlabeled regions are about 500 μm wide (see Fig. 9.5). Following monocular deprivation, the LGN afferents from the nondeprived eye come to occupy the majority of layer IV, while LGN afferents from the deprived eye occupy narrower regions (Fig. 9.8). This suggests that synapses from the nondeprived eye fail to undergo their normal process of elimination. In contrast, a greater than normal number of synapses from the deprived eye must be lost. The refinement of each eye's inputs into stripes can occur during binocular deprivation, although the stripes are somewhat obscured. This suggests that synapse elimination in layer IV can move forward in the absence of visually evoked activity (Fig. 9.9).

The majority of binocular neurons in the cortex are created by local projections from one cortical neuron to its neighbors, and these projections also become refined during development. Since neurons in all layers of the cortex are monocular following strabismus, it would be interesting to know what happens to these intracortical projections. Do they now become more segregated than normal, extending the striped pattern throughout the entire cortical depth? This seems to be precisely what happens. First, small injections of dye were made in the cortex, retrogradely labeling neurons that formed local projections to this area (Fig. 9.11). Then the animals were injected with 2-deoxyglucose (see Box: Watching Neurons Think) and stimulated through one eye to label all areas of cortex that were driven by that eye. With this double-labeling technique, one can learn whether local projection neurons are found exclusively in one ocular dominance column or both. In normal animals, the local projections come from both eye columns, and the cells that they innervate are binocularly driven. In strabismic cats, the local projections come exclusively from one eye (Löwel and Singer, 1992). Thus, activity influences the development of synaptic connections not only in ascending sensory projections but also in many of the intracortical projections as well.

These classic studies of developmental plasticity demonstrate that the strength of synaptic connections is modified by use. The central

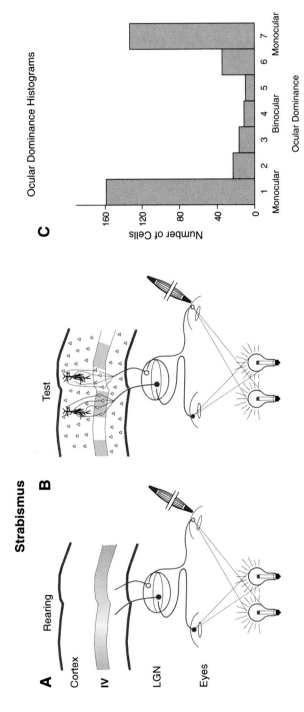

Figure 9.10 Response properties of visual cortex neurons in cats reared with artificial strabismus. (A) One eye (gray) was surgically deflected, such that a visual stimuli activated different topographic positions on each eye. Thus, cortical neurons were not activated by both eyes at the same time. (B) The terminal stripes from each eye occupied a similar amount of space. However, neurons outside of layer IV did not recieve convergent input from both eyes. (C) In strabismic cats, the vast majority of cortical neurons responded to one eye or the other. (Adapted from Hubel and Wiesel, 1965 with permission.)

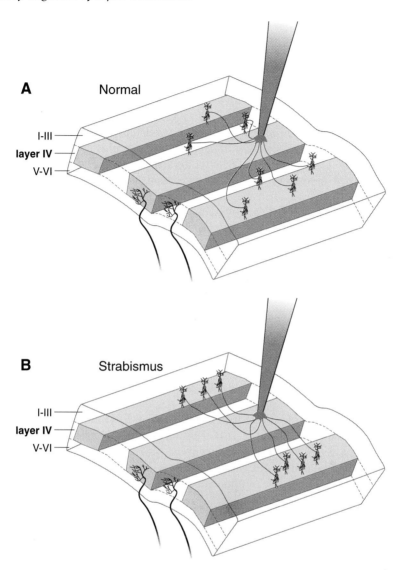

Figure 9.11 Visual experience influences intrinsic cortical projections. (A) When dye (red) injections were made into superficial layers of the visual cortex of normal cats, the label was retrogradely transported by neurons in both ocular dominance columns. (B) In cats reared with artificial strabismus, the label was retrogradely transported only by neurons that shared the same ocular dominance. (Adapted from Löwel and Singer, 1992.)

concept to emerge from these studies is that co-active synapses are stabilized, while inactive synapses, particularly those that are inactive while others are firing, become weakened and in many cases are eliminated. As one might expect, the development of a complicated structure such as the cortex is unlikely to be explained by one tidy

hypothesis. We have just learned that activity-dependent changes in connectivity are occurring at several locations. Functional and structural changes are also found in the LGN following lid suture or strabismus, and the extent to which these changes influence cortical development is not clear. Proprioceptive feedback from the eye

Watching Neurons Think:
Functional Properties of Neuron Ensembles

A major goal of neurophysiology is to demonstrate a causal relationship between CNS function and animal behavior. While our success has been limited, there are a number of exciting strategies that should bring us closer to that goal. For almost a century, neurophysiologists have been recording electrical activity from the nervous system, at first from large populations of cells with scalp electrodes (cf. electroencephalograms), and eventually with small extracellular electrodes that monitor the action potentials from a single neuron. For those interested in sensory coding and perception, the extracellular electrodes are usually lowered into the brain of an anesthetized animal, and a neuron's activity is recorded while stimuli are delivered to the ears, eyes, or other receptor populations. In this way, we learn how environmental stimuli are converted into a neuronal discharge pattern. For example, if an electrode is placed in the visual cortex and stimuli are delivered to each eye, we find that some neurons respond to bars of light that are vertically oriented whereas others are driven best by horizontal bars. The neurophysiologist would call this "orientation selectivity," and such response properties usually find their way into theories on the neural basis of visual perception. Therefore, single neuron recordings can provide an extremely sensitive measure of whether the correct synaptic connections have been established during development.

Of course, it would be most compelling to record neural activity while the animal is actually processing a stimulus or moving a limb. In an early approach, animals were injected with a tritium-labeled sugar molecule, [^{3}H]-2-deoxyglucose, that was taken up by active nerve cells (Kennedy *et al.*, 1975). It is now possible to measure neural activity and behavior simultaneously using several different techniques. Electrodes can be permanently mounted in the nervous system during an initial surgery, and these electrodes are then used to monitor neural activity when the animal recovers. Arrays of such electrodes are used to record from the hippocampus of freely moving rats as they explore their environment and learn new tasks. It is also possible to stimulate or inactivate a region of the brain in awake

muscles also contributes, and its blockade somehow prevents monocular deprivation from altering synaptic connections in the cortex.

Given the great complexity of cortex circuitry, it would be nice to have a simpler model system for synaptic plasticity. As we learned in the last chapter, the neuromuscular junction is the most accessible and well-studied of all synapses, and it has served as the mascot of synaptic plasticity studies for decades. In mammals, there is only a single type of synapse on fast muscle fibers, and only a single fiber ends up innervating each muscle cell in adults (above). If that were not good enough, it is also extremely easy

to record intracellularly from muscle cells, to manipulate the nerve or muscle cells, and to place the entire system in tissue culture. Of course, these advantages also serve as the limitations. For example, there are no inhibitory synapses and the postsynaptic cell does not have dendrites or spines, as found in many areas of the central nervous system.

Despite these differences, it is uncanny how much NMJ developmental plasticity resembles that found in the cortex. As we learned earlier, mammalian muscle cells are innervated by more than one axon at birth, but after synapse elimination only a single axon remains. When action

behaving animals, including humans, during the course of neurosurgical treatment, and to monitor the effects on motor function or sensory perception (Penfield and Rasmussen, 1950; Riquimaroux *et al.,* 1991).

There are now several ways to monitor brain activity in awake animals, particularly in humans, that can be performed without exposing the brain. While these techniques have not been applied widely to developing animals, they will probably play an important role in our future understanding of plasticity. One technique that offers 1 mm of spacial resolution, called function magnetic resonance imaging (fMRI), uses a very strong magnetic field (15,000 times the earth's magnetic field) to detect oxygen content. Since deoxyhemoglobin is paramagnetic relative to oxyhemoglobin and surrounding brain tissue, brain activity commonly produces a local increase in oxygen delivery. For example, it has recently been possible to visualize activity in a single barrel field in rat somatosensory cortex (Yang *et al.,* 1996). Another technique, magnetoencephalography (MEG), uses superconducting detectors to monitor the magnetic fields produced by a population of active neurons. This technique provides information about the timing, the location, and the magnitude of neural activity. For example, word-specific responses in the inferior temporooccipital cortex are slow or absent in dyslexic individuals compared to control subjects, suggesting a specific neural impairment in this developmental disorder (Salmelin *et al.,* 1996). Finally, there are changes in light absorbance that are well-correlated with neuronal activity, and it is possible to illuminate the surface of the brain and measure the reflected light while the system is processing information, referred to as differential optical imaging. Using these signals, many features of visual cortex development have been observed, including ocular dominance orientation selectivity (Blasdel *et al.,* 1995).

Obviously, the challenge to find causality between brain function and behavior is magnified during development when nonspecific behavioral factors (cf. level of arousal) and the fragility of nerve cell function (cf. rapid fatigue) introduce great restraints. However, the study of immature brains, and the behaviors that they manufacture, should prove useful because it allows one to correlate change in brain and behavior without imposing surgery, drugs, or bad genes on the nervous system.

potentials are blocked with TTX during the normal period of synapse elimination, muscle cells remain polyneuronally innervated (Fig. 9.12) (Thompson *et al.,* 1979). The same kind of results are obtained in the developing cat visual pathway, where TTX delays or blocks the segregation of retinal afferents in eye-specific layers of the LGN and also the segregation of LGN afferents in the cortex.

If too many synapses remain when activity is blocked, then we would predict that extra activity could speed up the process of synapse elimination. In fact, direct electrical stimulation of the *muscle* induces the loss of motor synapses

(Fig. 9.13). This result is particularly intriguing because it suggests that *postsynaptic* electrical activity can determine whether presynaptic terminals survive (O'Brien *et al.,* 1978). Together, these experiments show that synaptic transmission is necessary for the occurrence of synapse elimination at the developing NMJ. In fact, plasticity at the NMJ is a lifelong affair. Adult motor terminals will sprout to innervate adjacent muscle cells when neuromuscular transmission is blocked, and this polyneuronal innervation can be reduced when the muscle cells are stimulated directly (Jansen *et al.,* 1973; Holland and Brown, 1980).

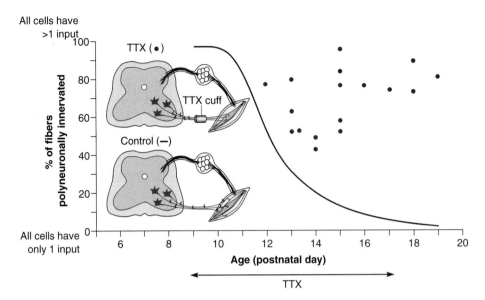

Figure 9.12 Decreased activity prevents synapse elimination. At the rat nerve–muscle junction, polyneuronal innervation declines between 10 and 15 days postnatal (line). When a TTX cuff was placed around the motor nerve root from Postnatal Day 9 to 19, and action potentials were eliminated, polyneuronal innervation remained high (red circles). (Adapted from Thompson *et al.,* 1979, with permission.)

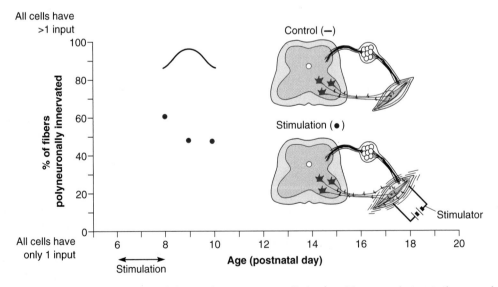

Figure 9.13 Increased muscle activity accelerates synapse elimination. Most rat soleus muscles are polyneuronally innervated between Postnatal Days 8 and 10 (line). When a stimulating electrode was implanted in the leg to activate the sciatic nerve and muscle from Postnatal Days 6–8, there was a severe decline in the number of polyneuronally innervated muscle cells (red circles). (Adapted from O'Brien *et al.,* 1978, with permission.)

Sensory Coding Properties Reflect Synapse Rearrangement

If synapse strength and elimination really depend on neural activity, then we might expect sensory coding properties to be influenced by the pattern of environmental stimulation during development (see Box: Watching Neurons Think). In fact, there are many examples of animals being raised in an altered sensory environment, that influences neuronal function. However, it is difficult to figure out what kind of neural activity pattern is produced by a given sensory environment. Nevertheless, this issue has been addressed successfully by two experiments in the central auditory system, one using sound stimulation and the other using electrical stimulation of the cochlea. Central auditory neurons usually respond to a limited range of frequencies because the auditory nerve fibers from the cochlea project topographically in the central nervous system (Chapter 6). A range of sound frequencies plotted against the sound intensities at which each frequency evokes a threshold response from a neuron, called a frequency tuning curve, provides a good measure of afferent innervation. When many areas of the cochlea project to a central neuron, then its frequency tuning curve is broad. When only a small region of the cochlea projects to a neuron, then its frequency tuning curve is narrow.

To test whether the temporal pattern of neural activity influences the development of frequency tuning, mice were reared in a sound environment consisting of repetitive clicks for a few weeks (Sanes and Constantine-Paton, 1985). This type of sound evokes synchronous activity in a large population of cochlear nerve axons. When frequency tuning curves are obtained from the inferior colliculus of normal mice and those reared in repetitive clicks, the latter group has significantly broader curves (Fig. 9.14). Therefore, when afferents all have the identical pattern of activity, they are apparently unable to segregate properly along the frequency axis.

A similar type of finding is obtained in cats that are deafened by damaging the inner hair cells. In this case, the dendritic endings of the cochlear neurons can be stimulated directly with an electrode that is implanted in the cochlea. In fact, human beings with profound hearing loss are now implanted with such cochlear prostheses, and these experiments were motivated by a desire to improve this technology (Snyder *et al.*, 1990). Animals are reared with repetitive electrical pulses to their cochlea, thus providing an activity pattern that is similar to that evoked by repetitive clicks in hearing animals. Since the animals are deaf, it is not possible to record frequency tuning curves. Therefore, a single position along the cochlea is stimulated electrically while an electrode is lowered through the inferior colliculus. In normal animals, a single point on the cochlea evokes a response within a limited region of tissue, referred to as a spacial tuning curve. In deafened stimulated animals, the spatial tuning curves are much broader, as if a single position in the cochlea now projects to a much wider area of the tonotopic map in the inferior colliculus (Fig. 9.14). Together, these two experiments support the idea that coactive synapses establish strong connections.

In the visual system, many cortical neurons respond to stimuli of a specific orientation or to stimuli that are moving in a specific direction. Several investigators have asked whether visually evoked synaptic activity influences the maturation of these complex response properties, although the actual activity pattern is unknown (Blakemore and Cooper, 1970; Cynader *et al.*, 1973). When kittens are reared in a visual environment consisting entirely of vertical or horizontal stripes, and neurons are subsequently recorded in the cortex, the majority of them respond selectively to the orientation that is present in the rearing environment (Fig. 9.15). To determine whether moving visual stimuli also influence the development of motion selectivity, kittens have been raised in stroboscopic light. As nightclub enthusiasts know, this stimulus permits one to see a full range of shapes and colors, but it eliminates smooth motion. When cortical neurons are recorded after a period of strobe-rearing, the majority can no longer respond

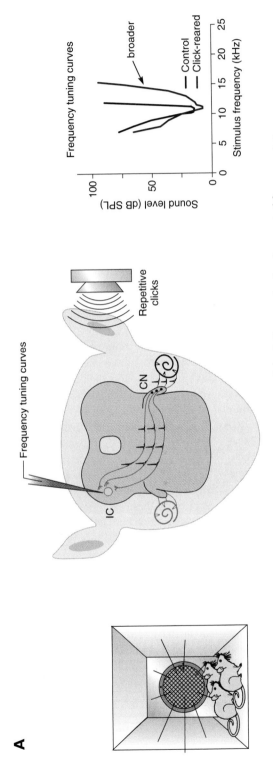

Figure 9.14 The temporal pattern of auditory nerve activity influences the development of frequency tuning. (A) Mice were reared with repetitive clicks that synchronized the activity of many auditory nerve fibers. Recordings were then obtained from single neurons in the inferior colliculus (IC), and frequency tuning curves were obtained from each one. As shown in the graph, neurons from click-reared mice were more broadly tuned (red), compared to those from controls (black). (B) Kittens were deafened by eliminating the cochlear hair cells, but leaving the auditory nerve fibers. A stimulating electrode was inserted in one ear, and repetitive electrical pulses were delivered to synchronize the activity of many auditory nerve fibers for about 3 months. To test for specificity, a single tonotopic position in the cochlea was stimulated while a recording electrode was advanced along the tonotopic axis of IC. As shown in the graph, a position in the cochlea activated a broader range of tissue in pulse-reared cats (red) than in controls (black). (Adapted from Sanes and Constantine-Paton, 1985; Snyder *et al.*, 1990.)

372

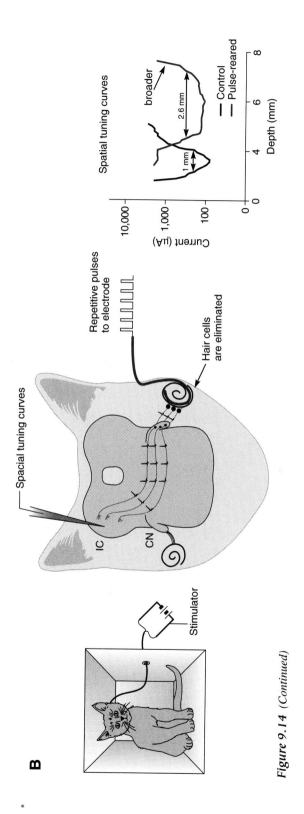

Figure 9.14 (Continued)

373

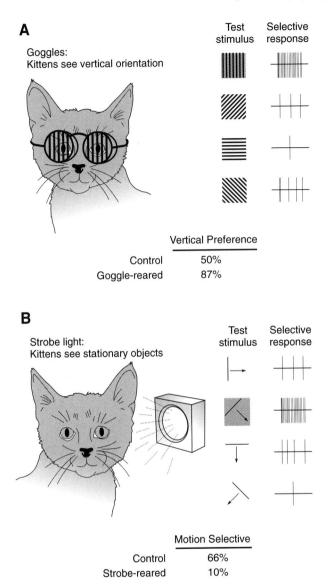

Figure 9.15 The visual environment influences orientation and motion processing. (A) Kittens were reared with goggles that permitted visual experience with only vertically oriented stimuli. The response to oriented stimuli was then obtained from single visual cortex neurons. The cell shown responds best to vertical stimuli (red). In goggle-reared cats, 87% of neurons were selective for vertical stimuli, compared to only 50% in controls. (B) Kittens were reared in stoboscopic light that permitted visual experience with only stationary objects. The response to moving stimuli was then obtained from single visual cortex neurons. The cell shown responds best to stimuli moving down and to the right (red). In strobe-reared cats, only 10% of neurons were motion selective, compared to 66% in controls. (Adapted from Stryker *et al.,* 1978; Pasternak *et al.,* 1985.)

selectively to the direction of movement (Fig. 9.15). These results, and many others like them, show that environmental stimuli influence a broad range of functional properties. Therefore, the presence or the strength of synapses is modified by experience.

Activity Contributes to the Alignment of Sensory Maps

When peripheral sensory axons reach the central nervous system, they usually innervate the target in an orderly manner, forming topographic maps. These sensory maps are quite accurate from the outset, and the precision is partly due to molecular gradients that direct axons to an approximate location within the target (see Chapter 6). However, synaptic activity also influences the development of topographic projections. This is particularly evident when two maps form in the same structure, and they must become aligned with one another. For example, neurons in the frog optic tectum are binocular, and they respond to the same visual position in space when activated through either eye. We have already studied the direct contralateral projection from retina to tectum in Chapter 6. The ipsilateral eye can also activate the tectum via an indirect projection. Tectal neurons project to a structure called the nucleus isthmus, and isthmal neurons project to the contralateral tectal lobe (Fig. 9.16A). Therefore, there are two maps of visual space in the tectum, one from the contralateral eye and one from the ipsilateral eye, and they are perfectly aligned. That is, a point in visual space activates a single position in the tectum via either eye.

To test whether visual activity plays a role in this precise alignment, animals were reared in the dark. The interesting result is that direct retinal projections from the contralateral eye continue to form a precise map, but the indirect projection via the nucleus isthmus is poorly organized (Keating and Feldman, 1975). That is, one map appears to form somewhat independent of activity, while the other map depends on it. The effect is so powerful that one can actually cause isthmal axons to move to a new location in the tectum when the contralateral map is disrupted. When the contralateral eye is rotated by 180° (Fig. 9.16B) a single point in space will activate different positions in the tectum via each eye. If this manipulation is done while the animals are still tadpoles, the isthmal projection to the tectum will shift so that the ipsilateral retinal map comes into register with the direct contralateral projection (Fig. 9.16C). Thus, isthmotectal axons can be induced to innervate a part of the tectum that they would not ordinarily contact (Udin and Keating, 1981).

In some cases, maps from two different sensory systems are found in the same structure and must also come into alignment during development. In the optic tectum of barn owls, there are maps of both the visual and the auditory world. The maps are aligned such that neurons respond to sound and light stimuli from the same position in space (Fig. 9.17). For example, neurons that respond to visual stimuli directly in front of the animal (0°) will also respond to sound that arrives at each ear simultaneously (0 μs interaural time difference). Neurons that respond to visual stimuli at 20° to the right will also respond to a sound stimulus that arrives first at the right ear and then at the left (40 μs interaural time difference). Does the alignment of these maps also depend on neural activity? To test this idea, owls were reared with prismatic glasses that displace visual stimuli by 23°. As in the retinotectal system, the physical connections between eye and tectum remained constant in prism-reared animals. If no compensation occurred, then visual stimuli and auditory stimuli from the same position in space would activate different positions in the tectum. That is, maps of auditory space and visual space would be out of alignment (Fig. 9.17). In fact, the auditory map adjusts to remain in register with the visual map. When the prisms are removed, tectal neurons that respond to visual stimuli directly in front of the animal (0°) are now found to respond to an auditory stimulus to one side (40 μs

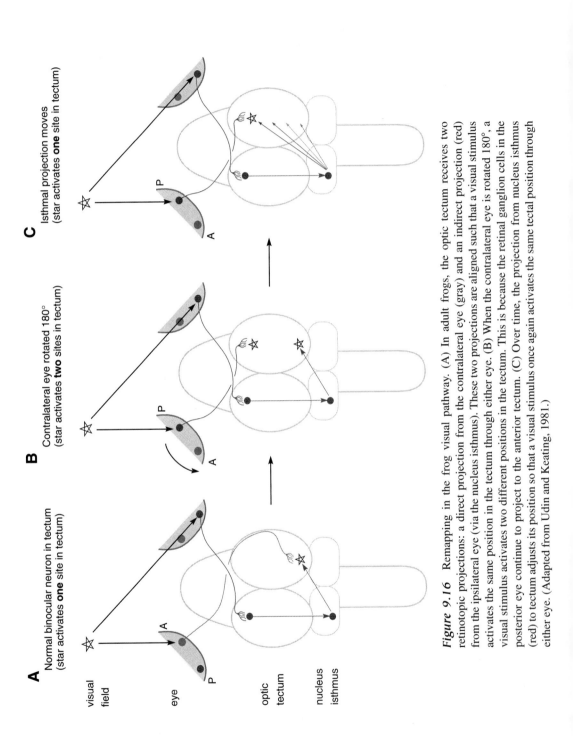

Figure 9.16 Remapping in the frog visual pathway. (A) In adult frogs, the optic tectum receives two retinotopic projections: a direct projection from the contralateral eye (gray) and an indirect projection (red) from the ipsilateral eye (via the nucleus isthmus). These two projections are aligned such that a visual stimulus activates the same position in the tectum through either eye. (B) When the contralateral eye is rotated 180°, a visual stimulus activates two different positions in the tectum. This is because the retinal ganglion cells in the posterior eye continue to project to the anterior tectum. (C) Over time, the projection from nucleus isthmus (red) to tectum adjusts its position so that a visual stimulus once again activates the same tectal position through either eye. (Adapted from Udin and Keating, 1981.)

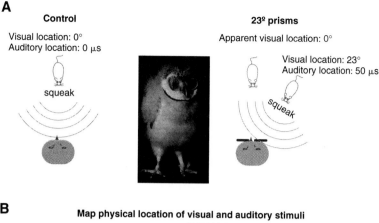

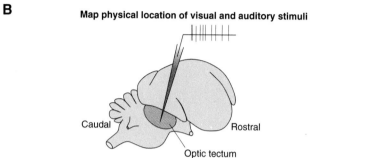

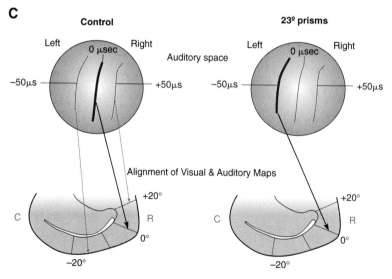

Figure 9.17 Remapping in the owl auditory pathway. (A) Barn owls were reared with prismatic goggles that shifted the visual field by 23°. In control animals, a squeaking mouse in front of the owl would appear 0° and the sound would reach both ears simultaneously (0 μs interaural time difference). With prisms in place, a squeaking mouse at 23° to the right would *appear* at 0°, and the squeak would reach the right ear first (50 μs interaural time difference). (B) Recordings from single neurons were made in the optic tectum, a structure that contains an auditory and visual map of space. (C) In control animals, the visual and auditory maps are well aligned. For example, visual stimuli at 0° and sound stimuli with a 0 μs time difference (corresponding to the midline in auditory space) map to the same position in the optic tectum (left, thick arrow). When the prisms were removed from experimental animals, the visual map was unchanged: visual stimuli at 0° still mapped to their original position in the tectum. However, the auditory map was reorganized: sound stimuli with a −40 μs time difference now mapped to the visual midline (right, thick arrow). Thus, the auditory map had compensated during prism rearing. (Adapted from Brainard and Knudsen, 1993 with permission.)

interaural time difference). Therefore, auditory connections change in response to visual activity (Brainard and Knudsen, 1993).

Spontaneous Activity and Afferent Segregation

When, exactly, do sensory coding properties reach maturity in normal animals? Orientation and motion selectivity mature rapidly from the onset of sight, and it is possible that normal neuronal activity simply maintains a precise but unstable set of connections (Blakemore and Van Sluyters, 1975). Alternatively, it is possible that the innervation patterns that underlie these coding properties do not attain their mature pattern without the proper stimulation. In simpler terms,

when does activity begin to influence neural development?

The answer to this question led down an unexpected path. Electrical activity is present in the nervous system even in the absence of visual or auditory stimulation, and this "spontaneous" activity has a profound influence on synapse formation and elimination. We previously learned that ocular dominance columns form in binocularly deprived cats. To test whether spontaneous retinal activity might be responsible for the segregation of thalamic afferents in the cortex, retinal activity was completely eliminated by injecting both eyes with TTX from about 2–6 weeks postnatal (Fig. 9.18). In TTX-reared cats, the LGN afferents fail to segregate into stripes in layer IV of the cortex (Stryker and Harris, 1986). Spontaneous activity may also play a role in the elimination of small retinal afferent side-

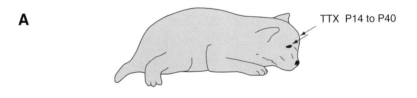

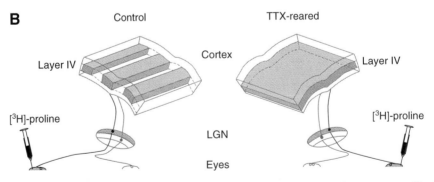

Figure 9.18 Spontaneous retinal activity regulates the formation of stripes. (A) Cats were reared in the dark, and [³H]-proline was injected into one eye to visualize ocular dominance columns. Although the columns were slightly degraded, they did form. (B) Bilateral intraocular TTX injections were performed beginning at Postnatal Day 14. When [³H]-proline was injected into one eye to visualize ocular dominance columns, it was found that segregation of geniculate afferents into stripes failed to occur. Thus, spontaneous retinal activity is sufficient to influence stripe formation. (Adapted from Stryker and Harris, 1986.)

branches in the inappropriate layer of LGN (see Fig. 9.6).

Since spontaneous activity can influence development, we should be able to record the amount that is present. For example, retinal ganglion cells fire action potentials before the system is activated by light. In the embryonic rat, single retinal neurons discharge about once every second, but occasionally fire short bursts of almost 100/s (Galli and Maffei, 1988). However, all of the work on environmental stimulation suggests that the pattern of activity is necessary for the modification or elimination of synapses (above). Is it possible that spontaneous activity has a temporal pattern? To address this question, the entire retina was isolated from an embryo and placed in a perfused recording chamber, where it is possible to record from many retinal ganglion cells at the same time (Fig. 9.19). Synchronous bursts of action potentials are recorded from many neurons about every minute or two, and regions of maximal activity move slowly across the retina (Meister *et al.,* 1991). Of course, the spontaneous action potentials in the retina would be of little value unless they elicit synaptic activity in the LGN (Fig. 9.19). In preparations containing both retina and thalamus, bursts of spontaneous excitatory currents are recorded from LGN neurons, and these bursts occur at the same frequency as retinal action potentials (Mooney *et al.,* 1996). Spontaneous action potentials have also been observed in the developing auditory system and the spinal cord, where bursting patterns of activity also seem to exist (Lippe, 1994; O'Donovan *et al.,* 1994; Kotak and Sanes, 1995). In the chick cochlear nucleus, a periodic waxing and waning of activity can be eliminated if the cochlea is removed, suggesting that spontaneous activity originates in the sensory epithelium, similar to the visual system.

While spontaneous activity may play a roll in synaptogenesis, it is also likely to influence synaptic maturation per se and the normal expression of various postsynaptic proteins. In Chapter 7, we learned that decreased synaptic activity leads to a rapid decline in postsynaptic protein synthesis. In fact, electrical activity can have a profound effect on the expression of neurotrophins and their receptors, molecules that could influence sprouting and synaptogenesis (see Chapter 7). Therefore, the presence of spontaneous electrical activity during early development may have a general effect on neuron growth and survival.

Some Forms of Plasticity Have a Time Limit

Synaptic activity begins to exert an influence soon after synaptogenesis, but how long does this process continue? If we embrace learning and memory in our definition, then it lasts for our entire lifetime (see Box: Remaining Flexible). However, there are certain significant changes in nervous system structure and function that occur most readily during a limited period of development. A common example is language acquisition, which is accomplished easily before age 10 and becomes a grueling task for most of us when attempted as adults (see Chapter 10). At least some forms of neuronal plasticity only last for a limited period during developmental, often called a critical period. The influence of visual experience on ocular dominance has been explored in older animals to determine whether cortical neuron function is always dependent on vision (Hubel and Wiesel, 1970). Ocular dominance is most susceptible to monocular deprivation after several weeks of sight. The visual environment influences cortical neuron function for roughly the first 3 months of life in cats, but this critical period does not apply to connections forming throughout the brain.

The term critical period is a very general expression, and the neuronal property under discussion should always be taken into account. In primates, monocular deprivation affects the segregation of LGN afferents in layer IV for about 2–3 months, but continues to produce severe weakening of intrinsic cortical synapses for up to a year (Fig. 9.20). Similarly, when retinal activity is blocked with TTX after ganglion cell arbors have segregated into eye-specific layers in the

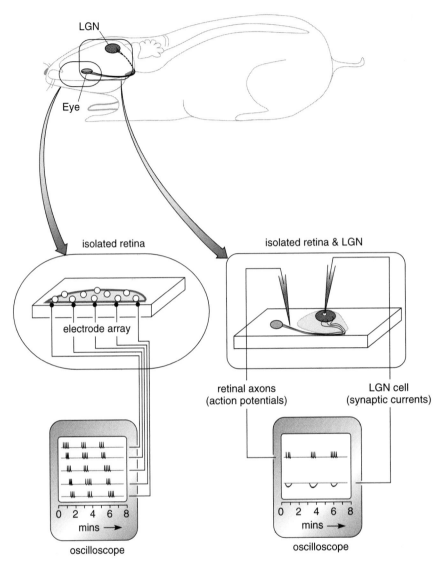

Figure 9.19   Spontaneous activity in the developing visual pathway. Explants of the retina (left) or the entire retinogeniculate pathway (right) were obtained from neonatal ferets. (Left) An array of electrodes was used to record bursts of activity from many retinal locations at the same time. These bursts of activity moved across the retina, as shown by the increasing response latency in each oscilloscope trace. (Right) Simultaneous recordings were made from retinal fibers and LGN neurons to show that bursts of presynaptic action potentials elicited long-lasting postsynaptic responses. (Adapted from Meister *et al.*, 1991; Mooney *et al.*, 1996.)

cat LGN, the response properties of LGN neurons are nonetheless altered (Dubin *et al.*, 1986). Therefore, activity-dependent mechanisms seem to be doing more than correcting a few minor errors of innervation. Even adult cortex can exhibit changes following deprivation. For example, monocular action potential blockade with TTX results in a decreased expression of GABAA receptor subunits in layer IV of primate cortex (Hendry *et al.*, 1994).

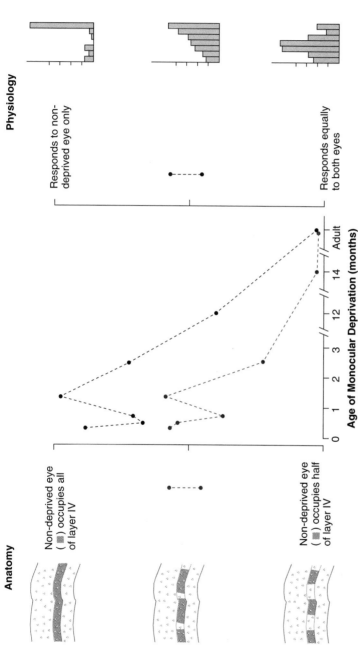

Figure 9.20 The effects of monocular deprivation are age dependent. One eye was sutured shut in macaque monkeys at different postnatal ages. The sutures were removed after several months and ocular dominance columns were examined with anatomical (left) and electrophysiological techniques (right). When deprivation began between 0 and 2 months of age, most neurons subsequently responded to the open eye only, and the open eye occupied much more of layer IV (red). After 3 months, the effects of deprivation declined with age. The effect of deprivation on ocular dominance columns seemed to decline more rapidly than the effect on ocular dominance histograms. (Adapted from LeVay et al., *J. Comp. Neurol.* **191:** 1–51, Copyright 1980. By permission of Wiley–Liss, Inc., a subsidiary of John Wiley & Sons, Inc.)

Cellular Events during Synapse Elimination

How does synaptic transmission regulate the strength or stability of neural connections? Studies of the molecular basis of developmental plasticity and adult learning have enjoyed a symbiotic relationship in recent years (see Box: Remaining Flexible). The modification of synapse function involves both pre- and postsynaptic signaling mechanisms, and the neurotransmitter itself is likely to initiate the biochemical cascade. But is it really possible that there is a single mechanism to account for synaptic plasticity? After all, most central neurons are innervated by a wide variety of synapses: some release glutamate, others GABA, still others release a neuromodulator such as serotonin. Moreover, a single glutamate-releasing synapse can activate receptors that open ion channels (cf. ionotropic) and others that activate second messenger systems (cf. metabotropic). Generalizations the cover the function of all these systems are clearly in short supply. Therefore, we focus on a few synapses that have been studied thoroughly, such as the nerve–muscle junction.

As we saw earlier, synapses fail to be eliminated when activity is blocked at the nerve–muscle junction. In fact, synapses capable of function can form in the absence of synaptic transmission (Cohen, 1972; Duxson, 1982). Presynaptic terminals are even able to differentiate in a zebrafish mutant lacking functional AChR clusters (Westerfield et al., 1990). In contrast, most sensory deprivation studies suggest that disuse of a synapse can lead to its weakening or elimination, especially if other synapses are active. When all terminals have equivalent activity levels, such as a nerve–muscle culture grown in the presence of curare, then many aspects of functional maturation continue. However, when terminals differ in their levels of activity, then synaptic transmission is pivotal to the maturation of synaptic efficacy. In the jargon of the field, synaptic terminals "compete" for the distinction of activating the postsynaptic neuron, and "stable" connections depend, in part, upon an active transmitter–receptor system. Therefore, the presence of synaptic transmission is not an absolute requirement for the initial formation of a synapse, but influences its subsequent development and stability.

Synapses Interact over a Short Distance

Synaptic terminals can influence neighboring contacts on the same postsynaptic cell, but only within a finite distance. When two motor nerves are grafted onto the same muscle in adult rats, both of them are able to maintain functional contacts over several months, even though muscles are normally innervated by a single axon. The trick is to place the two motor terminals at least several millimeters from one another (Kuffler et al., 1977). If the terminals are placed within a millimeter or two, then one of the contacts is eliminated within about 3 weeks (Fig. 9.21). In fact, some animals have muscle fibers that are normally innervated by more than one motor axon. In one polyneuronally innervated muscle in chicks, the distance between terminals can be reduced when synaptic transmission is blocked, presumably because competition between active terminals normally keeps them separated (Gordon et al., 1974).

The terminal endings from a single axonal arbor seem to innervate a continuous region of the postsynaptic cell, whether it is a primary dendrite or a small area of muscle cell (Forehand and Purves, 1984; Glanzman et al., 1991). For example, when sensory neurons from the sea slug *Aplysia* are grown in culture along with a common target motor neuron, their terminals come to occupy separate regions of the postsynaptic cell (Fig. 9.22). However, if the two sensory neurons are grown without a target, then they grow extensively along one another. That is, the sensory neurons are not simply exhibiting contact inhibition (see Chapter 4). Therefore, the antagonistic relationship between synapses must somehow be mediated by the postsynaptic neuron. Even if we know the amount and pattern of

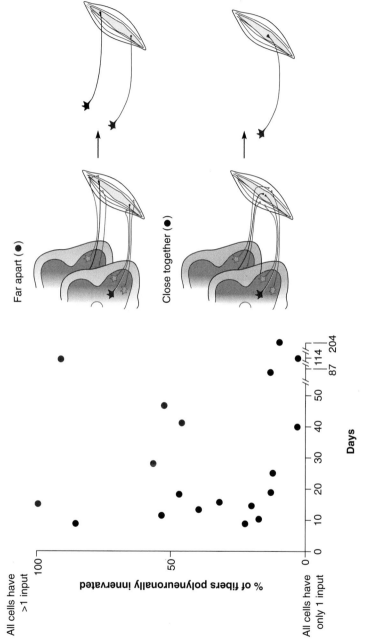

Figure 9.21 Synapse elimination depends on synapse distance. Two motor axons were positioned on the same muscle, either close to one another or at a distance. Intracellular recordings were made from muscle fibers to monitor polyneuronal innervation, as shown in Fig. 9.2. When the synapses were close together (black circles), synaptic elimination occurred within a few weeks. When the synapses were far apart (red circles), synaptic elimination failed to occur. (Adapted from *Brain Res.* **138**, Kuffler *et al.*, The elimination of synapses in multiply–innervated skeletal muscle fibers of the rat: dependence on distance between end plates, pp. 353–358, Copyright 1977 with permission from Elsevier Science.)

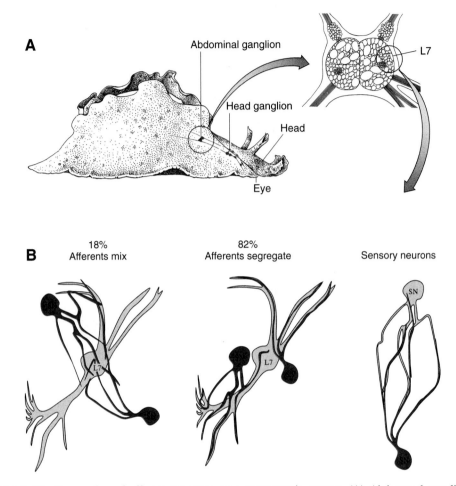

Figure 9.22 Segregation of afferent processes on a postsynaptic neuron. (A) Abdomenal ganglia were obtained from *Aplysia,* and sensory (SN) and motor (L7) neurons were placed in culture. (B) When two SN neurons (red) arborized on an L7 neuron (gray), the SN arbors intermingled in only 18% of the cases (left). In 82% of the cases, the SN neurons formed arbors on different L7 dendrites (middle). As a control, two SN neurons were grown together and formed arborizations on one another. (Adapted from Glanzman *et al.,* 1991.)

synaptic activity in a set of inputs, this may not be enough to predict whether one synapse will dislodge a second one. One must also know the spacial arrangement of these terminals.

Effect of Disuse

What is the evidence that synaptic strength decreases following a period of disuse? Surprisingly, there have been few direct measures of PSP amplitude after deprivation or denervation. John Eccles, who shared the 1970 Nobel prize for his work on synaptic transmission, provided the first test of synaptic strength following a period of disuse (Eccles *et al.,* 1959). It was possible to inactivate some of the sensory synapses onto spinal cord motor neurons by cutting their peripheral connection to the muscle. The sensory neurons do not die under these conditions, but they are no longer activated when the muscle contracts, and their central synapses are silenced.

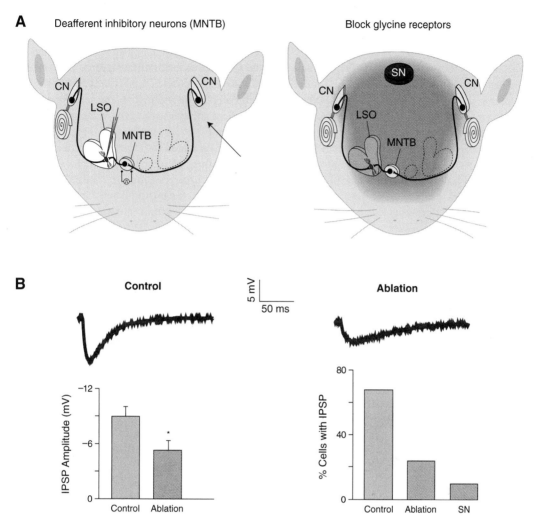

Figure 9.23 Disuse leads to weaker synapses. (A) During development, the activity of an inhibitory projection, from the MNTB to the LSO, was decreased in two ways. First, the MNTB neurons were functionally denervated (left) by removing the contralateral ear (arrow). Second, animals were reared with an agent (right), strychnine (SN), that blocked the inhibitory glycine receptors. (B) Within a few days, the inhibitory postsynaptic potentials (IPSPs) recorded in LSO were much reduced compared to controls (left). In fact, fewer LSO cells exhibited MNTB-evoked IPSPs following disuse (right). (Adapted from Kotak and Sanes, 1996 with permission.)

Intracellular recordings from motor neurons show that the inactivated sensory synapses are roughly half as strong as unmanipulated inputs, but this reduction in efficacy takes nearly 10 days to occur.

A much faster reduction in synaptic efficacy was observed in a developmental study. In the central auditory system, disuse of either inhibitory or excitatory synapses for as little as 1 day can decrease their strength (Kotak and Sanes, 1996, 1997). For example, a group of glycinergic synapses can be inactivated either by surgical removal of one cochlea or with the glycine receptor antagonist strychnine. The strength of synaptic transmission is then measured with whole-cell recordings using an acute brain slice preparation (Fig. 9.23). In normal animals, electrical stimulation of the glycinergic neurons produces large inhibitory postsynaptic potentials (IPSPs), but following a short period of disuse the IPSPs are small or absent. Similarly, denervation of glutamatergic afferents produces a reduction in evoked excitatory postsynaptic potentials (EPSPs). One problem with these studies is that several afferents innervate each postsynaptic cell, and a change in strength could reflect either a loss of some afferents, a decrease in the strength of each input without elimination, or a combination of both processes. To test whether the strength of single inputs is decreased, the stimulus level is adjusted to evoke the smallest unitary response, presumably due to a single axon. The size of these minimum synaptic responses is also smaller in denervated cells than in controls, suggesting that the strength of individual connections is weakened by disuse.

Disuse also affects the total number of connections that are made in the central nervous system. One region of rodent somatosensory cortex receives afferents from each of the facial whiskers and contains an array of barrel-shaped cell clusters that are activated selectively by each of the whiskers (Chapter 6). If the whiskers are destroyed before Postnatal Day 5, their associated barrels do not form, but if the whiskers are destroyed after that time then the manipulation has no effect (Van der Loos and Woolsey, 1973). There are also extensive intracortical connections between each of the whisker barrels, and this connectivity is dependent on continued use. When the sensory nerve to the whiskers is cut on Postnatal Day 7, after the barrel fields are formed, there is a dramatic reduction in the number of local projections (McCasland *et al.*, 1992).

Heterosynaptic Depression

Disuse of established synapses seems to impair their performance, yet we have also seen that the activity of a neighboring synapse can be even more harmful. This mechanism was tested at an unusual muscle in the rat foot, called the lumbrical muscle, which receives its innervation via two separate peripheral nerves (Fig. 9.24). It

is possible to electrically stimulate one group of motor axons during the normal period of synapse elimination and find out what happens to the synapses of unstimulated axons. The strength of the nerve–muscle connection was determined indirectly by measuring the size of nerve-evoked muscle contractions, where a larger contraction signifies a stronger connection. When one nerve is stimulated for about 6 days, the *unstimulated* axons are much less effective at producing a muscle contraction (Ridge and Betz, 1984). That is, the unstimulated axons are apparently eliminated from the muscle in disproportionate numbers, or the synapses become weaker than normal.

How long does it take for one synapse to destabilize its neighbor? The onset of synapse elimination was studied using a very simple culture system that contained two presynaptic neurons and one postsynaptic cell, a myocyte (Fig. 9.25). Whole-cell recordings were made from the myocyte while the activity of one or both presynaptic neurons was controlled with stimulating electrodes. In the first experiment, the synaptic currents elicited by each neuron were measured, and then one of the neurons was stimulated for several seconds. Within moments of this brief procedure, the unstimulated neuron produces much smaller synaptic currents, and the effect lasts for the duration of the experiment (Lo and Poo, 1991). When one synapse is able to modify the operation of a second one, the interaction is referred to as heterosynaptic.

Two additional observations seem to fit neatly into the puzzle. First, if the two synapses are separated from one another by >50 μm, then activation of one synapse is not able to suppress its neighbor. Two synapses can apparently compete for the right to activate a postsynaptic cell, but the interaction occurs over a very short distance, consistent with results from the adult NMJ and *Aplysia* cultures (Kuffler *et al.*, 1977; Glanzman *et al.*, 1991). Second, when both neurons are stimulated at the same time, there is no change in the strength of either synapse. That is, synaptic activity is able to *protect* a synapse from the ill effects of a noisy neighbor.

Synaptic terminals do not fight each other directly, but carry on their competition through

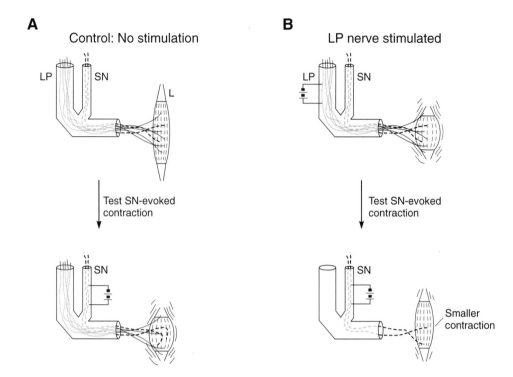

A Control: No stimulation

B LP nerve stimulated

Test SN-evoked contraction

Test SN-evoked contraction

Smaller contraction

Figure 9.24 Synaptic activity depresses less active inputs. The lumbrical muscle (L) in the rat foot is innervated by two physically separate motor nerve roots, LP and SN. (A) In control animals, the SN-evoked contraction of the lumbrical muscle is robust (bottom). (B) If the LP motor nerve root is repetitively stimulated during development, then the SN nerve root stimulation elicits a much weaker contraction of the lumbrical muscle. (Adapted from Ridge and Betz, 1984.)

an independent agent, the postsynaptic cell. It is a bit like choosing the winner of a boxing match by determining who punches the referee harder. The contribution of the postsynaptic cell to heterosynaptic depression can be demonstrated by activating it directly. When the muscle cell is activated with a puff of ACh from the tip of a pipet, then the size of synaptic responses declines by about 50% (Dan and Poo, 1992).

Of course, this begs the question of whether a depressed synapse is necessarily an eliminated synapse. Further, we have already learned that the rate of synapse elimination *in vivo* does not occur within minutes, but over a period of days. If synaptic depression really is the first hint of a retreating connection, then one might expect to record a synaptic response that gradually becomes smaller during development. This can be observed at the mammalian NMJ by measuring

the average number of ACh packets that are released by each synapse, called the quantal content (Fig. 9.26). Even at birth, one synapse is about twice as strong as the second, but over the next week one of the synapses becomes about four times stronger than the other (Colman *et al.,* 1997). That is, it releases four times as much transmitter. Therefore, the strength of one synapse apparently decreases with time, and it seems logical that it must be the one that is eventually eliminated.

Postsynaptic Receptors Are Eliminated

The postsynaptic cell probably plays an active role in causing extra synapses to withdraw.

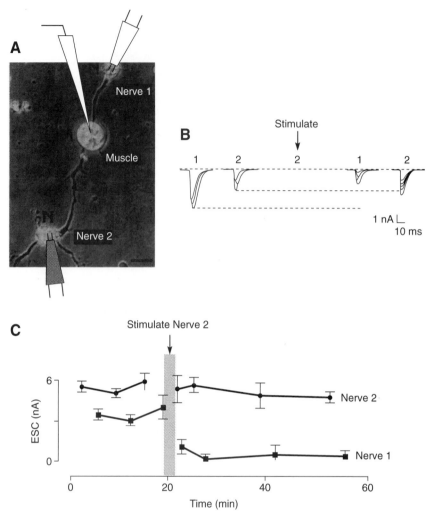

Figure 9.25 Heterosynaptic depression at the nerve–muscle synapse *in vitro*. (A) Whole-cell recordings were made from *Xenopus* muscle cells that were coinnervated by two neurons. (B) Evoked synaptic currents (ESCs) were measured in response to stimulation of each nerve. A strong stimulus was then applied to nerve 2, and the strength of each nerve was tested again. This procedure led to smaller evoked EPSCs from unstimulated nerve, but no change in nerve 2. (C) The graph of ESC amplitude before and after stimulation of nerve 2 shows that depression of the nerve 1-evoked response was long lasting. (Adapted from Lo and Poo, 1991.)

At the NMJ, postsynaptic AChR clusters are lost *before* nerve terminals withdraw from the muscle surface (Role *et al.,* 1987; Balice-Gordon and Lichtman, 1993). To demonstrate that the loss of AChRs is sufficient to produce synapse elimination, a small fraction of receptors was blocked by locally applying α-Btx. Over a number of days, the presynaptic terminal that is in contact with the inactivated region gradually withdraws (Balice-Gordon and Lichtman, 1994). However, it is critical that only a small fraction of neighboring receptors is blocked. If all the receptors are blocked, then the nerve terminal does not retract.

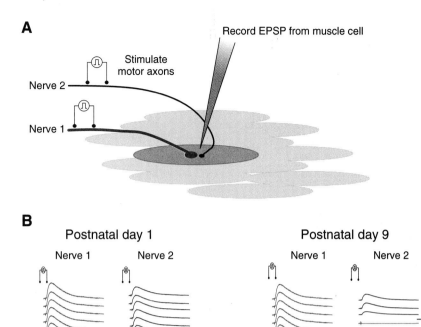

A

Record EPSP from muscle cell

Stimulate motor axons

Nerve 2

Nerve 1

B

Postnatal day 1   Postnatal day 9

Nerve 1   Nerve 2   Nerve 1   Nerve 2

Trials   Failures   Trials   Failures

40% failures   64% failures   16% failures   90% failures

Figure 9.26 Decrease in synaptic strength during the period of elimination. (A) Intracellular recordings were obtained from muscle cells and the response to stimulation of individual motor axons was obtained. (B) At Postnatal Day 1, stimulation of each motor axon demonstrated that one synapse was slightly stronger (red) than the other synapse (black). Stimulation of the weaker synapse produced more failures. At Postnatal Day 9, one of the synapses had become much stronger (red) than the other. (Adapted from Colman *et al.,* 1997.)

Involvement of Intracellular Calcium

Clearly, the presynaptic terminals are carrying on a rather hostile conversation through the postsynaptic cell, and there must be some molecular pathway that conveys the signal from one contact to another through the cytoplasm. One hypothesis is that depolarizing synaptic potentials open voltage-gated Ca^{2+} channels, and Ca^{2+}-dependent proteolytic enzymes are recruited to demolish the nonactive terminals, leading ul-

timately to their withdrawal (Fig. 9.27). A variety of proteolytic enzymes have been discovered in the nerve terminals and somata of developing neurons. This hypothesis was tested at the mammalian NMJ by decreasing extracellular Ca^{2+} or blocking specific Ca^{2+}-activated proteases, and both manipulations slow down the process of synapse elimination (Connold *et al.,* 1986).

Once again, there are important similarities between synapse elimination and heterosynaptic depression (above). First, it is possible to prevent heterosynaptic depression by injecting the

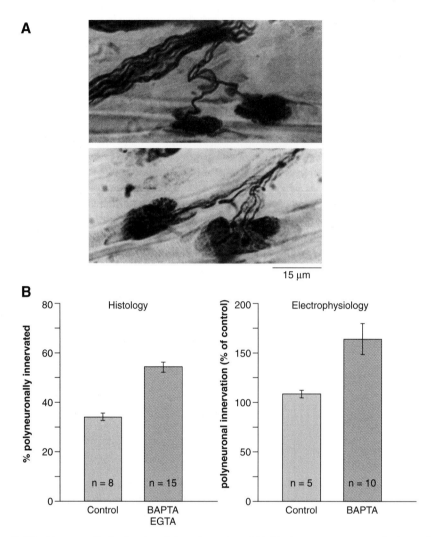

Figure 9.27 Synapse elimination is calcium dependent. (A) Single motor nerve terminals are found at the nerve–muscle junction (NMJ) of control rats (top), whereas the NMJ of BAPTA-treated animals was often multiply innervated (bottom). (B) Polyneuronal innervation was assessed by counting the number of silver-stained motor terminals per NMJ (left) and electrophysiologically (right) as described in Fig. 9.2. Both assays showed that calcium chelators prevented synapse elimination. (Adapted from *Dev. Brain Res.* **28,** Connold *et al.,* Effect of low calcium and protease inhibitors on synapse elimination during postnatal development in the rat soleus muscle, pp. 99–107, Copyright 1986, with permission from Elsevier Science.)

muscle cell with a Ca^{2+} chelator that sops up free Ca^{2+}, suggesting that a rise in postsynaptic calcium is necessary for depression to occur (Fig. 9.28). Second, it is possible to cause synaptic depression by momentarily raising postsynaptic calcium. This was accomplished by loading muscle cells with molecules of "caged" calcium, which can release the calcium into the cytoplasm when it is exposed to ultraviolet light. The synaptic responses at one muscle cell are recorded while a second neighboring muscle cell is exposed to a brief pulse of UV light, and synaptic transmission is depressed by 50% within seconds (Lo and Poo, 1994; Cash *et al.,* 1996).

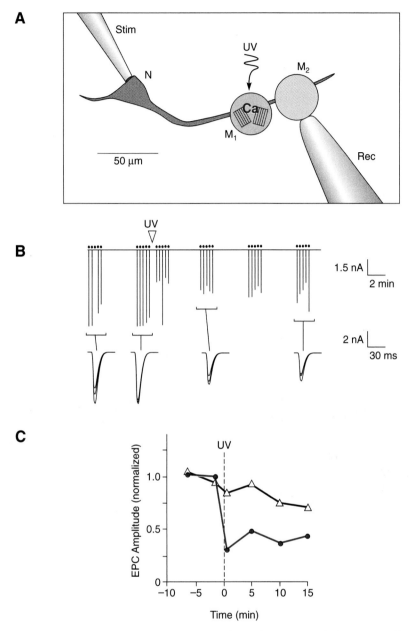

Figure 9.28 Synapse depression depends on postsynaptic calcium. (A) A whole-cell recording was made from an innervated myocyte (M_2) while the intracellular calcium was elevated in a second nearby myocyte (M_1). Calcium was elevated by first filling M_1 with caged calcium, and using UV light to release the calcium from its "cage." (B) Baseline nerve-evoked synaptic currents (downward deflections) were first recorded from M_2. When intracellular calcium was elevated in M_1 by exposure to UV light, the nerve-evoked synaptic currents became depressed within seconds. (C) Nerve-evoked synaptic currents in M_2 are plotted for control (open triangles, M_1 not loaded with caged calcium) and experimental (red circles, M_1 loaded with caged calcium) conditions. (Adapted from Cash *et al.*, 1996.)

Since synaptic activity leads to the depression and withdrawal of neighboring synapses, it follows that the active synapse must somehow be protected. To date, there is little information about what a protective mechanism might consist of at the molecular level. It is possible that the presynaptic rise in free calcium that accompanies each pulse of transmitter release might also activate a protective enzyme. An alternative idea is suggested by the observation that AChRs are removed *before* terminals are retracted. Perhaps active AChRs are protected from proteolytic enzymes, but inactive AChRs are more likely to be removed from the membrane.

NMDA Receptors and Calcium Signaling

Calcium signaling seems to play an important role in the stabilization of developing synapses, but how does calcium get into the neuron? One important pathway is through neurotransmitter receptor-coupled channels. As we learned in Chapter 8, NMDA-sensitive glutamate receptors (NMDAR) are highly expressed in the central nervous system during synaptogenesis. These receptors become active when glutamate and membrane depolarization are present at the same instant (Fig. 9.29A). When NMDARs are activated, they open a channel that permits Ca^{2+} to rush into the postsynaptic neuron. To find out whether NMDA receptors are involved in activity-dependent synapse plasticity, these receptors have been blocked in a number of developing systems. For example, we learned that monocular lid closure weakens cortical synapses that are driven by the deprived eye. However, when the same manipulation is performed during the chronic infusion of a NMDAR blocker, the strength of "deprived" synapses is preserved (Kleinschmidt *et al.,* 1987). Thus, synapses from the open eye activate NMDARs in the cortex, allowing calcium to enter postsynaptic neurons. We consider below what calcium might be doing once it enters

the postsynaptic neuron. Based on experiments at the neuromuscular junction, we might hypothesize that calcium entry leads to the removal of glutamate receptors from beneath "deprived" synapses, perhaps leading to the withdrawal of presynaptic terminals.

The NMDAR turns out to be broadly involved in the stability of developing excitatory synapses. In the cerebellum, where adult Purkinje cells are innervated by one climbing fiber, the chronic administration of AP5, a NMDAR blocker, results in 50% of Purkinje cells remaining multiply innervated (Rabacchi *et al.,* 1992). In frogs and rodents, AP5 can disrupt the innervation pattern of retinal afferents during the process of map formation (see Chapter 6). For example, when an extra eye is transplanted into a tadpole, the retinal axons project to the midbrain and form a "striped" innervation pattern, similar to the ocular dominance columns in mammalian visual cortex. The segregation of afferents into stripes is blocked completely in the presence of AP5 (Fig. 9.29C). Similarly, AP5 prevents maps from the two eyes from lining up with one another in the frog midbrain. This effect is reversible: when the the NMDAR blocker is removed, the fibers from each eye become segregated. In the mammalian superior colliculus, AP5 prevents the elimination of retinal projections that grow to the wrong topographic position during the first few postnatal weeks (Fig. 9.29B). These studies, and many others like them, show that the NMDAR plays a fundamental role in activity-dependent maturation of synaptic connections (Cline *et al.,* 1987; Scherer and Udin, 1989; Simon *et al.,* 1992). In this regard, it is interesting to recall that NMDARs are often expressed transiently during development, and the level of expression is, itself, regulated by activity (see Chapter 8). It is also significant that NMDARs play an important role in one neural analog of learning called long-term potentiation (see Box: Remaining Flexible). Therefore, NMDAR blockade commonly interferes with synapse elimination in the central nervous system, leading to less specific afferent projections.

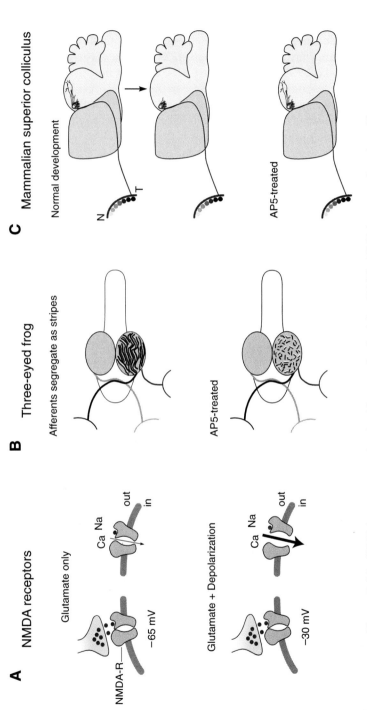

Figure 9.29 NMDA receptors are involved in synaptic plasticity. (A) The NMDA receptor is activated by a combination of glutamate binding and membrane depolarization, opening a channel that permits Ca^{2+} to enter the neuron. (B) When a third eye is implanted into frog embryos, the tectum becomes coinnervated by two eyes, and the terminals from each eye segregate into stripes, similar to primary visual cortex. When three-eyed frogs are treated with AP5, stripe formation is prevented. (C) Afferents from temporal retina are eliminated from the caudal superior colliculus (SC) during development. However, when NMDA receptors are blocked with AP5, these afferents remain in the caudal SC. (Adapted from Cline *et al.*, 1987; Simon *et al.*, 1992.)

The Role of Second Messenger Systems

We have seen that synaptic activity produces substantial changes in structure and expression of synapse-specific molecules in target neurons. How is synaptic activity transformed into a cytoplasmic signal for synapse elimination? Since we have already learned that calcium plays an important role in developmental plasticity, it is reasonable to ask what calcium interacts with. In fact, there are many calcium-binding proteins in the nervous system. One of these proteins, called calmodulin, is a major constituent of the postsynaptic density. Together with calcium, it serves to activate a cytoplasmic kinase called Ca^{2+}/calmodulin-dependent protein kinase II (CaMKII). Once activated, the CaMKII becomes autophosporylated, and its activity then becomes independent of Ca^{2+} and calmodulin binding.

To test the role of CaMKII, transgenic fruit flies were engineered to express an inhibitor of this enzyme during development. The motor nerve terminals of these transgenic animals have numerous sprouts, and there is a greater number of presynaptic sites compared to wild-type flies (Wang et al., 1994). The opposite effect is produced in the frog optic tectum by causing CaMKII to be expressed constitutively in postsynaptic neurons (Zou and Cline, 1996). Retinal axons make simpler arborizations when CaMKII is highly expressed, suggesting that connections are being eliminated more rapidly than normal. Thus, CaMKII participates in decisions about the number of connections to be made, making it a good candidate for the synapse elimination mechanism.

Another calcium- and calmodulin-dependent kinase, called eEF2 kinase, plays a significant role in controlling protein synthesis at developing synapses in the amphibian retinotectal system. In intact tadpole tecta, NMDA receptor activation leads eEF2 kinase to phosphorylate a protein called elongation factor II, which controls ribosomal movement along mRNA (Scheetz et al., 1997). In fact, one of the proteins whose local synthesis is controlled by NMDA receptor stimulation at young synapses is CaMKII.

There are several other protein kinases that may play a similar role during synaptogenesis. One kinase is partially dependent on intracellular calcium and phospholipid metabolites, protein kinase C (PKC). When mice are genetically engineered to be deficient in a neuron-specific form of PKC, synapse elimination is decreased in the cerebellum. About 40% of Purkinje neurons are innervated by more than one climbing fiber, while normal Purkinje cells are all innervated by a single axon (Kano et al., 1995). Other enzymes, such as protein kinase A (PKA), are activated by a rise in cAMP. A role for the cAMP and the PKA signaling pathway has been suggested by single gene mutant flies, called dunce (due to their poor learning abilities). The cAMP levels are persistently increased in dunce flies, and motor neuron terminals produce a greater number of contacts on muscle cells (Fig. 9.30). A similar effect is seen in the mutant ether-a-go-go, which displays increased neuromuscular activity. Interestingly, these phenotypes are similar to those seen in flies expressing the CaMKII inhibitor.

The cAMP/PKA signal can lead to changes in protein synthesis by phosphorylating specific activators or repressors of transcription (see Box: Remaining Flexible). In fact, the extra innervation produced in dunce flies can be eliminated if a second mutation is added that constitutively expresses a repressor of the cAMP response element (Davis et al., 1996). Thus, the quest for second messenger systems has clearly begun, and there is now good evidence that at least three types of protein kinase are involved. Recently, it has been found that the cAMP signal probably regulates the number of synaptic contacts by controlling a cell adhesion molecule, called Fas II, that is found both pre- and postsynaptically at the nerve–muscle junction of fruit flies (see Chapter 5). When dunce flies are engineered to carry a transgene that maintains high levels of fasII expression, the sprouting of motor terminals does not occur (Schuster et al., 1996b). It appears that synaptic activity may induce cAMP signaling, and cAMP may control the expression of a cell adhesion molecule, FasII (Fig. 9.30). Thus, one mechanism by which activity regulates synaptogenesis is through the control of CAMs.

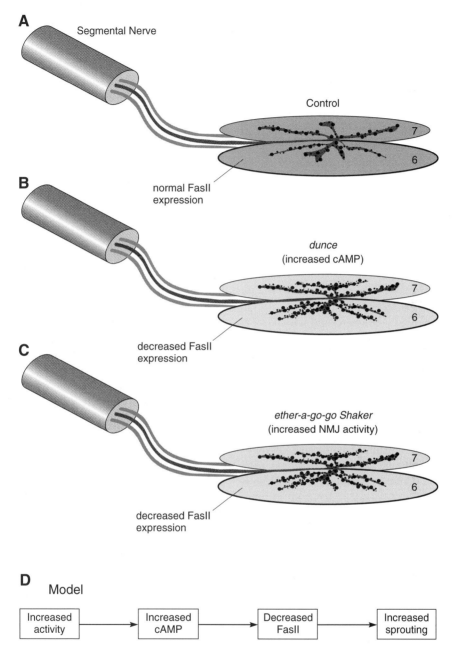

Figure 9.30 Activity-dependent synapse formation is mediated by cAMP. (A) In wild-type flies, muscles 6 and 7 are innervated by ~180 boutons, and the expression of FasII is relatively high. (B) In *dunce* flies, where cAMP levels are constitutively high, FasII levels are decreased, and ~70% more boutonal endings are made on muscle 6 and 7. (C) In double mutant *ether-a-go-go* Shaker flies, where synaptic activity is elevated at the neuromuscular synapse, FasII levels are lower, and ~55% more boutonal endings are made on muscles 6 and 7. (D) One model to explain these results is that synaptic activity increases postsynaptic cAMP which acts, perhaps via a cAMP-dependent transcription factor, to decrease FasII expression. Local sprouting then occurs due to the decreased adhesion. (Adapted from Budnik *et al.,* 1996; Zhong and Wu, 1991; Schuster *et al.,* 1996a.)

Metabotropic Receptors: The Plot Broadens

We have seen that mechanisms of synapse elimination are at least partially triggered by the primary transmitter and receptor. Nicotinic AChRs are likely to be involved in synapse elimination at the neuromuscular junction, and NMDARs appear to play an important role in the elimination of central glutamatergic synapses. Both of these signaling systems operate by opening an ion channel that is permeable to sodium, potassium, and/or calcium. However, mammalian central neurons express many different types of receptors, even within a single synapse. Are there other synaptic mechanisms involved besides ionotropic signaling? This question has been approached by examining synapse development in mice that are lacking specific receptor subunits. One interesting possibility is that glutamatergic transmission also activates metabotropic receptors (mGluRs). Rather than opening ion channels directly, mGluRs can activate either of two different signaling pathways: phospholipid metabolism or cAMP production.

One set of knockout mice that are deficient in a particular metabotropic glutamate receptor subunit, mGluR1, exhibits significantly less synapse elimination at cerebellar Purkinje cells compared to controls (Kano *et al.,* 1997). Furthermore, the metabotropic glutamate receptor may well act through a phospholipase (PLC) signaling pathway. In mice that are deficient in a specific isoform, PLCβ4, climbing fiber elimination is impaired in the rostral portion of the cerebellum where the mRNA for PLCβ4 is predominantly expressed (Kano *et al.,* 1998). Therefore, synapse elimination may involve the collaboration of more than one type of glutamate receptor and intracellular signaling cascade.

Neuromodulatory transmitters have also been shown to affect synaptic plasticity during development. For example, the effects of monocular deprivation are markedly reduced when cholinergic, noradrenergic, or serotonergic terminals are eliminated from the developing nervous system, although none of these afferents mediate visually evoked activity in the cortex (Kasamatsu and Pettigrew, 1976; Bear and Singer, 1986; Gu and Singer, 1995). Apparently, the projections from certain brain stem nuclei (e.g., the raphe, the locus coeruleus, and the nucleus basalis) arborize widely in the brain and can modify synaptic transmission in adult and developing animals. It is still unclear how these modulatory systems are activated during development or how they interact with the primary afferent transmitter system. However, such findings do suggest that our concept of synaptic plasticity in the central nervous sytem is rather rudimentary.

Gain Control

To this point, all of our discussion has focused on the concept that synapses can be weakened by the activity of neighboring connections. Is it also possible that synapses are strengthened or weakened by their own activity? To examine whether synaptic transmission can be strengthened in a developing system following a period of heightened use (see Box: Remaining Flexible), electrical stimuli are delivered to retinal afferents while recording from LGN neurons in a brain slice preparation. Following several bursts of high-frequency synaptic stimulation, 40% of the neurons exhibit enhanced synaptic transmission (Mooney *et al.,* 1993). That is, a test pulse to the afferent pathway evokes a larger excitatory synaptic current after the stimulation period, compared to the pretetanus interval. This phenomenon was called "long-term potentiation" (LTP) when it was first discovered in adult tissue (see Box: Remaining Flexible). Moreover, AP5 is able to block this activity-dependent potentiation of synaptic transmission in most neurons, indicating the involvement of NMDARs.

LTP has been found at other developing synapses, although it is most prominent in the cortex and the hippocampus. One possibility is that LTP is an important mechanism in the adult nervous system and simply appears during development without playing any particular role in synaptogenesis. However, LTP is particularly prominent during development in some areas of the cortex, suggesting that it plays a role in the selective survival or elimination of synaptic connections (Fig. 9.31). LTP has been studied at synapses between thalamic afferents and somatosensory barrel cortex, and it is only found before Postnatal Day 7 (Crair and Malenka, 1995). Moreover, manipulations of the sensory periphery (e.g., the whiskers) only produce structural changes in the cortex if they occur before Day 5, perhaps due to the downregulation of NMDA receptors after the first postnatal week.

Synaptic activity can also lead to a long-lasting decrease in EPSP amplitude, called long-term depression (LTD). In many areas of the brain, LTD is more prominent during early de-

velopment (Fig. 9.32). For example, LTD is present in layer IV of the visual cortex in juvenile cats and guinea pigs. However, it is virtually absent in adult animals (Dudek and Friedlander, 1996). Furthermore, LTD persists in other layers of the adult cortex. Therefore, LTD may play a role in the elimination of thalamocortical synapses, possibly contributing to the formation of ocular dominance columns.

How could LTP and LTD play a role in the selective stablization of inputs during development? To address this question, whole-cell recordings were obtained from frog tectal neurons *in vivo*. Small extracellular stimulating electrodes were placed at two positions within the

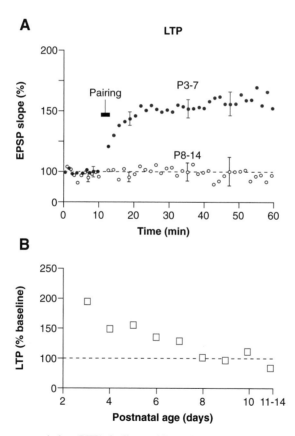

Figure 9.31   Long-term potentiation (LTP) declines with age in barrel cortex. (A) During the first postnatal week, there is an enhancement of excitatory synaptic transmission (red) when the neuron is depolarized during afferent stimulation at 1 Hz. The same stimulus does not enhance excitatory synaptic strength in tissue from P8 to P14 animals. (B) LTP gradually declines in magnitude during the first postnatal week. (Adapted from Crair and Malenka, with permission from *Nature* **375**: 325–328, Copyright 1995 Macmillan Magazines Limited.)

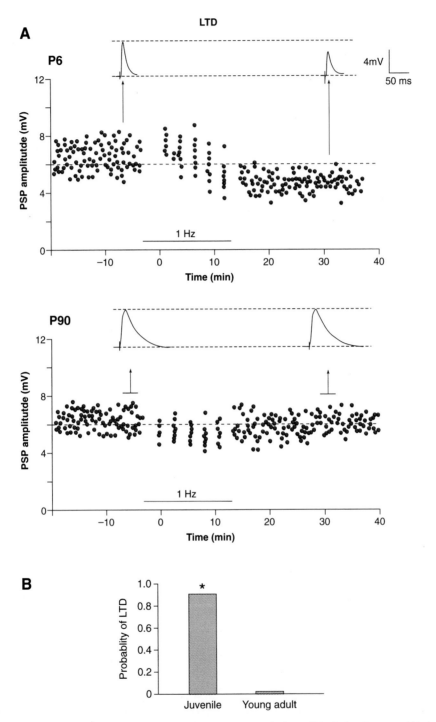

Figure 9.32 Long-term depression (LTD) declines with age in layer IV of visual cortex. (A) At Postnatal Day 6, low-frequency stimulation of the thalamic afferents leads to a long-lasting depression of excitatory synaptic currents. By P90, the same treatment has not. (B) The probability of detecting LTD is nearly 90% in tissue from juvenile animals, but is negligible in young adults. (Adapted from Dudek and Friedlander, Copyright 1996 Cell Press, with permission.)

retina, each of which projects to the recorded tectal neuron. Electrical stimulation of each position evokes an EPSC (Zhang *et al.,* 1998). Following synchronous stimulation of the two retinal positions for 20 s at 1 Hz, the EPSCs evoked by retinal stimulation at either site become larger. The situation is a bit more complicated when the two retinal sites are stimulated asynchronously. When stimulation of one retinal site produces an action potential and the other site produces a subthreshold excitatory synaptic event, the precise timing of the two inputs is crucial. If the subthreshold event leads the retinally evoked action potential by <20 ms, then it becomes potentiated. If the subthreshold event follows the retinally evoked action potential by <20 ms, then it becomes depressed. Thus, inputs that evoke subthreshold synaptic potentials can either be strengthened or weakened, depending on their activity with respect to other inputs, particularly those that evoke suprathreshold activity. These results may help to explain how LTP and LTD contribute to the refinement of retinal projections. As visual stimuli (or waves of spontaneous activity) sweep across the retina, a postsynaptic tectal neuron will be sequentially activated by a series of retinal ganglion cells. When the most effective retinal ganglion cell is activated, it will cause the tectal neuron to fire an action potential. Thus, any retinal ganglion cell that produces a subthreshold event within the next 20 ms may become depressed and subject to elimination.

Silent Synapses

An extreme case of synaptic potentiation occurs when the physical contacts between nerve cells display absolutely no transmission, yet can be turned on by using them. These so-called "silent synapses" have been observed in both young and adult animals. To demonstrate this directly in an adult fish, dual intracellular recordings were made in a glycinergic presynaptic neuron and the postsynaptic Mauthner neuron that it innervated. Direct current injection into the presynaptic neuron elicited an action potential, but there was no postsynaptic IPSP in about 25% of the pairs that were tested, even though the cells were labeled and found to be in contact with one another. These "silent synapses" can be turned on simply by stimulating the presynaptic neuron at a high rate (Charpier *et al.,* 1995).

Inactive contacts have also been observed in developing systems. When chick ciliary ganglion neurons and myotubes are cocultured, only 58% of the contacts are functional, despite their cholinergic phenotype (Dubinsky and Fischbach, 1990). However, after increasing cAMP levels in the cultures, 93% of contacts are functional, even though outgrowth and survival are uneffected. This result suggests that "silent" presynaptic terminals are activated by a cAMP signaling pathway.

It is possible that many glutamatergic synapses are silent during development because activation of NMDAR requires membrane depolarization. For example, intracellular recordings from the neonatal hippocampus show that most synapses have only NMDARs, and they do not respond when membrane potential is held at -60 mV. However, neural activity can enhance synaptic transmission by rapidly recruiting new functional AMPA-type glutamate receptors. If the postsynaptic neuron is depolarized by passing current through the recording electrode, and the synapses are stimulated simultaneously, then the size of the synaptic response increases dramatically (Durand *et al.,* 1996). The increased synaptic response can be blocked by CNQX, an AMPA-type glutamate receptor blocker. A similar observation was made in the optic tectum of developing tadpoles. When retinal afferents are stimulated electrically, most immature synapses do not exhibit a postsynaptic response if the cell is held near the resting potential. However, if the cell is depolarized to +55 mV, then the synapses immediately display a response. This is because the NMDAR is now able to open when bound by glutamate. As the synapses mature in this system, they begin to express a greater number of AMPA-type glutamate receptors. Furthermore, constitutive expression of CaMKII accelerates this transition (Wu *et al.,* 1996). Thus, CaMKII may actually serve as an activity-dependent mechanism for strengthening synapses by somehow recruiting functional AMPA-type receptors at the postsynaptic membrane.

Two experiments suggest that glutamate receptor turnover and modification are controlled by electrical activity. When primary cultures of spinal neurons are grown in the presence of the glutamate receptor blockers, a greater number of AMPA receptor subunits accumulate at synaptic contacts and spontaneous EPSCs are larger. Conversely, when excitatory synaptic activity is increased by growing the cultures in GABA and glycine receptor antagonists, synaptic AMPA receptors decline and spontaneous EPSCs are smaller (O'Brien et al., 1998). Apparently, synaptic transmission controls the number of synaptic AMPA receptors by regulating the half-life of the receptor subunits. The phosphorylation state of AMPA-type glutamate receptors can also be modified by activity of NMDA-type glutamate receptors. In this case, NMDAR activity leads to the dephosphorylation of a particular AMPA-type glutamate receptor called GluR1. When this happens, excitatory synaptic transmission is depressed (Lee et al., 1998). The relationship between these two results is far from clear. However, they do demonstrate that glutamate receptor accumulation and synaptic strength covary and that they can be regulated by use.

The ability of synapses to linger about, even though they provide little input to the postsynaptic cell, may be due to the presence of trophic substances. For example, when glial cell line-derived neurotrophic factor (GDNF) is overexpressed in the muscle cells of transgenic mice, the number of motor neuron terminals at each endplate is dramatically increased (Nguyen et al., 1998). The neurotrophin BDNF prolongs the multiple innervation of mammalian muscle cells in vivo, and this effect is far more prominent when assessed anatomically. At Postnatal Day 12, almost 80% of muscle cells are contacted by more than one nerve terminal, yet only about 25% of muscle cells display multiple EPSP amplitudes. This result suggests that many of the extra motor terminals must be functionally silent (Kwon and Gurney, 1996). Thus, synapse elimination may involve an intermediate state, one in which the synapse is anatomically present, but can not be detected with functional criteria.

Plasticity of Inhibitory Connections

At the nerve–muscle junction, where there is only a single type of synapse, it may soon be possible to explain synaptic competition and elimination at the level of molecular pathways. However, the typical central neuronal circuit has a variety of synapses that arise from different loci. For example, we have already discussed four types of inputs to a visual cortex neuron: ascending projections from the LGN, intrinsic or local projections, commissural projections from the other hemisphere, and modulatory afferents from brain stem nuclei. While it is possible that each type of synapse sets up shop independently of the others, this is not likely. Manipulations to one system inevitably affect the development of the others. Therefore, an important goal of synaptogenesis seems to be proper integration of different types of synapses. That is, the construction of a neural circuit. At the most basic level, we need to understand how inhibitory synapses affect the developmental plasticity of excitatory connections, and visa versa.

Although few studies have directly assessed the developmental plasticity of inhibitory synapses, there are some hints that the response may differ from excitatory afferents. For example, we have seen that monocular deprivation in kittens leads to a decreased efficacy of the "deprived" excitatory afferents in the visual cortex (see above). However, the inhibitory afferents that are activated by the deprived eye appear to be less affected by the manipulation (Singer, 1977b; Watkins et al., 1978). In fact, robust inhibition driven by the deprived eye might mask a weakened excitatory input (Kratz and Spear, 1976; Duffy et al., 1976). If the nondeprived eye is removed after a period of monocular deprivation, then within hours many cortical cells became responsive to the deprived eye. Similarly, if one injects the GABAergic antagonist bicuculline into monocularly deprived cats, then 50% of cells studied become responsive to the deprived eye.

There is also evidence suggesting that inhibitory transmission influences the formation or elimination of synaptic contacts. In the gerbil lateral superior olive (LSO), disruption of glycinergic transmission causes the inhibitory terminals to be more spread out and decreases the size of inhibitory synaptic potentials (Sanes and Takacs, 1993, Kotak and Sanes, 1996). A number of cellular mechanisms might allow inhibitory terminals to influence neuronal maturation. For example, recent studies suggest that inhibitory potentials are depolarizing during early postnatal development (Kandler and Friauf, 1995). These depolarizing responses may be able to activate voltage-gated calcium channels, thus raising intracellular free calcium (Obrietan and van den Pol, 1995). Moreover, inhibitory synapses also display long-term potentiation, similar to glutamatergic synapses, although the cellular mechanism is not yet clear (Komatsu, 1994).

Synaptic Influence on Neuron Morphology

Synaptic activity plays an extremely important role in regulating postsynaptic neuron morphology. During early development, even if denervation does not result in cell death (see Chapter 7), then it certainly leads to shrinkage of cell body size, atrophy of dendritic processes, or loss of dendritic spines in most areas of the central nervous system (Globus and Scheibel, 1966; Valverde, 1968; Rakic, 1972; Harris and Woolsey, 1981; Vaughn *et al.*, 1988). Furthermore, changes in the amount of sensory experience given to an animal during development (which presumably affects neural activity), also leads to measurable alterations in nerve cell morphology. Thus, young rats that are reared in an enriched, social environment have more dendritic branching than rats reared alone in an impoverished environment (Fiala *et al.*, 1978). More precise manipulations of the sensory en-

vironment, such as sound attenuation or vertical stripe rearing, have also been associated with specific changes in auditory or visual neuron morphology, respectively.

Although it is common to perform a manipulation and then wait days or weeks to look for a change in the central nervous system, the effects of denervation occur at a surprising rate. In the chick nucleus laminaris (NL), it is possible to denervate the ventral dendrites while leaving the dorsal dendrites untouched (Fig. 9.33). Thus, the entire NL dendritic arborization was visualized with a Golgi stain, beginning 1 h after the afferents to the ventral dendrites were cut. Even at this earliest time point, there is a 14% decrease in the ventral dendrites compared to the dorsal set (Deitch and Rubel, 1984). Since this is well before terminals are actually removed from the postsynaptic neuron, the dendritic atrophy probably results from the sudden cessation of synaptic activity. Electron microscopy revealed that this change in morphology correlates with a dramatic change in cytoskeletal structures, such as microtubules.

As with cell death, the effect of synaptic transmission can be tested directly by manipulations that block glutamate receptors. When chick embryos are treated with an NMDA receptor antagonist, cerebellar Purkinje cell dendrites do not develop as many branches and occupy a larger cross-sectional area (Vogel and Prittie, 1995). A similar effect has been observed in frog optic tectal neurons and in spinal motor neurons. In hippocampal cultures, the number of dendritic spines, but not the number of branches, is dependent on glutamatergic synaptic activity (Kossel *et al.*, 1997). It is also likely that other growth-promoting factors are coreleased with neurotransmitter. In organotypic cultures of visual cortex, function-blocking antibodies directed against the TrkB receptor decrease the amount of basal dendritic growth, indicating that endogenously released BDNF promotes postsynaptic growth (McAllister *et al.*, 1997).

Excitatory transmission may also constrain dendritic growth (Metzger *et al.*, 1998). When motor neurons are grown in dissociated culture, glutamate decreases the total length of processes

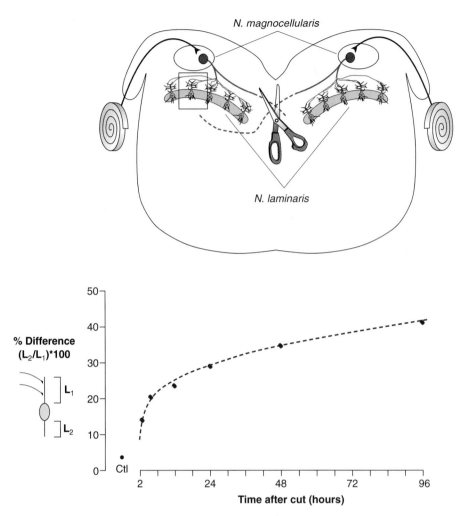

Figure 9.33 Synaptic activity regulates dendrite length in the chick auditory brain stem. (Top) Neurons of the nucleus laminaris (NL) receive afferents from ipsilateral nucleus magnocellularis (NM) to their dorsal dendrites and from the contralateral NM to their ventral dendrites. The ventral dendrites of NL neurons were denervated by cutting NM afferent axons at the midline. The dorsal dendrites remained fully innervated. (Bottom) When NL neurons were stained with the Golgi technique, the ventral dendrites were found to be significantly shorter than those on the dorsal side within 1 h of the manipulation. The ventral dendrites shrunk by almost 40% by 96 h after the lesion. (Adapted from Deitch and Rubel, Afferent influences on brain stem auditory nuclei of the chicken, *J. Comp. Neurol.,* Copyright 1984. By permission of Wiley–Liss, Inc., a subsidiary of John Wiley & Sons, Inc.)

that stain with a dendritic marker (MAP2), but not an axonal marker (tau). Furthermore, the effects of excitatory transmission can change during development as new signaling systems are added to the cytoplasm. For example, the decrease in the growth of optic tectum dendrites correlates with increased expression of the calcium-dependent protein kinase CaMKII. Furthermore, the rate of dendritic growth can be experimentally increased when animals are treated with a CaMKII inhibitor (Wu and Cline, 1998).

Given that the effects of excitatory denervation are so dramatic, it would be surprising if inhibitory synapses did not have a trophic influence on postsynaptic maturation. In fact, inhibitory terminals appear to have the opposite effect of excitatory terminals in a central auditory nucleus, the lateral superior olive (LSO). Neurons in the LSO can be selectively deprived of functional inhibition by removal of the contralateral cochlea, and this manipulation leads to a significant increase in dendritic branching. Furthermore, when organotypic cultures of the LSO are grown in the presence of the inhibitory antagonist strychnine, dendrites are twice as long as those grown in normal medium (Sanes and Hafidi, 1996). Thus, synaptic terminals do not provide a uniform signal to growing dendrites.

Conclusions

At one level, the purpose of synapse elimination seems perfectly obvious: to create the optimal connections between neurons based upon their use. Perhaps the nervous system cannot take full advantage of the plasticity mechanisms unless it generates extra cell bodies, a surplus of dendritic branches, and a profusion of presynaptic arbors. In reality, the purpose of synapse elimination will remain enigmatic until we can produce a specific alteration in a single set of adult connections, let's say two climbing fibers per Purkinje cell, and determine the exact behavioral outcome. Therefore, our understanding

of developmental plasticity is intimately tied to our insight into how the CNS encodes sensory information and controls movement. What is the optimal pattern of connectivity for running, singing, perfect pitch, speed reading, learning, and so forth? Is it even possible to have a nervous system that is optimized for diverse motor, sensory, and cognitive tasks? Unfortunately, we have yet to devise an experiment that tests whether extra cell bodies or small arborization errors actually affect animal behavior.

At present, we believe that synapses can be weakened or lost if they are not activated correctly during development. This might be particularly important for animals, such as humans, that inhabit a wide range of environments. For example, it is likely that our central auditory system is shaped by the spoken language(s) to which we are exposed as infants (see Chapter 10). However, the experimental manipulations that are used to demonstrate an influence of environment or neural activity remain rather extreme. For example, it is unlikely that any animal sees only vertical stripes during development. On the other hand, we know that developing humans do experience many "extreme" rearing environments (such as blindness, deafness, malnutrition, and many others) that result from genetic or epigenetic causes. Therefore, the clinical importance of understanding developmental plasticity is enormous.

Behavioral Development

Behavioral Ontogeny

We often think of animal behavior in terms of the complex motor tasks and perceptions that adults perform, but behavior actually begins well before birth. As a fetus, you were making coordinated, though perhaps not goal-directed, movements. You were kicking, swallowing, and responding to sounds and other sensory inputs. Techniques such as ultrasound have greatly expanded our observations of prenatal behavioral development. We can now see the emergence of normal behaviors in humans and even diagnose behavioral deficits prenatally. While still in its shell, a bird embryo also moves and makes peeping and clicking noises. Even fly embryos wiggle and squirm before they hatch. The first movements and motor responses that an animal makes are far simpler than the sophisticated movements of an adult. Do these embryonic behaviors serve any strategic purpose? Are they merely epiphenomena that arise while nerves become electrically active and connected to one

another? Which behaviors arise first in the embryo, how does the repertoire of behavior grow, and is there any logic in the sequence?

There are at least three basic opinions on these issues (for an excellent historical review, see Oppenheim, 1991). The first is that behaviors develop in an anticipatory manner, with forward reference to actions that will be of value in later life (Carmichael, 1954). For instance, prematurely born humans can respond to light although they would normally not be exposed to light in the womb. Since the nervous system is constructed over a period of time, adaptive behaviors can not be slapped together the moment they are needed, but arise as imperfect manifestations from the developing circuitry. In this view, embryonic behaviors are constrained by the way the nervous system is constructed. Some embryonic behaviors may also be constrained by evolution: inherited traits of an ancestral species that serve little function in the present environment. For example, the Babinski reflex of a human baby, the inward curling of the toes to pressure on the underside of the foot, is thought to be a relic of a more primitive primate nervous system in which feet were used for clinging.

A second view is that embryonic and juvenile behaviors are adaptive and serve specific functions (Oppenheim, 1982). For example, the rate of audible clicking noises that quail embryos produce and hear helps to synchronize hatching in the clutch (Vince and Salter, 1967; Vince, 1979). More frequent clicks accelerate hatching and less frequent clicks retard it. In reptiles, birds, and insects, hatching is composed of repeated movements. These movements are transient behaviors that are adaptive to one stage of life. It is important to recognize that embryonic and adult animals often live in very different environments. Each animal tends to exhibit stage-specific morphological, molecular, and behavioral adaptations to its environment. This is particularly obvious in the case of animals that go through metamorphosis, such as moths and frogs. Here, the larval and adult forms have a radically distinct appearance and behavior. The nervous systems of such animals undergo substantial modifications in response to metamorphic hormones (ecdysone for insects and thyroxine for amphibian), including death of many larval neurons and genesis of new adult neurons (Fig. 10.1).

A third view is that embryonic behaviors serve as an important substrate for building the nervous system (Carpenter, 1874). Neural circuits are built imperfectly, but through function they become finely tuned. The learning that we do as adults may be nothing more than a continuation of the mechanisms used to adjust the embryonic nervous system. The behavioral patterns that we see in embryonic and juvenile animals are the integrated beginnings of more complex patterns that continue to develop. Thus, we must necessarily crawl before we can walk. If this view is correct, disruption of early behaviors should have significant effects on the development of later behaviors. These three views are not mutually exclusive, and there is some truth in all of them, as we see in this chapter.

Cellular and Environmental Mechanisms

A key issue that we will address in this chapter concerns the cellular and genetic mechanisms that lead to neural circuits underlying specific behaviors. Donald Wilson, who worked on the neural basis of insect flight, was amazed that a locust spreading its wings for the first time could fly without practice and make appropriate adjustments to wind speed and visual signals (Wilson, 1968). "How perfect is the motor score that is built into the thoracic ganglion?" he wondered. It seemed to him that the CNS is genetically programmed to contain nearly everything that is necessary before actual flight occurs. Thirty years later, Michael Bate, who works on the development of the *Drosophila* nervous system, expressed a similar surprise, but for a different reason (Bate, 1998). Since genes that affect behaviors seem to function at a cellular level on the development and physiology of neurons, and since we have not found genes whose job it is to organize an entire neural circuit, it is difficult to comprehend the genetic basis of the neural circuits that underlie complicated behaviors. "How do we explain" Bate asks, "the remarkable fact that behavioral 'sense' of this kind is inherited and built into the nervous system as it develops?" In this chapter, we investigate the neural basis of the development of behavior, because all of the mechanisms that we have discussed in Chapters 1–9 lead toward a nervous system with functional circuits that orchestrate adaptive behavior.

Clearly, genetic factors are at the root of behavior in that flies and frogs do not behave as humans, no matter how similar their environment. Yet nervous systems in both insects and mammals are built of the same type of neurons, make the same type of synapses, use the same type of neurotransmitters, obey the same developmental rules, and often use homologous molecules. In the 1960s, Seymour Benzer began to address the question of behavior genetics by searching for single genes which, when mutated, lead to aberrant behaviors in fruit flies (Benzer,

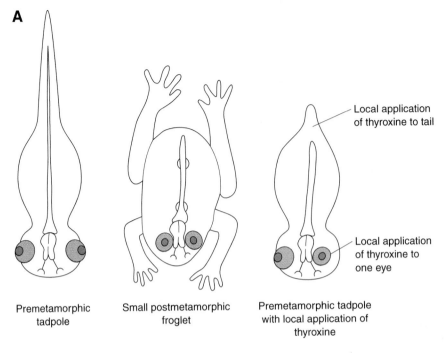

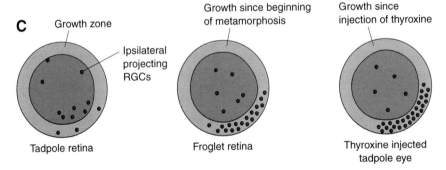

B Some thyroxine induced changes in frog nervous system
1) Massive cell death in tail spinal cord
2) Growth of brachial and lumbar enlargements by proliferation of motor and sensory neurons
3) Birth of new ipsilateral projections in ventral temporal retina (see below)

Figure 10.1 Changes in the nervous system caused by a metamorphic hormone. (A) In a normal *Xenopus* premetamorphic tadpole, the eyes are lateral, there are no limbs, and there is a tail. In a postmetamorphic adult, the eyes move dorsally and develop overlapping visual fields, the tail resorbs, and the limbs develop. Local application of the metamorphic hormone thyroxine to the eye of a tadpole causes it to migrate dorsally, while local application of thyroxine to the tail causes it to resorb even though the rest of the animal maintains the attributes of a tadpole. (B) Some other thyroxine inducible changes in the nervous system associated with metamorphosis. (C) An en face view of the retina in a tadpole (left), a metamorphic frog (middle), and a tadpole eye injected with thyroxine (right). In the normal tadpole eye only a few retinal ganglion cells have axons that project ipsilaterally as there is minimal binocular vision. In the metamorphosing frog, as binocular vision develops with the dorsal migration of the eye, many new ganglion cells are born in the ventrotemporal retina that project ipsilaterally and subserve binocular vision. The same effect is achieved when thyroxine is applied locally. (Adapted from Hoskins and Grobstein, 1984.)

1971). Surprisingly, many of the genes he and his colleagues discovered by this process are conserved among different species. For instance, the genes found to govern the 24-h circadian rhythm in flies have homologs that are involved in the same process in mammals (Ishida *et al.,* 1999). The genes that affect learning in flies are involved in mammalian learning (Dobnau and Tully, 1998). This is not to say that all the genes that influence fly behaviors are homologous to those that influence similar behaviors in mammals. However, one wonders how far these homologies extend. Are there, for example, genetically conserved programs that construct an entire neural circuit? If so, what molecular and genetic mechanisms modify these circuits to give species-specific behaviors?

Like other organs, the brain is built by gene products. Yet the nervous system is unique among organs in that it responds sensitively to a huge variety of environmental influences with structural and functional changes, even from an early age. Neural activity modulates the expression of many of the same structural and functional gene products that were used in the initial embryogenesis of the nervous system. This interplay between the environment and the genome continues throughout life. Because of this interplay, it is usually not reasonable to ascribe specific behaviors to purely genetic or environmental determinants. Yet, a genetic impact on behavior is as clear as an experiential one. The dysfunction of particular genes can have dramatic effects on behavior associated with congenital neurological diseases. Moreover, identical twins that are separated at birth and reared in different families may show amazing similarities in attitude and taste, compared to nonidentical twins reared together. The important point, often lost in such discussions, is that these two human beings usually also show an enormous array of dissimilarities reflecting lifelong interactions between environment and genome. In the following sections, it becomes apparent that our understanding of neural and behavioral development depends on the interaction between these two ingredients.

Environmental Determinants of Behavioral Development

From early embryonic stages of life, genetic influences operate in the context of a specific environment. This environment places selective pressures on the embryo and influences development. The most obvious examples come from studies of environmental hazards. Embryonic exposure to thalidomide was found to cause severe morphological birth defects in humans, and embryonic exposure to high levels of alcohol or heroine can lead to mental retardation (Johnson and Leff, 1999). In birds and mammals, embryonic exposure to sex-specific steroids can alter physical and or neural aspects of sexual maturation. In bird embryos, hearing a mother's call in the egg, can impose a preference for that call upon hatching. When a songbird learns to sing, it is strongly influenced by early auditory experience of its species-specific song, as we see below (Mooney, 1999).

Early deprivation of many kinds, visual, auditory, even emotional, is known to have permanent effects on behavioral development. Postnatal experiences in humans, of course, include education and training. Though we do not believe that human brains, or those of other animals, emerge as blank slates, it is nevertheless clear that experience shapes and adjusts the nervous system. An argument has been made that the brain is particularly adaptive, in the Darwinian sense, simply because it is an organ that learns how to modify behavior in order to improve survival in a changing environment. In fact, learning is one of the main functions of the nervous system, and this process probably begins in the embryo. In dealing with the genetic and environmental influences on behavior, we must address not only how genes control cellular and molecular events to construct the neural substrate of behavior but also how behavioral and sensory events feedback onto these molecular mechanisms.

The pure description of a developing behavior is valuable because it provides the most sensitive and inclusive indicator of a successfully assembled nervous system. Such an indicator is extremely sensitive to environmental or genetic influences on the cellular properties of neurons. Studies of human embryonic behavior reveal that a multitude of diseases have recognizable impacts on early behavior. For example, one of the earliest signs of fetal alcohol syndrome is the behavioral retardation of the fetus (Mulder *et al.,* 1986). By affecting the way neurons develop, environmental insults and genetic mutations have an enormous impact on the emergence of the functional circuitry underlying behavior, and this can severely restrict an organism's ability to perceive the world and to respond with coordinated movements.

Motor Behavior: The First Movements

The first simple twitch that an animal makes signals not only the beginning of an expanding repertoire of movements, but also the beginning of functional motor circuitry. The simplest form of such circuitry, as we have seen in Chapter 8, is the synapse formed between the motor neuron and a muscle fiber. In most species, the earliest skeletal movements are neurogenic. That is, movement is caused by synaptic activity at the nerve–muscle synapse. Thus, zebrafish mutants that fail to make functional neuromuscular junctions never begin to twitch either spontaneously or in response to stimuli (Westerfield *et al.,* 1990). In a few species, such as shark, the first embryonic movements are myogenic in that muscle cell activity is present without synaptic transmission. A different class of movements, those elicited by sensory stimulation, also emerges quite early in development. In this case, a synapse that completes a reflex arc between sensory and motor neurons must also be functional.

Are the First Behaviors Spontaneous or Reflexive?

One question that has intrigued those who study the origins of behavior is whether the very first skeletal movements of an animal are spontaneous and involve no sensory input or are reflexive movements in response to sensory stimulation. Sometimes it is difficult to tell when a movement is truly spontaneous. For example, "spontaneous" behaviors are found to increase in frequency during the later half of embryonic leech development (Reynolds *et al.,* 1998). This increase corresponds to the time of eye formation, suggesting that the embryos may actually be responding to light. In fact, if the embryos are observed in red light, rather than white light, this increase in spontaneous behavior is not observed. Thus, the spontaneous movements are stimulus induced. If the first behaviors are always reflexive, then sensory input must have a dominant role in establishing and refining behavior. If, however, truly spontaneous movements appear first, then the motor system is probably maturing independent of sensory input. Therefore, it is important to resolve this issue.

To address this question, observations have been made on several species. The behavior of chick embryos has proven most informative. By shining light through eggs, candling them as it is called, it is possible to see the embryo moving in its shell. If one observes the later stages of development, chick embryos are seen to move their wings and legs within their shells (Preyer, 1885). Careful studies of chick embryos raised in glass dishes, rather than shells, reveal that the undisturbed animal may exhibit a variety of behaviors (Fig. 10.2). These behaviors clearly occurred prior to the establishment of sensory input. For several days after their first occurrence, sensory stimulation did not change the frequency of these behaviors, nor is it able to evoke a motor response (Preyer, 1885). One could argue that there are, as in the leech, subtle stimuli to which the chick can respond. Perhaps, if all sensory stimuli are removed, the embryo will not move. To resolve this issue experimentally, chick embryos were surgically deafferented at early stages by removing the neural crest cells that give rise to sensory DRG cells (Hamburger *et al.,* 1966). In such embryos, movements began at the same stage as in unoperated controls and appeared indistinguishable

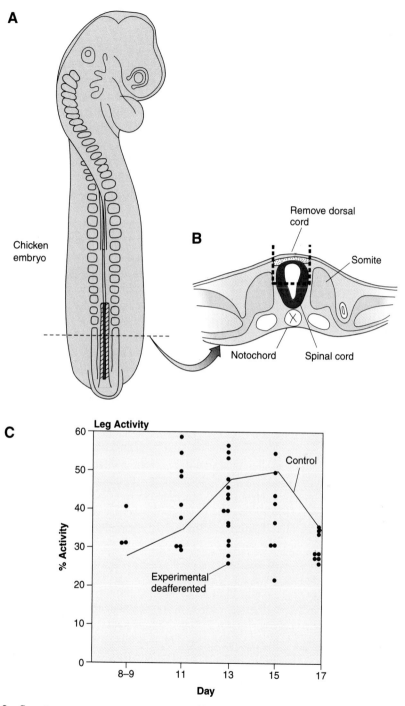

Figure 10.2 Spontaneous movements are generated in the absence of sensory input. (A) The cross-hatched region of the lumbar spinal cord (red) of this premotile chicken embryo is shown in cross section in B, which shows the operation done *in ovo;* the dorsal spinal cord and neural crest containing all the sensory neurons in this region are removed. (C) Activity monitor of average normal leg movements (line) and leg movements generated by legs without any sensory input in operated animals (circles). (Adapted from Hamburger *et al.,* Motility in the chick and embryo in the absence of sensory input, *J. Exp. Zool.,* Copyright 1966. By permission of Wiley–Liss, Inc., a subsidary of John Wiley & Sons, Inc.)

in frequency or quality for a number of days (Fig. 10.2). These experimental findings were further supported by anatomical and electrophysiological studies of the spinal cord in which it was seen that the motor system really does mature before the sensory system. There is no detectable physiological synaptic input onto motor neurons when sensory neurons are stimulated during this prereflexogenic period of behavior (Bekoff, 1976).

The Mechanism of Spontaneous Movements

If sensory stimulation is not involved in early motor behavior, then how are these spontaneous movements generated? Since embryonic spontaneous movements are often rhythmic and episodic in nature, this has led to the suggestion that there is a central generator that has input onto various motorpools. To study this, the chick embryonic spinal cord can be isolated and the nerve cell activity can be recorded (O'Donovan et al., 1998). The motor nerve roots of such isolated cords produce activity patterns that mimic closely their output in the intact animal (Fig. 10.3). In both cases, one observes alternating bursts of action potentials from extensor and flexor motor neurons. Electrophysiological records from the neurons themselves reveal that there are rich depolarizing synaptic inputs onto both sets of motor neurons simultaneously but that flexor and extensor motor neurons have different properties. While both neuronal populations begin to depolarize toward threshold at the same time and begin to fire synchronously, flexor motor neurons have a large shunt conductance due to GABAergic inputs, and these occur at the peak of the depolarization phase. As a result, flexor motor neurons stop firing just when the extensor motor neurons, whose excitation is due primarily to glutaminergic input, are firing most rapidly (Chub and O'Donovan, 1998). This synaptic activity leads to oscillations in flexor and extensor motor patterns, and these mechanisms are quite different from those governing coordinated movement in the adult. As the animal matures, a central pat-

tern generator drives a clear oscillation in the depolarization of both flexor and extensor motor neurons.

We are still left with the question of how such bursts of rhythmic activity first arise. This question can be addressed by dissecting the isolated spinal cord. Removing the dorsal half of the cord, where sensory axons travel, does not affect the rhythmic motor episodes, and the further dissection of the ventral cord shows that both the motor neurons in the lateral part and the ventral interneurons in the medial part fire in episodes (O'Donovan et al., 1998). This result is consistent with a scenario in which the embryonic neurons are connected to each other with a profusion of excitatory synapses. Thus, any depolarization leads to the profusion of excitatory activity amongst all the connected neurons. Although GABA is an inhibitory transmitter in most parts of the adult CNS, it can be excitatory early in spinal development (see Chapter 8). Blocking of both the GABAergic and glutaminergic synapses in the isolated cord stops the rhythmic activity. However, blocking either GABA or glutamate alone does not block the episodes of excitation. Thus, it is unlikely that there is a specific pattern generating circuitry in the cord. Rather, the rhythmic bursting pattern is an intrinsic property of this developing network. Similar waves of synchronized excitation appear to propagate in the ganglion cells of the retina far before light can evoke any activity, and these discharge patterns seem to influence synapse development (see Chapter 9). Motor neuron activity may also advance the process of neural maturation. In the Xenopus spinal neurons, both GABA expression and the appearance of a specific potassium channel depend on the spontaneous calcium waves (Spitzer and Ribera, 1998).

Embryonic Movements: Uncoordinated or Integrated?

How coordinated is embryonic motor behavior? Do the episodes of trunk and limb movement represent an integrated behavior that need only to be improved, or are the behaviors essentially spastic and random due to the immaturity

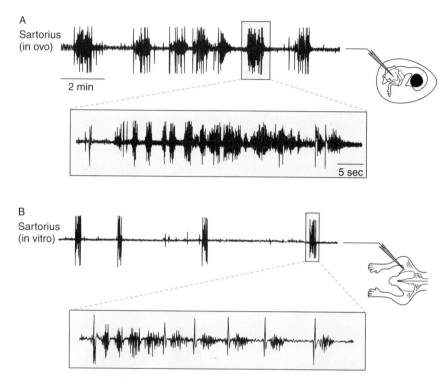

Figure 10.3 *In vitro* motor development physiology. (A) Electrographic recordings from the sartorius muscle of a chick embryo *in ovo*. (B) A piece of the embryo kept in a culture dish. Very similar spontaneous movements begin to occur in these two situations, although the bursts of activity in the *in vitro* preparation are shorter and less frequent. (Adapted from O'Donovan *et al.,* 1998.)

of the circuit? The pioneering work of Coghill in the 1920s favors the notion that behavior develops in an integrated fashion (Coghill, 1929). Behaviors build upon each other as the circuitry matures and new components are added. Coghill began to study the first movements of the salamander embryo because, like all amphibian embryos, they grow from shell-less eggs in water and are accessible for observation from the earliest stages of development. Also, there was an extensive history of embryological and neuranatomical studies on these animals. By looking at large numbers of such embryos, Coghill found that slow bending of the head to one side was the very first movement executed by the salamander embryo (Fig. 10.4). The movement involves the trunk muscles situated immediately behind the head. As development proceeds, muscles further and further down the body become involved and twitch more quickly so that

the "bend," which started as a slow movement at the neck region, becomes a quicker coiling of the entire body.

Careful examination of this behavior reveals that full coiling movements start at the neck region and then proceed down the body (Fig. 10.4), such that the sequence of each movement recapitulates the developmental progression of the movement as well as the progression of neuronal maturation (e.g., first in the hindbrain and then down the spinal cord). Both bending and coiling can be stimulated by a light touch of the skin on the side opposite the contraction. Coghill's anatomical explanation for this chronology is that sensory and motor neurons, which innervate the skin and muscles, are present in prereflexogenic stages. However, at the time bending away from a light touch emerges, a set of interneurons appear to form the first commissural pathways from sensory neurons on

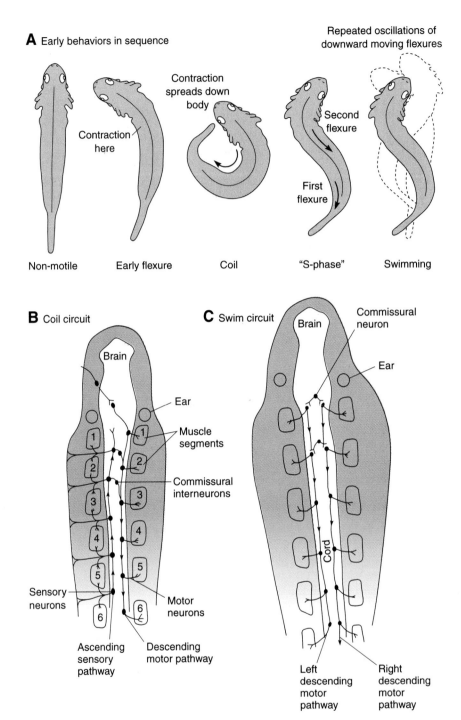

A Early behaviors in sequence

Repeated oscillations of downward moving flexures

Contraction spreads down body

Contraction here

Second flexure

First flexure

Non-motile   Early flexure   Coil   "S-phase"   Swimming

B Coil circuit

Brain

Ear

Muscle segments

Commissural interneurons

Sensory neurons

Motor neurons

Ascending sensory pathway   Descending motor pathway

C Swim circuit

Brain

Commissural neuron

Ear

Cord

Left descending motor pathway   Right descending motor pathway

Figure 10.4 Coghill's sequence of early amphibian behavior and the proposed neural basis. (A) An axolotl embryo at five stages of behavioral development. (B) The neural circuit for the coil response. A stimulus anywhere on one side of the body is transmitted to the contralateral spinal motor pathway by commissural cells in the anterior cord or hindbrain where it descends stimulating primary motorneurons of the cord. (C) The early swim circuit (the sensory mechanism is omitted but is the same as in B). Motor excitation travels down one side of the cord, but by this stage in development some reciprocally exciting commissural neurons that cross the floor plate in the hindbrain have developed so that excitation on one side at the neck region can crossover after a delay to excite the contralateral motor pathway, leading to coiling on one side being quickly followed by coiling on the other side. (Adapted from Coghill, 1929.)

one side to motor neurons on the other (Fig. 10.4). Longitudinal ipsilateral tracts extend down the motor columns and up the sensory columns while the commissural interneurons first appear only in the rostral cord and hindbrain. Thus a neural signal from a touch anywhere on the skin travels ipsilaterally up the sensory path, crosses over in the neck region, and stimulates motor neurons in that region of the other side causing a bending of the neck away. The signal then proceeds down the motor pathway on that side of the spinal cord involving successively more posterior segments.

Although coiling movements do not propel the animal forward, the rostrocaudal propagation of a contraction along the body is a progression that is seen in later stages of swimming. So how does swimming arise? After the animal is capable of coiling, the next component of new behavior is the "S" phase. This arises, as the coiling movements become faster and alternate from side to side. For example, if a right-hand coiling movement proceeds only half way down the body before a left-hand coiling movement starts at the neck region, the result is an S shaped wave proceeding caudally and the propagation of the animal forward: the beginning of swimming.

Coghill saw many behaviors develop in this integrated way, and one of his great contributions was his correlational of nervous system anatomy with the behavior: he attributed the origins of particular behaviors to the newly added neuronal connections. A classic modern example of such a correlation occurs for the Mauthner neurons, a pair of very large cells in the hindbrain of tadpoles and fish that receive auditory input ipsilaterally and project posteriorly onto contralateral motor neurons. This simple circuit is responsible for the rapid escape response. In the embryonic zebrafish, as early as 40 h after fertilization, the Mauthner cells can initiate an escape response, a directional jump away from the stimulus followed by a series of strong tail flexures. This system is probably involved in evoked hatching behavior, as the response is sufficient to rupture the egg membrane and allow the animal to escape. The Mauthner cell sometimes fires spontaneously, which suggests that it might function also in spontaneous hatching behavior. The Mauthner growth cone enters the spinal cord after all the primary motor neurons of the trunk spinal cord have begun axonal outgrowth and this temporal sequence of axonal outgrowth may play a role in defining the behavioral functionality of contacts between the Mauthner axon and the primary motor neurons. The transparency of larval zebrafish has enabled physiologists to use confocal calcium imaging in the intact fish to study the activity of the Mauthner cell during behavior (Fig. 10.5). Such work shows that during an escape, these cells are indeed activated in patterns that are exactly predicted by behavioral studies (O'Malley *et al.,* 1996). The development of descending pathways that integrate motor movements extends to voluntary movements initiated in the cerebral cortex of primates. Thus, it is not until the corticospinal tract develops fully that macaque monkeys are able to make fine finger movements and exhibit mature manual dexterity (Armand *et al.,* 1994).

The developmental neuroanatomy of behavior is not always so clearly integrated as it appeared in Coghill's salamanders. In the chick embryo, Hamburger (1963) describes the early movements as "uncoordinated twisting of the trunk, jerky flexions, extensions and kicking of the legs, gaping and later clapping of the beak, eye and eyelid movements and occasional wing-falling . . . performed in unpredictable combinations." Simple local reflexes could also be demonstrated in these animals, although the responses tended to be spastic. The integration of movements between limbs, such that the left leg alternates with the right during walking or the right and left wings beat synchronously during flight, does not emerge until later in development. Thus, the random thrashings and reflexes of individual parts of the chick embryo, as well as the mammalian embryo, are brought under control as the central circuitry develops. This imposed coordination of individual movements is carried out according to anatomically centralized pattern generators. So, if the brachial cord that drives wing movements in the chick embryo is exchanged with the lumbosacral cord that

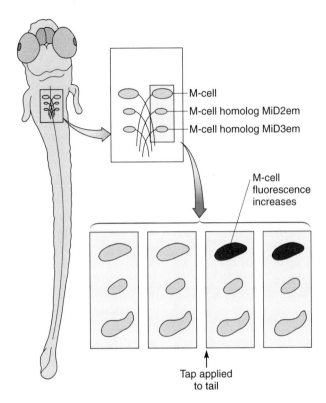

Figure 10.5 Visualizing the neural basis of behavior in zebrafish. In a newly posthatched zebrafish larva, the descending cells including the giant Mauthner neuron (M cell) and its two homologs in the hindbrain have been filled with a fluorescent calcium indicator. In the panel below, the four panels show successive time points about half a second apart. When a stimulus is applied to the tail, the M cell is activated (red), which initiates the escape behavior. (Adapted from O'Malley *et al.*, 1996.)

drives leg movements, then the wings begin to flap alternately and the legs hop synchronously (Fig. 10.6) (Straznicky, 1967; Narayanan and Hamburger, 1971). This is reminiscent of a more recent study in which certain parts of the brain were exchanged between chicks and quails. The result was that quails bobbed their heads like chickens (Balaban, 1997).

The Role of Activity in the Emergence of Coordinated Behavior

If the exchange of pieces of nervous system can lead to predictable abnormalities in behav-ior, then one wonders how much behavior is built into the nervous system. Are activity patterns and repetitive practice of simple movements important for the proper development of later movements? The deafferentation experiments mentioned above imply that sensory input is not necessary for the initiation of behavior. More remarkably, similar experiments show that sensory feedback is not involved in the coordination and maturation of motor behaviors. Perhaps the most revealing experiments having to do with the role of activity in the maturation of early motor behaviors are the ones done almost a century ago by Ross Harrison (1904). He raised some salamander embryos in an anesthetic solution throughout the period of bending and coiling and S movements. He then

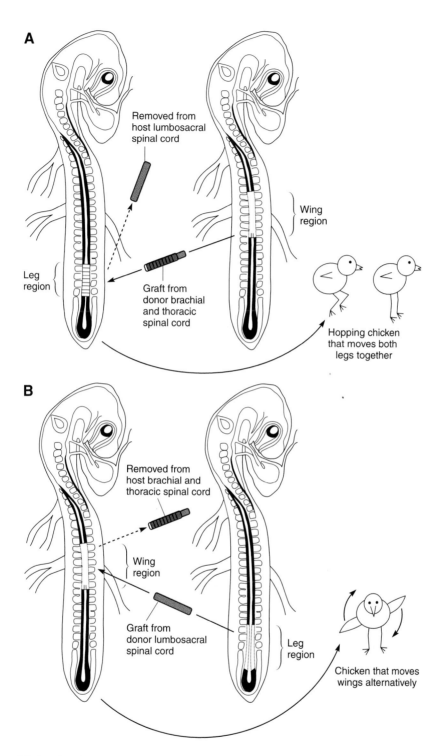

Figure 10.6 Flapping legs and walking arms. (A) The lumbar cord of one chick embryo is replaced by the brachial cord of a donor embryo. When the chick hatches, instead of walking, it jumps in the rhythm of flapping wings. (B) The reciprocal experiment leads to a chick that has alternating wing movements instead of normal flapping ones. (Adapted from Narayanan and Hamburger, Motility in chick embryos with substitution of lumbosacral by brachial and brachial by lumbrosacral spinal cord segments, *J. Exp. Zool.,* Copyright 1971. By permission of Wiley–Liss, Inc., a subsidiary of John Wiley & Sons, Inc.)

transferred the embryos to anesthetic-free solution when their control siblings had already proven themselves capable of sustained swimming. He found that the long-term anesthetized embryos were able to begin to swim as soon as the anesthetic was washed out. In a few minutes, they were behaviorally indistinguishable from the controls.

More recently, these types of experiments have been done with other drugs that block synaptic transmission or action potentials in combination with more quantitative behavioral measurements (Haverkamp and Oppenheim, 1986; Haverkamp, 1986). The results are essentially the same (Fig. 10.7). For the development of coordinated movements of the limbs in chicks or swimming movements in amphibians, activity in the nervous system is not crucial. In other words, the earliest movements that an animal makes are not a necessary stepping-stone to the development of at least some of the more sophisticated behaviors, even those that incorporate the early behaviors. Thus, it seems that many early motor patterns are hard-wired into the developing anatomy. These early behaviors, although serving as indicators of the development of certain connections, are no more than epiphenomena of the immature wiring pattern.

Embryo-Specific Behaviors

If some motor behaviors are epiphenomena and serve no particular purpose in the maturation

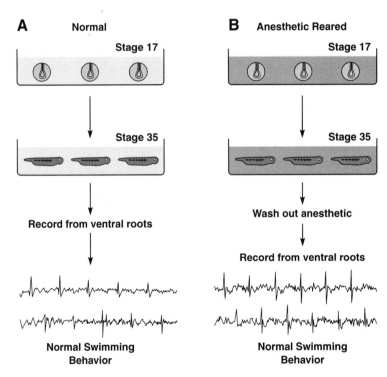

Figure 10.7 Swimming out of anesthesia. (A) A set of normal *Xenopus* embryos put in a culture dish at the late neural plate stage and raised till the swimming stage in normal pond water. They swim normally and electrophysiological records from ventral roots on opposite sides of the spinal cord show the expected alternating pattern of activity. (B) A set of sister embryos raised in an anesthetic solution until stage 35, at which point some the embryos were immediately put into a recording chamber. The pattern of activity of the swimming behavior looks essentially normal. (Adapted from Haverkamp, 1986.)

of the nervous system, then one might expect to see them only in the embryo. Indeed, several such embryo-specific behaviors are seen in the leech (Reynolds *et al.,* 1998). For example, one behavior is called lateral ridge formation and is the result of the contraction of dorsoventral "flattener" muscle at a time in development when the embryo is still essentially a germinal plate. The contraction of these muscles lifts the boundary of the future dorsal and ventral territories. Another embryo-specific behavior is called circumferential indentation and occurs when an embryonic leech is prodded on one side (Fig. 10.8). An adult leech, when presented with a similar stimulus, will usually exhibit a local

bend away from the stimulus, contracting muscles on one side and relaxing those on the other. However, the embryo excites all the muscles in those segments causing a circumferential contraction. It is likely that circumferential indentation is a behavior that simply occurs at an incomplete stage of neural circuit formation.

But not all transitory embryonic motor behaviors are useless or simply the result of partially completed neural circuitry. One behavior that serves a clear adaptational purpose is the hatching movements of bird embryos. Chicks, like many other shell bound embryos, go through a very specific motor behavior pattern just at hatching (Bekoff and Kauer, 1984). These behaviors

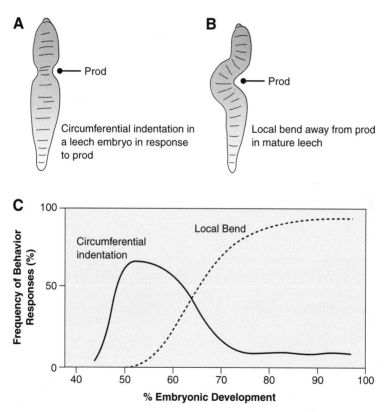

Figure 10.8 A transient embryo-specific behavior in a leech gets replaced. (A) At 50% of embryonic development, most prods to one side of the midbody of a leech embryo result in circumferential indentation of the body due to the contraction of muscles all around the body at the level of the poke. (B) At 80% of development, a similar prod leads to local bending away from the prod resulting from differential contraction of muscles on one side of the body versus the other. (C) Graphic illustration of the transitory embryonic behavior with the more mature behavior. (Adapted from Reynolds *et al.,* 1998.)

allow the embryo to get into the appropriate position for breaking open the shell. If one places a posthatch chick into the hatching position within a glass egg, the bird reinitiates its hatching behavior (Fig. 10.9). If sensory input from the neck is eliminated with a local anesthetic, then hatching behavior is suppressed (Bekoff and Sabichi, 1987). Therefore, it appears that sensory receptors located in the neck provide a specific input signal for initiating hatching

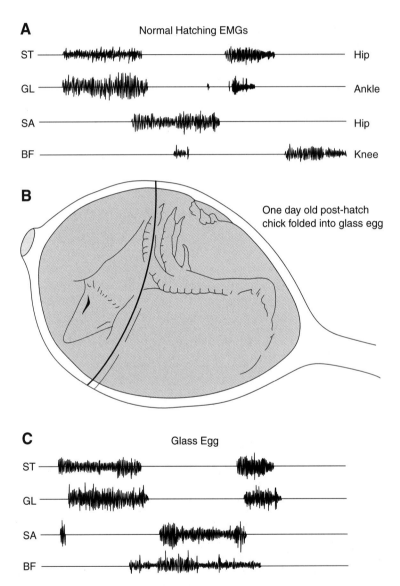

Figure 10.9   Chicken trying to hatch again in a glass egg. (A) Electromyographic (EMG) recordings of the normal hatching motor program in the chick embryo. ST and SA are hip muscles, GL is an ankle muscle, and BF is a knee muscle. Note the alternation between the activity of the hip and the lower leg. (B) A 1-day-old chick crammed back inside a glass egg. (C) EMG records from such a chick show that it reinitiates the hatching motor program. (Adapted from Bekoff and Kauer, 1984, with permission.)

behavior. Another example of a transient embryonic behavior is the migration that marsupial
embryos make from their womb to the mother's
pouch. Born at an extremely early phase of development with their hindlimbs little more than
buds, these tiny embryos use their forelimbs to
crawl tens of body lengths into the pouch where
they attach onto a nipple and suckle (another
transient but adaptive behavior of mammals) for
several months. During this time they complete
their embryonic development. Human infants
that do not suckle can be fed through a tube, and
the absence of these early suckling experiences
do not impair the development of adult eating.
This demonstrates, once again, that the juvenile
behavior is not a prerequisite for the adult motor
program, even though it is adaptive to the neonatal environment.

Metamorphosis signals a dramatic change
in lifestyle in holometabolic insects, such as
moths and flies, as well as amphibia, such as
frogs (Harris, 1990; Truman, 1992). The larval
behaviors of the swimming, filter-feeding tadpole are completely inappropriate for the land-
dwelling, bug-eating frog. The transition from
larval to adult state is activated by specific hormones, ecdysone for insects and thyroxine for
frogs. Each of these hormones has a widespread
effect on gene expression and cellular function.
Many very adaptive larval behaviors are lost at
this transition while new behaviors are gained.
As would be expected, there are also dramatic
changes in nervous system structure. In both
insects and amphibia, larval neurons die upon
exposure to metamorphic hormone, and some
neuroblasts that have been quiescent through larval life begin to proliferate. Some larval neurons
survive the transition to adult but are drastically
reorganized. For example, the motor neurons
that move the abdominal prolegs of the caterpillar do not die even though these appendages are
lost, but their axons and dendrites are remodeled
and old synapses are eliminated to support new
behaviors (Fig. 10.10).

In metamorphic insects, there are important
transitional behaviors associated with building
and emerging from the pupal state. In moths,
the adult motor system is constructed primarily
from remodeled larval components, whereas the
adult sensory system is primarily composed of
new neurons. Simple reflexes correlate these
neuronal changes with the acquisition or loss of
particular behaviors. For example, the loss of the
larval proleg retraction reflex is associated with
the loss of the dendrites of the proleg motor neurons. The adult stretch receptor reflex begins
when new adult-specific connections are added
to new dendritic growth in an adult neuron
(Levine and Weeks, 1990). Although humans do
not go through metamorphosis in the same way
as flies and frogs, the distinct behaviors of babies
and adults must be largely due to changes in the
nervous system that result not only from experience but also from a variety of intrinsic influences, such as hormones and growth factors that
are regulated throughout life.

Motor Learning

The emergence of motor behaviors is generally spontaneous and does not depend on
sensory input. The first coordination of motor
behavior also does not require neural activity.
Clearly, there are intrinsic mechanisms that re-
model the motor system and its attendant behavioral output through the developmental stages of
life. But throughout this discussion of motor development, we have neglected the importance
of learning mechanisms and sensory feedback.
Some simple coordinated movements, such as
larval swimming and limb synchronization, can
occur without feedback. However, humans do
not play Mozart on the piano without practice or
hit 70 home runs without some hand–eye coordination training. The beginning of hand–eye
coordination occurs in infancy, and observations
of babies show that they move the arm that is in
their visual field more than the other arm. This
suggests that babies may be trying to learn to
control their fine movements by visual feedback
(van der Meer *et al.,* 1995). Some obvious reflexes, such as blinking your eyes when objects
approach, are not native but are conditioned.

The cerebellar circuit is thought to have a
major role in motor learning. Damage to parts of

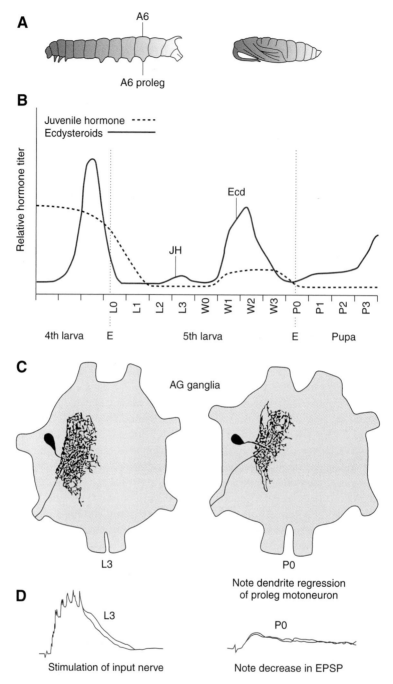

Figure 10.10 Changes in a single neuron during metamorphosis. (A) The caterpillar of the moth (*Maduca sexta*) showing abdominal segment 6 and the proleg associated with this segment. To the right is shown the pupal stage. (B) Profile of hormonal changes through larval life and the transition between the larval and the pupal development where ecdysone rises without an increase in juvenile hormone. (C) Remodeling of the A6 proleg motoneuron during metamorphosis. There is a dramatic pruning of the dendritic tree. (D) Correlated with this dendritic remodeling, there was a decrease in the activation of this neuron when the sensory input nerve was stimulated. These changes reflect the changing role of this neuron in postmetamorphic life where there are no prolegs. (Adapted from Streichert and Weeks, 1990, with permission.)

this circuit result in spastic movements and the inability to perform certain motor learning tasks. Mouse mutants born with defective cerebellar circuitry show unsteady gaits and have been given names like reeler, weaver, and staggerer in accordance with these pathologies. The vestibuloocular reflex (VOR) permits vertebrates to keep their eyes still when the head turns, thus allowing an object to remain stable in the field of view. This reflex is so strong that even with your eyes closed if you swivel 26° to the right your eyes will turn 26° to the left at the same velocity—the gain of this reflex is exactly −1. The multisynaptic reflex arc connects the sensory cells in the semicircular canal of the inner ear to the motor neurons that drive the extraocular muscles of the eye. If a person or an experimental animal puts on telescopic glasses that magnify the world or prisms that invert left and right, then a gain of −1 for this reflex is no longer appropriate. The visual world is destabilized and any turn of the head results in a slippage of the visual scene across the retina, usually leading to nausea. Over the course of a few days, however, the gain on the VOR is reset to be appropriate for the glasses or prisms, and the nausea stops until they are taken off (Fig. 10.11). Physiological work has shown that an error signal of retinal slippage is sent to the cerebellum and, as a result, the synaptic efficacy of the reflex arc is modified by heterosynaptic LTP-like mechanisms such as we have discussed in Chapter 9. There are different sites of plasticity within these circuits (Lisberger, 1988; Raymond *et al.,* 1996). One site of plasticity is in the vestibular nuclei, which receive inhibition from Purkinje cells of the cerebellar cortex. Another site of plasticity is in the cerebellar cortex itself. Damage to the cerebellum circuit interferes with the ability of the retinal signal to change the gain of the VOR. Cerebellar circuitry is not solely involved in motor learning. Certainly the cortex can encode new behaviors, and the sensory motor cortex in monkeys can undergo functional changes as these animals learn new fine motor tasks. Refinement of practiced motor behaviors probably continues throughout life, just as disused motor behaviors grow less precise.

Beginning to Make Sense of the World

The nervous system becomes active well before animals experience the world around them or move about in it. In fact, this "spontaneous" activity may initially be necessary for the survival and maturation of synapses or dendrites (see Chapter 9). At some point, however, the nervous system begins to sense the world, and some of the information is of immediate use. For example, neonatal mammals may be helpless in many ways, yet their survival depends on perceptual abilities that lead them toward their mothers nipples. Many animals begin to hear, smell, see, taste, and feel well before the sensory epithelia (e.g., hair cells, photoreceptors, etc.) and central nervous system connections are mature. Therefore, it is important to understand the relationship between neural tissue development and perception. How is visual detection limited by neonatal retinal ganglion cell physiology and morphology? Why do infants rarely enjoy espresso or extra hot salsa? Why can it take several seconds for a baby to determine the location of a speaker?

Studies of sensory perception are amongst the most difficult experiments in the field of neural development. Baby animals (especially human infants) tend to be slow, sleepy, cranky, unattentive, and/or forgetful. These are generally referred to as nonsensory factors. For example, adults pay better attention to novel stimuli than young animals. When adult primates are presented with two images, one of which they have never seen before, they spend about 70% of the time staring at this novel object. In contrast, infants spend an equal amount of time staring at the familiar and the novel objects (Bachevalier, 1990). Even though adults are more attentive to novel stimuli, they can also focus narrowly on a stimulus of interest and ignore novel stimuli that may be distracting. For example, when taking an examination, we tend to "block out" extraneous noise. This was demonstrated by asking people to detect a tone when it was presented on 75% of trials. Several other tones were presented on the other 25% of trials. Adults apparently come

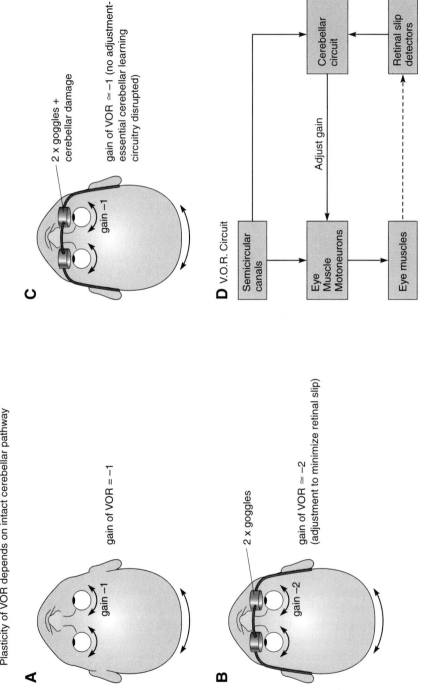

Figure 10.11 Adjusting the gain of the vestibuloocular reflex (VOR) and the role of the cerebellar pathway. (A) In a normal person, the eyes move in the opposite direction of the head at a gain of precisely −1 in order to stabilize the visual world on the retina. (B) When a person wears 2× magnifying goggles, he "learns" to adjust the gain of the VOR to −2 in order to avoid retinal slippage. (C) If cerebellar circuitry is disrupted, this learning does not occur and the gain does not readjust. (D) Proposed circuitry underlying this modifiable behavior. Input from both retinal slip detectors and the semicircular canal activity feeds into the cerebellar circuitry which adjusts the gain on the vestibular input onto the eye muscle motoneurons. If the gain is not perfect, the retinal slip detectors are activated again and the adjustment continues. (Adapted from Raymond *et al.*, 1996.)

to "expect" the tone that is presented 75% of the time, and they detect it quite well, whereas they are very poor at detecting the other tones (i.e., those presented on 25% of trials). Infants are remarkably different: they detect all of the tones equally well (Bargones and Werner, 1994). Thus, infants and adults experience the world in very different ways, and these nonsensory factors lurk in the background of all developmental studies of sensory perception.

Asking Babies Questions

How, then, can these uncooperative little animals tell us about their experiences? Various experimental tricks have been devised to determine how sensory information is being processed in young animals. In one scenario, the behavioral scientist watches for a motor reflex while presenting sensory stimuli. For example, we often respond to an unexpected noise with a startle, and this rapid muscle twitch provides a reliable measure that sound has been detected. We can also take advantage of the fact that animals tend to stop responding, or habituate, to the same stimulus presented many times. After the animal has habituated, we can present a new stimulus and ask whether the animal responds. This is a good way of determining how well an animal notices the difference between two similar stimuli (e.g., middle C versus C sharp).

A more difficult approach is to condition an animal to keep making a stereotyped behavior, such as a head turn, when a stimulus has been detected. Most animals will work for a reward, even human infants. Thus, the head turn that an infant makes to a sound can be reinforced by showing her an interesting toy (Fig. 10.12). The infant will then "work" for visual stimulation (that is, turn her head) when she hears a sound. Cheap pay, but it works. This procedure can be extended to very young infants (<6 months) by having an adult observer, who cannot hear the test sounds, watch the baby to determine when she makes a response to sound. The baby gets rewarded (with a viewing of the toy bear) whenever the observer determines that the baby has

responded. In this manner, any possible response that a baby might make to sound (for example, an eye movement or a tongue wag) can be conditioned. Of course, we believe that the baby is oblivious to this process, but she nonetheless ends up working for a reward and provides valuable information about sensory development along the way. Such training techniques assess far more than sensory skills, and one may well end up studying the development of attention or memory rather than the development of sensory perception.

Behavioral scientists tend to concentrate on two criteria: absolute sensitivity and discrimination. Absolute sensitivity measures the minimum amplitude stimulus that can be detected: the softest touch, the finest line, the quietest sound. Discrimination measures our ability to perceive a difference between two similar stimuli: sky blue versus turquoise, middle C versus C sharp, margarine versus butter. Of course, psychophysicists tend to measure our response to simpler stimuli. Below, we explore how developing animals first perceive their sensory world.

Sharp Eyesight

Human infants show clear evidence of being able to see at birth. For example, they stare for longer periods of time at a familiar face, such as their mother's. However, their visual skills appear to be very poor as compared to an adult. Visual acuity, or the the ability to detect fine detail, is almost entirely absent at birth. One measure of visual acuity is the number of black and white lines that can be observed per degree of visual space (The "rule of thumb" states that at arms distance your thumb occupies about one degree of visual space). Adults can see about 30 black and white lines per degree, but babies can only see about one. In the more common language of an eye doctor, the baby sees at 20 feet what a normal adult can see at 600 feet, and adult sensitivity is reached between 3 and 5 years of age (Birch *et al.,* 1983). In principle, this level of acuity would permit an infant to distinguish the fingers of a hand, but their actual

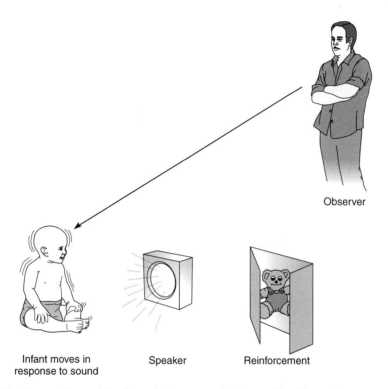

Observer

Infant moves in   Speaker   Reinforcement
response to sound

Figure 10.12 Determining an infant's sensitivity to sound. Infants will make small movements in response to a sound that they can hear, and this natural tendency has been exploited to measure the infant's ability to hear different sound frequencies. To improve the sensitivity of this procedure, an adult observer watched the infant and judged whether the infant saw the stimulus based on any motor response that the infant made. To increase the infant's responsiveness to sound, she can be reinforced for correct responses. In this case, the infant was rewarded with the appearance of a teddy bear.

abilities remain somewhat of a mystery. Our best ideas come from "preferential looking" studies that tell us what babies prefer to look at, given a choice (e.g., faces, curved lines, complex patterns), but not what they see.

The modest visual acuity of primates at birth is partly due to an immature retina. Photoreceptors are relatively short and wide at birth, meaning that less light is absorbed and a greater piece of visual real estate is viewed (Yuodelis and Hendrickson, 1986). Thalamic and cortical neurons may also impose limits on visual acuity. If one compares the theoretical acuity of the retina (based on the shape and density of photoreceptors) with the acuity of single cortex neurons, then the cortex neuron is found to be worse than expected in developing primates. Further-

more, the animal's acuity is worse than that of single cortical neurons (Fig. 10.13). Such results suggest that the development of accurate connections (see Chapters 5 and 6) may only create a minimal operating system, and optimal performance is acquired through detailed changes in synaptic architecture or function (see Chapter 9).

Binocular vision involves the coordinated use of both eyes to judge the distance of an object, and this requires both sensory and motor development. To look at an object close up, the eyes must be rotated toward one another (convergence) so that the visual image activates the correct portion of each retina. Similarly, the eyes must be rotated away from one another (divergence) to look at a distant object. Cruel as it sounds, one of the simplest ways to determine

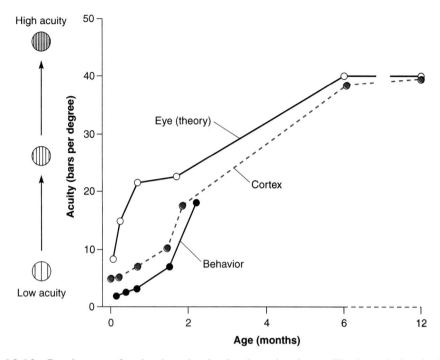

Figure 10.13 Development of acuity along the visual pathway in primates. The theoretical acuity (number of bars per degree) of retinal neurons improves more rapidly than the acuity of primary visual cortex neurons. The behavioral acuity of animals appears to track cortical development most closely, although there is still a disparity in performance. Therefore, it is possible that maturation of higher visual cortical areas is necessary for adult-like performance to emerge. (Adapted from *Vision Res.* **8,** Jacobs and Blakemore, Factors limiting the postnatal development of visual acuity in the monkey, pp. 947–958, Copyright 1988, with permission from Elsevier Science.)

whether depth perception is present in young animals is to ask whether they are willing to crawl off a "cliff." To do this safely, an infant is placed on an elevated glass surface that is patterned on one half and clear on the other. If an infant is willing to crawl out over the clear surface, off the "perceptual cliff," then one assumes poor depth perception. By the time that they crawl, most infants do avoid the cliff, indicating that depth perception is present (Walk and Gibson, 1961). More precise measurements of depth perception show a rather sudden improvement. For example, binocular perception in cats goes from being rather poor to almost adult-like between 4 and 6 weeks postnatal (Timney, 1981).

Why does binocular vision improve with age? Do neurons in the cortex suddenly become selective for binocular stimulation? In fact, several neural mechanisms may contribute to the

maturation of binocular vision (Daw, 1995). First, since the visual system detects smaller objects with age (discussed above), it is likely that it can also resolve smaller differences between the two eyes. Detecting differences between the two eyes is fundamental to depth perception. We also know that binocular information converges inappropriately in layer IV of neonatal cats and primates. Left and right eye afferents gradually segregate into eye-specific columns (see Chapter 9), and this tends to occur when binocular vision is improving. During the same period, neurons become more selective for the visual stimulus to which they will respond. For example, individual cortex neurons respond to a smaller range of bar orientations during development in cats and ferrets (Bonds, 1979; Chapman and Stryker, 1993). Thus, some interesting candidate mechanisms have been identified, but we have yet to design the experiments that will test their relationship to perception.

Acute Hearing

As is true of the visual system, the auditory system displays improved sensitivity and discrimination as an animal matures. Although kittens can hear at birth, they can only respond to extremely loud sounds, well above the level of city traffic (>100 dB sound pressure level), at 10 days postnatal. Their auditory thresholds gradually decrease such that they can detect sounds at the level of a whisper (30 dB SPL) by 1 month, and by adulthood they become even more sensitive than humans. A similar change is found in all developing animals. In humans, auditory thresholds drop rapidly during the first 6 months of life and are virtually adult-like by 2 years of age. Improved behavioral thresholds are well-correlated with a decrease in sound level needed to evoke an electrical potential from the cochlea, suggesting that the major factor limiting detection in young animals is the ear (Werner and Gray, 1998).

As thresholds decrease, most animals also respond to higher sound frequencies. This is probably due to a physical change in the cochlea because a single physical position along the cochlea responds to higher freqencies as the animal matures. Since the topographic projection from the cochlea to the central nervous system does not change significantly during this time, one might expect to find interesting changes in sound perception with development. In fact, 15-day-old rat pups can be trained to suppress activity when they hear a 8-kHz tone, but 3 days later they suppress activity to a higher frequency. That is, a higher sound frequency apparently sounds like the 8-kHz tone because the cochlear frequency map has shifted (Hyson and Rudy, 1987).

While the basic sensitivity and frequency range mature rapidly, several features of sound remain difficult to detect. This is well-illustrated for tasks in which one must detect a very brief event, often referred to as temporal processing

(Fig. 10.14). For example, adults are able to detect a 5 ms gap of silence in an ongoing sound. In contrast, one year old infants, who have already begun to process and produce speech sounds, can only detect gaps that are an order of magnitude longer (60 ms), and adult-like performance is not reached until about 5 years of age (Werner et al., 1992). Similarly, 4- to 5-year-old children are poorer than adults at detecting rapid modulation in sound level when the amplitude changes are relatively small.

These behavioral measures of temporal processing may be relevant to language development because human speech sounds are composed of rapidly changing frequency and intensity, including well-placed periods of silence. In fact, children with learning disabilities that are primarily due to a difficulty with spoken language also perform poorly on simple auditory discrimination tasks that require temporal processing. For example, when normal children are exposed sequentially to two tones, they can report the correct sequence with delays as small as 8 ms. In contrast, the language-impaired group required a silent interval of 300 ms in order to report the correct sequence. Recently, it has been found that performance can be improved when language-impaired children are trained to recognize speech sounds that are slowed down. Apparently, once the nervous system has learned to recognize this slower speech, it is better able to recognize the rapid temporal variations in normal speech (Tallal and Piercy, 1973; Tallal et al., 1996).

There are several candidate mechanisms that may explain poor temporal processing in young animals. For example, we have seen that synaptic potentials are usually of much longer duration in the neonatal central auditory system (see Chapter 8). We might suppose that long PSPs effectively limit the "clock speed" of the organism, or the fastest rate at which information can be processed. Thus, it will be interesting to learn more about the neural basis of temporal processing, particularly in the auditory system.

Perhaps the most useful information that a developing animal gets from its ears is the location of significant objects, such as its mother or

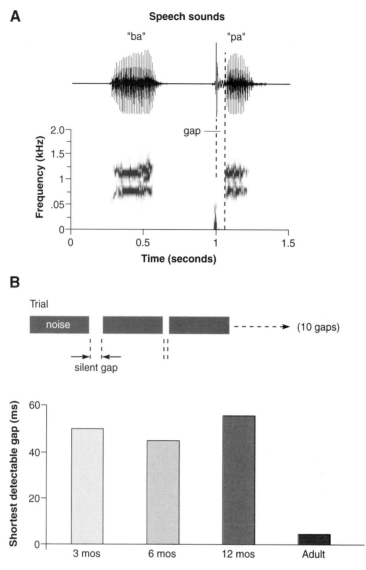

Figure 10.14 Development of temporal processing may affect speech perception. (A) An oscilloscope record of the human speech phonemes /ba/ and /pa/. Below each record is a spectrogram of the phoneme showing the sound frequencies that compose the phoneme and their relative intensity (darker is louder). Note that the /ba/ is a continuous sound, whereas /pa/ consists of a nonvoiced component (in this case, the p sound), followed by a brief gap, and then a voiced sound (the "a"). Perception of this brief gap is critical to word recognition. (B) The minimum gap that humans can perceive was assessed with a brief silent period embedded in a white noise stimulus. The bar graph shows that even at 12 months of age, humans are almost 10 times less sensitive at detecting a gap. (Adapted from Werner *et al.*, 1992.)

a predator. Although infants can tell whether a sound source is coming from the left or the right (sound lateralization), they are not able to make fine discrimations. Adult humans can detect a 1° change in the position of a speaker (recall the rule of thumb), but newborns can only detect a change of about 25°. In fact, even sound lateral-ization is fairly challanging to a newborn infant (Fig. 10.15). The sound stimulus must remain on for about 1 s if the infant is to make an appro-priate head orientation response, whereas adults need only about a millisecond of sound, such as a finger snap (Clarkson *et al.*, 1989). The ability of nonhuman mammals to lateralize sounds is also present even as the animal first experiences sound, yet we know little about the senstivity of the system. For example, rat pups suddenly be-gin to turn their heads toward a noise at 14 days

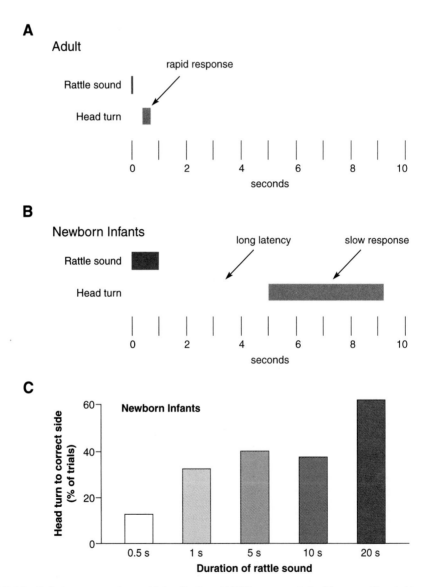

Figure 10.15   Infants are poor at sound lateralization. (A) When presented with a sound located to one size, adult humans turn their head quickly toward the sound source within a fraction of a second. (B) When human infants are presented with a sound to one side, they may take several seconds to respond, and the head movement can be quite slow. (C) For infants, a sound stimulus must be presented for a long time period in order to get accurate lateralization. Whereas adults can localize sounds that last for only a millisecond, newborn infants require at least 1 s of sound. (Adapted from Clarkson *et al.*, 1991.)

postnatal, a few days after the ear canal opens. However, the percentage of correct turns toward the sound continues to increase over the next 7 days (Kelly *et al.,* 1987).

The response of central neurons to sound is known to change during this period of development, and some of these alterations could help to explain immature sound localization. Maps of space are found in the superior colliculus (SC) of several mammals, and single SC neurons are selectively activated by sound (or visual and somatosensory stimuli) from a specific location. During the course of development, these SC neurons respond to a smaller part of the sensory world. In cats, the average size of a receptive field decreases about fourfold during the first 2 months after birth (Fig. 10.16). Furthermore, the visual receptive fields become adult-like a few weeks

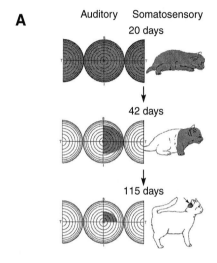

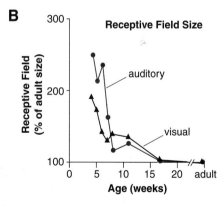

Figure 10.16 Single neuron receptive field sizes decrease dramatically during development. (A) Recording were made from single neurons in the superior colliculus that respond to more than one sensory modality. The auditory and somatosensory receptive fields are shown for three neurons from cats of increasing age. At 20 days, the neuron responded to auditory stimuli located anywhere in space and to touch on any area of skin. At 115 days, the neuron responded to a small area of auditory space (gray area) and to touch on a small area of skin under the right ear. (B) The relative sizes of auditory (red) and visual (black) receptive fields are plotted for neurons recorded throughout development. There is a dramatic decrease during the first 8 weeks, and mature properties are attained by the 17th week. (Adapted from Wallace and Stein, 1997, with permission.)

earlier than the auditory receptive fields in kittens (Wallace and Stein, 1997). In the guinea pig, an orderly map of auditory space is not apparent until Postnatal Day 32, even though hearing begins *in utero* (Withington-Wray *et al.,* 1990).

A second basis for immature processing is that sound-evoked discharge rates are extremely low in young animals, and they fatigue rapidly during stimulation. What does this mean for the performance of a developing nervous system? First, neurons have a poorer resolution: they devote few action potentials to a given change in the stimulus. For example, adult LSO neurons can devote twice as many action potentials to a given change of interaural level compared to juvenile animals (Sanes and Rubel, 1988). Therefore, either young animals make decisions based upon less neural information (e.g., fewer action potentials) or, more likely, they are not able to perform at adult levels because they have less neural information to work with. Striking as this result is, we still have little direct knowledge about the relationship between amount of neural activity and perception, even in adult animals.

Sex-Specific Behavior

The many differences between male and female behavior serve as a popular subject of conversation. They are also a source of considerable controversy, and the political stakes can be quite high. We primates tend to debate whether sex-specific behaviors are due to our "biology" or the social environment that we are raised in. While the debate is seductive, the relationship between brain development and sexual behavior varies tremendously from species to species. Since mating and maternity have been most thoroughly explored at the neural level, we mostly focus on these behaviors. However, it is worth mentioning some complex behaviors that differ between male and female animals. These differences in behavior are commonly referred to as sexual dimorphisms. Predatory behavior is sexually dimorphic in lions (females do more of it), urination posture is sexually dimorphic in dogs, and olfactory signaling is sexually dimor-

phic in moths. In both rats and monkeys, young animals engage in play behavior that differs between the sexes, at least in its frequency of occurrence. Males tend to have more play fights than females. These "fights" will typically begin with one animal jumping onto the other, and they end with one animal on top of the other. When testosterone is given to a pregnant monkey, the play behavior of her female offspring becomes more male-like.

Another behavioral sign of a sexually distinct nervous system comes from the male:female ratio of certain neurological and psychiatric diseases. For example, both dyslexia and schizophrenia are more prominant in males (about 75% of cases), while anorexia nervosa is exhibited primarily by females (over 90% of cases). Finally, many recent studies have focused on the cognitive abilities of adult humans (Kimura, 1996). When presented with two figures drawn at different orientation, males are better able to "mentally rotate" the objects to determine whether the two figures are the same. In contrast, when presented with a picture containing many objects, females are better able to say which objects have been moved in a second picture. While these results tend to fascinate us, the challenge will be to understand what exactly is being measured and what its relevance is to behavior.

Such differences in complex behavior patterns do raise a host of interesting questions: Are the differences due to biology or environment? If there is a biological signal, is it genetic or hormonal? Are the differences irretrievably established at birth or are they modifiable throughout life? Certain sexual characteristics emerge during early development, such as differentiation of the genitals and the motor neurons that innervate them (see Chapter 7). However, this is only the first step of a lifelong process. The nervous system continues to respond to steroid hormones throughout life, making it important to ask whether a behavior is determined by early exposure to a hormone or whether the behavior can be elicited in adults of either sex merely by adjusting the amount of circulating hormone. Therefore, we begin by discussing the early determinants of gender and then explore determinants of behavior and brain development.

Genetic Sex

Animals seem to have two general ways of establishing gender. In fruit flies and other insects, the genetic sex of each cell is the key determinant. If a cell has a single X, then it is male. If it has two Xs, then the cell expresses a protein called sex-lethal and becomes female. The nematode *C. elegans* also comes in two flavors, but they are male and hermaphrodite (i.e., an animal with both types of gonad). As with fruit flies, sex is determined by the ratio of X chromosomes to autosomes, and XO-lethal is the gene product that is activated in animals with a single X.

The genetic sex of each cell in a mammal is specified by the presence of either two X chromosomes or one X and one Y. However, the genetic sex of most somatic cells is not thought to have an immediate influence on their development. It is the genetic sex of gonadal tissue that really matters. Primary sex determination refers to differentiation of the gonadal tissue, and this is determined by the *SRY* gene on the Y chromosome that encodes a transription factor. If *SRY* is present, the gonads devolop into testes and secrete testosterone. If *SRY* is absent, the gonads develop into ovaries. The *SRY* gene product is a DNA-binding protein, and it probably controls the expression of downstream targets to prevent development along the female pathway. For example, a locus on the X chromosome, called *Dax-1,* is probably involved in ovary determination. Thus, it is thought that *SRY* represses *Dax-1* in genetic males. After primary sex determination is complete, all sex differences, including those of the nervous system, are thought to originate from the gonads. The possibility remains that the genetic sex of an individual somatic cell plays a role in maturation, as is discussed below.

Hormonal Signals

In most vertebrates, as the gonads differentiate and begin to secrete hormones, tissues throughout the body respond by adopting a male or a female phenotype. This is called secondary sex determination. The principal importance of gonadal hormones is powerfully demonstrated by removing the gonads before primary determination occurs (Jost, 1953). Without exception, animals develop as females (e.g., they have a vagina, a uterus, and oviducts). Furthermore, their sexual behavior is female-like, presumably because certain areas of the nervous system have developed female characteristics (Phoenix *et al.,* 1959). When genetically female (XX) rats are treated with testosterone within a few days of birth, they will not display female sexual behaviors as adults. That is, they will not arch their back (lordosis) when approached by a male, and they will mount a female rat if given another shot of testosterone. When genetically male rats (XY) are castrated soon after birth, they will not mount a female as an adult, even if given a shot of testosterone.

The testes masculinize the body by releasing the steroid hormone testosterone. The level first rises during the perinatal period, goes down after birth, and rises again at puberty. The testosterone must be converted to another compound in order to carry out some of its actions. For example, some members of a small community in the Domican Republic carry a disrupted form of the 5α-reductase gene and cannot convert testosterone to 5α-dihydrotestosterone (DHT). Although affected genetic males (XY) have functional testes and plenty of circulating testosterone, their external genitals are female (Imperato-McGinley *et al.,* 1979; Thigpen *et al.,* 1992). Interestingly, most of the individuals who were unambiguously raised as girls nonetheless chose to adopt a male identity during or after puberty. The results suggest that testosterone has a potent influence in determining gender identity, even overcoming the prolonged "environmental" influence of being raised as a female. Since DHT is probably not involved in gender identity (although it is involved in differentiation of external genetalia), how does testosterone masculinize the brain?

In the brains of mammals, testosterone is also converted to the estrogen hormone estradiol-17β, by an enzyme called aromatase. At first, this might seem puzzling because estradiol is secreted by the ovaries and promotes differentiation of the female reproductive organs.

However, testosterone is also an intermediate metabolite of estradiol in the ovaries. Thus, we should probably not think of hormones as being male or female. There are probably two factors that allow estradiol to act selectively on the brains of genetic males. First, aromatase activity is higher in the brains of male mice, particularly during the prenatal and neonatal periods (Hutchison, 1997). Second, the blood of young animals contains an estradiol-binding protein, called α-fetoprotein, that may prevent estrogen secreted by the ovaries from reaching the brain (Uriel *et al.,* 1976).

Since there are many different steroid hormones, and their actions are quite diverse, there must be specific transduction pathways. How do sex hormones influence neuron differentiation and function? Steroid receptors are cytoplasmic proteins with a steroid-binding domain and a DNA-binding domain. That is, they provide a very direct pathway to the genome (Beato *et al.,* 1995). When estradiol binds to its multisubunit receptor, it dissociates and the active DNA-binding complex enters the nucleus. Estradiol receptors are found in neurons of the hypothalamus and amygdala, and they are expressed transiently in the cortex and hypothalamus. Androgen receptors are also expressed at highest concentration in the hypothalamus and limbic structures.

Hormonal Control of Brain Gender

The hypothalamus is the most likely mammalian brain region to be a target of gonadal hormones during development. By lesioning or stimulating individual areas, it has been possible to show that some hypothalamic regions are involved directly in the production of sex-specific behaviors. For example, medial preoptic neurons fire rapidly just prior to male copulation, and copulatory behavior is disrupted when this area is lesioned. Medial preoptic neurons are also known to take up more testosterone than any other brain region in adult animals. One of the first studies to show that male and female brains actually differ in a measurable way was an ultrastructural study in the preoptic area (Raisman and Field, 1973b). A few years later, it was found that one part of the preoptic area, aptly named the sexual dimorphic nucleus of the preoptic area (SDN-POA), is so much larger in male rats than in females that one can actually see the difference in tissue sections without using a microscope (Fig. 10.17). A similar difference is found in the primate hypothalamus, including that of humans, but it is not yet clear whether the nuclei in each species are homologs of one another. Selective cell death may account for the sexual dimorphism in a human hypothalamic nucleus called INAH 1. Until age 5, the number of INAH 1 neurons is about the same in males and females, but the number of neurons then declines more rapidly in females (Swaab and Hofman, 1988).

The sexual dimorphism of SDN-POA is an example of secondary sex determination in the nervous system. The hormonal environment of developing males yields a larger nucleus, and the dimorphism can be greatly reduced by castrating genetic males within a few days of birth (Fig. 10.17). Furthermore, this nucleus can be enlarged in genetic females when they are treated with testosterone as neonates (Gorski *et al.,* 1978). Intracranial implants of estradiol turn out to be as effective as testosterone in masculinizing the SDN-POA and such estradiol-treated females fail to lordose or ovulate. Presumably, testosterone is normally converted to estradiol in the male SDN-POA, whereas the circulating estradiol in females is bound by α-fetoprotein (Naftolin *et al.,* 1975).

A second region of the hypothalamus, the ventromedial region (VMH), also participates in sexual behavior. Damage to this region disrupts female copulatory behaviors, such as lordosis in rats, and stimulation of the region seems to facilitate such behaviors. Lesions also have more profound effects on food intake, particularly in females. Neurons of the VMH are selectively activated by the ovarian hormone estrogen, and in female rats the cells respond by producing progesterone receptors. This does not occur in the male VMH. In primates, the hormonal signal may be somewhat different because loss of the

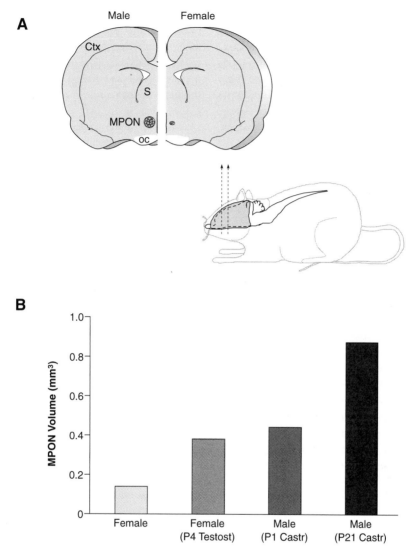

Figure 10.17 Sexual dimorphism in the mammalian brain. (A) A hypothalamic structure called the sexually dimorphic nucleus of the preoptic area (SDN-POA) is almost six times larger in male than in female rats. (B) In genetic females, the size of the SPN-POA can be increased by treatment with testosterone at Postnatal Day 4. In genetic males, the SPN-POA can be decreased in size by castration at Postnatal Day 1. (Adapted from Gorski *et al.,* 1978.)

adrenal glands, a source of androgen hormones, leads to reduction in copulatory behavior. Although there is little difference in the absolute size of the VMH, there is some reason to believe that it becomes sexually dimorphic during development (Sakuma, 1984). In fact, estradiol and testosterone have a dramatic effect on both neurite outgrowth and dendritic branching in organotypic cultures of the mouse hypothalamus (Toran-Allerand, 1980; Toran-Allerand *et al.,* 1983).

Sexual behavior in mice that have a disrupted estrogen receptor gene is signficantly attenuated. For example, females do not lordose. The males do initiate copulatory behavior, mounting females at a normal rate, but they rarely achieve an intromission or an ejaculation. Furthermore, the males are less aggressive than wild-type males, generally failing to attack an "intruder" mouse when it is placed in the male's home cage (Ogawa *et al.,* 1997). These results are interpreted to mean that estrogen receptor function is not necessary for the development of sexual "drive," but is necessary for the normal expression of other male-specific behaviors. However, until estrogen receptor function can be selectively disrupted in neonates, the relative effect of estradiol on neural development remains unknown.

Genetic Control of Brain Gender

Since the control of gender is cell autonomous in insects, sexual behavior has been explored from a genetic perspective. Male fruit flies recognize females based on an olfactory cue, called a contact pheromone, and males will perform a stereotyped courtship behavior when they receive this signal. The male will orient toward a female, tap her abdomen, flutter his wing in song, and place his proboscis (the mouthparts) on the female's genitals. If the female is receptive, the male will then mount her and copulate. How does the central nervous system create this complex set of behaviors? One approach to the problem is to create unusual flies, called mosaics, that have some cells that are genetically female (XX) and some cells that are genetically male (XO). By studying many of these animals, each one with a unique mosaic, it is possible to determine which brain cells must be male in order for male or female behaviors to occur (Hall, 1977).

In more recent studies, a genetic trick has been used to construct a line of animals in which a single part of the brain is female (Fig. 10.18). A piece of DNA, called PGAL4, is randomly inserted in the genome of many flies. By chance, it will occasionally insert next to an enhancer, and this enhancer will then activate the *GAL4* gene in the enhancer trap element. If the enhancer is only active in one part of the body, then *GAL4* will be expressed in that same part

of the body. How does this help feminize the brain? It turns out that *GAL4* can activate another promotor, called *upstream activating sequence* (UAS). If an experimenter can hook up a gene of interest to the *UAS* promotor, then the gene of interest will be expressed wherever *GAL4* expression occurs. This enhancer trap system was used to express the *transformer* gene, a feminizing signal, in olfactory neurons that might be processing the pheromonal signal (Ferveur *et al.,* 1995).

Transformed males were presented with flies of either sex to see whether they would selectively court the female. Surprisingly, some strains of flies courted males with as much vigor as they did females (Fig. 10.18). The behavior of transformed animals may be due to their failure in discriminating the female pheromone. In fact, when the enhancer trap technique is used to make male flies that secrete only female pheromones, these flies are courted as if they are females (Ferveur *et al.,* 1997). Thus, in flies, specific brain regions must have a gender if animals are to accurately interpret sensory information and produce sexually appropriate motor responses.

A separate tack has been to explore what kinds of genes must be expressed in male or female nerve cells in order for correct sexual behaviors to be produced (Hall, 1994). For example, a gene product called *fruitless* is expressed in about 500 neurons of male flies only, and mutations of this gene also cause males to court one another. A mutation of the *dissatisfaction* gene leads virgin females to resist males during courtship, and they fail to lay mature eggs (Finley *et al.,* 1997). Most mutations that effect sexual activity in flies are also found to effect other behaviors. Mutations of the *period* gene affect circadian rhythms, but they also change the temporal properties of the courtship song. Depending on the precise mutation, the interval between wing beats can be shorter or longer than normal. That is, the song will have a lower or higher frequency, respectively.

Despite the impressive molecular analyses in *Drosophila,* it is important to recognize that they are not genetic mating machines. Males and

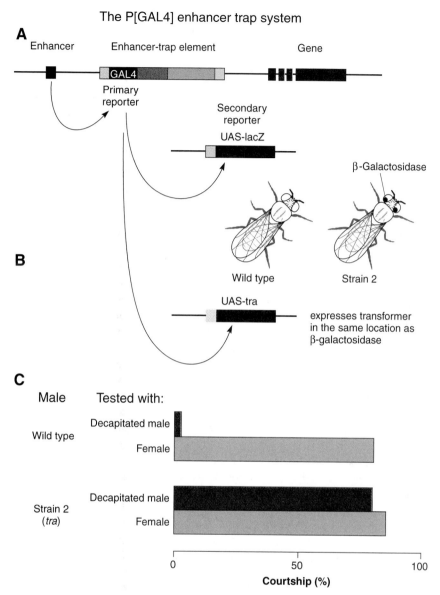

Figure 10.18 Enhancer traps and the expression of the *transformer* gene. (A) An enhancer trap element inserts into the fly genome between an enhancer region and the gene that it normally controls. Whenever the enhancer is activated by a transcription factor, a reporter gene within the enhancer trap is expressed. In this example, a yeast transcription factor called *GAL4* gene is expressed. To visualize the anatomical location of *GAL4* expression, the enhancer trap flies are crossed to flies that have a *UAS-lacZ* gene. Since *GAL4* is a transcription factor that activates *UAS*, the *lacZ* gene is expressed and it encodes a protein (β-galactosidase) that can be stained for. Thus, labeled cells are known to have *GAL4* expression. (B) The enhancer trap line can also be used to drive the expression of native genes, such as *transformer*. Expression occurs only in cells with an activated enhancer (red). (C) When an enhancer trap line was used to express *transformer* in olfactory neurons, the male flies courted males and females equally. Normal males only court females. (Adapted from Ferveur *et al.,* 1995.)

females can modify their behavior during the first date. For example, when a male is rejected by a nonvirgin female, he will lose interest in all females for a few hours. A genetic approach to vertebrate sexual behavior is still in its early stages. Many genetics laboratories seem to have focused on difficult concepts, such as gender "identity," rather than trying to understand the building blocks of sexual drive and copulation. In this sense, the fruit fly serves as a good paradigm for future research in all species.

Singing in the Brain

One of the most striking correlations between sexual behavior and brain anatomy is found amongst several species of songbirds. Male birds attract a mate of the same species with vocalizations, or songs, that are commonly learned during juvenile development (see below). Zebra finches learn one song during the first 80 days after hatching, while canaries add new phrases to their song each breeding season. When scientists first looked at the brains of these animals, they were startled to find brain regions of remarkably different size in each sex (Nottebohm and Arnold, 1976). The sexual dimorphism occurs in brain nuclei that are known to participate in song production (RA, HVc), and these structures are much larger in males (Fig. 10.19). Furthermore, when hatchling females are treated with estradiol, they can grow up to sing almost as adeptly as male birds (Gurney and Konishi, 1980; Simpson and Vicario, 1991). In male canaries, the size of vocal control nuclei changes during the course of a single breeding season, getting larger as testosterone levels rise (Nottebohm, 1981). Hormone treatment can apparently enhance the size of brain nuclei both by increasing afferent innervation and promoting dendritic growth (Fig. 10.19).

It seems odd that females do not vocalize, if only to facilitate the mating process. In fact, female tropical wrens do sing a "duet" with the males. Furthermore, when the song repertoire of a female wren is relatively large, then the size of its song control nuclei are similar to the size of those of males (Brenowitz and Arnold, 1986).

The vocal repertoire of the *Xenopus* females is also important in guaranteeing fertilized eggs. In this species, the male mating call has been well-characterized and, like birds, there is a sexual dimorphism of both neural and muscular components related to song production (Kelley, 1997). However, a newly discovered female vocal behavior, termed rapping, is thought to trigger the entire copulatory repertoire (Tobias *et al.*, 1998). When the female frog is unreceptive it produces a ticking sound, but when it is ready to lay eggs it begins to rap. This call stimulates males to vocalize even more vigorously and to attempt copulation. It is not yet known what the neural basis of ticking and rapping is or whether the female brain becomes specialized for this behavior during development.

From Gonads to Brain?

The simple hypothesis, then, is that testosterone is secreted by the testes, and this leads to a masculinized nervous system in male animals. A number of observations in birds and frogs suggest that other factors are involved (Wade and Arnold, 1996; Kelley, 1997). They raise the possibility that female and male brains differ from one another even in the absence of gonadal signals. First, the level of estradiol required to masculinize the nervous system of female birds is quite high, and even these high levels do not result in a fully masculinized phenotype. In frogs, the level of circulating androgen is quite similar in male and female animals during development. Second, it has not been possible to block masculine development of the nervous system in male birds by manipulations designed to decrease estrogen. Third, when genetic female zebra finches are pharmacologically engineered to develop with testes, and with little to no ovarian tissue, their vocal control nuclei continue to have a female phenotype (Fig. 10.19). Finally, female frogs that receive transplanted testes have a larger larynx and more laryngeal motor neurons than do females that are treated with a single androgen (Watson *et al.*, 1993).

These results suggest either that the gonads are a more complicated endocrine organ than we

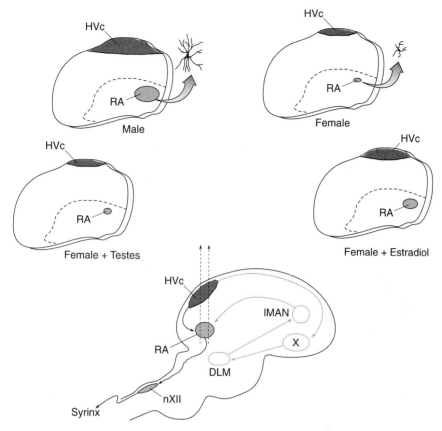

Figure 10.19 Sexual dimorphism in song production nuclei in birds. A sagittal section through the brain of songbirds shows major nuclei involved in the learning and production of vocalizations. The pathway from HVc to RA to nXII is the primary output pathway to the song production apparatus. Both HVc and RA are much larger in adult male birds (top left) compared to adult females (top right). In addition, neurons in the male RA nucleus have a more elaborate dendritic architecture compared to that in females. Female zebra finches can be engineered to develop with testes and little ovarian tissue, yet their HVc and RA nuclei do not become larger (bottom left). In contrast, when female birds are treated with estradiol during development, the HVc and RA nuclei do become masculinized. (Adapted from Schlinger, with permission, from the Annual Review of Physiology, Volume 61, © 1998, by Annual Reviews, http://www.AnnualReviews.org.)

suspect or that the nervous system contains intrinsic signals that bias its development in the absence of gonadal signals. For example, some rat diencephalic neurons express a sex-specific phenotype *in vitro* (Fig. 10.20). When explanted at E14–17, before the initial surge of testosterone, tyrosine hydroxylase-expressing neurons are 30% larger in male neurons, and the number of prolactin-expressing neurons is two to three times greater in female tissue, similar to adult animals (Kolbinger *et al.,* 1991; Beyer *et al.,* 1992). Therefore, it appears that the vertebrate

nervous system may also develop some sex characteristics independent of the gonads. In fact, the *SRY* gene is transcribed in the hypothalamus and midbrain of adult male mice, suggesting that these cells may be masculinized by a genetic signal.

Learning to Remember

Learning is often portrayed as an extension of neural development, and there are many

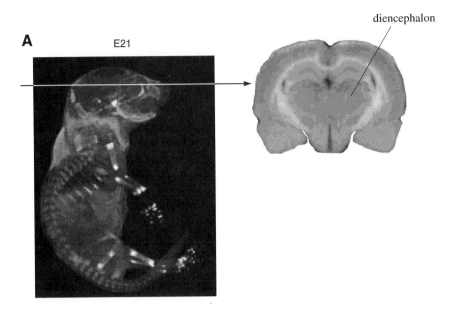

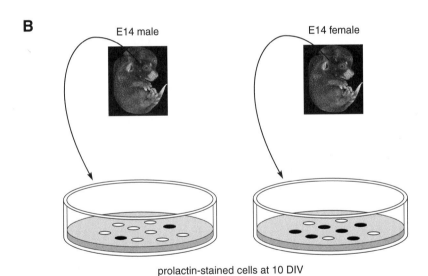

prolactin-stained cells at 10 DIV

Figure 10.20 Development of sexual dimorphism before gonadal development. (A) An image of a rat embryo at Embryonic Day 21 and a transverse section through the diencephalon. (B) When rat diencephalic neurons were explanted at Embryonic Day 14, the neurons from female embryos had two to three times more prolactin-expressing neurons (red) than males. (Adapted from Beyer *et al.,* 1992.)

similarities, particularly at the cellular level (see Box: Remaining Flexible in Chapter 9). But this portrait does not capture an important truth: learning and memory, themselves, change dur-

ing the course of development. Some forms of learning emerge during a limited period of development and then disappear. The filial imprinting of a baby duckling on its mother occurs during a brief time interval after hatching. Other forms of learning are robust in young animals, but gradually become less efficient. Humans retain the capacity to learn new vocabulary words throughout life, but there is a window of development when we learn words at a remarkable rate. Still other forms of learning seem to improve with time, perhaps due to the wealth of information already stored in a mature nervous system.

Memory is usually divided into two general types: recollection of facts (things that can be stated, or declarative memory) and recollection of skills (things that can be performed, or procedural memory). Humans with focal brain injuries are often found to have specific learning and memory deficits (Milner *et al.,* 1998). For example, people with extensive damage to the limbic system are completely unable to recall new facts, yet they can learn and remember new motor tasks. Exceptionally rapid learning or memorization has sometimes been mistaken for intelligence. In fact, human brilliance is often specialized: a knack for game theory coupled to rapid learning of spacial patterns might allow one person to be a champion bridge player, while a taste for chewing tobacco coupled to robust motor learning can produce a major league pitcher. Therefore, it is not too surprising that clinical measures of learning and memory are often difficult to reconcile with the broad patterns of human behavior.

The development of learning may also require a certain amount of practice, similar to many sensory and motor skills. For example, many animals build up a supply of provisions by hiding food in different locations. Of course, their spatial memory for the hiding places is crucial if they are to enjoy the fruits of their labor. When marsh tits are reared in captivity, they will continue to hide the sunflower seeds that they are fed. However, if the birds are given powdered seeds that can not be stored, they develop a smaller hippocampus (Clayton and Krebs, 1994). Thus, learning and memory skills require practice and this process may influence nervous system development. Since our immediate goal is to relate nervous system development to behavior, the following discussion focuses on reasonably simple forms of learning and procedural memory.

Where's Mamma?

Many vertebrates are born with an ability to obtain food and warmth from their mother, when offered. Nestling herring gulls peck at the tip of their mother's beak for food, neonatal rodents assume a specific position in order to suckle at a nipple, and newly hatched jewel fish have a natural tendency to approach objects that are colored like the broody adult. While these innate motor behaviors are very sophisticated in the apparent absence of any experience, many animals learn to recognize and respond selectively to their mother (Lorenz, 1937). Konrad Lorenz, a corecipient of the 1973 Nobel prize, made the rather dramatic observation that hatchling ducks and geese will follow the first moving object that they see, forming a very stable attachment. Ordinarily, the mother goose fills this role, but hatchlings can also learn to follow inanimate objects, and even the experimenter himself. This learned behavior is termed filial imprinting. While filial imprinting has the immediate advantage of keeping offspring with the provider, it can also have implications much later in life. When mature, the male birds will court a member of the species on which they imprinted, whether it is a bird, a dog, or a human.

Filial imprinting is not unique to birds. Tree shrew pups will imprint on the nursing mother during the second postnatal week. If removed from the nest during this period, a pup will not learn to follow its real mother, and it can be induced to follow a cloth permeated with the odor of a foster mother (Zippelius, 1972). Similarly, rat pups come to prefer their nest based on the mother's odor during the first few postnatal weeks, and this preference can be modified by providing a novel odorant during this period (Brunjes and Alberts, 1979). Newborn humans also display a preference for their mother. When infants are able to elicit either their mother's voice or the voice of another female by the rate at which they suck on a nipple, they preferentially activate their mother's voice (DeCasper and Fifer, 1980). What is the evidence that this preference is learned? When mothers read a story aloud during the last 6 weeks of pregnancy, their babies will subsequently prefer to hear that story over one that was not read aloud. Unexposed newborns display no preference between the two stories. Thus, even though an infant's hearing is quite limited *in utero,* he may already be forming certain auditory preferences (DeCasper and Spence, 1986).

What exactly is the nervous system learning during filial imprinting? Do infant animals simply learn their mother's smell or image? These questions have been explored in newly hatched ducklings, and the results suggest that several factors are necessary for filial imprinting to occur: visual cues, auditory cues, and social environment. When 1-day-old mallard ducklings are allowed to follow a stuffed mallard hen for 30 min, they develop a preference for this replica, presumably based on its visual appearance (Johnston and Gottlieb, 1981). However, mother ducks also produce an "assembly" vocalization, and this auditory cue maintains filial imprinting as the ducklings begin to grow. The assembly call is such a powerful signal that ducklings will preferentially follow an unfamiliar red-and-white striped box that is producing this call rather than a familiar mallard hen model.

Why is the mother's assembly call such a powerful cue? One possibility is that the mother's call is necessary to maintain her duckling's attachment when the entire family leaves the nest and begins to move about the environment. In fact, older ducklings become very attached to their siblings as they grow, and this "peer imprinting" can actually interfere with filial imprinting (Dyer *et al.,* 1989). For example, socially reared ducklings will not preferentially follow a silent, familiar mallard model, although individually reared ducklings will do so. However, the mallard maternal call will induce socially reared ducklings to follow a familiar mallard or an unfamiliar pintail model (Dyer and Gottlieb, 1990).

This raises an important question: Do ducklings respond innately to their mother's call or does their response depend on sensory experi-

ence? Interestingly, ducklings have an inborn preference for the mother's call rate, 4 notes/s. However, to maintain preference through hatching, the duckling must either hear its own "contentment" call or that of its siblings (Fig. 10.21). When ducklings are devocalized and reared in isolation with a contentment call that is slowed down to about 2 notes/s, they subsequently show no preference for the mothers assembly call (Gottlieb, 1980). Thus, imprinting is a far more elegant form of learning than was orginally suspected. Although ducks, geese, and chicks can visually imprint on an object after walking behind it, many other factors regulate this learning. By studying the animal in its natural setting, it becomes clear that developing animals are "prepared" to learn certain cues they will likely encounter, such as the vocalization of their siblings.

Fear and Loathing

Beyond the procurement of food and water, most animals need behavioral mechanisms to avoid danger, such as a poisonous plant or a predator. In fact, animals are born with the innate ability to avoid certain things. For example, several species of birds will run from a black hawk-shaped silhouette that is moved over their heads. This occurs even when the birds are reared in isolation with no chance to learn that the "hawk" image represents danger (Tinbergen, 1948). Many other dangers are not recognized at first, and animals must learn to avoid these stituations through some sort of experience. A well-studied form of learning, called fear conditioning, is probably responsible for much of our skill at avoiding danger. During fear conditioning, an animal learns to associate an unconditioned stimulus and response (e.g., a snake bite and the pain or fear it produces) with a neutral stimulus (e.g., the image of a snake). Obviously, an image of a snake can do no harm, but the animal has learned that if he sees a snake he may be bitten. Thus, the sight of a snake becomes a conditioned stimulus, and it produces a conditioned response (e.g., freezing). Although unethical by modern standards, a 9-month baby with no fear of animals was trained to fear rab-

Rearing

Testing

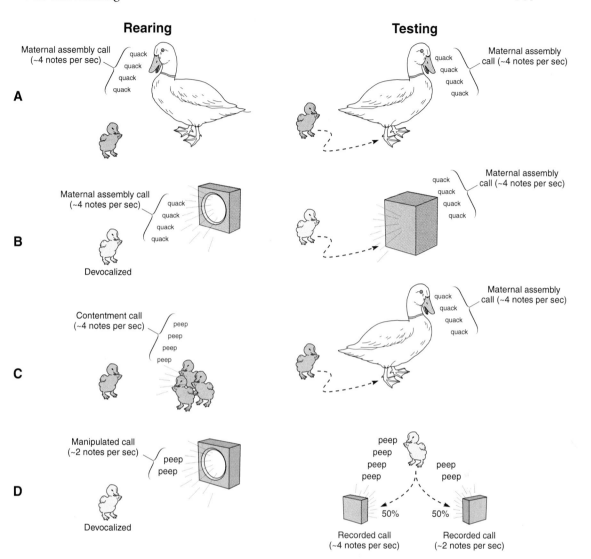

A

Maternal assembly call (~4 notes per sec)

quack
quack
quack
quack

quack
quack
quack
quack

Maternal assembly call (~4 notes per sec)

B

Maternal assembly call (~4 notes per sec)

quack
quack
quack
quack

Devocalized

quack
quack
quack
quack

Maternal assembly call (~4 notes per sec)

C

Contentment call (~4 notes per sec)

peep
peep
peep
peep

quack
quack
quack
quack

Maternal assembly call (~4 notes per sec)

D

Manipulated call (~2 notes per sec)

peep
peep

Devocalized

peep
peep
peep
peep

peep
peep

50%   50%

Recorded call (~4 notes per sec)

Recorded call (~2 notes per sec)

Figure 10.21 Maternal imprinting in ducklings. (A) When ducklings are exposed to the maternal vocalization (~4 notes/s), they will subsequently approach an assembly call (~4 notes/s). (B) Exposure to the assembly call alone is sufficient to promote auditory imprinting. (C) Exposure to the duckling's own contentment call, which is also ~4 notes/s, is sufficient to promote auditory imprinting. (D) When a duckling is exposed to an unnatural call (2 notes/s) during development, it is not able to recognize and respond to the assembly call when tested subsequently. (Adapted from Gottlieb, 1980.)

bits by pairing the rabbit with a startling noise (a hammer striking metal just behind the baby's head). This conditioning eventually caused the baby to cry every time he saw a rabbit (Watson and Raynor, 1920).

In a typical fear conditioning experiment, an animal is exposed to a frightening stimulus such as a mild foot shock and at the same time a pure tone is presented from a speaker. How do we know that the electric shock is frightening? Animals usually stop moving (i.e., they freeze) and their blood pressure goes up when they are in frightening situations, and this is precisely the response to mild foot shock. In contrast, the pure tone alone does not produce a change in movement or blood pressure. By presenting these stimuli together several times, the sound alone is able to elicit a "fear" response. Are developing animals able to form such associations? Actually, it seems to depend on the stimulus that the animal is asked to learn as well as the behavior that it is asked to perform. For example, rats pups at 15 days or older can learn to freeze in response to a tone that was paired previously with mild foot shock (Moye and Rudy, 1987).

For many learning tasks, animals improve with age. This was explored in rats by first pairing a brief loud sound that elicited a startle response (see Acute Hearing) with a long-lasting pure tone at moderate intensity (Fig. 10.22). Adult animals learn quickly that the pure tone predicts the arrival of the loud sound. During test trials they produce a much larger startle response when the pure tone is present, and this is referred to as fear-potentiated startle. Thus, if the pure tone enhances the startle response, then one concludes that the animal learned about a dangerous situation. When 16-day rat pups are trained in the same paradigm, they do not show any sign of learning (Hunt *et al.*, 1994). Their response to the tone plus noise is nearly identical to their response to noise alone (Fig. 10.22). For some learning tasks, neonates perform better than juvenile animals. Rat pups of 5–10 days can learn to avoid a sugar solution when it is paired with mild foot shock, yet 15-day pups fail to learn this task (Hoffmann and Spear, 1988). Thus, learning is not simply poor in young animals and robust in adults. Rather, it is a complex function of age, sensory modality, and the motor response that is being modified by training.

Even extremely simple forms of learning, such as habituation and sensitization, can emerge at different times during development. This has been studied at the level of both behavior and neurophysiology in the sea slug *Aplysia* (Rayport and Camardo, 1984; Rankin and Carew, 1988; Nolen and Carew, 1988). During habituation, animals produce a smaller reflexive response when they are exposed to repeated presentations of an identical stimulus. This form of learning can be demonstrated by squirting some seawater on the animal's siphon while monitoring its contraction. With each squirt of water the siphon withdrawal decreases, finally reaching about 30% of its initial amplitude. When stimulation ceases, the response gradually recovers over a few hours. Habituation can be observed in 5- to 10-day *Aplysia*, before most central neurons are born. However, the stimuli must be delivered with much shorter intervals to produce habituation in young animals. Consistent with these behavioral results, synaptic potentials that mediate the response decrease in size with repeated use in neurons from 5- to 10-day animals.

Do other simple forms of learning appear this early? This was assessed for sensitization, a form of nonassociative learning in which an animal produces a larger reflexive response when it is preceded by a strong, usually noxious stimulus. For example, when an electric shock is delivered to the tail, the same squirt of seawater evokes a much larger siphon withdrawal response. Sensitization was found to emerge quite late in development, almost 60 days after the appearance of habituation. Once again, a neural analog of sensitization was first observed at roughly the same time as the behavior. In adult animals, stimuli to the siphon nerve produce synaptic potentials in a neuron called R2, and the size of these synaptic potentials can be increased by delivering stimuli to the nerve emanating from the tail. However, this synaptic facilitation is observed only in animals >70 days. Thus, there is some reason to believe that specific forms of learning emerge at distinct periods of development due to the maturation of explicit neural mechanisms.

Complex Tasks

Studies that target simple forms of learning will be critical for linking behavior with underlying neural mechanisms. However, it is also interesting to ask how developing animals learn complex, multistep tasks, such as how to write a sentence or make a peanut butter sandwich. Of course, even sophisticated learning tasks are studied with a formal paradigm. For example, in

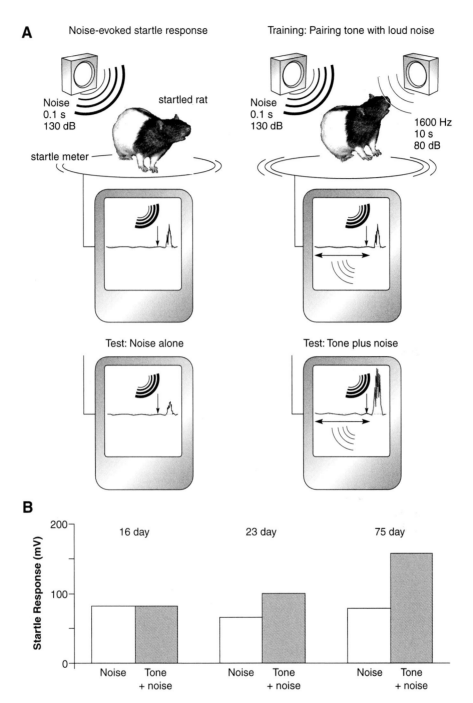

Figure 10.22 Emergence of fear-potentiated startle. (A) When rats are exposed to a loud sound, they make a sudden movement, called a startle response (left). This can be recorded by a platform on which the animal stands and it can be displayed on an oscilloscope. When a pure tone precedes the loud noise, the rats learn that the tone predicts the noise burst (right). In subsequent tests, they give a larger startle response to the paired tone plus noise, and this is called fear-potentiated startle. (B) When trained in this paradigm, 16-day rat pups display no potentiation, indicating that they have not learned to associate the two signals. At 23 days, the animals do display a potentiation due to pairing, although the potentiation displayed by adults is greater still. (Adapted from Hunt *et al.*, with permission. Copyright © 1994 by the American Psychological Association.)

a delayed nonmatch to sample task, a primate is first shown an object that can be moved to reveal a reward, such as a food pellet (Bachevalier, 1990). After a delay, the animal is next presented with two objects, one of which it saw previously. In this case, the animal must move the new object in order to obtain the reward (Fig. 10.23). The task can be made more complicated by in-

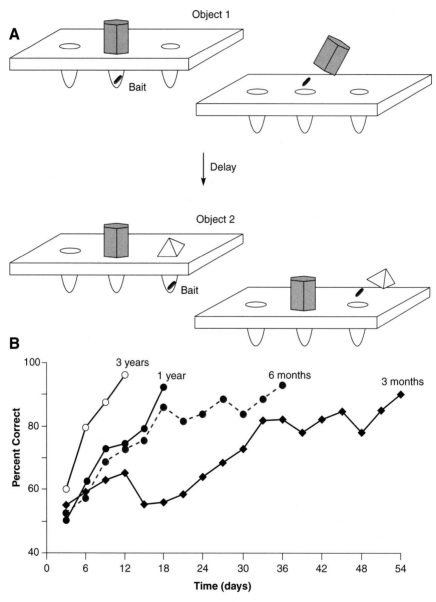

Figure 10.23 Development of memory in primates. (A) The delayed nonmatch to sample task involves remembering the object presented first and, after a delay, choosing the new object on a test trial. (B) The time to learn this task is shown for primates of different ages. At 2–3 years of age, animals learned the task within 8 days of training. However, 3-month-old monkeys did not reach criterion (90% correct responses) until they had received 36 days of training. (Adapted from Bachevalier, 1990, with permission.)

creasing the time between trials or by increasing the number of objects that must be memorized. Infant and adult primates were trained on a daily basis until they could perform the task correctly 90% of the time. Animal of 2–3 years of age reached criterion after 8 days of training, but 3-month-old monkeys required 36 days of training (Fig. 10.23). One possible limitiation for younger animals may be the amount of sensory activity entering the central nervous system (Bachevalier *et al.,* 1990). In 3-month animals, visually evoked activity is significantly lower in regions of the cortex thought to mediate this form of learning, as measured with the 2-deoxyglucose technique (see Box: Watching Neurons Think in Chapter 9).

When humans of different ages were challenged with a similar delayed nonmatch to sample task, they also displayed a gradual improvement with age (Overman, 1990). Yet children nearly 3 years of age take about 10 times longer to learn the task compared to adults. Furthermore, they forget things more quickly. The duration of time that children can retain a simple associative learning task gradually increases from 2 to 18 months of age (Hartshorn *et al.,* 1998). Complex learning tasks also emerge at different periods of development. As discussed above, memory is commonly divided into recollection of facts versus performance of skills. One type of factual ability is the recollection of the spacial environment. Spacial memory was tested in 2- and 4-year-old children by asking them to retrieve candy from eight different locations in an unfamiliar room. It was found that 2-year-olds revisited locations where they had already procured the candy more often than did 4-year-olds. That is, the younger subjects did not remember where they had been. In a different type of factual learning, children were asked to recall details of a story that they had been read and there was significant improvement between 5 and 10 years of age. Finally, children were asked to learn a complex motor task (i.e., a skill), and their performance was equivalent at 5 and 10 years of age (Foreman *et al.,* 1984; Hömberg *et al.,* 1993). These studies point out the diversity of complex associative learning. Presumably, the improvements that are observed with age result from the maturation of sensory function, motor skills, and learning and memory systems, themselves.

Getting Information from One Brain to Another

The development of animal communication is a fascinating mix of inherited traits and learning. For many of us animals, communication provides the foundation of our existence. Some might say that it forms the basis of our consciousness. Depending on our position in the food chain, it fetches us a mate, warns us of danger, informs of a food source, bonds us in society, and enriches us with artistry. Perhaps the best-studied communication system is that of songbirds, where adult males produce courtship vocalizations to attract conspecific females. While sex-specific behavior is explained in terms of genetic and epigenetic factors (above), the individual songs require learning and practice. When juvenile birds are reared in isolation such that they do not hear a normal adult song, they develop abnormal vocalizations. Yet the songs do contain some elements that are typical for the species.

When swamp sparrows or song sparrows are deafened at about 20 days after hatching, they produce extremely degraded vocalizations (Marler and Sherman, 1983). Yet these vocalizations still retain a few species-specific characteristics, such as song duration. Even relatively boring vocalizations such as the crow of a rooster may be affected by sensory experience. When a middle ear muscle is detached early in development, male chickens crow at a higher frequency than control animals, possibly because low-frequency sounds can no longer be dampled by the middle ear mechanism (Grassi *et al.,* 1990). These studies illustrate the role of learning, but suggest that there are intrinsic limitations on the song that any single species of bird is able to acquire.

More recently, scientists have settled on the zebra finch as a model for studies of song behavior and nervous system development. Juvenile birds leave the nest about 20 days after hatching and they begin to sing a few days later. As with sparrows, male zebra finches must be exposed to the species-specific song, and they must be able to hear themselves sing if they are to produce an accurate rendition as adults. When males reach about 90 days of age, they produce a stereotyped song that remains unchanged throughout life, providing they continue to hear themselves sing. Lesions of the vocal control nuclei, HVc or RA, have a devastating effect on song production in adults (Nottebohm and Arnold, *et al.,* 1976).

There is a second pathway from HVc to the anterior telencephalon, and this projection has been implicated in song learning. One indication of this special role in learning comes from the anatomy of the system (Herrmann and Arnold, 1991; Johnson *et al.,* 1995). The size of one of these telencephalic nuclei, IMAN, increases when birds first start to practice their tutor's song, and it eventually decreases in adulthood. The projection from IMAN to the motor output from the telencephalon, RA, is also greatest during the early stages of learning. Since degenerating nerve terminals can be stained within a few days of lesion, IMAN was lesioned at three different posthatch ages and the number of degenerating synapses within RA was assessed. The technique showed that the number of IMAN synapses decreases almost threefold during development (Fig. 10.24). The number of IMAN neurons that project to RA remains constant during this period, suggesting that terminals are being eliminated.

Interestingly, lesions to IMAN have no effect on song production in adult birds (Fig. 10.24). However, when IMAN is lesioned in animals before song learning has been completed, song learning and production are disrupted (Bottjer *et al.,* 1984). Together, these experiments suggest that certain nuclei participate in the learning of song, but not in its adult production. Does IMAN really play such a limited role in zebra finch behavior? One possibility is that IMAN participates in song recognition by adult females. Lesions of HVc are known to disrupt song recognition such that the females perform a precopulatory behavior in response to the song of another species (Brenowitz, 1991).

However, the role of IMAN in adult birds remains a small mystery.

Since IMAN seems to be essential for song learning, it would be interesting to know whether the cellular mechanisms are similar to other forms of plasticity. As discussed earlier, the NMDA receptor has a well-documented role in many forms of synaptic plasticity (see Chapter 9). In fact, the level of NMDA receptor expression is particularly high in IMAN during the period of song learning (Fig. 10.25). When tissue sections are labeled with an NMDA receptor antagonist (^{3}H-labeled MK-801), autoradiographic analysis shows that receptor number gradually declines over the first few months (Aamodt *et al.,* 1995). To test whether these receptors mediate song learning, the NMDA receptor antagonist AP5 was infused bilaterally into IMAN (Fig. 10.25). Beginning on Day 32, animals were presented with a tutor song every other day, and AP5 was infused either at the same time or on alternate days. Those animals receiving AP5 and training simultaneously performed very poorly at Day 90, only producing 20% of the tutor song. In contrast, the animals that had active NMDA receptors while receiving auditory training learned about 50% of the tutor song (Basham *et al.,* 1996). It is not yet known how AP5 affects synaptic activity in IMAN, but these results suggest that song learning in zebra finches shares one mechanism of synaptic plasticity with other forms of plasticity.

Language

Although human communication is far more complicated than bird song, there are some similarities. Learning is certainly involved at every stage of development, from the production and perception of vowels to the syntax of a sentence. Humans generally speak their first words between 9 and 12 months and slowly acquire about 50 single words, mostly nouns, over the next 8 months. As with birds, there is a period of development when communication skills are acquired most efficiently. From 2 to 6 years of age, children learn about 8 words per day. One indication

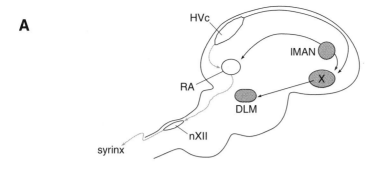

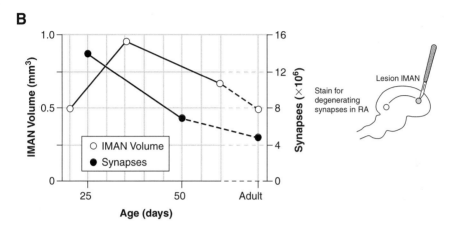

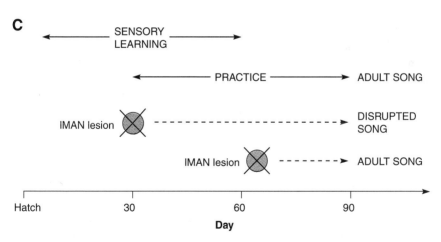

Figure 10.24 Song learning in birds. (A) The sagittal section through the songbird brain shows the major nuclei involved in song learning and production. (B) The projection from IMAN to RA was assessed by lesioning IMAN, waiting a day for the synapses to begin degenerating, and then staining the tissue degeneration. Thus, the greater the staining, the greater the innervation. The number of synapses begins to decline after Day 25. For comparison, the size of IMAN is plotted, and it also begins to decline after Day 35. (C) The telencephalic nucleus, IMAN, has been implicated in song learning by lesioning it at different ages. If lesioned at 30 days during sensory learning, the ability to produce song as an adult is disrupted. If IMAN is lesioned at around 60 days, then adult song is unaffected. (Adapted from Bottjer *et al.,* 1984; Herrmann and Arnold, 1991, with permission.)

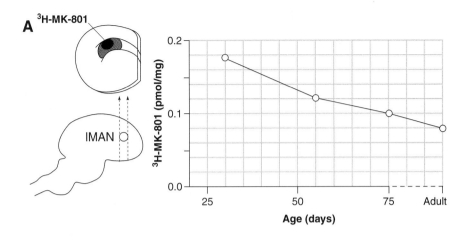

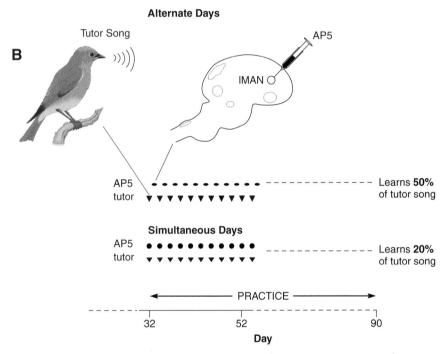

Figure 10.25 NMDA receptors are implicated in song learning. (A) The number of NMDA receptors was assessed by measuring the amount of a receptor antagonist (³H-labeled MK-801) that bound to IMAN during development. NMDA receptors began to decrease after Day 30. (B) The influence of NMDA receptors on song learning was tested by injecting an antagonist (AP5) into IMAN while the bird was being exposed to a tutor song. In control experiments, AP5 was injected on days when the birds were not exposed to the tutor song. When AP5 and exposure to tutor song were delivered simultaneously, the birds performed more poorly as adults, only producing 20% of the tutor song. (Adapted from Aamodt *et al.,* Early isolation from conspecific song does not affect the normal developmental decline of N-methyl-D-aspartate receptor binding in an avian song nucleus, *J. Neurobiol.,* Copyright © 1995. By permission of John Wiley & Sons, Inc.; Basham *et al.,* 1996.)

of a sensitive period for language development comes from studies of humans who learn to produce and understand a second language. When English language skills were analyzed in native Korean or Chinese speakers who arrived in the United States as children or adults, the youngest subjects performed best (Johnson and Newport, 1989). A second indication of a sensitive period comes from studies of deaf individuals who were exposed to sign language from birth to 1 year of age. Those individuals who are exposed to sign language from birth are more skilled than infants who are exposed even as early as 6 months of age (Newport, 1990).

In contrast to bird song, human communication is performed with equal precision in three sensory modilies. Those born with profound hearing loss can learn to communicate perfectly with their hands and visual system using sign language. Those born without sight can learn

to read with their somatosensory system using Braille. Furthermore, the development of language seems to be quite natural in any of these modalities. It has been known for some time that hearing infants begin to produce speech sounds well before they can understand words. These vocalizations, called "vocal babbling," are commonly made up of repeated syllables (e.g., da-dadada). Whereas deaf children are unable to produce perfect vocalizations as adults, similar to deafened songbirds, a remarkable thing happens: their language ability can be transferred to another sensory modality.

Early stages of language acquisition were studied in two infants who were deaf from birth, but were continually exposed to American Sign Language (ASL) by their deaf parents (Petitto and Marentette, 1991). To determine whether the infants would "babble" with their hands, the manual activity of each infant was codified in

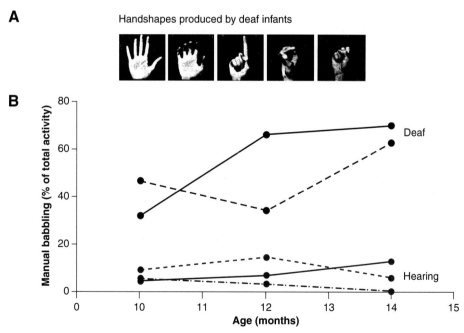

Figure 10.26 Manual communication by infants. (A) The hand signals produced by deaf infants were studied and codified in order to detect hand shapes that correspond to American Sign Language (ASL). (B) Deaf infants (black lines) produced hand shapes corresponding to ASL (manual babbling) more often than hearing infants (red lines) of the same age. (Adapted from Petitto and Marentette, 1991.)

some detail, and their production of ASL hand-shapes was analyzed (Fig. 10.26). Deaf children devote about 50% of their manual activity to ASL handshapes, while hearing children only produce about 10% of this activity, presumably by chance. Interestingly, the disparity between deaf and hearing children increases from 10 to 14 months of age, suggesting that deaf children learn language at the same stage of development as hearing children when given the opportunity to use their visual system. Finally, 98% of the manual babbling was performed in front of the body, presumably within the infant's visual field. Thus, imitation of a "tutor" and sensory feedback are important when learning to "speak" with ones hands, in general agreement with studies of bird song development.

Given the complexity of language, it is not surprising that we are only beginning to understand the neural mechanisms that support human communication and how it develops. The ability of infants from two countries to recognize their native vowel sounds was studied to find out whether early experience affects perception. Six-month-old infants from Sweden and the United States were asked to judge two vowel sounds, one from their own country and one from the other country (Kuhl *et al.,* 1992). The English vowel was a /i/ sound, as in the word "fee." The Swedish vowel was a front rounded vowel /y/ sound, as in the Swedish word "fy." Vowel sounds are composed of a unique set of frequencies, called formants, and the /i/ sound has slightly higher formants than the /y/ sound (Fig. 10.27). Most adult English speaking listeners can categorize a sound as being like a /i/ sound if the first and second formants are reasonably close to the ideal. This ability to generalize is thought to prevent confusion since individual voice quality varies a good deal, particularly between children, adult females, and adult males. To see whether infants are able to categorize vowel sounds, ideal /i/ and /y/ vowels, called prototypes, were generated, and slight variations were made to formant frequencies in order to produce variants (Fig. 10.27). Do infants treat the variants as a member of the group, as adults do? Infants were first exposed to the prototype vowel and then presented with a variant. If the infants perceived the variant to be different than the prototype, the infants were trained to turn their heads. The data show that American infants are more likely to treat variants of /i/ as a member of that group, but are less likely to treat variants of /y/ as members of that group. The opposite result is found for Swedish infants. These results suggest that experience with ones own language in the first 6 months of life allows for improved perception of unique speech sounds.

Summary

The great strides in molecular and cellular neurobiology have underscored the importance of revisiting behavioral research in animals, particularly during development. The maturation of neural processing, or the ability of a neuron to respond accurately to its synaptic inputs, clearly depends on all the building blocks being in place. What can be gained from studying the system as a whole? If we learn the alphabet, are we not automatically able to understand sentences? Of course, the blemish in this logic is simple to grasp: systems of molecules, or systems of nerve cells, take on new properties that were not expressed by the single molecule or nerve cell. While the genetic dissection of behavior is an important strategy, it should also be recognized that multiple gene products inevitably contribute to each phenotype, including behavior. Furthermore, the expression of many genes is influenced by the environment (i.e., neuronal activity). Therefore, a rich understanding of the relationship between brain and behavior is fundamental to interpreting all results. Studying animal behavior is one of the best ways to measure the properties of a system of nerve cells. It provides the most sensitive and universal indicator of a successfully assembled nervous system. All types of developmental errors (i.e., inappropriate fate, ion channel mutations, pathfinding errors, weak synapses) will affect the computational abilities of individual neurons. This is precisely why behavioral measures

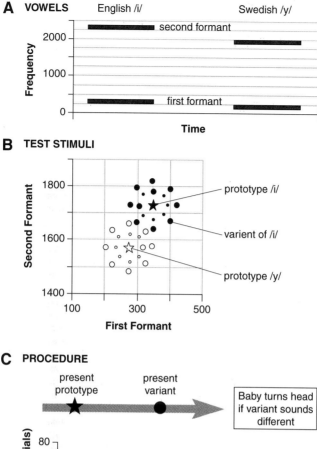

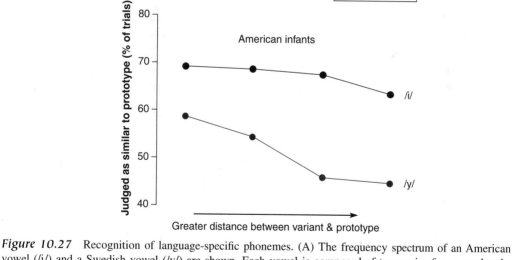

Figure 10.27 Recognition of language-specific phonemes. (A) The frequency spectrum of an American vowel (/i/) and a Swedish vowel (/y/) are shown. Each vowel is composed of two major frequency bands, called formants. (B) The ability of American and Swedish infants to recognize their native vowel sounds was examined with a range of computer-generated stimuli. An "ideal" version of each vowel, called a prototype, was produced, along with vowels with small changes to one of the formant frequencies (called variants). (C) Infants were trained to turned their head if the second of the two vowels sounded different than the first. The data for American infants show that their native /i/ sound can be recognized even when formant frequency changes a good deal. However, the same frequency changes for the Swedish /y/ led to decreased recognition. (Adapted from Kuhl *et al.*, 1992, Linguistic experience alters phonetic perception in infants by 6 months of age, *Science* **255**: 606–608, with permission.)

have long been used to tell clinicians when the nervous system is broken (e.g., schizophrenia, sleep apnea, delayed learning). It will, therefore, not be too great of a surprise when behavioral analyses reemerge this century as one of the most powerful tools available to developmental neuroscientists.

REFERENCES

Aamodt, S. M., Nordeen, E. J., and Nordeen, K. W. (1995). Early isolation from conspecific song does not affect the normal developmental decline of *N*-methyl-D-aspartate receptor binding in an avian song nucleus. *J. Neurobiol.* **27:** 76–84.

Acampora, D., Mazan, S., *et al.* (1995). Forebrain and midbrain regions are deleted in Otx2-/- mutants due to a defective anterior neuroectoderm specification during gastrulation. *Development* **121:** 3279–3290.

Adams, R. H., Sato, K., Shimada, S., Tohyama, M., Puschel, A. W., and Betz, H. (1995). Gene structure and glial expression of the glycine transporter GlyT1 embryonic and adult rodents. *J. Neurosci.* **15:** 2524–2532.

Agmon, A., Hollrigel, G., and O'Dowd, D. K. (1996). Functional GABAergic synaptic connection in neonatal mouse barrel cortex. *J. Neurosci.* **16:** 4684–4695.

Aguayo, A. J., Bray, G. M., Rasminsky, M., Zwimpfer, T., Carter, D., and Vidal-Sanz, M. (1990). Synaptic connections made by axons regenerating in the central nervous system of adult mammals. *J. Exp. Biol.* **153:** 199–224.

Allendoerfer, K. L., and Shatz, C. J. (1994). The subplate, a transient neocortical structure: its role in the development of connections between thalamus and cortex. *Annu. Rev. Neurosci.* **17:** 185–218.

Alonso, M. C., and Cabrera, C. V. (1988). The achaete–scute gene complex of *Drosophila melanogaster* comprises four homologous genes. *EMBO J.* **7:** 2585–2591.

Altman, J. (1969). Postnatal Neurogenesis and the Problem of Neural Plasticity. *In* "Developmental Neurobiology" (W. Himwich, Ed.). Charles Thomas, Springfield, IL.

Altman, J. (1972). Postnatal development of the cerebellar cortex in the rat. II. Phases in the maturation of Purkinje cells and of the molecular layer. *J. Comp. Neurol.* **145:** 399–463.

Altman, J., and Bayer, S. A. (1985). Embryonic development of the rat cerebellum. I. Delineation of the cerebellar primordium and early cell movements. *J. Comp. Neurol.* **231:** 1–26.

Alvarado-Mallart, R. M. (1993). Fate and potentialities of the avian mesencephalic/metencephalic neuroepithelium. *J. Neurobiol.* **24:** 1341–1355.

Alzheimer, C., Schwindt, P. C., and Crill, W. E. (1993). Postnatal development of a persistent Na$^+$ current in pyramidal neurons from rat sensorimotor cortex. *J. Neurophysiol.* **69:** 290–292.

Amati, B., and Land, H. (1994). Myc–Max–Mad: A transcription factor network controlling cell cycle progression, differentiation and death. *Curr. Opin. Genet. Dev.* **4:** 102–108.

Anchan, R. M., and Reh, T. A. (1995). Transforming growth factor-beta-3 is mitogenic for rat retinal progenitor cells in vitro. *J. Neurobiol.* **28:** 133–145.

Anchan, R. M., Reh, T. A., Angello, J., Balliet, A., and Walker, M. (1991). EGF and TGF-alpha stimulate retinal neuroepithelial cell proliferation in vitro. *Neuron* **6:** 923–936.

Anderson, D. J. (1997). Cellular and molecular biology of neural crest cell lineage determination. *Trends Genet.* **13:** 276–280.

Anderson, H. (1985). The development of projections and connections from transplanted locust sensory neurons. *J. Embryol. Exp. Morphol.* **85:** 207–224.

Anderson, H., and Bacon, J. (1979). Developmental determination of neuronal projection patterns from wind-sensitive hairs in the locust, *Schistocerca gregaria. Dev. Biol.* **72:** 364–373.

Anderson, M. J., and Cohen, M. W. (1977). Nerve-induced and spontaneous redistribution of acetylcholine receptors on cultured muscle cells. *J. Physiol.* **268:** 757–773.

Anderson, S. A., Eisenstat, D. D., Shi, L., and Rubenstein, J. L. (1997). Interneuron migration from basal forebrain to neocortex: Dependence on Dlx genes. *Science* **278:** 474–476.

Appel, B., Korzh, V., Glasgow, E., Thor, S., Edlund, T., Dawid, I. B., and Eisen, J. S. (1995). Motoneuron fate specification revealed by patterned LIM homeobox gene expression in embryonic zebrafish. *Development* **121:** 4117–4125.

Armand, J., Edgley, S. A., Lemon, R. N., and Olivier, E. (1994). Protracted postnatal development of corticospinal projections from the primary motor cortex to hand motoneurones in the macaque monkey. *Exp. Brain Res.* **101:** 178–182.

Armstrong, R. C., Aja, T. J., Hoang, K. D., Gaur, S., Bai, X., Alnemri, E. S., Litwack, G., Karanewsky, D. S., Fritz, L. C., and Tomaselli, K. J. (1997). Activation of the CED3/ICE-related protease CPP32 in cerebellar granule neurons undergoing apoptosis but not necrosis. *J. Neurosci.* **17:** 553–562.

Axel, R. (1995). The molecular logic of smell. *Sci. Am.* **273:** 154–159.

Axelsson, J., and Thesleff, F. (1959). A study of supersensitivity in denervated mammalian skeletal muscle. *J. Physiol. (London)* **147:** 178–193.

Baccaglini, P. I., and Spitzer, N. C. (1977). Developmental changes in the inward current of the action potential of Rohon–Beard neurones. *J. Physiol.* **271:** 93–117.

Bachevalier, J. (1990). Ontogenetic development of habit and memory formation in primates. *Ann. N. Y. Acad. Sci.* **608:** 457–477.

Bagust, J., Lewis, D. M., and Westerman, R. A. (1973). Polyneuronal innervation of kitten skeletal muscle. *J. Physiol.* **229:** 241–255.

Bahr, S., and Wolff, J. R. (1985). Postnatal development of axosomatic synapses in the rat visual cortex: Morphogenesis and quantitative evaluation. *J. Comp. Neurol.* **233:** 405–420.

Baier, H., and Bonhoeffer, F. (1992). Axon guidance by gradients of a target-derived component. *Science* **255:** 472–475.

Baier, H., Klostermann, S., Trowe, T., Karlstrom, R. O., Nusslein-Volhard, C., and Bonhoeffer, F. (1996). Genetic dissection of the retinotectal projection. *Development* **123:** 415–425.

Baier, H., and Korsching, S. (1994). Olfactory glomeruli in the zebrafish form an invariant pattern and are identifiable across animals. *J. Neurosci.* **14:** 219–230.

Bailey, A. M., and Posakony, J. W. (1995). Suppressor of hairless directly activates transcription of enhancer of split complex genes in response to Notch receptor activity. *Genes Dev.* **9:** 2609–2622.

Baird, D. H., Hatten, M. E., and Mason, C. A. (1992). Cerebellar target neurons provide a stop signal for afferent neurite extension *in vitro. J. Neurosci.* **2:** 619–634.

Balaban, E. (1997). Changes in multiple brain regions underlie species differences in a complex, congenital behavior. *Proc. Natl. Acad. Sci. USA* **94:** 2001–2006.

Balice-Gordon, R. J., and Lichtman, J. W. (1993). *In vivo* observations of pre- and postsynaptic changes during the transition from multiple to single innervation at developing neuromuscular junctions. *J. Neurosci.* **13:** 834–855.

Balice-Gordon, R. J., and Lichtman, J. W. (1994). Long-term synapse loss induced by focal blockade of postsynaptic receptors. *Nature* **372:** 519–524.

Bamji, S. X., Majdan, M., Pozniak, C. D., Belliveau, D. J., Aloyz, R., Kohn, J., Causing, C. G., and Miller, F. D. (1998). The p75 neurotrophin receptor mediates neuronal apoptosis and is essential for naturally occurring sympathetic neuron death. *J. Cell. Biol.* **140:** 911–923.

Banerjee, U., and Zipursky, S. L. (1990). The role of cell–cell interaction in the development of the *Drosophila* visual system. *Neuron* **4:** 177–187.

Banker, G., and Goslin, K. (1991). Rat hippocampal neurons in low density culture. *In* "Culturing Nerve Cells." (G. Banker and K. Goslin, Eds.), pp. 251–281. MIT Press, Cambridge, MA.

Barbacid, M. (1994). The Trk family of neurotrophin receptors. *J. Neurobiol.* **25:** 1386–1403.

Bargones, J. Y., and Werner, L. A. (1994). Adults listen selectively: Infants do not. *Psychol. Sci.* **5:** 170–174.

Barish, M. E. (1986). Differentiation of voltage-gated potassium current and modulation of excitability in cultured amphibian spinal neurones. *J. Physiol.* **375:** 229–250.

Barres, B. A., Hart, I. K., Coles, H. S., Burne, J. F., Voyvodic, J. T., Richardson, W. D., and Raff, M. C. (1992). Cell death and control of cell survival in the oligodendrocyte lineage. *Cell* **70:** 31–46.

Barres, B. A., and Raff, M. C. (1994). Control of oligodendrocyte number in the developing rat optic nerve. *Neuron* **12:** 935–942.

Barres, B. A., Silverstein, B. E., Corey, D. P., and Chun, L. L. Y. (1988). Immunological, morphological, and electrophysiological variation among retinal ganglion cells purified by panning. *Neuron* **1:** 791–803.

Barrett, G. L., and Bartlett, P. F. (1994). The p75 nerve growth factor receptor mediates survival or death depending on the stage of sensory neuron development. *Proc. Natl. Acad. Sci. USA* **91:** 6501–6505.

Basham, M. E., Nordeen, E. J., and Nordeen, K. W. (1996). Blockade of NMDA receptors in the anterior forebrain impairs sensory acquisition in the zebra finch (*Poephila guttata*). *Neurobiol. Learn. Mem.* **66:** 295–304.

Bastiani, M. J., and Goodman, C. S. (1986). Guidance of neuronal growth cones in the grasshopper embryo. III. Recognition of specific glial pathways. *J. Neurosci.* **6:** 3542–3551.

Bastiani, M. J., Harrelson, A. L., Snow, P. M., and Goodman, C. S. (1987). Expression of fasciclin I and II glycoproteins on subsets of axon pathways during neuronal development in the grasshopper. *Cell* **48:** 745–755.

Bastmeyer, M., Bahr, M., and Stuermer, C. A. (1993). Fish optic nerve oligodendrocytes support axonal regeneration of fish and mammalian retinal ganglion cells. *Glia* **8:** 1–11.

Bate, M. (1998). Making sense of behavior. *Int. J. Dev. Biol.* **42:** 507–509.

Bayliss, D. A., Viana, F., Bellingham, M. C., and Berger, A. J. (1994). Characteristics and postnatal development of a hyperpolarization-activated inward current in rat hypoglossal motoneurons *in vitro*. *J. Neurophysiol.* **71:** 119–128.

Bear, M. F., and Singer, W. (1986). Modulation of visual cortical plasticity by acetylcholine and noradrenaline. *Nature* **320:** 172–176.

Beard, J. (1896). The history of a transient nervous apparatus in certain Ichthyopsida. An account of the development and degeneration of ganglion-cells and nerve fibers. *Zool Jahrbücher Abt Morphol* **9:** 1–106.

Beato, M., Herrlich, P., and Schütz, G. (1995). Steroid hormone receptors: Many actors in search of a plot. *Cell* **83:** 851–857.

Becker, C.-M., Hoch, W., and Betz, H. (1988). Glycine receptor heterogeneity in rat spinal cord during postnatal development. *EMBO J.* **7:** 3717–3726.

Beggs, H. E., Soriano, P., and Maness, P. F. (1994). NCAM-dependent neurite outgrowth is inhibited in neurons from Fyn-minus mice. *J. Cell. Biol.* **127:** 825–833.

Bekoff, A. (1976). Ontogeny of leg motor output in the chick embryo: A neural analysis. *Brain Res.* **106:** 271–291.

Bekoff, A., and Kauer, J. A. (1984). Neural control of hatching: Fate of the pattern generator for the leg movements of hatching in post-hatching chicks. *J. Neurosci.* **4:** 2659–2666.

Bekoff, A., and Sabichi, A. L. (1987). Sensory control of the initiation of hatching in chicks: Effects of a local anesthetic injected into the neck. *Dev. Psychobiol.* **20:** 489–495.

Ben-Ari, Y., Cherubini, E., Corradetti, R., and Gaiarsa, J. L. (1989). Giant synaptic potentials in immature rat CA3 hippocampal neurones. *J. Physiol.* **416:** 303–325.

Ben-Ari, Y., Cherubini, E., and Krnjevic, K. (1988). Changes in voltage dependence of NMDA currents during development. *Neruosci. Lett.* **94:** 88–92.

Bennett, M. R., and Pettigrew, A. G. (1974). The formation of synapses in reinnervated and cross-reinnervated striated muscle during development. *J. Physiol. (London)* **241:** 547–573.

Bentley, D., and Caudy, M. (1983). Pioneer axons lose directed growth after selective killing of guidepost cells. *Nature* **304:** 62–65.

Bentley, D., and O'Connor, T. P. (1994). Cytoskeletal events in growth cone steering. *Curr. Opin. Neurobiol.* **4:** 43–48.

Bentley, D., and Toroian-Raymond, A. (1986). Disoriented pathfinding by pioneer neurone growth cones deprived of filopodia by cytochalasin treatment. *Nature* **323:** 712–715.

Benzer, S. (1971). From the gene to behavior. *JAMA* **218:** 1015–1022.

Berg, D. K., and Hall, Z. W. (1975). Increased extrajunctional acetylcholine sensitivity produced by chronic postsynatpic neuromuscular blockade. *J. Physiol.* **244:** 659–676.

Bevan, S., and Steinbach, J. H. (1977). The distribution of α-bungarotoxin binding sites on mammalian skeletal muscle developing *in vivo*. *J. Physiol.* **267:** 195–213.

Beyer, C., Kolbinger, W., Froehlich, U., Pilgrim, C., and Reisert, I. (1992). Sex differences of hypothalamic prolactin cells develop independently of the presence of sex steroids. *Brain Res.* **593:** 253–256.

Biggin, M. D., and McGinnis, W. (1997). Regulation of segmentation and segmental identity by *Drosophila* homeoproteins: The role of DNA binding in functional activity and specificity. *Development* **124:** 4425–4433.

Birch, E. E., Gwiazda, J., Bauer, J. A., Jr., Naegele, J., and Held, R. (1983). Visual acuity and its meridional variations in children aged 7–60 months. *Vision Res.* **23:** 1019–1024.

Birren, S. J., Verdi, J. M., and Anderson, D. J. (1992). Membrane depolarization induces p140trk and NGF responsiveness, but not p75LNGFR, in MAH cells. *Science* **257:** 395–397.

Bixby, J. L., and Harris, W. A. (1991). Molecular mechanisms of axon growth and guidance. *Annu. Rev. Cell. Biol.* **7:** 117–159.

Bixby, J. L., Pratt, R. S., Lilien, J., and Reichardt, L. F. (1987). Neurite outgrowth on muscle cell surfaces involves extracellular matrix receptors as well as Ca^{2+}-dependent and -independent cell adhesion molecules. *Proc. Natl. Acad. Sci. USA* **84:** 2555–2559.

Bixby, J. L., and Spitzer, N. C. (1982). The appearance and development of chemosensitivity in Rohon–Beard neurones of the *Xenopus* spinal cord. *J. Physiol.* **330:** 513–536.

Blair, L. A. C. (1983). The timing of protein synthesis required for the development of the sodium action potential in embryonic spinal neurons. *J. Neurosci.* **3:** 1430–1436.

Blakely, R. D., Clark, J. A., Pacholczyk, T., and Amara, S. G. (1991). Distinct, developmentally regulated brain mRNAs direct the synthesis of neurotransmitter transporters. *J. Neurochem.* **56:** 860–871.

Blakemore, C., and Cooper, G. F. (1970). Development of the brain depends on the visual environment. *Nature* **228:** 477–478.

Blakemore, C., and Van Sluyters, R. C. (1975). Innate and environmental factors in the development of the kitten's visual cortex. *J. Physiol.* **248:** 663–716.

Blaschke, A. J., Staley, K., and Chun, J. (1996). Widespread programmed cell death in proliferative and postmitotic regions of the fetal cerebral cortex. *Development* **122:** 1165–1174.

Blasdel, G., Obermayer, K., and Kiorpes, L. (1995). Organization of ocular dominance and orientation columns in the striate cortex of neonatal macaque monkeys. *Vis. Neurosci.* **12:** 589–603.

Bliss, T. V. P., and Lømo, T. (1973). Long-lasting potentiation of synaptic transmission in the dentate area of the anesthtized rabbit following stimulation of the perforant path. *J. Physiol.* **232:** 331–356.

Bloch, R. J., and Steinbach, J. H. (1981). Reversible loss of acetylcholine receptor clusters at the developing rat neuromuscular junction. *Dev. Biol.* **81:** 386–391.

Bonds, A. B. (1979). Development of orientation tuning in the visual cortex of kittens. *In* "Developmental Neurobiology of Vision" (R. D. Freeman, Ed.), pp. 31–41. Plenum, New York.

Bonhoeffer, F., and Huf, J. (1985). Position-dependent properties of retinal axons and their growth cones. *Nature* **315:** 409–410.

Bonni, A., Frank, D. A., Schindler, C., and Greenberg, M. E. (1993). Characterization of a pathway for ciliary neurotrophic factor signaling to the nucleus. *Science* **262:** 1575–1579.

Bonni, A., Sun, Y., Nadal-Vicens, M., Bhatt, A., Frank, D. A., Rozovsky, I., Stahl, N., Yancopoulos, G. D., and Greenberg, M. E. (1997). Regulation of gliogenesis in the central nervous system by the JAK-STAT signaling pathway. *Science* **278:** 477–483.

Borasio, G. D., John, J., Wittinghofer, A., Barde, Y. A., Sendtner, M., and Heumann, R. (1989). ras p21 protein promotes survival and fiber outgrowth of cultured embryonic neurons. *Neuron* **2:** 1087–1096.

Born, D. E., and Rubel, E. W. (1985). Afferent influences on brain stem auditory nuclei of the chicken: Neuron number and size following cochlea removal. *J. Comp. Neurol.* **22:** 435–445.

Born, D. E., and Rubel, E. W. (1988). Afferent influences on brain stem auditory nuclei of the chicken: Presynaptic action potentials regulate protein synthesis in nucleus magnocellularis neurons. *J. Neurosci.* **8:** 901–919.

Bottjer, S. W., Miesner, E. A., and Arnold, A. P. (1984). Forebrain lesions disrupt development but not maintenance of song in passerine birds. *Science* **224:** 901–903.

Bovolenta, P., and Mason, C. (1987). Growth cone morphology varies with position in the developing mouse visual pathway from retina to first targets. *J. Neurosci.* **7:** 1447–1460.

Bowe, M. A., Deyst, K. A., Leszyk, J. D., and Fallon, J. R. (1994). Identification and purification of an agrin receptor from Torpedo postsynaptic membranes: A heteromeric complex related to the dystroglycans. *Neuron* **12:** 1173–1180.

Bowe, M. A., and Nadler, J. V. (1990). Developmental increase in the sensitivity to magnesium of NMDA receptors on CA1 hippocampal pyramidal cells. *Dev. Brain Res.* **56:** 55–61.

Bradley, P., and Berry, M. (1978). The Purkinje cell dendritic tree in mutant mouse cerebellum. A quantitative Golgi study of Weaver and Staggerer mice. *Brain. Res.* **142:** 135–141.

Brainard, M. S., and Knudsen, E. I. (1993). Experience-dependent plasticity in the inferior colliculus: A site for visual calibration of the neural representation of auditory space in the barn owl. *J. Neurosci.* **13:** 4589–4608.

Braisted, J. E., McLaughlin, T., Wang, H. U., Friedman, G. C., Anderson, D. J., and O'Leary, D. D. (1997). Graded and lamina-specific distributions of ligands of EphB receptor tyrosine kinases in the developing retinotectal system. *Dev. Biol.* **191:** 14–28.

Brandt, P., and Neve, R. L. (1992). Expression of plasma membrane calcium pumping ATPase mRNAs in developing rat brain and adult brain subregions: Evidence for stage-specific expression. *J. Neurochem.* **59:** 1566–1569.

Bray, D. (1979). Mechanical tension produced by nerve cells in tissue culture. *J. Cell. Sci.* **37:** 391–410.

Bray, D., and Hollenbeck, P. J. (1988). Growth cone motility and guidance. *Annu. Rev. Cell. Biol.* **4:** 43–61.

Breedlove, S. M., and Arnold, A. P. (1983). Hormonal control of a developing neuromuscular system. I. Complete demasculinization of the male rat spinal nucleus of the bulbocavernosus using the anti-androgen flutamide. *J. Neurosci.* **3:** 417–423.

Bregman, B. S., and Goldberger, M. E. (1983). Infant lesion effect. III. Anatomical correlates of sparing and recovery of function after spinal cord damage in newborn and adult cats. *Brain Res.* **285:** 137–154.

Bregman, B. S., Kunkel-Bagden, E., Schnell, L., Dai, H. N., Gao, D., and Schwab, M. E. (1995). Recovery from spinal cord injury mediated by antibodies to neurite growth inhibitors [see comments]. *Nature* **378:** 498–501.

Brenner, S. (1974). The genetics of *Caenorhabditis elegans*. *Genetics* **77:** 71–94.

Brenowitz, E. A. (1991). Altered perception of species-specific song by female birds after lesions of a forebrain nucleus. *Science* **251:** 303–305.

Brenowitz, E. A., and Arnold, A. P. (1986). Interspecific comparisons of the size of neural song control regions and song complexity in duetting birds: Evolutionary implications. *J. Neurosci.* **6:** 2875–2879.

Briscoe, J., Sussel, L., Serup, P., Hartigan-O'Connor, D., Jessell, T. M., Rubenstein, J. L., and Ericson, J. (1999). Homeobox gene Nkx2.2 and specification of neuronal identity by graded sonic hedgehog signaling. *Nature* **398:** 622–677.

Broadie, K. S., and Bate, M. (1993a). Development of the embryonic neuromuscular synapse of *Drosophila melanogaster. J. Neurosci.* **13:** 144–166.

Broadie, K. S., and Bate, M. (1993b). Innervation directs receptor synthesis and localization in *Drosophila* embryo synaptogenesis. *Nature* **361:** 350–353.

Broadie, K., Sink, H., Van Vactor, D., Fambrough, D., Whitington, P. M., Bate, M., and Goodman, C. S. (1993). From growth cone to synapse: The life history of the RP3 motor neuron. *Dev. Suppl.:* 227–238.

Bronner-Fraser, M., Stern, C. D., and Fraser, S. (1991). Analysis of neural crest cell lineage and migration. *J. Craniofac. Genet. Dev. Biol.* **11:** 214–222.

Brose, K., Bland, K. S., Wang, K. H., Arnott, D., Henzel, W., Goodman, C. S., Tessier-Lavigne, M., and Kidd, T. (1999). Slit proteins bind Robo receptors and have an evolutionarily conserved role in repulsive axon guidance. *Cell* **96:** 795–806.

Brown, A., Slaughter, T., and Black, M. M. (1992). Newly assembled microtubules are concentrated in the proximal and distal regions of growing axons. *J. Cell. Biol.* **119:** 867–882.

Brunjes, P. C., and Alberts, J. R. (1979). Olfactory stimulation induces filial preferences for huddling in rat pups. *J. Comp. Physiol. Psychol.* **93:** 548–555.

Brunso-Bechtold, J. K., Henkel, C. K., and Linville, C. (1992). Ultrastructural development of the medial superior olive (MSO) in the ferret. *J. Comp. Neurol.* **324:** 539–556.

Buchanan, J., Sun, Y.-a., and Poo, M.-m. (1989). Studies of nerve–muscle interactions in *Xenopus* cell culture: Fine structure of early functional contacts. *J. Neurosci.* **9:** 1540–1554.

Buck, L., and Axel, R. (1991). A novel multigene family may encode odorant receptors: A molecular basis for odor recognition. *Cell* **65:** 175–187.

Budnik, V., Koh, Y.-H., Guan, B., Hartmann, B., Hough, C., Woods, D., and Gorczyca, M. (1996). Regulation of synapse structure and function by the *Drosophila* tumor suppressor gene dlg. *Neuron* **17:** 627–640.

Bueker, E. D. (1948). Implantation of tumors in the hind limb field of the embryonic chick and the developmental response of the lumbosacral nervous system. *Anat. Rec.* **102:** 369–390.

Bunge, R. P. (1975). Changing uses of nerve tissue culture. *In* "The Nervous System," Vol. 1, "The Basic Neurosciences" (D. B. Tower, Ed.), pp. 31–42. Raven Press, New York.

Burden, S. (1977a). Development of the neuromusclular junction in the chick embryo: The number, distribution, and stability of acetylcholine receptors. *Dev. Biol.* **57:** 317–329.

Burden, S. (1977b). Acetylcholine receptors at the neuromuscular junction: Developmental change in receptor turnover. *Dev. Biol.* **61:** 79–85.

Burden, S. J., Sargent, P. B., and McMahon, U. J. (1979). Acetylcholine receptors in regenerating muscle accumulate at original synaptic sites in the absence of the nerve. *J. Cell. Biol.* **82:** 412–425.

Burgard, E. C., and Hablitz, J. J. (1993). Developmental changes in NMDA and non-NMDA receptor-mediated synaptic potentials in rat neocortex. *J. Neurophysiol.* **69:** 230–240.

Burmeister, M., Novak, J., Liang, M. Y., Basu, S., Ploder, L., Hawes, N. L., Vidgen, D., Hoover, F., Goldman, D., Kalnins, V. I., Roderick, T. H., Taylor, B. A., Hankin, M. H., and McInnes, R. R. (1996). Ocular retardation mouse caused by Chx10 homeobox null allele: Impaired retinal progenitor proliferation and bipolar cell differentiation. *Nat. Genet.* **12:** 376–384.

Burr, H. S. (1916). The effects of the removal of the nasal pits in *Amblystoma* embryos. *J. Exp. Zool.* **20:** 27–57.

Burrill, J. D., and Easter, S. S., Jr. (1995). The first retinal axons and their microenvironment in zebrafish: Cryptic pioneers and the pretract. *J. Neurosci.* **15:** 2935–2947.

Cabrera, C. V., Martinez-Arias, A., and Bate, M. (1987). The expression of three members of the achaete–scute gene complex correlates with neuroblast segregation in *Drosophila. Cell* **50:** 425–433.

Callahan, C. A., Muralidhar, M. G., Lundgren, S. E., Scully, A. L., and Thomas, J. B. (1995). Control of neuronal pathway selection by a *Drosophila* receptor protein–tyrosine kinase family member. *Nature* **376:** 171–174.

Calof, A. L., and Reichardt, L. F. (1984). Motoneurons urified by cell sorting respond to two distinct activities in myotube-conditioned medium. *Dev. Biol.* **106:** 194–210.

Cameron, H. A., Hazel, T. G., and McKay, R. D. (1998). Regulation of neurogenesis by growth factors and neurotransmitters. *J. Neurobiol.* **36:** 287–306.

Cameron, J. S., Lhuillier, L., Subramony, P., and Dryer, S. E. (1998). Developmental regulation of neuronal K$^+$ channels by target-derived TGFβ *in vivo* and *in vitro. Neuron* **21:** 1045–1053.

Campanelli, J. T., Roberds, S. L., Campbell, K. P., and Scheller, R. H. (1994). A role for dsytrophin-associated glycoproteins and utrophin in agrin-induced AchR clustering. *Cell* **77:** 663–674.

Campbell, G., and Shatz, C. J. (1992). Synapses formed by identified retinogeniculate axons during segregation of eye input. *J. Neurosci.* **12:** 1847–1858.

Campenot, R. B. (1977). Local control of neurite development by nerve growth factor. *Proc. Natl. Acad. Sci. USA* **74:** 4516–4519.

Campenot, R. B. (1982). Development of sympathetic neurons in compartmentalized cultures. II. Local control of neurite survival by nerve growth factor. *Dev. Biol.* **93:** 13–21.

Campos-Ortega, J. A. (1998). The genetics of the *Drosophila* achaete–scute gene complex: A historical appraisal. *Int. J. Dev. Biol.* **42:** 291–297.

Carmichael, L. (1954). The onset and early development of behavior. *In* "Manual of Child Psychology" (L. Carmichael, Ed.), pp. 60–214. Wiley, New York.

Carney, P. R., and Silver, J. (1983). Studies on cell migration and axon guidance in the developing distal auditory system of the mouse. *J. Comp. Neurol.* **215:** 359–369.

Carpenter, W. B. (1874). "Principles of Mental Physiology." King, London.

Carr, V. M., and Simpson, S. B. (1978). Proliferative and degenerative events in the early development of chick dorsal root ganglia. II. Responses to altered peripheral fields. *J. Comp. Neurol.* **182:** 741–755.

Casaccia-Bonnefil, P., Carter, B. D., Dobrowsky, R. T., and Chao, M. V. (1996). Death of oligodendrocytes mediated by the interaction of nerve growth factor with its receptor p75. *Nature* **383:** 716–719.

Cash, S., Zucker, R. S., and Poo, M.-m. (1996). Spread of synaptic depression mediated by presynaptic cytoplasmic signaling. *Science* **272:** 998–1001.

Castellani, V., and Bolz, J. (1997). Membrane-associated molecules regulate the formation of layer-specific cortical circuits. *Proc. Natl. Acad. Sci. USA* **94:** 7030–7035.

Castellani, V., Yue, Y., Gao, P. P., Zhou, R., and Bolz, J. (1998). Dual action of a ligand for Eph receptor tyrosine kinases on specific populations of axons during the development of cortical circuits. *J. Neurosci.* **18:** 4663–4672.

Casticas, S., Thanos, S., and Clarke, P. G. H. (1987). Major role for neuronal death during brain development: Refinement of topographic connections. *Proc. Natl. Acad. Sci. USA* **84:** 8165–8168.

Catalano, S. M., Messersmith, E. K., Goodman, C. S., Shatz, C. J., and Chedotal, A. (1998). Many major CNS axon projections develop normally in the absence of semaphorin III. *Mol. Cell. Neurosci.* **11:** 173–182.

Catsicas, M., Péquignot, Y., and Clarke, P. G. H. (1992). Rapid onset of neuronal death induced by blockade of either axoplasmic transport or action potentials in afferent fibers during brain development. *J. Neurosci.* **12:** 4642–4650.

Caudy, M., and Bentley, D. (1986). Pioneer growth cone steering along a series of neuronal and non-neuronal cues of different affinities. *J. Neurosci.* **6:** 1781–1795.

Caudy, M., Vassin, H., Brand, M., Tuma, R., Jan, L. Y., and Jan, Y. N. (1988). Daughterless, a *Drosophila* gene essential for both neurogenesis and sex determination, has sequence similarities to myc and the achaete–scute complex. *Cell* **55:** 1061–1067.

Caviness, V. S., Jr., and Takahashi, T. (1995). Proliferative events in the cerebral ventricular zone. *Brain. Dev.* **17:** 159–163.

Cepko, C. L., Austin, C. P., Yang, X., Alexiades, M., and Ezzeddine, D. (1996). Cell fate determination in the vertebrate retina. *Proc. Natl. Acad. Sci. USA* **93:** 589–595.

Chalepakis, G., Stoykova, A., *et al.* (1993). Pax: Gene regulators in the developing nervous system. *J. Neurobiol.* **24:** 1367–1384.

Chalfie, M. (1993). Touch receptor development and function in *Caenorhabditis elegans*. *J. Neurobiol.* **24:** 1433–1441.

Chalfie, M., and Au, M. (1989). Genetic control of differentiation of the *Caenorhabditis elegans* touch receptor neurons. *Science* **243:** 1027–1033.

Chambon, P. (1996). A decade of molecular biology of retinoic acid receptors. *FASEB J.* **10:** 940–954.

Chan, S. S., Zheng, H., Su, M. W., Wilk, R., Killeen, M. T., Hedgecock, E. M., and Culotti, J. G. (1996). UNC-40, a *C. elegans* homolog of DCC (deleted in colorectal cancer), is required in motile cells responding to UNC-6 netrin cues. *Cell* **87:** 187–195.

Chang, H. C., Karim, F. D., O'Neill, E. M., Rebay, I., Solomon, N. M., Therrien, M., Wassarman, D. A., Wolff, T., and Rubin, G. M. (1994). Ras signal transduction pathway in *Drosophila* eye development. *Cold Spring Harbor Symp. Quant. Biol.* **59:** 147–153.

Chao, M. V. (1994). The p75 neurotrophin receptor. *J. Neurobiol.* **25:** 1373–1385.

Chapman, B., and Stryker, M. P. (1993). Development of orientation selectivity in ferret visual cortex and effects of deprivation. *J. Neurosci.* **13:** 5251–5262.

Charpier, S., Behrends, J. C., Triller, A., Faber, D. S., and Korn, H. (1995). "Latent" inhibitory connections become functional during activity-dependent plasticity. *Proc. Natl. Acad. Sci. USA* **92:** 117–120.

Chen, Q. X., Stelzner, A., Kay, A. R., and Wong, R. K. S. (1990). GABA$_A$ receptor function is regulated by phosphorylation in acutely dissociated guinea-pig hippocampal neurones. *J. Physiol.* **420:** 207–221.

Cheng, E. H., Kirsch, D. G., Clem, R. J., Ravi, R., Kastan, M. B., Bedi, A., Ueno, K., and Hardwick, J. M. (1997). Conversion of Bcl-2 to a Bax-like death effector by caspases. *Science* **278:** 1966–1968.

Cheng, H. J., Nakamoto, M., Bergemann, A. D., and Flanagan, J. G. (1995). Complementary gradients in expression and binding of ELF-1 and Mek4 in development of the topographic retinotectal projection map. *Cell* **82:** 371–381.

Chiba, A., Shepherd, D., and Murphey, R. K. (1988). Synaptic rearrangement during postembryonic development in the cricket. *Science* **240:** 901–905.

Chien, C. B., Rosenthal, D. E., Harris, W. A., and Holt, C. E. (1993). Navigational errors made by growth cones without filopodia in the embryonic *Xenopus* brain. *Neuron* **11:** 237–251.

Chitnis, A. B., Patel, C. K., Kim, S., and Kuwada, J. Y. (1992). A specific brain tract guides follower growth cones in two regions of the zebrafish brain. *J. Neurobiol.* **23:** 845–854.

Cho, K. O., Hunt, C. A., and Kennedy, M. B. (1992). The rat brain postsynaptic density fraction contains a homolog of the *Drosophila* discs-large tumor suppressor protein. *Neuron* **9:** 929–942.

Chow, I., and Cohen, M. W. (1983). Developmental changes in the distribution of acetylcholine receptors in the myotomes of *Xenopus laevis*. *J. Physiol.* **339:** 553–571.

Chub, N., and O'Donovan, M. J. (1998). Blockade and recovery of spontaneous rhythmic activity after application of neurotransmitter antagonists to spinal networks of the chick embryo. *J. Neurosci.* **18:** 294–306.

Chu-Wang, I. W., and Oppenheim, R. W. (1978). Cell death of motoneurons in the chick embryo spinal cord. II. A quantitative and qualitative analysis of degeneration in the ventral root, including evidence for axon outgrowth and limb innervation prior to cell death. *J. Comp. Neurol.* **177:** 59–85.

Clarke, J. D., and Lumsden, A. (1993). Segmental repetition of neuronal phenotype sets in the chick embryo hindbrain. *Development* **118:** 151–162.

Clarkson, M. G., Clifton, R. K., Swain, I. U., and Perris, E. E. (1989). Stimulus duration and repetition rate influences newborns' head orientation towards sound. *Dev. Psychobiol.* **22:** 683–705.

Clarkson, M. G., Swain, I. U., Clifton, R. K., and Cohen, K. (1991). Newborns' head orientation toward trains of brief sounds. *J. Acoust. Soc. Am.* **89:** 2411–2420.

Clayton, N. C., and Krebs, J. R. (1994). Hippocampal growth and attrition in birds affected by experience. *Proc. Natl. Acad. Sci. USA* **91:** 7410–7414.

Clendening, B., and Hume, R. I. (1990). Cell interactions regulate dendritic morphology and responses to neurotransmitters in embryonic chick sympathetic preganglionic neurons *in vitro*. *J. Neurosci.* **10:** 3992–4005.

Cline, H. T., Debski, E. A., and Constantine-Paton, M. (1987). *N*-Methyl-D-aspartate receptor antagonist desegregates eye-specific stripes. *Proc. Natl. Acad. Sci.* **84:** 4342–4345.

Coghill, G. E. (1929). "Anatomy and the Problem of Behaviour." Cambridge Univ. Press, London.

Cohen, J., and Johnson, A. R. (1991). Differential effects of laminin and merosin on neurite outgrowth by developing retinal ganglion cells. *J. Cell. Sci. Suppl.* **15:** 1–7.

Cohen, M. W. (1972). The development of neuromuscular connexions in the presence of D-tubocurarine. *Brain Res.* **41:** 457–463.

Cohen, M. W., Anderson, M. J., Zorychta, E., and Weldon, P. R. (1979). Accumulation of acetylcholine receptors at nerve–muscle contacts in culture. *Prog. Brain Res.* **49:** 335–349.

Cohen, M. W., and Weldon, P. R. (1980). Localization of acetylcholine receptors and synaptic ultrastructure at nerve–muscle contacts in culture: Dependence on nerve type. *J. Cell. Biol.* **86:** 388–401.

Cohen, N. A., Brenman, J. E., Snyder, S. H., and Bredt, D. S. (1996). Binding of the inward rectifier K+ channel Kir 2.3 to PSD-95 is regulated by protein kinase A phosphorylation. *Neuron* **17:** 759–767.

Cohen, S., and Levi-Montalcini, R. (1956). A nerve growth-stimulating factor isolated from snake venom. *Proc. Natl. Acad. Sci. USA* **42:** 571–574.

Colamarino, S. A., and Tessier-Lavigne, M. (1995a). The axonal chemoattractant netrin-1 is also a chemorepellent for trochlear motor axons. *Cell* **81:** 621–629.

Colamarino, S. A., and Tessier-Lavigne, M. (1995b). The role of the floor plate in axon guidance. *Annu. Rev. Neurosci.* **18:** 497–529.

Colman, H., Nabekura, J., and Lichtman, J. W. (1997). Alterations in synaptic strength preceding axon withdrawal. *Science* **275:** 356–361.

Condron, B. G., Patel, N. H., and Zinn, K. (1994). Engrailed controls glial/neuronal cell fate decisions at the midline of the central nervous system. *Neuron* **13:** 541–554.

Condron, B. G., and Zinn, K. (1994). The grasshopper median neuroblast is a multipotent progenitor cell that generates glia and neurons in distinct temporal phases. *J. Neurosci.* **14:** 5766–5777.

Condron, B. G., and Zinn, K. (1995). Activation of cAMP-dependent protein kinase triggers a glial to neuronal cell-fate switch in an insect neuroblast lineage. *Curr. Biol.* **5:** 51–61.

Connold, A. L., Evers, J. V., and Vrbova, G. (1986). Effect of low calcium and protease inhibitors on synapse elimination during postnatal development in the rat soleus muscle. *Dev. Brain Res.* **28:** 99–107.

Connors, B. W., Ransom, B. R., Kunis, D. M., and Gutnick, M. J. (1982). Activity dependent K+ accumulation in the developing rat optic nerve. *Science* **216:** 1341–1343.

Conradi, S., and Ronnevi, L.-O. (1975). Spontaneous elimination of synapses on cat spinal motoneurons after birth: Do half of the synapses on the cell bodies disappear? *Brain Res.* **92:** 505–510.

Cook, J. E., and Rankin, E. C. (1986). Impaired refinement of the regenerated retinotectal projection of the goldfish in stroboscopic light: A quantitative WGA-HRP study. *Exp. Brain Res.* **63:** 421–430.

Corfas, G., and Fischbach, G. D. (1993). The number of Na+ channels in cultured chick muscle is increased by ARIA, an acetylcholine receptor-inducing activity. *J. Neurosci.* **13:** 2118–2125.

Cornel, E., and Holt, C. (1992). Precocious pathfinding: Retinal axons can navigate in an axonless brain. *Neuron* **9:** 1001–1011.

Corriveau, R. A., and Berg, D. K. (1993). Coexpression of multiple acetylcholine receptor genes in neurons: Quantification of transcripts during development. *J. Neurosci.* **13:** 2662–2671.

Covault, J., and Sanes, J. R. (1985). Neural cell adhesion molecule (N-CAM) accumulates in denervated and paralyzed skeletal muscles. *Proc. Natl. Acad. Sci. USA* **82:** 4544–4548.

Cragg, B. G. (1975). The development of synapses in the visual system of the cat. *J. Comp. Neurol.* **160:** 147–166.

Craig, A. M., and Banker, G. (1994). Neuronal polarity. *Annu. Rev. Neurosci.* **17:** 267–310.

Craig, A. M., Blackstone, C. D., Huganir, R. L., and Banker, G. (1993). The distribution of glutamate receptors in cultured rat hippocampal neurons: Postsynaptic clustering of AMPA-selective subunits. *Neuron* **10:** 1055–1068.

Crair, M. C., and Malenka, R. C. (1995). A critical period for long-term potentiation at thalamocortical synapses. *Nature* **375:** 325–328.

Crossley, P. H., Martinez, S., *et al.* (1996). Midbrain development induced by FGF8 in the chick embryo. *Nature* **380:** 66–68.

Crowley, C., Spencer, S. D., Nishimura, M. C., Chen, K. S., Pitts-Meek, S., Armanini, M. P., Ling, L. H., MacMahon, S. B., Shelton, D. L., Levinson, A. D., and Phillips, H. S. (1994). Mice lacking nerve growth factor display perinatal loss of sensory and sympathetic neurons yet develop basal forebrain cholinergic neurons. *Cell* **76:** 1001–1011.

Culotti, J. G. (1994). Axon guidance mechanisms in *Caenorhabditis elegans*. *Curr. Opin. Genet. Dev.* **4:** 587–595.

Cynader, M., Berman, N., and Hein, A. (1973). Cats reared in stroboscopic illumination: Effects of receptive fields in visual cortex. *Proc. Natl. Acad. Sci.* **70:** 1353–1354.

Dahm, L. M., and Landmesser, L. T. (1991). The regulation of synaptogenesis during normal development and following activity blockade. *J. Neurosci.* **11:** 238–255.

Dai, J., and Sheetz, M. P. (1995). Axon membrane flows from the growth cone to the cell body. *Cell* **83:** 693–701.

Dai, Z., and Peng, H. B. (1993). Elevation in presynaptic Ca^{2+} accompanying initial nerve–muscle contact in tissue culture. *Neuron* **10:** 827–837.

Dan, Y., and Poo, M.-m. (1992). Hebbian depression of isolated neuromuscular synapses *in vitro*. *Science* **256:** 1570–1573.

Danielian, P. S., and McMahon, A. P. (1996). Engrailed-1 as a target of the Wnt-1 signalling pathway in vertebrate midbrain development. *Nature* **383:** 332–334.

D'Arcangelo, G., Miao, G. G., Chen, S. C., Soares, H. D., Morgan, J. I., and Curran, T. (1995). A protein related to extracellular matrix proteins deleted in the mouse mutant reeler. *Nature* **374:** 719–723.

Darnell, D. K., and Schoenwolf, G. C. (1995). Dorsoventral patterning of the avian mesencephalon/metencephalon: Role of the notochord and floor plate in suppressing Engrailed-2. *J. Neurobiol.* **26:** 62–74.

Davenport, R. W., Dou, P., Mills, L. R., and Kater, S. B. (1996). Distinct calcium signaling within neuronal growth cones and filopodia. *J. Neurobiol.* **31:** 1–15.

David, S., and Aguayo, A. J. (1981). Axonal elongation into peripheral nervous system bridges after central nervous system injury in adult rats. *Science* **214:** 931–933.

Davies, A. M., Bandtlow, C., Heumann, R., Korsching, S., Rohrer, H., and Thoenen, H. (1987). Timing and site of nerve growth factor synthesis in developing skin in relation to innervation and expression of the receptor. *Nature* **326:** 353–358.

Davies, A. M., Lee, K. F., and Jaenisch, R. (1993). p75-deficient trigeminal sensory neurons have an altered response to NGF but not to other neurotrophins. *Neuron* **11:** 565–574.

Davies, K. E., Tinsley, J. M., and Blake, D. J. (1995). Molecular analysis of Duchenne muscular dystrophy: Past, present, and future. *Ann. N.Y. Acad. Sci.* **758:** 287–296.

Davis, A. A., and Temple, S. (1994). A self-renewing multipotential stem cell in embryonic rat cerebral cortex. *Nature* **372:** 263–266.

Davis, G. W., Schuster, C. M., and Goodman, C. S. (1996). Genetic dissection of structural and functional components of synaptic plasticity. III. CREB is necessary for presynaptic functional plasticity. *Neuron* **17:** 669–679.

Davis, P. K., Carlini, W. G., Ransom, B. R., Black, J. A., and Waxman, S. G. (1987). Carbonic anhydrase activity develops postnatally in the rat optic nerve. *Dev. Brain Res.* **31:** 291–298.

Daw, N. W. (1995). "Visual Development." Plenum, New York.

Daw, N. W., Fox, K., Sato, H., and Czepita, D. (1992). Critical period for monocular deprivation in the cat visual cortex. *J. Neurophysiol.* **67:** 197–202.

DeCasper, A. J., and Fifer, W. P. (1980). Of human bonding: Newborns prefer their mothers' voices. *Science* **208:** 1174–1176.

DeCasper, A. J., and Spence, M. J. (1986). Prenatal maternal speech influences newborns' perception of speech sounds. *Infant Behav. Dev.* **9:** 133–150.

DeChiara, T. M., Bowen, D. C., Valenzuela, D. M., Simmons, M. V., Poueymirou, W. T., Thomas, S., Kinetz, E., Compton, D. L., Rojas, E., Park, J. S., Smith, C., DiStefano, P. S., Glass, D. J., Burden, S. J., and Yancopoulos, G. D. (1996). The receptor tyrosine kinase MuSK is required for neuromuscular junction formation *in vivo*. *Cell* **85:** 501–512.

DeChiara, T. M., Vejsada, R., Poueymirou, W. T., Acheson, A., Suri, C., Conover, J. C., Friedman, B., McClain, J., Pan, L., Stahl, N., Ip, N. Y., Kato, A., and Yancopoulos, G. D. (1995). Mice lacking the CNTF receptor, unlike mice lacking CNTF, exhibit profound motor neuron deficits at birth. *Cell* **83:** 313–322.

Decker, R. S. (1976). Influence of thyroid hormones on neuronal death and differentiation in larval *Rana pipiens*. *Dev. Biol.* **49:** 101–118.

Decker, R. S. (1977). Lysosomal properties during thyroxine-induced lateral motor column neurogenesis. *Brain Res.* **132:** 407–422.

Deitch, J. S., and Rubel, E. W. (1984). Afferent influences on brain stem auditory nuclei of the chicken: Time course and specificity of dendritic atrophy following deafferentation. *J. Comp. Neurol.* **229:** 66–79.

Del Rio, J. A., Heimrich, B., Borrell, V., Forster, E., Drakew, A., Alcantara, S., Nakajima, K., Miyata, T., Ogawa, M., Mikoshiba, K., Derer, P., Frotscher, M., and Soriano, E. (1997). A role for Cajal-Retzius cells and reelin in the development of hippocampal connections [see comments]. *Nature* **385:** 70–74.

Dent, M. A., Raisman, G., and Lai, F. A. (1996). Expression of type 1 inositol 1,4,5-trisphosphate receptor during axogenesis and synaptic contact in the central and peripheral nervous system of developing rat. *Development* **122:** 1029–1039.

DeRobertis, E. M., and Sasai, Y. (1996). A common plan for dorsoventral patterning in *Bilateria*. *Nature* **380:** 37–40.

Desai, C., Garriga, G., McIntire, S. L., and Horvitz, H. R. (1988). A genetic pathway for the development of the

Caenorhabditis elegans HSN motor neurons. *Nature* **336:** 638–646.

Desai, C., and Horvitz, H. R. (1989). *Caenorhabditis elegans* mutants defective in the functioning of the motor neurons responsible for egg laying. *Genetics* **121:** 703–721.

Desai, C. J., Gindhart, J. G., Jr., Goldstein, L. S., and Zinn, K. (1996). Receptor tyrosine phosphatases are required for motor axon guidance in the *Drosophila* embryo. *Cell* **84:** 599–609.

Desarmenien, M. G., and Spitzer, N. C. (1991). Role of calcium and protein kinase C in development of the delayed rectifier potassium current in *Xenopus* spinal neurons. *Neuron* **7:** 797–805.

Detwiler, S. R. (1936). "Neuroembryology. An Experimental Study." MacMillan, New York.

Diamond, J., and Miledi, R. (1962). A study of fetal and new-born rat muscle fibres. *J. Physiol. (London)* **162:** 393–408.

Dietrich, W. D., Durham, D., Lowry, O. H., and Woolsey, T. A. (1981). Quantitative histochemical effects of whisker damage on single identified cortical barrels in the adult mouse. *J. Neurosci.* **1:** 929–935.

Dobzhansky, T. (1951). Genetics and the Origin of Species. Columbia Univ. Press, New York.

Doe, C. (1992a). The Generation of Neuronal Diversity in the *Drosohila* Embryonic Central Nervous System: Determinants of Neuronal Identity. (M. Shankland and E. Macagno, Eds.), pp. 119–154. Academic Press, San Diego.

Doe, C. Q. (1992b). Molecular markers for identified neuroblasts and ganglion mother cells in the *Drosophila* central nervous system. *Development* **116:** 855–863.

Doe, C. Q., Chu-LaGraff, Q., Wright, D. M., and Scott, M. P. (1991). The prospero gene specifies cell fates in the *Drosophila* central nervous system. *Cell* **65:** 451–464.

Doherty, P., Ashton, S. V., Moore, S. E., and Walsh, F. S. (1991). Morphoregulatory activities of NCAM and N-cadherin can be accounted for by G protein-dependent activation of L- and N-type neuronal Ca^{2+} channels. *Cell* **67:** 21–33.

Doniach, T. (1995). Basic FGF as an inducer of anteroposterior neural pattern. *Cell* **83:** 1067–1070.

Donoghue, M. J., Merlie, J. P., Rosenthal, N., and Sanes, J. R. (1991). Rostrocaudal gradient of transgene expression in adult skeletal muscle. *Proc. Natl. Acad. Sci. USA* **88:** 5847–5851.

Dorsky, R. I., Chang, W. S., Rapaport, D. H., and Harris, W. A. (1997). Regulation of neuronal diversity in the *Xenopus* retina by Delta signalling. *Nature* **385:** 67–70.

Dourado, M. M., Dryer, S. E. (1992). Changes in the electrical properties of chick ciliary ganglion neurones during embryonic development. *J. Physiol.* **449:** 411–428.

Dourado, M. M., Brumwell, C., Wisgirda, M. E., Jacob, M. H., and Dryer, S. E. (1994). Target tissues and innervation regulate the characteristics of K^+ currents in chick ciliary ganglion neurons developing *in situ. J. Neurosci.* **14:** 3156–3165.

Dowsing, B., Puche, A., Hearn, C., and Key, B. (1997). Presence of novel N-CAM glycoforms in the rat olfactory system. *J. Neurobiol.* **32:** 659–670.

Drager, U. C., and Hubel, D. H. (1975). Responses to visual stimulation and relationship between visual, auditory, and somatosensory inputs in mouse superior colliculus. *J. Neurophysiol.* **38:** 690–713.

Drager, U. C., and Hubel, D. H. (1978). Studies of visual function and its decay in mice with hereditary retinal degeneration. *J. Comp. Neurol.* **180:** 85–114.

Drescher, U., Kremoser, C., Handwerker, C., Loschinger, J., Noda, M., and Bonhoeffer, F. (1995). *In vitro* guidance of retinal ganglion cell axons by RAGS, a 25 kDa tectal protein related to ligands for Eph receptor tyrosine kinases. *Cell* **82:** 359–370.

Driever, W., and Nusslein-Volhard, C. (1988). The bicoid protein determines position in the *Drosophila* embryo in a concentration-dependent manner. *Cell* **54:** 95–104.

Driscoll, M., and Chalfie, M. (1992). Developmental and abnormal cell death in *C. elegans. Trends Neurosci.* **15:** 15–19.

Dubin, M. W., Stark, L. A., and Archer, S. M. (1986). A role for action potential activity in the development of neuronal connections in the kitten retinogeniculate pathway. *J. Neurosci.* **6:** 1021–1036.

Dubinsky, J. M., and Fischbach, G. D. (1990). A role for cAMP in the development of functional neuromuscular transmission. *J. Neurobiol.* **21:** 414–426.

Dubinsky, J. M., Loftus, D. J., Fischbach, G. D., and Elson, E. L. (1989). Formation of acetylcholine receptor clusters in chick myotubes: Migration or new insertion? *J. Cell Biol.* **109:** 1733–1743.

Dubnau, J., and Tully, T. (1998). Gene discovery in *Drosophila:* New insights for learning and memory. *Annu. Rev. Neurosci.* **21:** 407–444.

Duboule, D., and Morata, G. (1994). Colinearity and functional hierarchy among genes of the homeotic complexes. *Trends Genet* **10:** 358–364.

Dudek, S. M., and Friedlander, M. J. (1996). Developmental down-regulation of LTD in cortical layer IV and its independence of modulation by inhibition. *Neuron* **16:** 1097–1106.

Duffy, F. H., Burchfiel, J. L., and Conway, J. L. (1976). Bicuculline reversal of deprivation amblyopia in the cat. *Nature* **260:** 256–257.

Durand, G. M., Kovalchuk, Y., and Konnerth, A. (1996). Long-term potentiation and functional synapse induction in developing hippocampus. *Nature* **381:** 71–75.

Durston, A. J., Timmermans, J. P., *et al.* (1989). Retinoic acid causes an anteroposterior transformation in the developing central nervous system. *Nature* **340:** 140–144.

Duxson, M. J. (1982). The effect of postsynaptic block on the development of the neuromuscular junction in postnatal rats. *J. Neurocytol.* **11:** 395–408.

Dyer, A. B., and Gottlieb, G. (1990). Auditory basis of maternal attachment in ducklings (Anas platyrhynchos) under simulated naturalistic imprinting conditions. *J. Comp. Psychol.* **104:** 190–194.

Dyer, A. B., Lickliter, R., and Gottlieb, G. (1989). Maternal and peer imprinting in mallard ducklings under experimentally simulated natural social conditions. *Dev. Psychobiol.* **22:** 463–475.

Dyson, S. E., and Jones, D. G. (1980). Quantitation of terminal parameters and their interrelationships in maturing central synapses: A perspective for experimental studies. *Brain Res.* **183:** 43–59.

Eagleson, G. W., and Harris, W. A. (1990). Mapping of the presumptive brain regions in the neural plate of *Xenopus laevis. J. Neurobiol.* **21:** 427–440.

Easter, S. S., Jr., Burrill, J., Marcus, R. C., Ross, L. S., Taylor, J. S., and Wilson, S. W. (1994). Initial tract formation in the vertebrate brain. *Prog. Brain Res.* **102:** 79–93.

Easter, S. S., Jr., and Stuermer, C. A. (1984). An evaluation of the hypothesis of shifting terminals in goldfish optic tectum. *J. Neurosci.* **4:** 1052–1063.

Ebens, A., Brose, K., Leonardo, E. D., Hanson, M. G., Jr., Bladt, F., Birchmeier, C., Barres, B. A., and Tessier-Lavigne, M. (1996). Hepatocyte growth factor/scatter factor is an axonal chemoattractant and a neurotrophic factor for spinal motor neurons. *Neuron* **17:** 1157–1172.

Eccles, J. C., Krnjevic, K., and Miledi, R. (1959). Delayed effects of peripheral severance of afferent nerve fibres on the efficacy of their central synapses. *J. Physiol.* **145:** 204–220.

Edelman, G. M. (1984). Modulation of cell adhesion during induction, histogenesis, and perinatal development of the nervous system. *Annu. Rev. Neurosci.* **7:** 339–377.

Edmonson, J. C., and Hatten, M. E. (1987). Glial guided granule neuron migration *in vitro:* A high resolution time-lapse video microscopic study. *J. Neurosci.* **7:** 1928–1934.

Eisen, J. S. (1991a). Determination of primary motoneuron identity in developing zebrafish embryos. *Science* **252:** 569–572.

Eisen, J. S. (1991b). Motoneuronal development in the embryonic zebrafish. *Development Suppl:* 141–147.

Elkins, T., Zinn, K., McAllister, L., Hoffmann, F. M., and Goodman, C. S. (1990). Genetic analysis of a *Drosophila* neural cell adhesion molecule: Interaction of fasciclin I and Abelson tyrosine kinase mutations. *Cell* **60:** 565–575.

ElShamy, W. M., Linnarsson, S., Lee, K. F., Jaenisch, R., and Ernfors, P. (1996). Prenatal and postnatal requirements of NT-3 for sympathetic neuroblast survival and innervation of specific targets. *Development* **122:** 491–500.

Ericson, J., Briscoe, J., Rashbass, P., van Heyningen, V., and Jessell, T. M. (1997). Graded sonic hedgehog signaling and the specification of cell fate in the ventral neural tube. *Cold Spring Harbor Symp. Quant. Biol.* **62:** 451–466.

Erkman, L., McEvilly, R. J., Luo, L., Ryan, A. K., Hooshmand, F., O'Connell, S. M., Keithley, E. M. Rapaport, D. H., Ryan, A. F., and Rosenfeld, M. G. (1996). Role of

transcription factors Brn-3.1 and Brn-3.2 in auditory and visual system development. *Nature* **381:** 603–606.

Ernfors, P., Lee, K.-F., and Jaenisch, R. (1994). Mice lacking brain-derived neurotrophic factor develop with sensory deficits. *Nature* **368:** 147–150.

Ernfors, P., Van De Water, T., Loring, J., and Jaenisch, R. (1995). Complementary roles of BDNF and NT-3 in vestibular and auditory development. *Neuron* **14:** 1153–1164.

Ernst, M. (1926). Ueber Untergang von Zellen während der normalen Entwicklung bei Wirbeltieren. *Z. Anat. Entwicklungsgesch.* **79:** 228–262.

Evers, J., Laser, M., Sun, Y.-a., Xie, Z.-p., and Poo, M.-m. (1989). Studies of nerve–muscle interactions in *Xenopus* cell culture: Analysis of early synaptic currents. *J. Neurosci.* **9:** 1523–1539.

Fahrbach, S. E., Choi, M. K., and Truman, J. W. (1994). Inhibitory effects of actinomycin D and cycloheximide on neuronal death in adult *Manduca sexta. J. Neurobiol.* **25:** 59–69.

Fallon, J. R., and Gelfman, C. E. (1989). Agrin-related molecules are concentrated at acetylcholine receptor clusters in normal and aneural developing muscle. *J. Cell Biol.* **108:** 1527–1535.

Falls, D. L., Rosen, K. M., Corfas, G., Lane, W. S., and Fischbach, G. D. (1993). ARIA, a protein that stimulates acetylcholine receptor synthesis, is a member of the neu ligand family. *Cell* **72:** 801–815.

Fan, J., and Raper, J. A. (1995). Localized collapsing cues can steer growth cones without inducing their full collapse. *Neuron* **14:** 263–274.

Fannon, A. M., and Colman, D. R. (1996). A model for central synaptic junctional complex formation based on the differential adhesive specificities of the cadherins. *Neuron* **17:** 423–434.

Fantl, V., Stamp, G., Andrews, A., Rosewell, I., and Dickson, C. (1995). *Genes Dev.* **9:** 2364–2372.

Fatt, P., and Katz, B. (1951). Spontaneous subthreshold activity at motor nerve endings. *J. Physiol. (London)* **117:** 109–128.

Fawcett, J. W. (1997). Astrocytic and neuronal factors affecting axon regeneration in the damaged central nervous system. *Cell Tissue Res.* **290:** 371–377.

Fawcett, J. W., and Gaze, R. M. (1982). The retinotectal fibre pathways from normal and compound eyes in *Xenopus. J. Embryol. Exp. Morphol.* **72:** 19–37.

Fehon, R. G., Kooh, P. J., Rebay, I., Regan, C. L., Xu, T., Muskavitch, M. A., and Artavanis-Tsakonas, S. (1990). Molecular interactions between the protein products of the neurogenic loci Notch and Delta, two EGF-homologous genes in *Drosophila. Cell* **61:** 523–534.

Feldman, J. D., Gaze, R. M., and Keating, M. J. (1971). The post-metamorphic innervation by optic fibres of a virgin tectum in *Xenopus laevis. J. Physiol. (London)* **213:** 34P.

Ferns, M. J., Campanelli, J. T., Hoch, W., Scheller, R. H., and Hall, Z. (1993). The ability of agrin to cluster

AChRs depends on alternative splicing and on cell surface proteoglycans. *Neuron* **11:** 491–502.

Ferns, M., Deiner, M., and Hall, Z. (1996). Agrin-induced acetylcholine receptor clustering in mammalian muscle requires tyrosine phosphorylation. *J. Cell Biol.* **132:** 937–944.

Ferns, M. J., Hoch, W., Campanelli, J. T., Rupp, F., Hall, Z. W., and Scheller, R. H. (1992). RNA splicing regulates agrin-mediated acetylcholine receptor clustering activity on cultured myotubes. *Neuron* **8:** 1079–1086.

Ferreira, A., Han, H.-Q., Greengard, P., and Kosik, K. S. (1995). Suppression of synapsin II inhibits the formation and maintenance of synapses in hippocampal culture. *Proc. Natl. Acad. Sci. USA* **92:** 9225–9229.

Fertuck, H. C., and Salpeter, M. (1976). Quantitation of junctional and extrajunctional acetylcholine receptors by electron microscopic autoradiography after ^{125}I-α-bungarotoxin binding at mouse neuromuscular junctions. *J. Cell Biol.* **69:** 144–158.

Ferveur, J. F., Savarit, F., O'Kane, C. J., Sureau, G., Greenspan, R. J., and Jallon, J. M. (1997). Genetic feminization of pheromones and its behavioral consequences in *Drosophila* males. *Science* **276:** 1555–1558.

Ferveur, J. F., Störtkuhl, K. F., Stocker, R. F., and Greenspan, R. J. (1995). Genetic feminization of brain structures and changed sexual orientation in male *Drosophila*. *Science* **267:** 902–905.

Fiala, B. A., Joyce, J. N., and Greenough, W. T. (1978). Environmental complexity modulates growth of granule cell dendrites in developing but not adult hippocampus of rats. *Exp. Neurol.* **59:** 372–383.

Finley, K. D., Taylor, B. J., Milstein, M., and McKeown, M. (1997). dissatisfaction, a gene involved in sex-specific behavior and neural development of *Drosophila* melanogaster. *Proc. Natl. Acad. Sci. USA* **94:** 913–918.

Fischbach, G. D., and Cohen, S. A. (1973). The distribution of acetylcholine sensitivity over uninnervated and innervated muscle fibers grown in cell culture. *Dev. Biol.* **31:** 147–162.

Fishman, M. C. (1996). GAP-43: Putting constraints on neuronal plasticity. *Perspect. Dev. Neurobiol.* **4:** 193–198.

Flanagan, J. G., and Vanderhaeghen, P. (1998). The ephrins and Eph receptors in neural development. *Annu. Rev. Neurosci.* **21:** 309–345.

Florence, S. L., and Casagrande, V. A. (1990). Development of geniculocortical axon arbors in a primate. *Vision Neurosci.* **5:** 291–309.

Florence, S. L., Taub, H. B., and Kaas, J. H. (1998). Large-scale sprouting of cortical connections after peripheral injury in adult macaque monkeys [see Comments]. *Science* **282:** 1117–1121.

Fode, C., Gradwohl, G., Morim, X., Dierich, A., LeMeur, M., Goridis, C., and Guillemont, F. (1998). The bHLH protein Neurogenin 2 is a determination factor for epibranchial placode-derived sensory neurons. *Neuron* **20:** 483–494.

Ford-Holevinski, T. S., Hopkins, J. M., McCoy, J. P., and Agranoff, B. W. (1986). Laminin supports neurite outgrowth from explants of axotomized adult rat retinal neurons. *Brain Res.* **393:** 121–126.

Forehand, C. J., and Purves, D. (1984). Regional innervation of rabbit ciliary ganglion cells by the terminals of preganglionic axons. *J. Neurosci.* **4:** 1–12.

Foreman, N., Arber, M., and Savage, J. (1984). Spatial memory in preschool infants. *Dev. Psychobiol.* **17:** 129–137.

Forscher, P., Kaczmarek, L. K., Buchanan, J. A., and Smith, S. J. (1987). Cyclic AMP induces changes in distribution and transport of organelles within growth cones of Aplysia bag cell neurons. *J. Neurosci.* **7:** 3600–3611.

Fortini, M. E., and Artavanis-Tsakonas, S. (1994). The suppressor of hairless protein participates in notch receptor signaling. *Cell* **79:** 273–282.

Fox, K., Daw, N., Sato, H., and Czepita, D. (1992). The effect of visual experience on development of NMDA receptor synaptic transmission in kitten visual cortex. *J. Neurosci.* **12:** 2672–2684.

Frade, J. M., Rodríguez-Tébar, A., and Barde, Y. A. (1996). Induction of cell death by endogenous nerve growth factor through its p75 receptor. *Nature* **383:** 166–168.

Frank, E., and Wenner, P. (1993). Environmental specification of neuronal connectivity. *Neuron* **10:** 779–785.

Fraser, S. E., and Bronner-Fraser, M. (1991). Migrating neural crest cells in the trunk of the avian embryo are multipotent. *Development* **112:** 913–920.

Fredette, B. J., Miller, J., and Ranscht, B. (1996). Inhibition of motor axon growth by T-cadherin substrata. *Development* **122:** 3163–3171.

French, K., and Kristan, W. (1992). Intrinsic and extrinsic factors influencing the development of Retzius neurons in the leech nervous system. *In* "Determinants of Neuronal Identity" (M. Shankland and E. Macagno, Eds.), pp. 97–117. Academic Press, San Diego.

Freund, C. L., Gregory-Evans, C. Y., Furukawa, T., Papaioannou, M., Looser, J., Ploder, L., Bellingham, J., Ng, D., Herbrick, J. A., Duncan, A., Scherer, S. W., Tsui, L. C., Loutradis Anagnostou, A., Jacobson, S. G., Cepko, C. L., Bhattacharya, S. S., and McInnes, R. R. (1997). Cone rod dystrophy due to mutations in a novel photoreceptor-specific homeobox gene (CRX) essential for maintenance of the photoreceptor. *Cell* **91:** 543–553.

Friedman, G. C., and O'Leary, D. D. (1996). Retroviral misexpression of engrailed genes in the chick optic tectum perturbs the topographic targeting of retinal axons. *J. Neurosci.* **16:** 5498–5509.

Friedrich, R. W., and Korsching, S. I. (1997). Combinatorial and chemotopic odorant coding in the zebrafish olfactory bulb visualized by optical imaging. *Neuron* **18:** 737–752.

Frisen, J., Yates, P. A., McLaughlin, T., Friedman, G. C., O'Leary, D. D., and Barbacid, M. (1998). Ephrin-A5 (AL-1/RAGS) is essential for proper retinal axon guidance and topographic mapping in the mammalian visual system. *Neuron* **20:** 235–243.

Frohner, S. C., Luetje, C. W., Scotland, P. B., and Patrick, J. (1990). The postsynaptic 43K protein clusters muscle nicotinic acetylcholine receptors in *Xenopus* oocytes. *Neuron* **5:** 403–410.

Fu, W.-m., and Lin, J.-L. (1993). Activation of protein kinase C potentiates postsynaptic acetylcholine response at developing neuromuscular synapses. *Br. J. Pharmacol.* **110:** 707–712.

Fuerstenberg, S., Broadus, J., and Doe, C. Q. (1998). Asymmetry and cell fate in the *Drosophila* embryonic CNS. *Int. J. Dev. Biol.* **42:** 379–383.

Fujisawa, H. (1981). Retinotopic analysis of fiber pathways in the regenerating retinotectal system of the adult newt cynops *Pyrrhogaster. Brain Res.* **206:** 27–37.

Fukuda, A., and Prince, D. A. (1992). Postnatal development of electrogenic sodium pump activity in rat hippocampal pyramidal neurons. *Dev. Brain Res.* **65:** 101–114.

Funte, L. R., and Haydon, P. G. (1993). Synaptic target contact enhances presynaptic calcium influx by activating cAMP-dependent protein kinase during synaptogenesis. *Neuron* **10:** 1069–1078.

Gage, F. H., Armstrong, D. M., Williams, L. R., and Varon, S. (1988). Morphological response of axotomized septal neurons to nerve growth factor. *J. Comp. Neurol.* **269:** 147–155.

Gagliardini, V., Fernandez, P. A., Lee, R. K., Drexler, H. C., Rotello, R. J., Fishman, M. C., and Yuan, J. (1994). Prevention of vertebrate neuronal death by the crmA gene. *Science* **263:** 826–828.

Gähwiler, B. H., Thompson, S. M., Audinat, E., and Robertson, R. T. (1991). Organotypic slice cultures of nerual tissue. *In* "Culturing Nerve Cells" (G. Banker and K. Goslin, Eds.), pp. 379–411. MIT Press, Cambridge, MA.

Galli, L., and Maffei, L. (1988). Spontaneous impulse activity of rat retinal ganglion cells in prenatal life. *Science* **242:** 90–91.

Gan, L., Xiang, M., Zhou, L., Wagner, D. S., Klein, W. H., and Nathans, J. (1996). POU domain factor Brn-3b is required for the development of a large set of retinal ganglion cells. *Proc. Natl. Acad. Sci. USA* **93:** 3920–3925.

Garcia-Verdugo, J. M., Doetsch, F., Wichterle, H., Lim, D. A., and Alvarez-Buylla, A. (1998). Architecture and cell types of the adult subventricular zone: In search of the stem cells. *J. Neurobiology* **36:** 234–248.

Gardette, R., Listerud, M. D., Brussaard, A. B., and Role, L. W. (1991). Developmental changes in transmitter sensitivity and synaptic transmission in embryonic chicken sympathetic neurons innervated *in vitro. Dev. Biol.* **147:** 83–95.

Garthwaite, G., Yamini, B., Jr., and Garthwaite, J. (1987). Selective loss of Purkinje and granule cell responsiveness to *N*-Methyl-D-aspartate in rat cerebellum during development. *Brain Res.* **433:** 288–292.

Gautam, M., Noakes, P. G., Moscoso, L., Rupp, F., Scheller, R. H., Merlie, J. P., and Sanes, J. R. (1996). Defective neuromuscular synaptogenesis in agrin-deficient mutant mice. *Cell* **85:** 525–535.

Gautam, M., Noakes, P. G., Mudd, J., Nichol, M., Chu, G. C., Sanes, J. R., and Merlie, J. P. (1995). Failure of postsynaptic specialization to develop at neuromuscular junctions of rapsyn-deficient mice. *Nature* **377:** 232–236.

Gavalas, A., Studer, M., Lumsden, A., Rijli, F. M., Krumlauf, R., Chambon, P. (1998). Hoxa1 and Hoxb1 synergize in patterning the hindbrain, cranial nerves and second pharyngeal arch. *Development* **125:** 1123–1136.

Gaze, R. M., Keating, M. J., Ostberg, A., and Chung, S. H. (1979). The relationship between retinal and tectal growth in larval *Xenopus:* Implications for the development of the retino-tectal projection. *J. Embryol. Exp. Morphol.* **53:** 103–143.

Gee, S. H., Montanaro, F., Lindenbaum, M. H., and Carbonetto, S. (1994). Dystroglycan-α, a dystrophin-associated glycoprotein, is a functional agrin receptor. *Cell* **77:** 675–686.

Gehart, J., and Kirschner, M. (1997). Cells, Embryos, and Evolution. Blackwell Sciences, Oxford, England.

Gehring, W. J. (1993). Exploring the homeobox. *Gene* **135:** 215–221.

Ghosh, A., Carnahan, J., and Greenberg, M. E. (1994). Requirement for BDNF in activity-dependent survival of cortical neurons. *Science* **263:** 1618–1623.

Ghosh, A., and Greenberg, M. E. (1995). Distinct roles for bFGF and NT-3 in the regulation of cortical neurogenesis. *Neuron* **15:** 89–103.

Ghysen, A., and Dambly-Chaudiere, C. (1992). Development of the peripheral nervous system in *Drosophila. In* "Determinants of Neuronal Identity" (M. Shankland and E. Macagno, Eds.), pp. 225–292. Academic Press, San Diego.

Giesen, K., Hummel, T., Stollewerk, A., Harrison, S., Travers, A., and Klambt, C. (1997). Glial development in the *Drosophila* CNS requires concomitant activation of glial and repression of neuronal differentiation genes. *Development* **124:** 2307–2316.

Gilbert, S., and Raunio, A. M. (1997). "Embryology: Constructing the Organism." Sinauer, Sunderland, MA.

Gillespie, S. K. H., Balasubramanian, S., Fung, E. T., and Huganir, R. L. (1996). Rapsyn clusters and activates the synapse-specific receptor tyrosine kinase MuSK. *Neuron* **16:** 953–962.

Glanzman, D. L., Kandel, E. R., and Schacher, S. (1991). Target-dependent morphological segregation of *Aplysia* sensory outgrowth *in vitro. Neuron* **7:** 903–913.

Glass, D. J., Bowen, D. C., Stitt, T. N., Radziejewski, C., Bruno, J., Ryan, T. E., Gies, D. R., Shah, S., Mattsson, K., Burden, S. J., DiStefano, P. S., Valenzuela, D. M., DeChiara, T. M., and Yancopoulos, G. D. (1996). Agrin acts via a musk receptor complex. *Cell* **85:** 513–523.

Globus, A., and Scheibel, A. B. (1966). Loss of dendritic spines as an index of presynaptic terminal patterns. *Nature (London)* **212:** 463–465.

Glover, J. C., Petursdottir, G., and Jansen, J. K. S. (1986). Fluorescent dextran-amines used as axonal tracers in the nervous system of the chicken embryo. *J. Neurosci. Methods* **18:** 243–254.

Godfrey, E. W., Nitkin, R. M., Wallace, B. G., Rubin, L. L., and McMahon, U. J. (1984). Components of Torpedo electric organ and muscle that cause aggregation of acetylcholine receptors in cultured muscle cells. *J. Cell Biol.* **99:** 615–627.

Godsave, S. F., and Slack, J. M. (1989). Clonal analysis of mesoderm induction in *Xenopus laevis. Dev. Biol.* **134:** 486–490.

Goldberg, D. J., and Wu, D. Y. (1996). Tyrosine phosphorylation and protrusive structures of the growth cone. *Perspect. Dev. Neurobiol.* **4:** 183–192.

Goldman, D., Carlson, B. M., and Staple, J. (1991). Induction of adult-type nicotinic acetylcholine receptor gene expression in noninnervated regenerating muscle. *Neuron* **7:** 649–658.

Goodearl, A. D., Yee, A. G., Sandrock, A. W., Jr., Corfas, G., and Fischbach, G. D. (1995). ARIA is concentrated in the synaptic basal lamina of the developing chick neuromuscular junction. *J. Cell Biol.* **130:** 1423–1434.

Goodkin, F. (1980). The development of mature patterns of head-eye coordination in the human infant. *Early Hum. Dev.* **4:** 373–386.

Goodman, C. S. (1996). Mechanisms and molecules that control growth cone guidance. *Annu. Rev. Neurosci.* **19:** 341–377.

Goodman, C. S., Bastiani, M. J., Doe, C. Q., du Lac, S., Helfand, S. L., Kuwada, J. Y., and Thomas, J. B. (1984). Cell recognition during neuronal development. *Science* **225:** 1271–1279.

Goodman, C. S., Raper, J. A., Chang, S., and Ho, R. (1983). Grasshopper growth cones: Divergent choices and labeled pathways. *Prog. Brain Res.* **58:** 283–304.

Gordon, T., Perry, R., Tuffery, A. R., and Vrbova, G. (1974). Possible mechanisms determining synapses formation in developing skeletal muscles of the chick. *Cell Tissue Res.* **155:** 13–25.

Gorski, R. A., Gordon, J. H., Shryne, J. E., and Southam, A. M. (1978). Evidence for a morphological sex difference within the medial preoptic area of the rat brain. *Brain Res.* **148:** 333–346.

Goslin, K., and Banker, G. (1989). Experimental observations on the development of polarity by hippocampal neurons in culture. *J. Cell Biol.* **108:** 1507–1516.

Gottlieb, G. (1980). Development of species identification in ducklings. VI. Specific embryonic experience required to maintain species-typical perception in ducklings. *J. Comp. Physiol. Psychol.* **94:** 579–587.

Gottmann, K., Dietzel, I. D., Lux, H. D., Huck, S., and Rohrer, H. (1988). Development of inward currents in chick sensory and autonomic neuronal precurser cells in culture. *J. Neurosci.* **8:** 3722–3732.

Gould, S. J. (1970). "Ontogeny and Phylogeny." Harvard Univ. Press, Cambridge, MA.

Grandori, C., and Eisenman, R. N. (1997). Mye target genes. *Trends in Biochem. Sci.* **22:** 177–181.

Grassi, S., Ottaviani, F., and Bambagioni, D. (1990). Vocalization-related stapedius muscle activity in different age chickens (*Gallus gallus*) and its role in vocal development. *Brain Res.* **529:** 158–164.

Grenningloh, G., Rehm, E. J., and Goodman, C. S. (1991). Genetic analysis of growth cone guidance in *Drosophila*: Fasciclin II functions as a neuronal recognition molecule. *Cell* **67:** 45–57.

Grens, A., Mason, E., Marsh, J. L., and Bode, H. R. (1995). Evolutionary conservation of a cell fate specification gene: The *Hydra* achaete–scute homolog has proneural activity in *Drosophila. Development* **121:** 4027–4035.

Grillenzoni, N., van Helden, J., Dambly-Chaudiere, C., and Ghysen, A. (1998). The iroquois complex controls the somatotopy of *Drosophila* notum mechanosensory projections. *Development* **125:** 3563–3569.

Gross, R. E., Mehler, M. F., Mabie, P. C., Zang, Z., Santschi, L., and Kessler, J. A. (1996). Bone morphogenetic proteins promote astroglial lineage commitment by mammalian subventricular zone progenitor cells. *Neuron* **17:** 595–606.

Groves, A. K., and Anderson, D. J. (1996). Role of environmental signals and transcriptional regulators in neural crest development. *Dev. Genet.* **18:** 64–72.

Grunz, H., and Tacke, L. (1989). Neural differentiation of *Xenopus laevis* ectoderm takes place after disaggregation and delayed reaggregation without inducer. *Cell Differ. Dev.* **28:** 211–217.

Gu, Q., and Singer, W. (1995). Involvement of serotonin in developmental plasticity of kitten visual cortex. *Eur. J. Neurosci.* **7:** 1146–1153.

Gu, Y., and Hall, Z. W. (1988). Immunological evidence for a change in subunits of the acetylcholine receptor in developing and denervated rat muscle. *Neuron* **1:** 117–125.

Gundersen, R. W., and Barrett, J. N. (1979). Neuronal chemotaxis: Chick dorsal–root axons turn toward high concentrations of nerve growth factor. *Science* **206:** 1079–1080.

Guo, X., Metzler-Northrup, J., Lein, P., Rueger, D., and Higgins, D. (1997). Leukemia inhibitory factor and ciliary neurotrophic factor regulate dendritic growth in cultures of rat sympathetic neurons. *Brain Res. Dev. Brain Res.* **104:** 101–110.

Guo, X., Rueger, D., and Higgins, D. (1998). Osteogenic protein-1 and related bone morphogenetic proteins regulate dendritic growth and the expression of microtubule-associated protein-2 in rat sympathetic neurons. *Neurosci. Lett.* **245:** 131–134.

Gurney, M. E. (1981). Hormonal control of cell form and number in the zebra finch song system. *J. Neurosci.* **1:** 658–673.

Gurney, M. E., and Konishi, M. (1980). Hormone-induced sexual differentiation of brain and behavior in zebra finches. *Science* **208:** 1380–1383.

Hafidi, A., Moore, T., and Sanes, D. H. (1996). Regional distribution of neurotrophin receptors in the developing auditory brainstem. *J. Comp. Neurol.* **367:** 454–464.

Halder, G., Callaerts, P., *et al.* (1995). Induction of ectopic eyes by targeted expression of the eyeless gene in *Drosophila* [see Comments]. *Science* **267**: 1788–1792.

Hall, J. C. (1977). Portions of the central nervous system controlling reproductive behavior in *Drosophila melanogaster. Behav. Genet.* **7**: 291–312.

Hall, J. C. (1994). The mating of a fly. *Science* **264**: 1702–1714.

Halpern, M. E., Chiba, A., Johansen, J., and Keshishian, H. (1991). Growth cone behavior underlying the development of stereotypic synaptic connections in *Drosophila* embryos. *J. Neurosci.* **11**: 3227–3238.

Halter, D. A., Urban, J., Rickert, C., Ner, S. S., Ito, K., Travers, A. A., and Technau, G. M. (1995). The homeobox gene repo is required for the differentiation and maintenance of glia function in the embryonic nervous system of *Drosophila melanogaster. Development* **121**: 317–332.

Ham, J., Babij, C., Whitfield, J., Pfarr, C. M., Lallemand, D., Yaniv, M., and Rubin, L. L. (1995). A c-Jun dominant negative mutant protects sympathetic neurons against programmed cell death. *Neuron* **14**: 927–939.

Hamburger, V. (1934). The effects of wing bud extirpation on the development of the central nervous system in chick embryos. *J. Exp. Zool.* **68**: 449–494.

Hamburger, V. (1943). The effects of wing bud extirpation on the development of the central nervous system in chick embryos. *J. Exp. Zool.* **68**: 449–494.

Hamburger, V. (1963). Some aspects of the embryology of behavior. *Q. Rev. Biol.* **38**: 342–365.

Hamburger, V. (1969). Hans Spemann and the organizer concept. *Experientia* **25**: 1121–1125.

Hamburger, V., and Levi-Montalcini, R. (1949). Proliferation, differentiation and degeneration in the spinal ganglia of the chick embryo under normal and experimental conditions. *J. Exp. Zool.* **111**: 457–501.

Hamburger, V., Wenger, E., and Oppenhein, R. W. (1966). Motility in the chick and embryo in the absence of sensory input. *J. Exp. Zool.* **162**: 133–160.

Hamill, O. P., Marty, A., Neher, E., Sakmann, B., and Sigworth, F. J. (1981). Improved patch-clamp techniques for high-resolution current recording from cell and cell-free membrane patches. *Pflüegers Arch.* **391**: 85–100.

Hammarback, J. A., Palm, S. L., Furcht, L. T., and Letourneau, P. C. (1985). Guidance of neurite outgrowth by pathways of substratum-adsorbed laminin. *J. Neurosci. Res.* **13**: 213–220.

Han, H.-Q., Nichols, R. A., Rubin, M. R., Bähler, M., and Greengard, P. (1991). Induction of formation of presynaptic terminals in neuroblastoma cells by synapsin IIb. *Nature* **349**: 697–700.

Harish, O. E., and Poo, M.-m. (1992). Retrograde modulation at developing neuromuscular synapses: Involvement of G protein and arachidonic acid cascade. *Neuron* **9**: 1201–1209.

Harris, D. A., Falls, D. L., Dill-Devor, R. M., and Fischbach, G. D. (1988). Acetylcholine receptor-inducing factor from chicken brain increases the level of mRNA encoding the receptor a subunit. *Proc. Natl. Acad. Sci. USA* **85**: 1983–1987.

Harris, R. M., and Woolsey, T. A. (1981). Dendritic plasticity in mouse barrel cortex following postnatal vibrissa follicle damage. *J. Comp. Neurol.* **196**: 357–376.

Harris, W. (1997). Cellular diversification in the vertebrate retina. *Curr. Opin. Genet. Dev.* **7**: 651–658.

Harris, W., and Hartenstein, V. (1999). Cellular determination. *In* "Fundamental Neuroscience" (M. Zigmond, F. Bloom, S. Landis, J. Roberst, and L. Squire, Eds.), pp. 481–517. Academic Press, San Diego.

Harris, W. A. (1982). The transplantation of eyes to genetically eyeless salamanders: Visual projections and somatosensory interactions. *J. Neurosci.* **2**: 339–353.

Harris, W. A. (1986). Homing behaviour of axons in the embryonic vertebrate brain. *Nature* **320**: 266–269.

Harris, W. A. (1989). Local positional cues in the neuroepithelium guide retinal axons in embryonic *Xenopus* brain. *Nature* **339**: 218–221.

Harris, W. A. (1990). Neurometamorphosis. *J. Neurobiol.* **21**: 953–957.

Harris, W. A., Holt, C. E., and Bonhoeffer, F. (1987). Retinal axons with and without their somata, growing to and arborizing in the tectum of *Xenopus* embryos: A time-lapse video study of single fibres *in vivo. Development* **101**: 123–133.

Harrison, R. G. (1904). An experimental study of the relation of the nervous system to the developing musculature in the embryo of the frog. *Am. J. Anat.* **3**: 197–220.

Harrison, R. G. (1907). Observations on the living developing nerve fiber. *Anat. Rec.* **1**: 116–118.

Harrison, R. G. (1910). The outgrowth of the nerve fiber as a mode of protoplasmic movement. *J. Exp. Zool.* **9**: 787–846.

Hartenstein, V. (1989). Early neurogenesis in *Xenopus*: The spatio-temporal pattern of proliferation and cell lineages in the embryonic spinal cord. *Neuron* **3**: 399–411.

Hartenstein, V., and Posakony, J. W. (1990). A dual function of the Notch gene in *Drosophila sensillum* development. *Dev. Biol.* **142**: 13–30.

Hartley, D. A., Xu, T. A., and Artavanis-Tsakonas, S. (1987). The embryonic expression of the Notch locus of *Drosophila melanogaster* and the implications of point mutations in the extracellular EGF-like domain of the predicted protein. *EMBO J.* **6**: 3407–3417.

Hartshorn, K., Rovee-Collier, C., Gerhardstein, P., Bhatt, R. S., Wondoloski, T. L., Klein, P., Gilch, J., Wurtzel, N., and Campos-de-Carvalho, M. (1998). The ontogeny of long-term memory over the first year-and-a-half of life. *Dev. Psychobiol.* **32**: 69–89.

Hatini, V., Tao, W., and Lai, E. (1994). Expression of winged helix genes, BF-1 and BF-2, define adjacent domains within the developing forebrain and retina. *J. Neurobiol.* **25**: 1293–1309.

Hatten, M. E. (1985). Neuronal regulation of astroglial morphology and proliferation *in vitro. J. Cell Biol.* **100**: 384–396.

Hatten, M. E. (1993). The role of migration in central nervous system neuronal development. *Curr. Opin. Neurobiol.* **3:** 38–44.

Haverkamp, L. J. (1986). Anatomical and physiological development of the *Xenopus* embryonic motor system in the absence of neural activity. *J. Neurosci.* **6:** 1338–1348.

Haverkamp, L. J., and Oppenheim, R. W. (1986). Behavioral development in the absence of neural activity: Effects of chronic immobilization on amphibian embryos. *J. Neurosci.* **6:** 1332–1337.

Haydon, P. G., McCobb, D. P., and Kater, S. B. (1984). Serotonin selectively inhibits growth cone motility and synaptogenesis of specific identified neurons. *Science* **226:** 561–564.

Hayes, B. P., and Roberts, A. (1973). Synaptic junction development in the spinal cord of an amphibian embryo: An electron microscope study. *Z. Zellforsch.* **137:** 251–269.

Heidemann, S. R. (1996). Cytoplasmic mechanisms of axonal and dendritic growth in neurons. *Int. Rev. Cytol.* **165:** 235–296.

Heidemann, S. R., Lamoureux, P., and Buxbaum, R. E. (1995). Cytomechanics of axonal development. *Cell Biochem. Biophys.* **27:** 135–155.

Held, H. (1897). Beiträge zur Structur der Nervenzellen und ihrer Fortädtze. *Arch. Anat. Physiol. Anat. Abt.* **21:** 204–294.

Hemmati-Brivanlou, A., Kelly, O. G., *et al.* (1994). Follistatin, an antagonist of activin, is expressed in the Spemann organizer and displays direct neuralizing activity. *Cell* **77:** 283–295.

Hemmati-Brivanlou, A., and Melton, D. A. (1994). Inhibition of activin receptor signaling promotes neuralization in *Xenopus*. *Cell* **77:** 273–281.

Hendrikson, C. K., and Vaughn, J. E. (1974). Fine structural relationships between neurites and radial glial processes in developing mouse spinal cord. *J. Neurocytol.* **3:** 659–675.

Hendry, I. A., Stöckel, K., Thoenen, H., and Iversen, L. L. (1974). The retrograde axonal transport of nerve growth factor. *Brain Res.* **68:** 103–121.

Hendry, S. H., Huntsman, M. M., Vinuela, A., Mohler, H., de Blas, A. L., and Jones, E. G. (1994). GABAA receptor subunit immunoreactivity in primate visual cortex: Distribution in macaques and humans and regulation by visual input in adulthood. *J. Neurosci.* **14:** 2383–2401.

Hengartner, M. O., Ellis, R. E., and Horvitz, H. R. (1992). *Caenorhabditis elegans* gene ced-9 protects cells from programmed cell death. *Nature* **356:** 494–499.

Henrique, D., Hirsinger, E., Adam, J., Le Roux, I., Pourquie, O., Ish-Horowicz, D., and Lewis, J. (1997). Maintenance of neuroepithelial progenitor cells by Delta–Notch signalling in the embryonic chick retina. *Curr. Biol.* **7:** 661–670.

Herrmann, K., and Arnold, A. P. (1991). The development of afferent projections to the robust archistriatal nucleus in male zebra finches: A quantitative electron microscopic study. *J. Neurosci.* **11:** 2063–2074.

Hestrin, S. (1992). Developmental regulation of NMDA receptor-mediated synaptic currents at a central synapse. *Nature* **357:** 686–689.

Heumann, R., Schwab, M., Merkl, R., and Thoenen, H. (1984). Nerve growth factor-mediated induction of choline acetyltransferase in PC12 cells: Evaluation of the site of action of nerve growth factor and the involvement of lysosomal degradation products of nerve growth factor. *J. Neurosci.* **4:** 3039–3050.

Hibbard, E. (1965). Orientation and directed growth of Mauthner's cell axons from duplicated vestibular nerve roots. *J. Exp. Neurol.* **13:** 289–301.

Hinds, J. W., and Hinds, P. A. (1976a). Synapse formation in the mouse olfactory bub. I. Quantitative studies. *J. Comp. Neurol.* **169:** 15–40.

Hinds, J. W., and Hinds, P. A. (1976b). Synapse formation in the mouse olfactory bub. II. Morphogenesis. *J. Comp. Neurol.* **169:** 41–62.

Hoffmann, H., and Spear, N. E. (1988). Ontogenetic differences in conditioning of an aversion to a gustatory CS with a peripheral US. *Behav. Neural Biol.* **50:** 16–23.

Holash, J. A., Soans, C., Chong, L. D., Shao, H., Dixit, V. M., and Pasquale, E. B. (1997). Reciprocal expression of the Eph receptor Cek5 and its ligand(s). in the early retina. *Dev. Biol.* **182:** 256–269.

Holland, R. L., and Brown, M. C. (1980). Postsynaptic transmission block can cause terminal sprouting of a motor nerve. *Science* **207:** 649–651.

Hollenbeck, P. J., and Bray, D. (1987). Rapidly transported organelles containing membrane and cytoskeletal components: Their relation to axonal growth. *J. Cell Biol.* **105:** 2827–2835.

Holley, S. A., Jackson, P. D., *et al.* (1995). A conserved system for dorsal–ventral patterning in insects and vertebrates involving sog and chordin [see Comments]. *Nature* **376:** 249–253.

Hollyday, M., and Hamburger, V. (1976). Reduction of the naturally occurring motor neuron loss by enlargement of the periphery. *J. Comp. Neurol.* **170:** 311–320.

Hollyfield, J. G. (1968). Differential addition of cells to the retina in *Rana pipiens* tadpoles. *Dev. Biol.* **18:** 163–179.

Holt, C. E. (1984). Does timing of axon outgrowth influence initial retinotectal topography in *Xenopus*? *J. Neurosci.* **4:** 1130–1152.

Holt, C. E., Bertsch, T. W., Ellis, H. M., and Harris, W. A. (1988). Cellular determination in the *Xenopus* retina is independent of lineage and birth date. *Neuron* **1:** 15–26.

Holt, C. E., and Harris, W. A. (1983). Order in the initial retinotectal map in *Xenopus*: A new technique for labelling growing nerve fibres. *Nature* **301:** 150–152.

Holt, C. E., and Harris, W. A. (1998). Target selection: Invasion, mapping and cell choice. *Curr. Opin. Neurobiol.* **8:** 98–105.

Holtfreter, J. (1939). Studien zur Ermittlung der Gestaltlungsfaktoren in der Organentwicklung der Amphibien. *Roux' Arch. Entwicklungsmech. Org.* **139:** 227–273.

Holtfreter, J., and Hamburger, V. (1955). "Amphibians in

Analysis of Development'' (Willer, Weiss, and Hamburger, Eds.). Saunders, Philadelphia.

Hömberg, V., Bickmann, U., and Müller, K. (1993). Ontogeny is different for explicit and implicit memory in humans. *Neurosci. Lett.* **150:** 187–190.

Honig, M. G., and Hume, R. I. (1986). Fluorescent carbocyanine dyes allow living neurons of identified origin to be studied in long-term cultures. *J. Cell Biol.* **103:** 171–187.

Hopf, C., and Hoch, W. (1996). Agrin binding to alpha-dystroglycan. Domains of agrin necessary to induce acetylcholine receptor clustering are overlapping but not identical to the alpha-dystroglycan-binding region. *J. Biol. Chem.* **271:** 5231–5236.

Hoppe, P. E., and Greenspan, R. J. (1986). Local function of the Notch gene for embryonic ectodermal pathway choice in *Drosophila. Cell* **46:** 773–783.

Horan, G. S., Ramírez-Solis, R., Featherstone, M. S., Wolgemuth, D. J., Bradley, A., and Behringer, R. R. (1995). Compound mutants for the paralogous hoxa-4, hoxb-4, and hoxd-4 genes show more complete homeotic transformations and a dose-dependent increase in the number of vertebrae transformed. *Genes Dev.* **9:** 1667–1677.

Hoskins, S. G., and Grobstein, P. (1984). Induction of the ipsilateral retinothalamic projection in *Xenopus laevis* by thyroxine. *Nature* **307:** 730–733.

Hosoya, T., Takizawa, K., Nitta, K., and Hotta, Y. (1995). Glial cells missing: A binary switch between neuronal and glial determination in *Drosophila. Cell* **82:** 1025–1036.

Hoyle, G. W., Mercer, E. H., Palmiter, R. D., and Brinster, R. L. (1993). Expression of NGF in sympathetic neurons leads to excessive axon outgrowth from ganglia but decreased terminal innervation within tissues. *Neuron* **10:** 1019–1034.

Huang, C. F., Tong, J., and Schmidt, J. (1992). Protein kinase C couples membrane excitation to acetylcholine receptor gene inactivation in chick skeletal muscle. *Neuron* **9:** 671–678.

Hubel, D. H., and Wiesel, T. N. (1965). Binocular interaction in striate cortex of kittens reared with artificial squint. *J. Neurophysiol.* **28:** 1041–1059.

Hubel, D. H., and Wiesel, T. N. (1970). The period of susceptibility to the physiological effects of unilateral eye closure in kittens. *J. Physiol.* **206:** 419–436.

Huganir, R. L., and Greengard, P. (1983). cAMP-dependent protein kinase phosphorylates the nicotinic acetylcholine receptor. *Proc. Natl. Acad. Sci.* **80:** 1130–1134.

Huganir, R. L., Miles, K., and Greengard, P. (1984). Phosphorylation of the nicotinic acetylcholine receptor by an endogenous tyrosine-specific protein kinase. *Proc. Natl. Acad. Sci. USA* **81:** 6968–6972.

Hughes, A. F. (1961). Cell degeneration in the larval ventral horn of *Xenopus laevis. J. Embryol. Exp. Morphol.* **9:** 269–284.

Huguenard, J. R., Hamill, O. P., and Prince, D. A. (1988). Developmental changes in Na^+ conductances in rat neocortical neurons: Appearance of a slowly inactivating component. *J. Neurophysiol.* **9:** 778–795.

Hume, R. I., Role, L. W., and Fischbach, G. D. (1983). Acetylcholine release from growth cones detected with patches of acetylcholine receptor rich membranes. *Nature* **305:** 632–634.

Hunt, P. S., Richardson, R., and Campbell, B. A. (1994). Delayed development of fear-potentiated startle in rats. *Behav. Neurosci.* **108:** 69–80.

Hunt, R. K., and Jacobson, M. (1974). Specification of positional information in retinal ganglion cells of *Xenopus laevis*: Intra-ocular control of the time of specification. *Proc. Natl. Acad. Sci. USA* **71:** 3616–3620.

Hurlin, P. J., Queva, C., Koskinen, P. J., Steingrimsson, E., Ayer, D. E., Copeland, N. G., Jenkins, N. A., and Eisenman, R. N. (1995). Mad3 and Mad4: Novel Max-interacting transcriptional repressors that suppress c-myc dependent transformation and are expressed during neural and epidermal differentiation. *EMBO J.* **14:** 5646–5659.

Hutchison, J. B. (1997). Gender-specific steroid metabolism in neural differentiation. *Cell. Mol. Neurobiol.* **17:** 603–626.

Huttenlocher, P. R., and de Courten, C. (1987). The development of synapses in striate cortex of man. *Human Neurobiol.* **6:** 1–9.

Hyatt, G. A., Schmitt, E. A., Marsh-Armstrong, N., McCaffery, P., Drager, U. C., and Dowling, J. E. (1996). Retinoic acid establishes ventral retinal characteristics. *Development* **122:** 195–204.

Hyson, R. L., and Rubel, E. W. (1989). Transneuronal regulation of protein synthesis in the brain-stem auditory system of the chick requires synaptic activation. *J. Neurosci.* **9:** 2835–2845.

Hyson, R. L., and Rudy, J. W. (1987). Ontogenetic change in the analysis of sound frequency in the infant rat. *Dev. Psychobiol.* **20:** 189–207.

Ibanez, C. F. (1994). Structure-function relationships in the neurotrophin family. *J. Neurobiol.* **25:** 1349–1361.

Igarashi, M., Strittmatter, S. M., Vartanian, T., and Fishman, M. C. (1993). Mediation by G proteins of signals that cause collapse of growth cones. *Science* **259:** 77–79.

Imperato-McGinley, J., Peterson, R. E., Gautier, T., and Sturla, E. (1979). Male pseudohermaphroditism secondary to 5 alpha-reductase deficiency—a model for the role of androgens in both the development of the male phenotype and the evolution of a male gender identity. *J. Steroid Biochem.* **11:** 637–645.

Innocenti, G. M., Fiore, L., and Caminiti, R. (1977). Exuberent projection into the corpus callosum from the visual cortex of newborn cats. *Neurosci. Lett.* **4:** 237–242.

Inoue, A., and Sanes, J. R. (1997). Lamina-specific connectivity in the brain: Regulation by N-cadherin, neurotrophins, and glycoconjugates. *Science* **276:** 1428–1431.

Inoué, S. (1981). Video image processing greatly enhances contrast, quality, and speed in polarization-based microscopy. *J. Cell Biol.* **89:** 346–356.

Inoué, S. (1989). Foundations of confocal scanning imaging in light microscopy. *In* "The Handbook of Biological Confocal Microscopy" (Pawley, Ed.), pp. 1–14. IMR Press, Madison, WI.

Ishida, N., Kaneko, M., and Allada, R. (1999). Biological clocks. *Proc. Natl. Acad. Sci. USA* **96:** 8819–8820.

Itasaki, N., Ichijo, H., Hama, C., Matsuno, T., and Nakamura, H. (1991). Establishment of rostrocaudal polarity in tectal primordium: Engrailed expression and subsequent tectal polarity. *Development* **113:** 1133–1144.

Itasaki, N., and Nakamura, H. (1992). Rostrocaudal polarity of the tectum in birds: Correlation of en gradient and topographic order in retinotectal projection. *Neuron* **8:** 787–798.

Itasaki, N., and Nakamura, H. (1996). A role for gradient en expression in positional specification on the optic tectum. *Neuron* **16:** 55–62.

Iwasato, T., Erzurumlu, R. S., Huerta, P. T., Chen, D. F., Sasaoka, T., Ulupinar, E., and Tonegawa, S. (1997). NMDA receptor-dependent refinement of somatotopic maps. *Neuron* **19:** 1201–1210.

Jablonska, B., Gierdalski, M., Kossut, M., and Skangiel-Kramska, J. (1999). Partial blocking of NMDA receptors reduces plastic changes induced by short-lasting classical conditioning in the SI barrel cortex of adult mice. *Cereb. Cortex* **9:** 222–231.

Jackson, H., and Parks, T. N. (1982). Functional synapse elimination in the developing avian cochlear nucleus with simultaneous reduction in cochlear nerve axon branching. *J. Neurosci.* **2:** 1736–1743.

Jacobs, D. S., and Blakemore, C. (1988). Factors limiting the postnatal development of visual acuity in the monkey. *Vision Res.* **8:** 947–958.

Jacobson, M. (1991). "Developmental Neurobiology." Plenum, New York.

Jan, Y. N., and Jan, L. Y. (1998). Asymmetric cell division. *Nature* **392:** 775–778.

Jansen, J. K. S., Lømo, T., Nicolaysen, K., and Westgaard, R. H. (1973). Hyperinnervation of skeletal muscle fibers: Dependence on muscle activity. *Science* **181:** 559–561.

Jarman, A. P., Grau, Y., Jan, L. Y., and Jan, Y. N. (1993). Atonal is a proneural gene that directs chordotonal organ formation in the *Drosophila* peripheral nervous system. *Cell* **73:** 1307–1321.

Jarman, A. P., Grell, E. H., Ackerman, L., Jan, L. Y., and Jan, Y. N. (1994). Atonal is the proneural gene for *Drosophila* photoreceptors. *Nature* **369:** 398–400.

Jendelová, P., and Syková, E. (1991). The role of glia in K^+ and pH homeostasis in the neonatal rat spinal cord. *Glia* **4:** 56–63.

Jessell, T. M., Bovolenta, P., Placzek, M., Tessier-Lavigne, M., and Dodd, J. (1989). Polarity and patterning in the neural tube: The origin and function of the floor plate. *Ciba Found. Symp.* **144:** 255–276.

Jessell, T. M., Siegel, R. E., and Fischbach, G. D. (1979). Induction of acetylcholine receptors on cultured skeletal muscle by a factor extracted from brain and spinal cord. *Proc. Natl. Acad. Sci. USA* **76:** 5397–5401.

Jessen, K. R., and Mirsky, R. (1994). Neural development: Fate diverted. *Curr. Biol.* **4:** 824–827.

Johns, P. R., and Fernald, R. D. (1981). Genesis of rods in teleost fish retina. *Nature* **293:** 141–142.

Johnson, D., Lanahan, A., Buck, C. R., Sehgal, A., Morgan, C., Mercer, E., Bothwell, M., and Chao, M. (1986). Expression and structure of the human NGF receptor. *Cell* **47:** 545–554.

Johnson, E. M., Jr. (1978). Destruction of the sympathetic nervous system in neonatal rats and hamsters by vinblastine: Prevention by concomitant administration of nerve growth factor. *Brain Res.* **141:** 105–118.

Johnson, E. M., Jr., Andres, R. Y., and Bradshaw, R. A. (1978). Characterization of the retrograde transport of nerve growth factor (NGF). using high specific activity [^{125}I] NGF. *Brain Res.* **150:** 319–331.

Johnson, F., Sablan, M. M., and Bottjer, S. W. (1995). Topographic organization of a forebrain pathway involved with vocal learning in zebra finches. *J. Comp. Neurol.* **358:** 260–278.

Johnson, J. L., and Leff, M. (1999). Children of substance abusers: Overview of research findings. *Pediatrics* **103:** 1085–1099.

Johnson, J. S., and Newport, E. L. (1989). Critical period effects in second language learning: The influence of maturational state on the acquisition of English as a second language. *Cognit. Psychol.* **21:** 60–99.

Johnston, T. D., and Gottlieb, G. (1981). Visual preferences of imprinted ducklings are altered by the maternal call. *J. Comp. Physiol. Psychol.* **95:** 663–675.

Jones, B. W., Fetter, R. D., Tear, G., and Goodman, C. S. (1995). Glial cells missing: A genetic switch that controls glial versus neuronal fate. *Cell* **82:** 1013–1023.

Jones, E. G., and Pons, T. P. (1998). Thalamic and brainstem contributions to large-scale plasticity of primate somatosensory cortex [see Comments]. *Science* **282:** 1121–1125.

Jost, A. (1953). Problems of fetal endocrinology: The gonadal and hypophyseal hormones. *Recent Prog. Horm. Res.* **8:** 379–418.

Kaang, B.-K., Kandel, E. R., and Grant, S. G. N. (1993). Activation of cAMP-responsive genes by stimuli that produce long-term facilitation in *Aplysia* sensory neurons. *Neuron* **10:** 427–435.

Kaethner, R. J., and Stuermer, C. A. (1992). Dynamics of terminal arbor formation and target approach of retinotectal axons in living zebrafish embryos: A time-lapse study of single axons. *J. Neurosci.* **12:** 3257–3271.

Kalil, K., and Reh, T. (1982). A light and electron microscopic study of regrowing pyramidal tract fibers. *J. Comp. Neurol.* **211:** 265–275.

Kandel, E. R., and Tauc, L. (1965). Mechanism of heterosynaptic facilitation in the giant cell of the abdominal ganglion of *Aplysia depilans*. *J. Physiol.* **181:** 28–47.

Kandler, K., and Friauf, E. (1995). Development of glycinergic and glutamatergic synaptic transmission in the auditory brainstem of perinatal rats. *J. Neurosci.* **15:** 6890–6904.

Kane, C. J., Brown, G. J., and Phelan, K. D. (1996). Transforming growth factor-β_2 both stimulates and inhibits neurogenesis of rat cerebellar granule cells in culture. *Brain Res.* **96:** 46–51.

Kano, M., Hashimoto, K., Chen, C., Abeliovich, A., Aiba, A., Kurihara, H., and Tonegawa, S. (1995). Impaired synapse elimination during cerebellar development in PKCg mutant mice. *Cell* **83:** 1223–1231.

Kano, M., Hashimoto, K., Kurihara, H., Watanabe, M., Inoue, Y., Aiba, A., and Tonegawa, S. (1997). Persistent multiple climbing fiber innervation of cerebellar Purkinje cells in mice lacking mGluR1. *Neuron* **18:** 71–79.

Kano, M., Hashimoto, K., Watanabe, M., Kurihara, H., Offermanns, S., Jiang, H., Wu, Y., Jun, K., Shin, H. S., Inoue, Y., Simon, M. I., and Wu, D. (1998). Phospholipase cβ4 is specifically involved in climbing fiber synapse elimination in the developing cerebellum. *Proc. Natl. Acad. Sci. USA* **95:** 15,724–15,729.

Kapfhammer, J. P., and Raper, J. A. (1987a). Collapse of growth cone structure on contact with specific neurites in culture. *J. Neurosci.* **7:** 201–212.

Kapfhammer, J. P., and Raper, J. A. (1987b). Interactions between growth cones and neurites growing from different neural tissues in culture. *J. Neurosci.* **7:** 1595–1600.

Kaplan, D. R., Hempstead, B. L., Martin-Zanca, D., Chao, M. V., and Parada, L. F. (1991a). The *trk* proto-oncogene product: A signal transducing receptor for nerve growth factor. *Science* **252:** 554–558.

Kaplan, D. R., Martin-Zanca, D., and Parada, L. F. (1991b). Tyrosine phosphorylation and tyrosine kinase activity of the *trk* proto-oncogene product induced by NGF. *Nature* **350:** 158–160.

Kaprielian, Z., Cho, K. O., Hadjiargyrou, M., and Patterson, P. H. (1995). CD9, a major platelet cell surface glycoprotein, is a ROCA antigen and is expressed in the nervous system. *J. Neurosci.* **15:** 562–573.

Kaprielian, Z., and Patterson, P. H. (1993). Surface and cytoskeletal markers of rostrocaudal position in the mammalian nervous system. *J. Neurosci.* **13:** 2495–2508.

Karlstrom, R. O., Trowe, T., Klostermann, S., Baier, H., Brand, M., Crawford, A. D., Grunewald, B., Haffter, P., Hoffmann, H., Meyer, S. U., Muller, B. K., Richter, S., van Eeden, F. J., Nusslein-Volhard, C., and Bonhoeffer, F. (1996). Zebrafish mutations affecting retinotectal axon pathfinding. *Development* **123:** 427–438.

Kasamatsu, T., and Pettigrew, J. D. (1976). Depletion of brain chatecholamines: Failure of ocular dominance shift after monocular occlusion in kittens. *Science* **194:** 206–209.

Kater, S., and Letourneau, P. (1985). "Biology of the Nerve Growth Cone." A. R. Liss, New York.

Kater, S. B., and Mills, L. R. (1991). Regulation of growth cone behavior by calcium. *J. Neurosci.* **11:** 891–899.

Keating, M. J., and Feldman, J. (1975). Visual deprivation

and intertectal neuronal connections in *Xenopus laevis.* *Proc. R. Soc. London Ser. B* **191:** 467–474.

Keino-Masu, K., Masu, M., Hinck, L., Leonardo, E. D., Chan, S. S., Culotti, J. G., and Tessier-Lavigne, M. (1996). Deleted in colorectal cancer (DCC). encodes a netrin receptor. *Cell* **87:** 175–185.

Keller, R., Shih, J., and Sater, A. (1992). The cellular basis of the convergence and extension of the *Xenopus* neural plate. *Dev. Dyn.* **193:** 199–217.

Kelley, D. B. (1997). Generating sexually differentiated songs. *Curr. Opin. Neurobiol.* **7:** 839–843.

Kelley, M. W., Turner, J. K., and Reh, T. A. (1994). Retinoic acid promotes differentiation of photoreceptors *in vitro.* *Development* **120:** 2091–2102.

Kelly, J. B., Judge, P. W., and Fraser, I. H. (1987). Development of the auditory orientation response in the albino rat (*Rattus norvegicus*). *J. Comp. Psychol.* **101:** 60–66.

Kengaku, M., and Okamoto, H. (1995). bFGF as a possible morphogen for the anteroposterior axis of the central nervous system in *Xenopus. Development* **121:** 3121–3130.

Kennedy, C., Des Rosiers, M. H., Jehle, J. W., Reivich, M., Sharpe, F., and Sokoloff, L. (1975). Mapping of functional neural pathways by autoradiographic survey of local metabolic rate with [^{14}C]deoxyglucose. *Science* **7:** 850–853.

Kennedy, T. E., Serafini, T., de la Torre, J. R., and Tessier-Lavigne, M. (1994). Netrins are diffusible chemotropic factors for commissural axons in the embryonic spinal cord. *Cell* **78:** 425–435.

Keshishian, H., and Bentley, D. (1983a). Embryogenesis of peripheral nerve pathways in grasshopper legs. I. The initial nerve pathway to the CNS. *Dev. Biol.* **96:** 89–102.

Keshishian, H., and Bentley, D. (1983b). Embryogenesis of peripheral nerve pathways in grasshopper legs. III. Development without pioneer neurons. *Dev. Biol.* **96:** 116–124.

Keynes, R., Tannahill, D., Morgenstern, D. A., Johnson, A. R., Cook, G. M., and Pini, A. (1997). Surround repulsion of spinal sensory axons in higher vertebrate embryos. *Neuron* **18:** 889–897.

Keynes, R. J., and Stern, C. D. (1984). Segmentation in the vertebrate nervous system. *Nature* **310:** 786–789.

Kidd, T., Bland, K. S., and Goodman, C. S. (1999). Slit is the midline repellent for the robo receptor in *Drosophila.* *Cell* **96:** 785–794.

Kidd, T., Russell, C., Goodman, C. S., and Tear, G. (1998). Dosage-sensitive and complementary functions of roundabout and commissureless control axon crossing of the CNS midline. *Neuron* **20:** 25–33.

Kidokoro, Y., Anderson, M. J., and Gruener, R. (1980). Changes in synaptic potential properties during acetylcholine receptor accumulation and neurospecific interactions in *Xenopus* nerve–muscle cell cultures. *Dev. Biol.* **78:** 464–483.

Kidokoro, Y., and Yeh, E. (1982). Initial synaptic transmission at the growth cone in *Xenopus* nerve–muscle cultures. *Proc. Natl. Acad. Sci. USA* **79:** 6727–6731.

Killackey, H. P., Rhoades, R. W., and Bennett-Clarke, C. A. (1995). The formation of a cortical somatotopic map. *Trends Neurosci.* **18:** 402–407.

Killisch, I., Dotti, C. G., Laurie, D. J., Luddens, H., and Seeburg, P. H. (1991). Expression patterns of GABAA receptor subtypes in developing hippocampal neurons. *Neuron* **7:** 927–936.

Kim, E., Niethammer, M., Rothschild, A., Jan, Y. N., and Sheng, M. (1995). Clustering of Shaker-type K$^+$ channels by interaction with a family of membrane-associated guanylate kinases. *Nature* **378:** 85–88.

Kim, E., and Sheng, M. (1996). Differential K$^+$ channel clustering activity of PSD-95 and SAP-97, two related membrane-associated putative guanylate kinases. *Neuropharmacology* **35:** 993–1000.

Kim, J., Jones, B. W., Zock, C., Chen, Z., Wang, H., Goodman, C. S., and Anderson, D. J. (1998). Isolation and characterization of mammalian homologs of the *Drosophila* gene glial cells missing. *Proc. Natl. Acad. Sci. USA* **95:** 12,364–12,369.

Kimura, D. (1996). Sex, sexual orientation and sex hormones influence human cognitive function. *Curr. Opin. Neurobiol.* **6:** 259–263.

King, A. J., Hutchings, M. E., Moore, D. R., and Blakemore, C. (1988). Developmental plasticity in the visual and auditory representations in the mammalian superior colliculus. *Nature* **332:** 73–76.

Kirn, J. R., and DeVoogd, T. J. (1989). Genesis and death of vocal control neurons during sexual differentiation in the zebra finch. *J. Neurosci.* **9:** 3176–3187.

Kirsh, J., Malosio, M.-L., Wolters, I., and Betz, H. (1993a). Distribution of gephyrin transcripts in the adult and developing rat brain. *Eur. J. Neurosci.* **5:** 1109–1117.

Kirsh, J., Wolters, I., Triller, A., and Betz, H. (1993b). Gephyrin antisense oligonucleotides prevent glycine receptor clustering in spinal neurons. *Nature* **366:** 745–748.

Kistner, U., Wenzel, B. M., Veh, R. W., Cases-Langhoff, C., Garner, A. M., Appeltauer, U., Voss, B., Gundelfinger, E. D., and Garner, C. C. (1993). SAP90, a rat presynaptic protein related to the product of the *Drosophila* tumor suppressor gene dlg-A. *J. Biol. Chem.* **268:** 4580–4583.

Klambt, C., and Goodman, C. S. (1991). Role of the midline glia and neurons in the formation of the axon commissures in the central nervous system of the *Drosophila* embryo. *Ann. N.Y. Acad. Sci.* **633:** 142–159.

Klarsfeld, A., Bessereau, J. L., Salmon, A. M., Triller, A., Babinet, C., and Changeux, J. P. (1991). An acetylcholine receptor alpha-subunit promoter conferring preferential synaptic expression in muscle of transgenic mice. *EMBO J.* **10:** 625–632.

Klarsfeld, A., Laufer, R., Fontaine, B., Devillers-Thiery, A., Dubreuil, C., and Changeux, J. P. (1989). Regulation of muscle AChR alpha subunit gene expression by electrical activity: Involvement of protein kinase C and Ca^{2+}. *Neuron* **2:** 1229–1236.

Klein, R., Silos-Santiago, I., Smeyne, R. J., Lira, S. A., Brambilla, R., Bryant, S., Zhang, L., Snider, W. D., and Barbacid, M. (1994). Disruption of the neurotrophin-3 receptor gene trkC eliminates la muscle afferents and results in abnormal movements. *Nature* **368:** 249–2451.

Klein, R., Smeyne, R. J., Wurst, W., Long, L. K., Auerbach, B. A., Joyner, A. L., and Barbacid, M. (1993). Targeted disruption of the trkB neurotrophin receptor gene results in nervous system lesions and neonatal death. *Cell* **8:** 113–122.

Kleinschmidt, A., Bear, M. F., and Singer, W. (1987). Blockade of "NMDA" receptors disrupts experience-dependent plasticity of kitten striate cortex. *Science* **238:** 355–358.

Knox, R. J., Quattrocki, E. A., Connor, J. A., and Kaczmarek, L. K. (1992). Recruitment of Ca^{2+} channels by protein kinase C during rapid formation of putative neuropeptide release sites in isolated *Aplysia* neurons. *Neuron* **8:** 883–889.

Knudsen, E. I. (1991). Dynamic space codes in the superior colliculus. *Curr. Opin. Neurobiol.* **1:** 628–632.

Knudsen, E. I. (1985). Experience alters the spatial tuning of auditory units in the optic tectum during a sensitive period in the barn owl. *J. Neurosci.* **5:** 3094–3109.

Knudsen, E. I., du Lac, S., and Esterly, S. D. (1987). Computational maps in the brain. *Annu. Rev. Neurosci.* **10:** 41–65.

Kobayashi, H., Koppel, A. M., Luo, Y., and Raper, J. A. (1997). A role for collapsin-1 in olfactory and cranial sensory axon guidance. *J. Neurosci.* **17:** 8339–8352.

Kolbinger, W., Trepel, M., Beyer, C., Pilgrim, C., and Reisert, I. (1991). The influence of genetic sex on sexual differentiation of diencephalic dopaminergic neurons *in vitro* and *in vivo*. *Brain Res.* **544:** 349–352.

Kolodkin, A. L. (1996). Growth cones and the cues that repel them. *Trends Neurosci.* **19:** 507–513.

Kolodkin, A. L., Matthes, D. J., and Goodman, C. S. (1993). The semaphorin genes encode a family of transmembrane and secreted growth cone guidance molecules. *Cell* **75:** 1389–1399.

Kolodziej, P. A., Timpe, L. C., Mitchell, K. J., Fried, S. R., Goodman, C. S., Jan, L. Y., and Jan, Y. N. (1996). Frazzled encodes a *Drosophila* member of the DCC immunoglobulin subfamily and is required for CNS and motor axon guidance. *Cell* **87:** 197–204.

Komatsu, Y. (1994). Age-dependent long-term potentiation of inhibitory synaptic transmission in rat visual cortex. *J. Neurosci.* **14:** 6488–6499.

Komatsu, Y., and Iwakiri, M. (1991). Postnatal development of neuronal connections in cat visual cortex studied by intracellular recording in slice preparation. *Brain Res.* **540:** 14–24.

Kornau, H. C., Schenker, L. T., Kennedy, M. B., and Seeburg, P. H. (1995). Domain interaction between NMDA receptor subunits and the postsynaptic density protein PSD-95. *Science* **269:** 1737–1740.

Kossel, A. H., Williams, C. V., Schweizer, M., and Kater, S. B. (1997). Afferent innervation influences the development of dendritic branches and spines via both activity-dependent and non-activity-dependent mechanisms. *J. Neurosci.* **17:** 6314–6324.

Kotak, V. C., and Sanes, D. H. (1995). Synaptically evoked prolonged depolarizations in the developing auditory system. *J. Neurophysiol.* **74:** 1611–1620.

Kotak, V. C., and Sanes, D. H. (1996). Developmental influence of glycinergic inhibition: Regulation of NMDA-mediated EPSPs. *J. Neurosci.* **16:** 1836–1843.

Kotak, V. C., and Sanes, D. H. (1997). Deafferentation of glutamatergic afferents weakens synaptic strength in the developing auditory system. *Eur. J. Neurosci.* **9:** 2340–2347.

Kratz, K. E., and Spear, P. D. (1976). Postcritical-period reversal of effects of monocular deprivation on striate cortex cells in the cat. *J. Neurophysiol.* **39:** 501–511.

Kuang, R. Z., Merline, M., and Kalil, K. (1994). Topographic specificity of corticospinal connections formed in explant coculture. *Development* **120:** 1937–1947.

Kuffler, D., Thompson, W., and Jansen, J. K. S. (1977). The elimination of synapses in multiply innervated skeletal muscle fibres of the rat: Dependence on distance between end-plates. *Brain Res.* **138:** 353–358.

Kuhl, P. K., Williams, K. A., Lacerda, F., Stevens, K. N., and Lindblom, B. (1992). Linguistic experience alters phonetic perception in infants by 6 months of age. *Science* **255:** 606–608.

Kuhn, H. G., Winkler, J., Kempermann, G., Thal, L. J., and Gage, F. H. (1997). Epidermal growth factor and fibroblast growth factor-2 have different effects on neural progenitors in the adult rat brain. *Neuroscience* **17:** 5820–5829.

Kuida, K., Zheng, T. S., Na, S., Kuan, C., Yang, D., Karasuyama, H., Rakic, P., and Flavell, R. A. (1996). Decreased apoptosis in the brain and premature lethality in CPP32-deficient mice. *Nature* **384:** 368–372.

Kullberg, R. W., Lentz, T. L., and Cohen, M. W. (1977). Development of the myotomal neuromuscular junction in *Xenopus laevis*: An electrophysiological and fine-structural study. *Dev. Biol.* **60:** 101–129.

Kwon, Y. W., and Gurney, M. E. (1996). Brain-derived neurotrophic factor transiently stabilizes silent synapses on developing neuromuscular junctions. *J. Neurobiol.* **29:** 503–516.

Lahey, T., Gorczyca, M., Jia, X. X., and Budnik, V. (1994). The *Drosophila* tumor suppressor gene dlg is required for normal synaptic bouton structure. *Neuron* **13:** 823–835.

Lamb, T. M., Knecht, A. K., Smith, W. C., Stachel, S. E., Economides, A. N., Stahl, N., Yancopolous, G. D., and Harland, R. M. (1993). Neural Induction by the secreted polypeptide noggin. *Science* **262:** 713–718.

Lander, A. D., Tomaselli, K., Calof, A. L., and Reichardt, L. F. (1983). Studies on extracellular matrix components that promote neurite outgrowth. *Cold Spring Harbor Symp. Quant. Biol.* **48:** 611–623.

Landis, S. (1992). Cellular and molecular mechanisms determining neurotransmitter phenotypes in sympathetic

neurons. *In* "Determinants of Neuronal Identity" (M. Shankland and E. Macagno, Eds.), pp. 497–523. Academic Press, San Diego.

Landis, S. C. (1983). Neuronal growth cones. *Annu. Rev. Physiol.* **45:** 567–580.

Landmesser, L., and Pilar, G. (1972). The onset and development of transmission in the chick ciliary ganglion. *J. Physiol. (London)* **222:** 691–713.

Langley, J. N. (1895). Note on regeneration of pre-ganglionic fibres of the sympathetic. *J. Physiol. (London)* **18:** 280–284.

Langley, J. N. (1897). On the regeneration of pre-ganglionic amd post-ganglionic visceral nerve fibres. *J. Physiol. (London)* **22:** 215–230.

Lankford, K. L., and Letourneau, P. C. (1991). Roles of actin filaments and three second-messenger systems in short-term regulation of chick dorsal root ganglion neurite outgrowth. *Cell Motil. Cytoskeleton* **20:** 7–29.

Larmet, Y., Dolphin, A. C., and Davies, A. M. (1992). Intracellular calcium regulates the survival of early sensory neurons before they become dependent on neurotrophic factors. *Neuron* **9:** 563–574.

Larrabee, M. G., and Bronk, D. W. (1947). Prolonged facilitation of synaptic excitation in sympathetic ganglia. *J. Neurophysiol.* **10:** 139–154.

Larsell, O. (1931). The effect of experimental excision of one eye on the development of the optic lobe and opticus layer in larvae of the tree-frog. *J. Exp. Zool.* **58:** 1–20.

Laufer, R., Klarsfeld, A., and Changeux, J. P. (1991). Phorbol esters inhibit the activity of the chicken acetylcholine receptor alpha-subunit gene promoter. Role of myogenic regulators. *Eur. J. Biochem.* **202:** 813–818.

Laurie, D. J., Wisden, W., and Seeburg, P. H. (1992). The distribution of 13 GABA^A receptor subunit mRNAs in the rat brain. III. Embryonic and postnatal development. *J. Neurosci.* **12:** 4151–4172.

Lazebnik, Y. A., Kaufmann, S. H., Desnoyers, S., Poirier, G. G., and Earnshaw, W. C. (1994). Cleavage of poly(ADP-ribose) polymerase by a proteinase with properties like ICE. *Nature* **371:** 346–347.

Leber, S. M., Breedlove, S. M., and Sanes, J. R. (1990). Lineage, arrangement, and death of clonally related motoneurons in chick spinal cord. *J. Neurosci.* **10:** 2451–2462.

Le Douarin, N. (1982). "The Neural Crest." Cambridge Univ. Press, New York.

Lee, H.-K., Kameyama, K., Huganir, R. L., and Bear, M. F. (1998). NMDA induces long-term synaptic depression and dephosphorylation of the Glur1 subunit of AMPA receptors in hippocampus. *Neuron* **21:** 1151–1162.

Lee, J. E., Hollenberg, S. M., Snider, L., Turner, D. L., Lipnick, N., and Weintraub, H. (1995). Conversion of *Xenopus* ectoderm into neurons by Neuro D, a basic helix-loop-helix protein. *Science* **268:** 836–844.

Lee, K. F., Li, E., Huber, L. J., Landis, S. C., Sharpe, A. H., Chao, M. V., and Jaenisch, R. (1992). Targeted mutation of the gene encoding the low affinity NGF receptor p75 leads to deficits in the peripheral sensory nervous system. *Cell* **69:** 737–749.

Leibrock, J., Lottspeich, F., Hohn, A., Hofer, M., Gengerer, B., Masiakowski, P., Thoenen, H., and Barde, Y. (1989). Molecular cloning and expression of brain-derived neurotrophic factor. *Nature* **341:** 149–152.

Lemmon, V., Burden, S. M., Payne, H. R., Elmslie, G. J., and Hlavin, M. L. (1992). Neurite growth on different substrates: Permissive versus instructive influences and the role of adhesive strength. *J. Neurosci.* **12:** 818–826.

Le Roux, P. D., and Reh, T. A. (1994). Regional differences in glial-derived factors that promote dendritic outgrowth from mouse cortical neurons *in vitro. J. Neurosci.* **14:** 4639–4655.

Le Roux, P. D., and Reh, T. A. (1996). Reactive astroglia support primary dendritic but not axonal outgrowth from mouse cortical neurons *in vitro. Exp. Neurol.* **137:** 49–65.

Letourneau, P., Kater, S., and Macagno, E. (1991). "The Growth Cone." Raven Press, New York.

Letourneau, P. C. (1975). Cell-to-substratum adhesion and guidance of axonal elongation. *Dev. Biol.* **44:** 92–101.

Letourneau, P. C. (1996). The cytoskeleton in nerve growth cone motility and axonal pathfinding. *Perspect. Dev. Neurobiol.* **4:** 111–123.

LeVay, S., Stryker, M. P., and Shatz, C. J. (1978). Ocular dominance columns and their development in layer IV of the cat's visual cortex. *J. Comp. Neurol.* **179:** 223–244.

LeVay, S., Wiesel, T. N., and Hubel, D. H. (1980). The development of ocular dominance columns in normal and visually deprived monkeys. *J. Comp. Neurol.* **191:** 1–51.

Levi-Montalcini, R. (1949). The development of the acoustico-vestibular centers in the chick embryo in the absence of the afferent root fibers and of descending fiber tracts. *J. Comp. Neurol.* **91:** 209–241.

Levi-Montalcini, R., and Booker, B. (1960). Destruction of the sympathetic ganglia in mammals by an antiserum to a nerve growth protein. *Proc. Natl. Acad. Sci. USA* **46:** 384–391.

Levi-Montalcini, R., and Cohen, S. (1956). *In vitro* and *in vivo* effects of a nerve growth-stimulating agent isolated from snake venom. *Proc. Natl. Acad. Sci. USA* **42:** 695–699.

Levi-Montalcini, R., and Hamburger, V. (1951). Selective growth stimulating effects of mouse sarcoma on the sensory and sympathetic nervous system of the chick embryo. *J. Exp. Zool.* **116:** 321–361.

Levi-Montalcini, R., and Hamburger, V. (1953). A diffusible agent of mouse sarcoma, producing hyperplasia of sympathetic ganglia and hyperneurotization of viscera on the chick embryo. *J. Exp. Zool.* **123:** 233–287.

Levi-Montalcini, R., and Levi, G. (1942). Les consequences de la destruction d'un territoire d'innervation peripheique sur le développements des centres nerveux correspondents dans l'embryon de poulet. *Arch. Biol. (Liege)* **53:** 537–545.

Levine, E. M., Roelink, H., Turner, J., and Reh, T. A. (1997). Sonic hedgehog promotes rod photoreceptor differentiation in mammalian retinal cells *in vitro. J. Neurosci.* **17:** 6277–6288.

Levine, R. B., and Weeks, J. C. (1990). Hormonally mediated changes in simple reflex circuits during metamorphosis in *Manduca. J. Neurobiol.* **21:** 1022–1036.

Lewis, C. A., Ahmed, Z., and Faber, D. S. (1990). Developmental changes in the regulation of glycine-activated Cl⁻ channels of cultured rat medullary neurons. *Dev. Brain Res.* **51:** 287–290.

Lewis, E. B. (1978). A gene complex controlling segmentation in *Drosophila. Nature* **276:** 565–570.

Li, H. S., Chen, J. H., Wu, W., Fagaly, T., Zhou, L., Yuan, W., Dupuis, S., Jiang, Z. H., Nash, W., Gick, C., Ornitz, D. M., Wu, J. Y., and Rao, Y. (1999). Vertebrate slit, a secreted ligand for the transmembrane protein roundabout, is a repellent for olfactory bulb axons. *Cell* **96:** 807–818.

Li, P., Nijhawan, D., Budihardjo, I., Srinivasula, S. M., Ahmad, M., Alnemri, E. S., and Wang, X. (1997). Cytochrome c and dATP-dependent formation of Apaf-1/caspase-9 complex initiates an apoptotic protease cascade. *Cell* **91:** 479–489.

Lichtman, J. W. (1977). The reorganization of synaptic connexions in the rat submandibular ganglion during postnatal development. *J. Physiol.* **273:** 155–177.

Lichtman, J. W., and Purves, D. (1980). The elimination of redundant preganglionic innervation to hamster sympathetic ganglion cells in early post-natal life. *J. Physiol.* **301:** 213–228.

Liem, K. F., Jr., Tremml, G., *et al.* (1995). Dorsal differentiation of neural plate cells induced by BMP-mediated signals from epidermal ectoderm. *Cell* **82:** 969–979.

Lillien, L. E., and Raff, M. C. (1990). Differentiation signals in the CNS: Type-2 astrocyte development *in vitro* as a model system. *Neuron* **5:** 111–119.

Lin, C. H., Espreafico, E. M., Mooseker, M. S., and Forscher, P. (1996). Myosin drives retrograde F-actin flow in neuronal growth cones. *Neuron* **16:** 769–782.

Lin, J. H., Saito, T., Anderson, D. J., Lance-Jones, C., Jessell, T. M., and Arber, S. (1998). Functionally related motor neuron pool and muscle sensory afferent subtypes defined by coordinate ETS gene expression [see Comments]. *Cell* **95:** 393–407.

Lin, L.-F. H., Doherty, D. H., Lile, J. D., Bektesh, S., and Collins, F. (1993). GDNF: A glial cell line-derived neruotrophic factor for midbrain dopaminergic neurons. *Science* **260:** 1130–1132.

Linden, R. (1994). The survival of developing neurons: A review of afferent control. *Neurosci.* **58:** 671–682.

Linsdell, P., and Moody, W. J. (1995). Electrical activity and calcium influx regulate ion channel development in embryonic *Xenopus* skeletal muscle. *J. Neurosci.* **15:** 4507–4514.

Lippe, W. R. (1994). Rhythmic spontaneous activity in the developing avian auditory system. *J. Neurosci.* **14**: 1486–1495.

Lisberger, S. G. (1988). The neural basis for learning of simple motor skills. *Science* **242**: 728–735.

Liu, C., and Chambers, W. (1958). Intraspinal sprouting of dorsal root axons. *Arch. Neurol. Psychiatry* **79**: 46–61.

Lloyd, D. P. C. (1949). Post-tetanic potentiation of response in monosynaptic reflex pathways of the spinal cord. *J. Gen. Physiol.* **33**: 147–170.

Lo, Y.-j., and Poo, M.-m. (1991). Activity-dependent synaptic competition *in vitro*: Heterosynaptic supression of developing synapses. *Science* **254**: 1019–1022.

Lo, Y.-j., and Poo, M.-m. (1994). Heterosynaptic supression of developing neruomuscular synapses in culture. *J. Neurosci.* **14**: 4684–4693.

Loeb, D. M., Maragos, J., Martin-Zanca, D., Chao, M. V., Parada, L. F., and Greene, L. A. (1991). The trk proto-oncogene rescues NGF responsiveness in mutant NGF-nonresponsive PC12 cell lines. *Cell* **66**: 961–966.

Loetscher, H., Deuschle, U., Brockhaus, M., Reinhardt, D., Nelboeck, P., Mous, J., Grünberg, J., Haass, C., and Jacobsen. H. (1997). Presenilins are processed by caspase-type proteases. *J. Biol. Chem.* **272**: 20,655–20,659.

Logan, C., Wizenmann, A., Drescher, U., Monschau, B., Bonhoeffer, F., and Lumsden, A. (1996). Rostral optic tectum acquires caudal characteristics following ectopic engrailed expression. *Curr. Biol.* **6**: 1006–1014.

Lohnes, D., Mark, M., Mendelsohn, C., Dollé, P., Decimo, D., LeMeur, M., Dierich, A., Gorry, P., and Chambon, P. (1995). Developmental roles of the retinoic acid receptors. *J. Steroid Biochem. Mol. Biol.* **53**:1–6, 475–486.

Lohoff, A. M., Quillan, M., Dan, Y., and Poo, M.-m. (1992). Asymmetric modulation of cytosolic cAMP activity induces growth cone turning. *J. Neurosci.* **12**: 1253–1261.

Lois, C., and Alvarez-Buylla, A. (1993). Proliferating subventricular zone cells in the adult mammalian forebrain can differentiate into neurons and glia. *Proc. Natl. Acad. Sci. USA* **90**: 2074–2077.

Lois, C., Garcia-Verdugo, J. M., and Alvarez-Buylla, A. (1996). Chain migration of neuronal precursors. *Science* **271**: 978–981.

Lømo, T., and Rosenthal, J. (1972). Control of ACh sensitivity by muscle activity in the rat. *J. Physiol.* **221**: 493–513.

Lorenz, K. (1937). The companion in the bird's world. *Auk.* **54**: 245–273.

Löwel, S., and Singer, W. (1992). Selection of intrinsic horizontal connections in the visual cortex by correlated neuronal activity. *Science* **255**: 209–212.

Lu, B., Fu, W.-m., Greengard, P., and Poo, M.-m. (1993). CGRP enhances nicotinic ACh channel activity at developing neuromuscular synapses through cAMP-dependent protein kinase. *Nature* **363**: 76–79.

Lu, J., Karadsheh, M., and Delpire, E. (1999). Developmental regulation of the neuronal-specific isoform of the K-Cl cotransporter KCC2 in postnatal rat brains. *J. Neurobiol.* **39**: 558–568.

Luhmann, H. J., and Prince, D. A. (1991). Postnatal maturation of the GABAergic system in rat neocortex. *J. Neurophysiol.* **65**: 247–263.

Lumsden, A. G., and Davies, A. M. (1983). Earliest sensory nerve fibres are guided to peripheral targets by attractants other than nerve growth factor. *Nature* **306**: 786–788.

Lumsden, A. G., and Davies, A. M. (1986). Chemotropic effect of specific target epithelium in the developing mammalian nervous system. *Nature* **323**: 538–539.

Lumsden, A., and Keynes, R. (1989). Segmental patterns of neuronal development in the chick hindbrain. *Nature* **337**: 424–428.

Luo, L., Jan, L., and Jan, Y. N. (1996). Small GTPases in axon outgrowth. *Perspect. Dev. Neurobiol.* **4**: 199–204.

Luo, Y., Raible, D., and Raper, J. A. (1993). Collapsin: A protein in brain that induces the collapse and paralysis of neuronal growth cones. *Cell* **75**: 217–227.

Luskin, M. B. (1993). Restricted proliferation and migration of postnatally generated neurons derived from the forebrain subventricular zone. *Neuron* **11**: 173–189.

Lytton, W. W., and Kristan, W. B. (1989). Localization of a leech inhibitory synapse by photo-ablation of individual dendrites. *Brain Res.* **504**: 43–48.

Ma, Q., Chen, Z., del Barco Barrantes, I., de la Pompa, J. L., and Anderson, D. J. (1998). Neurogenin 1 is essential for the determination of neuronal precursors for proximal cranial sensory ganglia. *Neuron* **20**: 469–482.

Maderdrut, J. L., Oppenheim, R. W., and Prevette, D. (1988). Enhancement of naturally occurring cell death in the sympathetic and parasympathetic ganglia of the chicken embryo following blockade of ganglionic transmission. *Brain Res.* **444**: 189–194.

Magill-Solc, C., and McMahon, U. J. (1988). Motor neurons contain agrin-like molecules. *J. Cell Biol.* **107**: 1825–1833.

Maher, P. A. (1988). Nerve growth factor induces protein tyrosine phosphorylation. *Proc. Natl. Acad. Sci. USA* **85**: 6788–6791.

Manns, M., and Fritzsch, B. (1991). The eye in the brain: Retinoic acid effects morphogenesis of the eye and pathway selection of axons but not the differentiation of the retina in *Xenopus laevis. Neurosci. Lett.* **127**: 150–154.

Mariani, J., and Changeux, J.-P. (1981). Ontogenesis of olivocerebellar relationships. I. Studies by intracellular recordings of the multiple innervation of Pukinje cells by climbing fibers in the developing rat cerebellum. *J. Neurosci.* **1**: 696–702.

Marin-Padilla, M. (1998). Cajal–Retzius cells and the development of the neocortex. *Trends Neurosci.* **21**: 64–71.

Markus, A., von Holst, A., Rohrer, H., and Heumann, R. (1997). NGF-mediated survival depends on p21ras in chick sympathetic neurons from the superior cervical but not from lumbosacral ganglia. *Dev. Biol.* **191**: 306–310.

Marler, P., and Sherman, V. (1983). Song structure without auditory feedback: Emendations of the auditory template hypothesis. *J. Neurosci.* **3**: 517–531.

Maroney, A. C., Glicksman, M. A., Basma, A. N., Walton, K. M., Knight, E., Jr., Murphy, C. A., Bartlett, B. A., Finn, J. P., Angeles, T., Matsuda, Y., Neff, N. T., and Dionne, C. A. (1998). Motoneuron apoptosis is blocked by CEP-1347 (KT 7515), a novel inhibitor of the JNK signaling pathway. *J. Neurosci.* **18**: 104–111.

Marshall, H., Nonchev, S., *et al.* (1992). Retinoic acid alters hindbrain Hox code and induces transformation of rhombomeres 2/3 into a 4/5 identity [see Comments]. *Nature* **360**: 737–741.

Marshall, H., Studer, M., *et al.* (1994). A conserved retinoic acid response element required for early expression of the homeobox gene Hoxb-1. *Nature* **370**: 567–571.

Marsh-Armstrong, N., McCaffery, P., Gilbert, W., Dowling, J. E., and Drager, U. C. (1994). Retinoic acid is necessary for development of the ventral retina in zebrafish. *Proc. Natl. Acad. Sci. USA* **91**: 7286–7290.

Martin, D. P., Schmidt, R. E., DiStefano, P. S., Lowry, O. H., Carter, J. G., and Johnson, E. M., Jr. (1988). Inhibitors of protein synthesis and RNA synthesis prevent neuronal death caused by nerve growth factor deprivation. *J. Cell Biol.* **106**: 829–844.

Martinez, S., and Alvarado-Mallart, R. (1990). Expression of the homeobox Chick-en gene in chick/quail chimeras with inverted mes-metencephalic grafts. *Dev. Biol.* **139**: 432–436.

Martinez, S., Wassef, M., and Alvarado, M. R. (1991). Induction of a mesencephalic phenotype in the 2-day-old chick prosencephalon is preceded by the early expression of the homeobox gene en. *Neuron* **6**: 971–981.

Martinou, J. C., Dubois-Dauphin, M., Staple, J. K., Rodriguez, I., Frankowski, H., Missotten, M., Albertini, P., Talabot, D., Catsicas, S., Pietra, C., and Huarte, J. (1994). Overexpression of BCL-2 in transgenic mice protects neurons from naturally occurring cell death and experimental ischemia. *Neuron* **13**: 1017–1030.

Martinou, J. C., Falls, D. L., Fischbach, G. D., and Merlie, J. P. (1991). Acetylcholine receptor-inducing acitivity stimulates expression of the e-subunit gene of the muscle acetylcholine receptor. *Proc. Natl. Acad. Sci. USA* **88**: 7669–7673.

Martin-Zanca, D., Barbacid, M., and Parada, L. F. (1990). Expression of the trk proto-oncogene is restricted to the sensory cranial and spinal ganglia of neural crest origin in mouse development. *Genes Dev.* **4**: 683–694.

Martin-Zanca, D., Hughes, S. H., and Barbacid, M. (1986). A human oncogene formed by the fusion of truncated tropomyosin and protein tyrosine kinase sequences. *Nature* **319**: 743–748.

Matthes, D. J., Sink, H., Kolodkin, A. L., and Goodman, C. S. (1995). Semaphorin II can function as a selective inhibitor of specific synaptic arborizations. *Cell* **81**: 631–639.

Mattson, M. P., and Kater, S. B. (1987). Calcium regulation of neurite elongation and growth cone motility. *J. Neurosci.* **7**: 4034–4043.

Mattson, M. P., and Kater, S. B. (1989). Excitatory and inhibitory neurotransmitters in the generation and degeneration of hippocampal neuroarchitecture. *Brain Res.* **478**: 337–348.

Mattson, M. P., Taylor-Hunter, A., and Kater, S. B. (1988). Neurite outgrowth in individual neurons of a neuronal population is differentially regulated by calcium and cyclic AMP. *J. Neurosci* **8**: 1704–1711.

McAllister, A. K., Katz, L. C., and Lo, D. C. (1997). Opposing roles for endogenous BDNF and NT-3 in regulating cortical dendritic growth. *Neuron* **18**: 767–778.

McCaffery, P., and Drager, U. C. (1993). Retinoic acid synthesis in the developing retina. *Adv. Exp. Med. Biol.* **328**: 181–190.

McCasland, J. S., Bernardo, K. L., Probst, K. L., and Woolsey, T. A. (1992). Cortical local circuit axons do not mature after early deafferentation. *Proc. Natl. Acad. Sci. USA* **89**: 1832–1836.

McCobb, D. P., Best, P. M., and Beam, K. G. (1989). Development alters the expression of calcium currents in chick limb motoneurons. *Neuron* **2**: 1633–1643.

McCobb, D. P., Best, P. M., and Beam, K. G. (1990). The differentiation of excitability in embryonic chick limb motoneurons. *J. Neurosci.* **10**: 2974–2984.

McCobb, D. P., Haydon, P. G., and Kater, S. B. (1988). Dopamine and serotonin inhibition of neurite elongation of different identified neurons. *J. Neurosci. Res.* **19**: 19–26.

McConnell, S. K. (1988). Development and decision-making in the mammalian cerebral cortex. *Brain Res.* **472**: 1–23.

McConnell, S. K. (1995). Constructing the cerebral cortex: Neurogenesis and fate determination. *Neuron* **15**: 761–768.

McFarlane, S., Cornel, E., Amaya, E., and Holt, C. E. (1996). Inhibition of FGF receptor activity in retinal ganglion cell axons causes errors in target recognition. *Neuron* **17**: 245–254.

McFarlane, S., McNeill, L., and Holt, C. E. (1995). FGF signaling and target recognition in the developing *Xenopus* visual system. *Neuron* **15**: 1017–1028.

McKenna, M. P., and Raper, J. A. (1988). Growth cone behavior on gradients of substratum bound laminin. *Dev. Biol.* **130**: 232–236.

McKerracher, L., Chamoux, M., and Arregui, C. O. (1996). Role of laminin and integrin interactions in growth cone guidance. *Mol. Neurobiol.* **12**: 95–116.

McMahon, A. P., and Bradley, A. (1990). The Wnt-1 (int-1) proto-oncogene is required for development of a large region of the mouse brain. *Cell* **62**: 1073–1085.

Meadows, L. A., Gell, D., Broadie, K., Gould, A. P., and White, R. A. (1994). The cell adhesion molecule, connectin, and the development of the *Drosophila* neuromuscular system. *J. Cell Sci.* **107**: 321–328.

Mears, S. C., and Frank, E. (1997). Formation of specific

monosynaptic connections between muscle spindle afferents and motoneurons in the mouse. *J. Neurosci.* **17**: 3128–3135.

Meier, T., Gesemann, M., Cavalli, V., Ruegg, M. A., and Wallace, B. G. (1996). AChR phosphorylation and aggregation induced by an agrin fragment that lacks the binding domain for α-dystroglycan. *EMBO J.* **15**: 2625–2631.

Meister, M., Wong, R. O. L., Baylor, D. A., and Shatz, C. J. (1991). Synchronous bursts of action potentials in ganglion cells of the developing mammalian retina. *Science* **252**: 939–943.

Merlie, J. P., Isenberg, K. E., Russell, S. D., and Sanes, J. R. (1984). Denervation supersensitivity in skeletal muscle: Analysis with a cloned cDNA probe. *J. Cell Biol.* **99**: 332–335.

Merlie, J. P., and Sanes, J. R. (1985). Concentration of acetylcholine receptor mRNA in synaptic regions of adult muscle fibres. *Nature* **317**: 66–68.

Merzenich, M. (1998). Long-term change of mind [Comment]. *Science* **282**: 1062–1063.

Merzenich, M. M., and Jenkins, W. M. (1993). Reorganization of cortical representations of the hand following alterations of skin inputs induced by nerve injury, skin island transfers, and experience. *J. Hand Ther.* **6**: 89–104.

Messersmith, E. K., Leonardo, E. D., Shatz, C. J., Tessier-Lavigne, M., Goodman, C. S., and Kolodkin, A. L. (1995). Semaphorin III can function as a selective chemorepellent to pattern sensory projections in the spinal cord. *Neuron* **14**: 949–959.

Metin, C., and Frost, D. O. (1989). Visual responses of neurons in somatosensory cortex of hamsters with experimentally induced retinal projections to somatosensory thalamus. *Proc. Natl. Acad. Sci. USA* **86**: 357–361.

Metzger, F., Wiese, S., and Sendtner, M. (1998). Effect of glutamate on dendritic growth in embryonic rat motoneurons. *J. Neurosci.* **18**: 1735–1742.

Meyer, R. L., and Wolcott, L. L. (1987). Compression and expansion without impulse activity in the retinotectal projection of goldfish. *J. Neurobiol.* **18**: 549–567.

Meyer-Franke, A., Kaplan, M. R., Pfrieger, F. W., and Barres, B. A. (1995). Characterization of the signaling interactions that promote the survival and growth of developing retinal ganglion cells in culture. *Neuron* **15**: 805–819.

Milligan, C. E., Prevette, D., Yaginuma, H., Homma, S., Cardwell, C., Fritz, L. C., Tomaselli, K. J., Oppenheim, R. W., and Schwartz, L. M. (1995). Peptide inhibitors of the ICE protease family arrest programmed cell death of motoneurons *in vivo* and *in vitro*. *Neuron* **15**: 385–393.

Milner, B., Squire, L. R., and Kandel, E. R. (1998). Cognitive neuroscience and the study of memory. *Neuron* **20**: 445–468.

Ming, G. L., Song, H. J., Berninger, B., Holt, C. E., Tessier-Lavigne, M., and Poo, M. M. (1997). cAMP-dependent growth cone guidance by netrin-1. *Neuron* **19**: 1225–1235.

Miskevich, F., Zhu, Y., Ranscht, B., and Sanes, J. R. (1998). Expression of multiple cadherins and catenins in the chick optic tectum. *Mol. Cell Neurosci.* **12**: 240–255.

Mitchell, K. J., Doyle, J. L., Serafini, T., Kennedy, T. E., Tessier-Lavigne, M., Goodman, C. S., and Dickson, B. J. (1996). Genetic analysis of Netrin genes in *Drosophila*: Netrins guide CNS commissural axons and peripheral motor axons. *Neuron* **17**: 203–215.

Miyata, T., Nakajima, K., Mikoshiba, K., and Ogawa, M. (1997). Regulation of Purkinje cell alignment by reelin as revealed with CR-50 antibody. *J. Neurosci.* **17**: 3599–3609.

Molnar, Z., and Blakemore, C. (1991). Lack of regional specificity for connections formed between thalamus and cortex in coculture. *Nature* **351**: 475–477.

Mombaerts, P., Wang, F., Dulac, C., Chao, S. K., Nemes, A., Mendelsohn, M., Edmondson, J., and Axel, R. (1996). Visualizing an olfactory sensory map. *Cell* **87**: 675–686.

Monschau, B., Kremoser, C., Ohta, K., Tanaka, H., Kaneko, T., Yamada, T., Handwerker, C., Hornberger, M. R., Loschinger, J., Pasquale, E. B., Siever, D. A., Verderame, M. F., Muller, B. K., Bonhoeffer, F., and Drescher, U. (1997). Shared and distinct functions of RAGS and ELF-1 in guiding retinal axons. *EMBO J.* **16**: 1258–1267.

Moody, S. (1999). "Cell Lineage and Determination." Academic Press, San Diego.

Mooney, R. (1999). Sensitive periods and circuits for learned birdsong. *Curr. Opin. Neurobiol.* **9**: 121–127.

Mooney, R., Madison, D. V., and Shatz, C. J. (1993). Enhancement of transmission at the developing retinogeniculate synapse. *Neuron* **10**: 815–825.

Mooney, R., Penn, A. A., Gallego, R., and Shatz, C. J. (1996). Thalamic relay of spontaneous retinal activity prior to vision. *Neuron* **17**: 863–874.

Mori-Okamoto, J., Ashida, H., Maru, E., and Tatsuno, J. (1983). The development of action potentials in cultures of explanted cortical neurons from chick embryos. *Dev. Biol.* **97**: 408–416.

Moscoso, L. M., Cremer, H., and Sanes, J. R. (1998). Organization and reorganization of neuromuscular junctions in mice lacking neural cell adhesion molecule, tenascin-C, or fibroblast growth factor-5. *J. Neurosci.* **18**: 1465–1477.

Moss, B. L., and Role, L. W. (1993). Enhanced ACh sensitivity is accompanied by changes in ACh receptor channel properties and segregation of ACh receptor subtypes on sympathetic neurons during innervation *in vivo*. *J. Neurosci.* **13**: 13–28.

Motoyama, N., Wang, F., Roth, K. A., Sawa, H., Nakayama, K., Nakayama, K., Negishi, I., Senju, S., Zhang, Q., Fujii, S., and Loh, D. Y. (1995). Massive cell death of immature hematopoietic cells and neurons in Bcl-x-deficient mice. *Science* **267**: 1506–1510.

Moury, J. D., and Jacobson, A. G. (1990). The origins of neural crest cells in the axolotl. *Dev. Biol.* **141**: 243–253.

Moye, T. B., and Rudy, J. W. (1987). Ontogenesis of trace conditioning in young rats: Dissociation of associative and memory processes. *Dev. Psychobiol.* **20:** 405–414.

Mueller, A. L., Chesnut, R. M., and Schwartzkroin, P. A. (1983). Actions of GABA in developing rabbit hippocampus: An *in vitro* study. *Neurosci. Lett.* **39:** 193–198.

Mueller, A. L., Taube, J. S., and Schwartzkroin, P. A. (1984). Development of hyperpolarizing inhibitory postsynaptic potentials and hyperpolarizing responses to γ-aminobutyric acid in rabbit hippocampus studied *in vitro. J. Neurosci.* **4:** 860–867.

Mulder, E. J., Kamstra, A., O'Brien, M. J., Visser, G. H., and Prechtl, H. F. (1986). Abnormal fetal behavioural state regulation in a case of high maternal alcohol intake during pregnancy. *Early Hum. Dev.* **14:** 321–326.

Muller, B. K., Jay, D. G., and Bonhoeffer, F. (1996). Chromophore-assisted laser inactivation of a repulsive axonal guidance molecule. *Curr. Biol.* **6:** 1497–1502.

Muller, U., and Kypta, R. (1995). Molecular genetics of neuronal adhesion. *Curr. Opin. Neurobiol.* **5:** 36–41.

Mutani, R., Futamachi, K., and Prince, D. A. (1974). Potassium activity in immature cortex. *Brain Res.* **75:** 27–39.

Naftolin, F., Ryan, K. J., Davies, I. J., Reddy, V. V., Flores, F., Petro, Z., Kuhn, M., White, R. J., Takaoka, Y., and Wolin, L. (1975). The formation of estrogens by central neuroendocrine tissues. *Recent Prog. Horm. Res.* **31:** 295–319.

Nakayama, K., Ishida, N., Shirane, M., Inomata, A., Inoue, T., Shishido, N., Horii, I., Loh, D. Y., and Nakayama, K. (1996). Mice lacking p27(Kip1) display increased body size, multiple organ hyperplasia, retinal dysplasia, and pituitary tumors. *Cell* **85:** 707–720.

Narayanan, C. H., and Hamburger, V. (1971). Motility in chick embryos with substitution of lumbosacral by brachial and brachial by lumbosacral spinal cord segments. *J. Exp. Zool.* **178:** 415–431.

Nardi, J. B. (1983). Neuronal pathfinding in developing wings of the moth *Manduca sexta. Dev. Biol.* **95:** 163–174.

Nardi, J. B., and Vernon, R. A. (1990). Topographical features of the substratum for growth of pioneering neurons in the *Manduca* wing disc. *J. Neurobiol.* **21:** 1189–1201.

Nedivi, E., Wu, G. Y., and Cline, H. T. (1998). Promotion of dendritic growth by CPG15, an activity-induced signaling molecule. *Science* **281:** 1863–1866.

Newman-Gage, H., Westrum, L. E., and Bertrum, J. F. (1987). Stereological analysis of synaptogenesis in the molecular layer of piriform cortex in the prenatal rat. *J. Comp. Neurol.* **261:** 295–305.

Newport, E. (1990). Maturational constraints on language learning. *Cognit. Sci.* **14:** 11–28.

Nguyen, Q. T., Parsadanian, A. S., Snider, W. D., and Lichtman, J. W. (1998). Hyperinnervation of neuromuscular junctions caused by GDNF overexpression in muscle. *Science* **279:** 1725–1729.

Nicholls, J. G., and Hernandez, U. G. (1989). Growth and synapse formation by identified leech neurones in culture: A review. *Q. J. Exp. Physiol.* **74:** 965–973.

Niethammer, M., Kim, E., and Sheng, M. (1996). Interaction between the C terminus of NMDA receptor subunits and multiple members of the PSD-95 family of membrane-associated guanylate kinases. *J. Neurosci.* **16:** 2157–2163.

Nieuwkoop, P. D. (1973). The organization center of the amphibian embryo: Its origin, spatial organization, and morphogenetic action. *Adv. Morphog.* **10:** 1–39.

Nieuwkoop, P. D. (1985). Inductive interactions in early amphibian development and their general nature. *J. Embryol. Exp. Morphol. (Suppl.)* **89:** 333–347.

Nitkin, R. M., Smith, M. A., Magill, C., Fallon, J. R., Yao, M., Wallace, B. G., and McMahon, U. J. (1987). Identification of agrin, a synaptic organizing protein from *Torpedo* electric organ. *J. Cell Biol.* **105:** 2471–2478.

Njå, A., and Purves, D. (1977). Specific innervation of guinea-pig superior cervical ganglion cells by preganglionic fibres arising from different levels of the spinal cord. *J. Physiol.* **264:** 565–583.

Noakes, P. G., Gautam, M., Mudd, J., Sanes, J. R., and Merlie, J. P. (1995). Aberrant differentiation of neuromuscular junctions in mice lacking s-laminin/laminin β$_2$. *Nature* **374:** 258–262.

Noakes, P. G., Phillips, W. D., Hanley, T. A., Sanes, J. R., and Merlie, J. P. (1993). 43K protein and acetylcholine receptors colocalize during the initial stages of neuromuscular synapse formation *in vivo. Dev. Biol.* **155:** 275–280.

Nolen, T. G., and Carew, T. J. (1988). The cellular analog of sensitization in *Aplysia* emerges at the same time in development as behavioral sensitization. *J. Neurosci.* **8:** 212–222.

Nordeen, E. J., and Nordeen, K. W. (1988). Sex and regional differences in the incorporation of neurons born during song learning in zebra finches. *J. Neurosci.* **8:** 2869–2874.

Nordeen, E. J., Nordeen, K. W., Sengelaub, D. R., and Arnold, A. P. (1985). Androgens prevent normally occurring cell death in a sexually dimorphic spinal nucleus. *Science* **229:** 671–673.

Nose, A., Mahajan, V. B., and Goodman, C. S. (1992). Connectin: A homophilic cell adhesion molecule expressed on a subset of muscles and the motoneurons that innervate them in *Drosophila. Cell* **70:** 553–567.

Nose, A., Takeichi, M., and Goodman, C. S. (1994). Ectopic expression of connectin reveals a repulsive function during growth cone guidance and synapse formation. *Neuron* **13:** 525–539.

Nose, A., Van Vactor, D., Auld, V., and Goodman, C. S. (1992). Development of neuromuscular specificity in *Drosophila. Cold Spring Harbor Symp. Quant. Biol.* **57:** 441–449.

Nottebohm, F. (1980). Testosterone triggers growth of brain vocal control nuclei in adult female canaries. *Brain Res.* **189:** 429–436.

Nottebohm, F. (1981). A brain for all seasons: Cyclical anatomical changes in song control nuclei of the canary brain. *Science* **214:** 1368–1370.

Nottebohm, F., and Arnold, A. P. (1976). Sexual dimorphism in vocal control areas of the songbird brain. *Science* **194:** 211–213.

Nusslein-Volhard, C., and Wieschaus, E. (1980). Mutations affecting segment number and polarity in *Drosophila*. *Nature* **287:** 795–801.

Oakley, R. A., and Tosney, K. W. (1993). Contact-mediated mechanisms of motor axon segmentation. *J. Neurosci.* **13:** 3773–3792.

Obata, K., Oide, M., and Tanaka, H. (1978). Excitatory and inhibitory actions of GABA and glycine on embryonic chick spinal neurons in culture. *Brain Res.* **144:** 179–184.

O'Brien, R. A. D., Östberg, A. J. C., and Vrbová, G. (1978). Observations on the elimination of polyneuronal innervation in developing mammalian skeletal muscle. *J. Physiol.* **282:** 571–582.

O'Brien, R. A. D., Östberg, A. J. C., and Vrbová, G. (1984). Protease inhibitors reduce the loss of nerve terminals induced by activity and calcium in developing rat soleus muscles *in vitro*. *Neuroscience* **12:** 637–646.

O'Brien, R. J., and Fischbach, G. D. (1986a). Isolation of embryonic chick motoneurons and their survival *in vitro*. *J. Neurosci.* **6:** 3265–3274.

O'Brien, R. J., and Fischbach, G. D. (1986b). Modulation of embryonic chick motoneuron glutamate sensitivity by interneurons and agonists. *J. Neurosci.* **6:** 3290–3296.

O'Brien, R. J., Kamboz, S., Ehlers, M. D., Rosen, K. R., Fischbach, G. D., and Huganir, R. L. (1998). Activity-dependent modulation of synaptic AMPA receptor accumulation. *Neuron* **21:** 1067–1078.

Obrietan, K., and van den Pol, A. N. (1995). GABA neurotransmission in the hypothalamus: Developmental reversal from Ca^{2+} elevating to depressing. *J. Neurosci.* **15:** 5065–5077.

O'Connor, L. T., Lauterborn, J. C., Gall, C. M., and Smith, M. A. (1994). Localization and alternative splicing of agrin mRNA in adult rat brain: Transcripts encoding isoforms that aggregate acetylcholine receptors are not restricted to cholinergic regions. *J. Neurosci.* **14:** 1141–1152.

O'Connor, T. P., Duerr, J. S., and Bentley, D. (1990). Pioneer growth cone steering decisions mediated by single filopodial contacts *in situ*. *J. Neurosci.* **10:** 3935–3946.

O'Donovan, M., Ho, S., and Yee, W. (1994). Calcium imaging of rhythmic network activity in the developing spinal cord of the chick embryo. *J. Neurosci.* **14:** 6354–6369.

O'Donovan, M. J., Wenner, P., Chub, N., Tabak, J., and Rinzel, J. (1998). Mechanisms of spontaneous activity in the developing spinal cord and their relevance to locomotion. *Ann. N. Y. Acad. Sci.* **860:** 130–141.

O'Dowd, D. K. (1983). RNA synthesis dependence of action potential development in spinal cord neurones. *Nature* **303:** 619–621.

O'Dowd, D. K., Ribera, A. B., and Spitzer, N. C. (1988). Development of voltage-dependent calcium, sodium, and potassium currents in *Xenopus* spinal neurons. *J. Neurosci.* **8:** 792–805.

Ogawa, S., Lubahn, D. B., Korach, K. S., Pfaff, D. W. (1997). Behavioral effects of estrogen receptor gene disruption in male mice. *Proc. Natl. Acad. Sci. USA* **94:** 1476–1481.

O'Leary, D. D., Heffner, C. D., Kutka, L., Lopez-Mascaraque, L., Missias, A., and Reinoso, B. S. (1991). A target-derived chemoattractant controls the development of the corticopontine projection by a novel mechanism of axon targeting. *Development* **Suppl. 2:** 123–130.

O'Leary, D. D. M., Stanfield, B. B., and Cowan, W. M. (1981). Evidence that the early postnatal restriction of the cells or origin of the callosal projection is due to the elimination of axonal collatorals rather than to the death of the neurons. *Dev. Brain Res.* **1:** 607–617.

Olsen, C. R., and Pettigrew, J. D. (1974). Single units in the visual cortex of kittens reared in stroboscopic illumination. *Brain Res.* **70:** 189–204.

O'Malley, D. M., Kao, Y. H., and Fetcho, J. R. (1996). Imaging the functional organization of zebrafish hindbrain segments during escape behaviors. *Neuron* **17:** 1145–1155.

Oppenheim, R. W. (1982). The neuroembryological study of behavior: Progress, problems, perspectives. *Curr. Top. Dev. Biol.* **17:** 257–309.

Oppenheim, R. W. (1989). The neurotrophic theory and naturally occurring motoneuron death. *Trends Neurosci.* **12:** 252–255.

Oppenheim, R. W. (1991). Cell death during development in the nervous system. *Annu. Rev. Neurosci.* **14:** 453–501.

Oppenheim, R. W. (1992). Pathways in the emergence of developmental neuroethology: Antecedents to current views of neurobehavioral ontogeny. *J. Neurobiol.* **23:** 1370–1403.

Oppenheim, R. W., Chu-Wang, I.-W., and Foelix, R. F. (1975). Some aspects of synaptogenesis in the spinal cord of the chick embryo: A quantitative electron microscopic study. *J. Comp. Neurol.* **161:** 383–418.

Oppenheim, R. W., Houenou, L. J., Johnson, J. E., Lin, L. F., Li, L., Lo, A. C., Newsome, A. L., Prevette, D. M., and Wang, S. (1995). Developing motor neurons rescued from programmed and axotomy-induced cell death by GDNF. *Nature* **373:** 344–346.

Oppenheim, R. W., Prevette, D., Tytell, M., and Homma, S. (1990). Naturally occurring and induced neuronal death in the chick embryo *in vivo* requires protein and RNA synthesis: Evidence for the role of cell death genes. *Dev. Biol.* **138:** 104–113.

Oppenheim, R. W., Prevette, D., Yin, Q. W., Collins, F., and MacDonald, J. (1991). Control of embryonic motoneuron survival *in vivo* by ciliary neurotrophic factor. *Science* **29:** 1616–1618.

Oppenheim, R. W., and Reitzel, J. (1975). Ontogeny of behavioral sensitivity to strychnine in the chick embryo:

Evidence for the early onset of CNS inhibition. *Brain Behav. Evol.* **11:** 130–159.

Oppenheim, R. W., Yin, Q. W., Prevette, D., and Yan, Q. (1992). Brain-derived neurotrophic factor rescues developing avian motoneurons from cell death. *Nature* **360:** 755–757.

O'Rourke, N. A., Chenn, A., and McConnell, S. K. (1997). Postmitotic neurons migrate tangentially in the cortical ventricular zone. *Development* **124:** 997–1005.

Overman, W. H. (1990). Performance on traditional matching to sample, non-matching to sample, and object discrimination tasks by 12- and 32-month-old children. *Ann. N. Y. Acad. Sci.* **608:** 365–385.

Owens, D. F., Boyce, L. H., Davis, M. B. E., and Kriegstein, A. R. (1996). Excitatory GABA responses in embryonic and neonatal cortical slices demonstrated by gramicidin perforated-patch recordings and calcium imaging. *J. Neurosci.* **16:** 6414–6423.

Palade, G. E., and Palay, S. L. (1954). Electron microscope observations of interneuronal and neuromuscular synapses. *Anat. Rec.* **118:** 335–336.

Palca, J. (1991). Famous monkeys provide surprising results [News]. *Science* **252:** 1789.

Pappas, G. D., and Purpura, D. P. (1964). Electron microscopy of immature human and feline hippocampus. *Prog. Brain Res.* **4:** 176–186.

Parks, T. N. (1979). Afferent influences on the development of the brain stem auditory nuclei of the chicken: Otocyst ablation. *J. Comp. Neurol.* **183:** 665–678.

Parnavelas, J. G., Barfield, J. A., Franke, E., and Luskin, M. B. (1991). Separate progenitor cells give rise to pyramidal and nonpyramidal neurons in the rat telencephalon. *Cereb. Cortex* **1:** 463–468.

Pasternak, T., Schumer, R. A., Gizzi, M. S., and Movshon, J. A. (1985). Abolition of visual cortical direction selectivity affects visual behavior in cats. *Exp. Brain Res.* **61:** 214–217.

Penfield, W. (1954). "The Excitable Cortex in Conscious Man." Liverpool Univ. Press, Liverpool.

Penfield, W., and Rasmussen, T. (1950). "The Cerebral Cortex of Man: A Clinical Study of Localization of Function." Macmillan Co., New York.

Péquignot, Y., and Clarke, P. G. (1992). Changes in lamination and neuronal survival in the isthmo-optic nucleus following the intraocular injection of tetrodotoxin in chick embryos. *J. Comp. Neurol.* **321:** 336–350.

Peterson, E. R., and Crain, S. M. (1981). Preferential growth of neurites from isolated fetal mouse dorsal root ganglia in relation to specific regions of co-cultured spinal cord explants. *Brain Res.* **254:** 363–382.

Petitto, L. A., and Marentette, P. F. (1991). Babbling in the manual mode: Evidence for the ontogeny of language. *Science* **251:** 1493–1496.

Phelan, P., Nakagawa, M., Wilkin, M. B., Moffat, K. G., O'Kane, C. J., Davies, J. A., and Bacon, J. P. (1996). Mutations in shaking-B prevent electrical synapse formation in the *Drosophila* giant fiber system. *J. Neurosci.* **16:** 1101–1113.

Phillips, W. D., Kopta, C., Blount, P., Gardner, P. D., Steinbach, J. H., and Merlie, J. P. (1991). ACh receptor-rich domains organized in fibroblasts by recombinant 43-kilodalton protein. *Science* **251:** 568–570.

Phoenix, C. H., Goy, R. W., Gerall, A. A., and Young, A. C. (1959). Organizing action of prenatally administered testosterone propionate on the tissues mediating mating behavior in the female guinea pig. *Endocrinol.* **65:** 369–382.

Piatt, J. (1955). Regeneration of the spinal cord in the salamander. *J. Exp. Zool.* **129:** 177–207.

Piccolo, S., Sasai, Y., *et al.* (1996). Dorsoventral patterning in *Xenopus*: Inhibition of ventral signals by direct binding of chordin to BMP-4. *Cell* **86:** 589–598.

Pilar, G., Landmesser, L., and Burstein, L. (1980). Competition for survival among developing ciliary ganglion cells. *J. Neurophysiol.* **43:** 233–254.

Pimenta, A. F., Zhukareva, V., Barbe, M. F., Reinoso, B. S., Grimley, C., Henzel, W., Fischer, I., and Levitt, P. (1995). The limbic system-associated membrane protein is an Ig superfamily member that mediates selective neuronal growth and axon targeting. *Neuron* **15:** 287–297.

Pini, A. (1993). Chemorepulsion of axons in the developing mammalian central nervous system. *Science* **261:** 95–98.

Pittman, R., and Oppenheim, R. W. (1979). Cell death of motoneurons in the chick embryo spinal cord. IV. Evidence that a functional neuromuscular interaction is involved in the regulation of naturally occurring cell death and the stabilization of synapses. *J. Comp. Neurol.* **187:** 425–446.

Pittman, R. N. (1985). Release of plasminogen activator and a calcium-dependent metalloprotease from cultured sympathetic and sensory neurons. *Dev. Biol.* **110:** 91–101.

Plotkin, M. D., Snyder, E. Y., Hebert, S. C., Delpire, E. (1997). Expression of the Na-K-2Cl cotransporter is developmentally regulated in postnatal rat brains: A possible mechanism underlying GABA's excitatory role in immature brain. *J. Neurobiol.* **33:** 781–795.

Plunkett, J. A., Simmons, R. B., and Walthall, W. W. (1996). Dynamic interactions between nerve and muscle in *Caenorhabditis elegans*. *Dev. Biol.* **175:** 154–165.

Pons, T. P., Garraghty, P. E., Ommaya, A. K., Kaas, J. H., Taub, E., and Mishkin, M. (1991). Massive cortical reorganization after sensory deafferentation in adult macaques [see Comments]. *Science* **252:** 1857–1860.

Poo, M.-m. (1982). Rapid lateral diffusion of functional ACh receptors in embryonic muscle cell membrane. *Nature* **295:** 332–334.

Porter, B. E., Weis, J., and Sanes, J. R. (1995). A motoneuron-selective stop signal in the synaptic protein s-laminin. *Neuron* **14:** 549–559.

Preyer, W. (1885). "Specielle Physiologie des Embryo." Grieben, Leipzig.

Prokop, A., Landgraf, M., Rushton, E., Broadie, K., and Bate, M. (1996). Presynaptic development at the neuromuscular junction: Assembly and localization of presynaptic active zones. *Neuron* **17:** 617–626.

Puche, A. C., Poirier, F., Hair, M., Bartlett, P. F., and Key, B. (1996). Role of galectin-1 in the developing mouse olfactory system. *Dev. Biol.* **179:** 274–287.

Puelles, L., and Rubenstein, J. L. (1993). Expression patterns of homeobox and other putative regulatory genes in the embryonic mouse forebrain suggest a neuromeric organization. *Trends Neurosci.* **16:** 472–479.

Purves, D., and Lichtman, J. W. (1985). Geometrical differences among homologous neurons in mammals. *Science* **228:** 298–302.

Purves, D., Thompson, W., and Yip, J. W. (1981). Re-innervation of ganglia transplanted to the neck from different levels of the guinea-pig sympathetic chain. *J. Physiol.* **313:** 49–63.

Qian, X., Davis, A. A., Goderie, S. K., and Temple, S. (1997). FGF2 concentration regulates the generation of neurons and glia from multipotent cortical stem cells. *Neuron* **18:**81–93.

Qu, Z., and Huganir, R. L. (1994). Comparison of innervation and agrin-induced tyrosine phosphorylation of the nicotinic acetylcholine receptor. *J. Neurosci.* **14:** 6834–6841.

Rabacchi, S., Bailly, Y., Delhaye-Bouchaud, N., and Mariani, J. (1992). Involvement of the *N*-methyl D-aspartate receptor in synapse elimination during cerebellar development. *Science* **256:** 1823–1825.

Rabizadeh, S., Oh, J., Zhong, L. T., Yang, J., Bitler, C. M., Butcher, L. L., and Bredesen, D. E. (1993). Induction of apoptosis by the low-affinity NGF receptor. *Science* **261:** 345–348.

Radel, J. D., Hankin, M. H., and Lund, R. D. (1990). Proximity as a factor in the innervation of host brain regions by retinal transplants. *J. Comp. Neurol.* **300:** 211–229.

Raff, M. C. (1989). Glial cell diversification in the rat optic nerve. *Science* **243:** 1450–1455.

Raghavan, S., and White, R. A. (1997). Connectin mediates adhesion in *Drosophila. Neuron* **18:** 873–880.

Raisman, G., and Field, P. M. (1973a). A quantitative investigation of the development of collateral reinnervation after partial deafferentation of the septal nuclei. *Brain Res.* **50:** 241–264.

Raisman, G., and Field, P. M. (1973b). Sexual dimorphism in the neuropil of the preoptic area of the rat and its dependence on neonatal androgen. *Brain Res.* **54:** 1–29.

Rajan, I., and Cline, H. T. (1998). Glutamate receptor activity is required for normal development of tectal cell dendrites *in vivo. J. Neurosci.* **18:** 7836–7846.

Rajan, P., and McKay, R. D. (1998). Multiple routes to astrocytic differentiation in the CNS. *Neuroscience* **18:** 3620–3629.

Rakic, P. (1971). Neuron–glia relationship during granule cell migration in developing cerebellar cortex: A Golgi and electron microscopic study in *Macaques rhesus. J. Comp. Neurol.* **141:** 283–312.

Rakic, P. (1972). Extrinsic cytological determinants of bas-

ket and stellate cell dendritic pattern in the cerebellar molecular layer. *J. Comp. Neurol.* **146:** 335–354.

Ramoa, A. S., and McCormick, D. A. (1994). Developmental changes in electrophysiological properties of LGNd neurons during reorganization of retinogeniculate connections. *J. Neurosci.* **14:** 2089–2097.

Ramon y Cajal, S. (1890). A quelle epoque aparaissent les expansions des cellule nerveuses de la moelle epinere du poulet. *Anat. Anz.* **5:** 609–613.

Ramon y Cajal, S. (1905). Genèse des fibres nerveuses de l'embryon et observations contraires à la thérie catenaire. *Trab Lab Invest. Biol., Univ. Madrid* **4:** 219–284.

Ramon y Cajal, S. (1928). "Degeneration and Regeneration of the Nervous System." Hafner, New York.

Ramon y Cajal, S. (1929). Studies on Vertebrate Neurogenesis. Charles Thomas, Springfield, IL.

Ramon y Cajal, S. (1937). "Recollections of My Life." MIT Press, Cambridge, MA.

Ramos, R. G., Igloi, G. L., Lichte, B., Baumann, U., Maier, D., Schneider, T., Brandstatter, J. H., Frohlich, A., and Fischbach, K. F. (1993). The irregular chiasm C-roughest locus of *Drosophila,* which affects axonal projections and programmed cell death, encodes a novel immunoglobulin-like protein. *Genes Dev.* **7:** 2533–2547.

Rankin, C. H., and Carew, T. J. (1988). Dishabituation and sensitization emerge as separate processes during development in *Aplysia. J. Neurosci.* **8:** 197–211.

Raper, J. A., Bastiani, M. J., and Goodman, C. S. (1984). Pathfinding by neuronal growth cones in grasshopper embryos. IV. The effects of ablating the A and P axons upon the behavior of the G growth cone. *J. Neurosci.* **4:** 2329–2345.

Raven, C. P., and Kloos, J. (1945). Induction by medial and lateral pieces of the archenteron roof, with special reference to the determination of the neural crest. *Acta Neerl. Morphol.* **5:** 348–362.

Raynaud, A., Clairambault, P., Renous, S., and Gasc, J. P. (1977). Organisation des cornes ventrales de la moelle epiniere, dans les regions brachiale et lombiare, chez les embryons de Reptiles serpentiformes et de Reptiles a membres bien developpes. *C. R. Acad. Sci. Hebd. Seances Acad. Sci. D.* **19:** 1507–1509.

Rayport, S. G., and Camardo, J. S. (1984). Differential emergence of cellular mechanisms and mediating habituation and sensitization in the developing *Aplysia* nervous system. *J. Neurosci.* **4:** 2528–2532.

Ready, D. F. (1989). A multifaceted approach to neural development. *Trends Neurosci.* **12:** 102–110.

Ready, D. F., Hanson, T. E., and Benzer, S. (1976). Development of the *Drosophila* retina, a neurocrystalline lattice. *Dev. Biol.* **53:** 217–240.

Recanzone, G. H., Merzenich, M. M., and Jenkins, W. M. (1992). Frequency discrimination training engaging a restricted skin surface results in an emergence of a cutaneous response zone in cortical area 3a. *J. Neurophysiol.* **67:** 1057–1070.

Redfern, P. A. (1970). Neuromuscular transmission in new-born rats. *J. Physiol.* **209:** 701–709.

Redies, C. (1997). Cadherins and the formation of neural circuitry in the vertebrate CNS. *Cell Tissue Res.* **290:** 405–413.

Redies, C., and Takeichi, M. (1996). Cadherins in the developing central nervous system: An adhesive code for segmental and functional subdivisions. *Dev. Biol.* **180:** 413–423.

Rees, R. P., Bunge, M. B., and Bunge, R. P. (1976). Morphological changes in the neuritic growth cone and target neuron during synaptic junction development in culture. *J. Cell Biol.* **68:** 240–246.

Reh, T. A., and Cagan, R. L. (1994). Intrinsic and extrinsic signals in the developing vertebrate and fly eyes: Viewing vertebrate and invertebrate eyes in the same light. *Perspect. Dev. Neurobiol.* **2:** 183–190.

Reh, T. A., and Constantine-Paton, M. (1984). Retinal ganglion cell terminals change their projection sites during larval development of *Rana pipiens*. *J. Neurosci.* **4:** 442–457.

Reichling, D. B., Kyrozis, A., Wang, J., and MacDermott, A. B. (1994). Mechanisms of GABA and glycine depolarization-induced calcium transients in rat dorsal horn neurons. *J. Physiol.* **476:** 411–421.

Reiness, C. G., and Hall, Z. W. (1981). The developmental change in immunological properties of the acetylcholine receptor in rat muscle. *Dev. Biol.* **81:** 324–331.

Reiness, C. G., and Weinberg, C. B. (1981). Metabolic stabilization of acetylcholine receptors at newly formed neuromuscular junctions in rat. *Dev. Biol.* **84:** 247–254.

Reinsch, S. S., Mitchison, T. J., and Kirschner, M. (1991). Microtubule polymer assembly and transport during axonal elongation. *J. Cell Biol.* **115:** 365–379.

Reissmann, E., Ernsberger, U., Francis-West, P. H., Rueger, D., Brickell, P. M., and Rohrer, H. (1996). Involvement of bone morphogenetic protein-4 and bone morphogenetic protein-7 in the differentiation of the adrenergic phenotype in developing sympathetic neurons. *Development* **122:** 2079–2088.

Reist, N. E., Magill, C., and McMahon, U. J. (1987). Agrin-like molecules at synaptic sites in normal, denervated, and damaged skeletal muscles. *J. Cell Biol.* **105:** 2457–2469.

Reist, N. E., Werle, M. J., and McMahon, U. J. (1992). Agrin released by motor neurons induces the aggregation of acetylcholine receptors at neuromuscular junctions. *Neuron* **8:** 865–868.

Ressler, K. J., Sullivan, S. L., and Buck, L. B. (1993). A zonal organization of odorant receptor gene expression in the olfactory epithelium. *Cell* **73:** 597–609.

Retaux, S., and Harris, W. A. (1996). Engrailed and retinotectal topography. *Trends Neurosci.* **19:** 542–546.

Reynolds, B. A., and Weiss, S. (1992). Generation of neurons and astrocytes from isolated cells of the adult mammalian central nervous system. *Science* **255:** 1707–1710.

Reynolds, S. A., French, K. A., Baader, A., and Kristan, W. B., Jr. (1998). Development of spontaneous and evoked behaviors in the medicinal leech. *J. Comp. Neurol.* **402:** 168–180.

Ribera, A. B., and Spitzer, N. C. (1989). A critical period of transcription required for differentiation of the action potential of spinal neurons. *Neuron* **2:** 1055–1062.

Richardson, P. M., McGuinness, U. M., and Aguayo, A. J. (1980). Axons from CNS neurons regenerate into PNS grafts. *Nature* **284:** 264–265.

Ridge, R. M. A. P., and Betz, W. J. (1984). The effect of selective, chronic stimulation on motor unit size in developing rat muscle. *J. Neurosci.* **4:** 2614–2620.

Riehl, R., Johnson, K., Bradley, R., Grunwald, G. B., Cornel, E., Lilienbaum, A., and Holt, C. E. (1996). Cadherin function is required for axon outgrowth in retinal ganglion cells *in vivo*. *Neuron* **17:** 837–848.

Rio, C., Rieff, H. I., Qi, P., Khurana, T. S., and Corfas, G. (1997). Neuregulin and erbB receptors play a critical role in neuronal migration. *Neuron* **19:** 39–50.

Riquimaroux, H., Gaioni, S. J., and Suga, N. (1991). Cortical computational maps control auditory perception. *Science* **1:** 565–568.

Rivera, C., Voipio, J., Payne, J. A., Ruusuvuori, E., Lahtinen, H., Lamsa, K., Pirvola, U., Saarma, M., and Kaila, K. (1999). The K+/Cl- cotransporter KCC2 renders GABA hyperpolarizing during neuronal maturation. *Nature* **397:** 251–255.

Robinow, S., Talbot, W. S., Hogness, D. S., and Truman, J. W. (1993). Programmed cell death in the *Drosophila* CNS is ecdysone-regulated and coupled with a specific ecdysone receptor isoform. *Development* **119:** 1251–1259.

Roe, A. W., Pallas, S. L., Kwon, Y. H., and Sur, M. (1992). Visual projections routed to the auditory pathway in ferrets: Receptive fields of visual neurons in primary auditory cortex. *J. Neurosci.* **12:** 3651–3664.

Roelink, H., Augsburger, A., *et al.* (1994). Floor plate and motor neuron induction by vhh-1, a vertebrate homolog of hedgehog expressed by the notochord. *Cell* **76:** 761–775.

Roessler, E., Belloni, E., Gaudenz, K., Jay, P., Berta, P., Scherer, S. W., Tsui, L. C., and Muenke, M. (1996). Mutations in the human Sonic Hedgehog gene cause holoprosencephaly. *Nat. Genetics* **14:** 357–360.

Rohrbough, J., and Spitzer, N. C. (1996). Regulation of intracellular Cl⁻ levels by Na(⁺)-dependent Cl⁻cotransport distinguishes depolarizing from hyperpolarizing GABAA receptor-mediated responses in spinal neurons. *J. Neurosci.* **16:** 82–91.

Role, L. W. (1985). Neural regulation of acetylcholine sensitivity in embryonic sympathetic neurons. *Proc. Natl. Acad. Soc. USA* **85:** 2825–2829.

Role, L. W., Matossian, V. R., O'Brien, R. J., and Fischbach, G. D. (1985). On the mechanism of acetylcholine receptor accumulation at newly formed synapses on chick myotubes. *J. Neurosci.* **5:** 2197–2204.

Role, L. W., Roufa, D. G., and Fischbach, G. D. (1987). The distribution of acetylcholine receptor clusters and sites of transmitter release along chick ciliary ganglion neurite-myotube contacts in culture. *J. Cell Biol.* **104:** 371–379.

Roskies, A. L., and O'Leary, D. D. (1994). Control of topographic retinal axon branching by inhibitory membrane-bound molecules. *Science* **265:** 799–803.

Ross, L. S., Parrett, T., and Easter, S. S., Jr. (1992). Axonogenesis and morphogenesis in the embryonic zebrafish brain. *J. Neurosci.* **12:** 467–482.

Rotzler, S., Schramek, H., and Brenner, H. R. (1991). Metabolic stabilization of endplate acetylcholine receptors regulated by Ca^{2+} influx associated with muscle activity. *Nature* **349:** 337–339.

Roy, N., Mahadevan, M. S., McLean, M., Shutler, G., Yaraghi, Z., Farahani, R., Baird, S., Besner-Johnston, A., Lefebvre, C., Kang, X., Salih, M., Arbry, H., Tamai, K., Guan, X., Ioannon, P., Crawford, T. O., deJong, P. J., Surh, L., Ikeda, J.-E., Korneluk, R. G., and MacKenzie, R. G. (1995). The gene for neuronal apoptosis inhibitory protein is partially deleted in individuals with spinal muscular atrophy. *Cell* **80:** 167–178.

Rubel, E. W., Smith, D. J., and Miller, L. C. (1976). Organization and development of brain stem auditory nuclei of the chicken: Ontogeny of n. magnocellularis and n. laminaris. *J. Comp. Neurol.* **166:** 469–489.

Ruegg, M. A., Tsim, K. W. K., Horton, S. E., Kroger, S., Escher, G., Gensch, E. M., and McMahan, U. J. (1992). The agrin gene codes for a family of basal lamina proteins that differ in function and distribution. *Neuron* **8:** 691–699.

Ruiz i Altaba, A. (1992). Planar and vertical signals in the induction and patterning of the *Xenopus* nervous system. *Development* **116:** 67–80.

Rupp, F., Payan, D. G., Magill-Solc, C., Cowan, D. M., and Scheller, R. H. (1992). Structure and expression of a rat agrin. *Neuron* **6:** 811–823.

Sabry, J. H., O'Connor, T. P., Evans, L., Toroian-Raymond, A., Kirschner, M., and Bentley, D. (1991). Microtubule behavior during guidance of pioneer neuron growth cones *in situ*. *J. Cell Biol.* **115:** 381–395.

Sakaguchi, D. S., and Murphey, R. K. (1985). Map formation in the developing *Xenopus* retinotectal system: An examination of ganglion cell terminal arborizations. *J. Neurosci.* **5:** 3228–3245.

Sakaguchi, D. S. (1989). The development of retinal ganglion cells deprived of their targets. *Dev. Biol.* **134:** 103–111.

Sakuma, Y. (1984). Influences of neonatal gonadectomy or androgen exposure on the sexual differentiation of the rat ventromedial hypothalamus. *J. Physiol. (London)* **349:** 273–286.

Salmelin, R., Service, E., Kiesila, P., Uutela, K., and Salonen, O. (1996). Impaired visual word processing in dyslexia revealed with magnetoencephalography. *Ann. Neurol.* **40:** 157–162.

Salpeter, M. M., and Harris, R. (1983). Distribution and turnover rate of acetylcholine receptors throughout the junction folds at a vertebrate neuromuscular junction. *J. Cell Biol.* **96:** 1781–1785.

Sánchez, M. P., Silos-Santiago, I., Frisén, J., He, B., Lira, S. A., and Barbacid, M. (1996). Renal agenesis and the absence of enteric neurons in mice lacking GDNF. *Nature* **382:** 70–73.

Sandrock, A. W., Jr., Dryer, S. E., Rosen, K. M., Gozani, S. N., Kramer, R., Theill, L. E., and Fischbach, G. D. (1997). Maintenance of acetylcholine receptor number by neuregulins at the neuromuscular junction *in vivo*. *Science* **276:** 599–603.

Sandrock, A. W., Jr., Goodearl, A. D., Yin, Q. W., Chang, D., and Fischbach, G. D. (1995). ARIA is concentrated in nerve terminals at neuromuscular junctions and at other synapses. *J. Neurosci.* **15:** 6124–6136.

Sanes, D. H. (1993). The development of synaptic function and integration in the central auditory system. *J. Neurosci.* **13:** 2627–2637.

Sanes, D. H., and Constantine-Paton, M. (1985). The sharpening of frequency tuning curves requires patterned activity during development in the mouse, *Mus musculus*. *J. Neurosci.* **5:** 1152–1166.

Sanes, D. H., and Hafidi, A. (1996). Glycinergic transmission regulates dendrite size in organotypic culture. *J. Neurobiol.* **4:** 503–511.

Sanes, D. H., and Rubel, E. W. (1988). The ontogeny of inhibition and excitation in the gerbil lateral superior olive. *J. Neurosci.* **8:** 682–700.

Sanes, D. H., and Siverls, V. (1991). Development and specificity of inhibitory terminal arborizations in the central nervous system. *J. Neurobiol.* **22:** 837–854.

Sanes, D. H., and Takacs, C. (1993). Activity-dependent refinement of inhibitory connections. *Eur. J. Neurosci.* **5:** 570–574.

Sanes, J. R., Johnson, Y. R., Kotzbauer, P. T., Mudd, J., Hanley, T., Martinou, J. C., and Merlie, J. P. (1991). Selective expression of an acetylcholine receptor–lacZ transgene in synaptic nuclei of adult muscle fibers. *Development* **113:** 1181–1191.

Sanes, J. R., and Yamagata, M. (1999). Formation of lamina-specific synaptic connections. *Curr. Opin. Neurobiol.* **9:** 79–87.

Sasai, Y., Lu, B., *et al.* (1994). *Xenopus* chordin: A novel dorsalizing factor activated by organizer-specific homeobox genes. *Cell* **79:** 779–790.

Sasai, Y., Lu, B., Steinbeisser, H., and De Robertis, E. M. (1995). Regulation of neural induction by the Chd and Bmp-4 antagonistic patterning signals in *Xenopus*. *Nature*. **376:** 333–336.

Scheetz, A. J., Nairn, A. C., and Constantine-Paton, M. (1997). *N*-methyl-D-aspartate receptor activation and visual activity induce elongation factor-2 phosphorylation in amphibian tecta: A role for *N*-methyl-D-aspartate receptors in controlling protein synthesis. *Proc. Natl. Acad. Sci. USA* **94:** 14,770–14,775.

Scherer, W. J., and Udin, S. B. (1989). *N*-methyl-D-aspartate antagonists prevent interaction of binocular maps in *Xenopus* tectum. *J. Neurosci.* **9:** 3837–3843.

Schlinger, B. A. (1998). Sexual differentiation of avian brain and behavior: Current views on gonadal hormone-dependent and independent mechanisms. *Annu. Rev. Physiol.* **60:** 407–429.

Schmidt, J., and Coen, T. (1995). Changes in retinal arbors in compressed projections to half tecta in goldfish. *J. Neurobiol.* **28:** 409–418.

Schmidt, J. T. (1978). Retinal fibers alter tectal positional markers during the expansion of the retinal projection in goldfish. *J. Comp. Neurol.* **177:** 279–295.

Schmidt, J. T., and Buzzard, M. (1990). Activity-driven sharpening of the regenerating retinotectal projection: Effects of blocking or synchronizing activity on the morphology of individual regenerating arbors. *J. Neurobiol.* **21:** 900–917.

Schmidt, J. T., and Eisele, L. E. (1985). Stroboscopic illumination and dark rearing block the sharpening of the regenerated retinotectal map in goldfish. *Neuroscience* **14:** 535–546.

Schmidt, T. A., Larsen, J. S., and Kjeldsen, K. (1992). Quantification of rat cerebral cortex Na$^+$,K($^+$)-ATPase: Effect of age and potassium depletion. *J. Neurochem.* **59:** 2094–2104.

Schneiderman, A. M., Hildebrand, J. G., Brennan, M. M., and Tumlinson, J. H. (1986). Trans-sexually grafted antennae alter pheromone-directed behaviour in a moth. *Nature* **323:** 801–803.

Schotzinger, R., Yin, X., and Landis, S. (1994). Target determination of neurotransmitter phenotype in sympathetic neurons. *J. Neurobiol.* **25:** 620–639.

Schreiber, J., Sock, E., and Wegner, M. (1997). The regulator of early gliogenesis glial cells missing is a transcription factor with a novel type of DNA-binding domain. *Proc. Natl. Acad. Sci. USA* **94:** 4739–4744.

Schulte-Merker, S., Lee, K. J., *et al.* (1997). The zebrafish organizer requires chordino [Letter]. *Nature* **387:** 862–863.

Schuster, C. M., Davis, G. W., Fetter, R. D., and Goodman, C. S. (1996a). Genetic dissection of structural and functional components of synaptic plasticity. I. Fasciclin II controls synaptic stabilization and growth [see Comments]. *Neuron* **17:** 641–654.

Schuster, C. M., Davis, G. W., Fetter, R. D., and Goodman, C. S. (1996b). Genetic dissection of structural and functional components of synaptic plasticity. II. Fasciclin II controls presynaptic structural plasticity. *Neuron* **17:** 655–667.

Schwab, M. E., and Bartholdi, D. (1996). Degeneration and regeneration of axons in the lesioned spinal cord. *Physiol. Rev.* **76:** 319–370.

Schwartz, I. R., Pappas, G. D., and Purpura, D. P. (1968). Fine structure of neurons and synapses in the feline hippocampus during postnatal ontogenesis. *Exp. Neurol.* **22:** 394–407.

Sealock, R., Wray, B. E., and Froehner, S. C. (1984). Ultra-structural localization of the M_r 43,000 protein and the acetylcholine receptor in *Torpedo* postsynaptic membranes using monoclonal antibodies. *J. Cell Biol.* **98:** 2239–2244.

Seebach, B. S., and Ziskind-Conhaim, L. (1994). Formation of transient inappropriate sensorimotor synapses in developing rat spinal cords. *J. Neurosci.* **14:** 4520–4528.

Seeger, M., Tear, G., Ferres-Marco, D., and Goodman, C. S. (1993). Mutations affecting growth cone guidance in *Drosophila*: Genes necessary for guidance toward or away from the midline. *Neuron* **10:** 409–426.

Selleck, M. A., and Bronner-Fraser, M. (1995). Origins of the avian neural crest: The role of neural plate-epidermal interactions. *Development* **121:** 525–538.

Serafini, T., Kennedy, T. E., Galko, M. J., Mirzayan, C., Jessell, T. M., and Tessier-Lavigne, M. (1994). The netrins define a family of axon outgrowth-promoting proteins homologous to *C. elegans* UNC-6. *Cell* **78:** 409–424.

Shah, N. M., Marchionni, M. A., Isaacs, I., Stroobant, P., and Anderson, D. J. (1994). Glial growth factor restricts mammalian neural crest stem cells to a glial fate. *Cell* **77:** 349–360.

Shainberg, A., and Burstein, M. (1976). Decrease of acetylcholine receptor synthesis in muscle cultures by electrical stimulation. *Nature* **264:** 368–369.

Shankland, M., and Macagno, E. (Eds.) (1992). "Determinants of Neural Identity." Academic Press, San Diego.

Sharma, S. C., and Hollyfield, J. G. (1980). Specification of retinotectal connexions during development of the toad *Xenopus laevis. J. Embryol. Exp. Morphol.* **55:** 77–92.

Sherman, S. M., and Spear, P. D. (1982). Organization of visual pathways in normal and visually deprived cats. *Physiol. Rev.* **62:** 738–855.

Sherrington, C. S. (1906). "The Integrative Action of the Nervous System." Scribner's, New York.

Shitaka, Y., Matsuki, N., Saito, H., and Katsuki, H. (1996). Basic fibroblast growth factor increases functional L-type Ca^{2+} channels in fetal hippocampal neurons: Implications for neurite morphogenesis *in vitro. J. Neurosci.* **16:** 6476–6489.

Shyng, S.-L., Xu, R., and Salpeter, M. M. (1991). cAMP stabilizes the degradation of original junctional acetylcholine receptors in denervated muscle. *Neuron* **6:** 469–475.

Si, J., Luo, Z., and Mei, L. (1996). Induction of acetylcholine receptor gene expression by ARIA requires activation of mitogen-activated protein kinase. *J. Biol. Chem.* **16:** 19,752–19,759.

Sidman, R. L. (1961). Histogenesis of the mouse retina studied with thymidine ^{3}H. *In* "The Structure of the Eye" (G. K. Smelser, Ed.), pp. 487–506. Academic Press, New York.

Sidman, R. L., Miale, I. L., and Feder, N. (1959). Cell proliferation and migration in the primitive ependymal zone: An autoradiographic study of histogenesis in the nervous system. *Exp. Neurol.* **1:** 322–333.

Siegelbaum, S. A., Trautmann, A., and Koenig, J. (1984). Single acetylcholine-activated channel currents in developing muscle cells. *Dev. Biol.* **104:** 366–379.

Silver, J. (1984). Studies on the factors that govern directionality of axonal growth in the embryonic optic nerve and at the chiasm of mice. *J. Comp. Neurol.* **223:** 238–251.

Silver, J., and Ogawa, M. Y. (1983). Postnatally induced formation of the corpus callosum in acallosal mice on glia-coated cellulose bridges. *Science* **220:** 1067–1069.

Simeone, A., Acampora, D., *et al.* (1991). Differential regulation by retinoic acid of the homeobox genes of the four HOX loci in human embryonal carcinoma cells. *Mech. Dev.* **33:** 215–227.

Simon, A. M., Hoppe, P., and Burden, S. J. (1992). Spatial restriction of AChR gene expression to subsynaptic nuclei. *Development* **114:** 545–553.

Simon, D. K., and O'Leary, D. D. (1992). Responses of retinal axons *in vivo* and *in vitro* to position-encoding molecules in the embryonic superior colliculus. *Neuron* **9:** 977–989.

Simon, D. K., Prusky, G. T., O'Leary, D. D. M., and Constantine-Paton, M. (1992). N-methyl-D-aspartate receptor antagonists disrupt the formation of a mammalian neural map. *Proc. Natl. Acad. Sci. USA* **89:** 10,593–10,597.

Simons, D. J., Durham, D., and Woolsey, T. A. (1984). Functional organization of mouse and rat SmI barrel cortex following vibrissal damage on different postnatal days. *Somatosens. Res.* **1:** 207–245.

Simpson, H. B., and Vicario, D. S. (1991). Early estrogen treatment alone causes female zebra finches to produce learned, male-like vocalizations. *J. Neurobiol.* **22:** 755–776.

Singer, M. A., O'Connor, T. P., and Bentley, D. (1995). Pioneer growth cone migration in register with orthogonal epithelial domains in the grasshopper limb bud. *Int. J. Dev. Biol.* **39:** 965–973.

Singer, W. (1977a). Control of thalamic transmission by corticofugal and ascending reticular pathways in the visual system. *Physiol. Rev.* **57:** 386–420.

Singer, W. (1977b). Effects of monocular deprivation on excitatory and inhibitory pathways in cat striate cortex. *Exp. Brain Res.* **24:** 25–41.

Singson, A., Leviten, M. W., Bang, A. G., Hua, X. H., and Posakony, J. W. (1994). Direct downstream targets of proneural activators in the imaginal disc include genes involved in lateral inhibitory signaling. *Genes Dev.* **8:** 2058–2071.

Skeath, J. B, and Carroll, S. B. (1992). Regulation of proneural gene expression and cell fate during neuroblast segregation in the *Drosophila* embryo. *Development* **114:** 939–946.

Skeath, J. B., Panganiban, G., Selegue, J., and Carroll, S. B. (1992). Gene regulation in two dimensions: The proneural achaete and scute genes are controlled by combinations of axis-patterning genes through a common intergenic control region. *Genes Dev.* **6:** 2606–2619.

Skene, J. H., Jacobson, R. D., Snipes, G. J., McGuire, C. B., Norden, J. J., and Freeman, J. A. (1986). A protein induced during nerve growth (GAP-43) is a major component of growth-cone membranes. *Science* **233:** 783–786.

Skoff, R. P., Price, D. L., and Stocks, A. (1976). Electron microscopic autoradiographic studies of gliogenesis in rat optic nerve. II. Time of origin. *J. Comp. Neurol.* **169:** 313–334.

Small, S., and Levine, M. (1991). The initiation of pair-rule stripes in the *Drosophila* blastoderm. *Curr. Opin. Genet. Dev.* **1:** 255–260.

Smart, I. (1961). The subependymal layer of the mouse brain and its cell production as shown by radioautography after thymidine-H3 injection. *J. Comp. Neurol.* **116:** 325–347.

Smeyne, R. J., Klein, R., Schnapp, A., Long, L. K., Bryant, S., Lewin, A., Lira, S. A., and Barbacid, M. (1994). Severe sensory and sympathetic neuropathies in mice carrying a disrupted Trk/NGF receptor gene. *Nature* **368:** 246–249.

Smith, W. C., Knecht, A. K., Wu, M., and Harland, R. M. (1993). Secreted *noggin* protein mimics the Spemann organizer in dorsalizing *Xenopus* mesoderm. *Nature* **361:** 547–549.

Smolen, A. J. (1981). Postnatal development of ganglionic neurons in the absence of preganglionic input: Morphological observations on synapse formation. *Dev. Brain Res.* **1:** 49–58.

Snyder, R. L., Rebscher, S. J., Cao, K., Leake, P. A., and Kelly, K. (1990). Chonic intracochlear electrical stimulation in the neonatally deafened cat. I. Expansion of central representation. *Hearing Res.* **50:** 7–34.

So, K. L., Pun, S., Wan, D. C., and Tsim, K. W. (1996). Cerebellar granule cells express a specific isoform of agrin that lacks the acetylcholine receptor aggregating activity. *FEBS Lett.* **379:** 63–68.

Solum, D., Hughes, D., Major, M. S., and Parks, T. N. (1997). Prevention of normally occurring and deafferentation-induced neuronal death in chick brainstem auditory neurons by periodic blockade of AMPA/kainate receptors. *J. Neurosci.* **17:** 4744–4751.

Song, H., Ming, G., He, Z., Lehmann, M., Tessier-Lavigne, M., and Poo, M. (1998). Conversion of neuronal growth cone responses from repulsion to attraction by cyclic nucleotides [see Comments]. *Science* **281:** 1515–1518.

Song, H. J., Ming, G. L., and Poo, M. M. (1997). cAMP-induced switching in turning direction of nerve growth cones. *Nature* **388:** 275–279. Erratum (1997). *Nature* **389:** 412.

Speidel, C. C. (1941). Adjustments of nerve endings. *Harvey Lect.* **36:** 126–158.

Sperry, R. W. (1943). Effect of 180 degree rotation of the retinal field on visuomotor coordination. *J. Exp. Zool.* **92:** 263–279.

Sperry, R. W. (1963). Chemoaffinity in the orderly growth of nerve fiber patterns and connections. *Proc. Natl. Acad. Sci. USA* **50:** 703–710.

Spitzer, N. C. (1981). Development of membrane properties in vertebrates. *Trends Neurosci.* **4**: 169–172.

Spitzer, N. C. (1994). Spontaneous Ca^{2+} spikes and waves in embryonic neurons: Signaling systems for differentiation. *Trends Neurosci.* **17**: 115–118.

Spitzer, N. C., and Lamborghini, J. E. (1976). The development of the action potential mechanism of amphibian neurons isolated in cell culture. *Proc. Natl. Acad. Sci. USA* **73**: 1641–1645.

Spitzer, N. C., and Ribera, A. B. (1998). Development of electrical excitability in embryonic neurons: Mechanisms and roles. *J. Neurobiol.* **37**: 190–197.

Sretavan, D. W., and Shatz, C. J. (1986). Prenatal development of retinal ganglion cell axons: Segregation into eye-specific layers within the cat's lateral geniculate nucleus. *J. Neurosci.* **6**: 234–251.

Sretavan, D. W., Shatz, C. J., and Stryker, M. P. (1988). Modification of retinal ganglion cell axon morphology by prenatal infusion of tetrodotoxin. *Nature* **336**: 468–471.

Stahl, B., Muller, B., von Boxberg, Y., Cox, E. C., and Bonhoeffer, F. (1990). Biochemical characterization of a putative axonal guidance molecule of the chick visual system. *Neuron* **5**: 735–743.

Stahl, N., and Yancopolous, G. D. (1994). The tripartite CNTF receptor complex: Activation and signaling involves components shared with other cytokines. *J. Neurobiol.* **25**: 1454–1466.

Stephens, R. M., Loeb, D. M., Copeland, T. D., Pawson, T., Greene, L. A., and Kaplan, D. R. (1994). Trk receptors use redundant signal transduction pathways involving SHC and PLC-γ1 to mediate NGF responses. *Neuron* **12**: 691–705.

Steward, O. (1994). Dendrites as compartments for macromolecular synthesis. *Proc. Natl. Acad. Sci. USA* **91**: 10,766–10,768.

Stoeckli, E. T., and Landmesser, L. T. (1995). Axonin-1, Nr-CAM, and Ng-CAM play different roles in the *in vivo* guidance of chick commissural neurons. *Neuron* **14**: 1165–1179.

Stoeckli, E. T., Sonderegger, P., Pollerberg, G. E., and Landmesser, L. T. (1997). Interference with axonin-1 and NrCAM interactions unmasks a floor-plate activity inhibitory for commissural axons. *Neuron* **18**: 209–221.

Stoop, R., and Poo, M.-m. (1996). Synaptic modulation by neurotrophic factors: Differential and synergistic effects of brain-derived neurotrophic factor and ciliary neurotrophic factor. *J. Neurosci.* **16**: 3256–3264.

Stoppini, L., Buchs, P. A., and Muller, D. (1991). A simple method for organotypic cultures of nervous tissue. *J. Neurosci. Methods* **37**: 173–182.

Straznicky, K. (1967). The development of the innervation and the musculature of wings innervated by thoracic nerves. *Acta Biol. Acad. Sci. Hung.* **18**: 437–448.

Strittmatter, S. M., Fankhauser, C., Huang, P. L., Mashimo, H., and Fishman, M. C. (1995). Neuronal pathfinding is abnormal in mice lacking the neuronal growth cone protein GAP-43. *Cell* **80**: 445–452.

Strittmatter, S. M., and Fishman, M. C. (1991). The neuronal growth cone as a specialized transduction system. *Bioessays* **13**: 127–134.

Stryker, M. P., and Harris, W. A. (1986). Binocular impulse blockade prevents the formation of ocular dominance columns in the cat visual cortex. *J. Neurosci.* **6**: 2117–2133.

Stryker, M. P., Sherk, H., Levinthal, A. G., and Hirsch, H. V. B. (1978). Physiological consequences for the cat's visual cortex of effectively restricting early visual experience with oriented contours. *J. Neurophysiol.* **41**: 896–909.

Stuart, J. J., Brown, S. J., Beeman, R. W., and Denell, R. E. (1993). The *Tribolium* homeotic gene Abdominal is homologous to abdominal-A of the *Drosophila* bithorax complex. *Development* **117**: 233–243.

Studer, M., Popperl, H., *et al.* (1994). Role of a conserved retinoic acid response element in rhombomere restriction of Hoxb-1. *Science* **265**: 1728–1732.

Stuermer, C. A. (1988). Retinotopic organization of the developing retinotectal projection in the zebrafish embryo. *J. Neurosci.* **8**: 4513–4530.

Stuermer, C. A., and Easter, S. S., Jr. (1984). Rules of order in the retinotectal fascicles of goldfish. *J. Neurosci.* **4**: 1045–1051.

Subramony, P., Raucher, S., Dryer, L., and Dryer, S. E. (1996). Posttranslational regulation of Ca^{2+}-activated K^+ currents by a target-derived factor in developing parasympathetic neurons. *Neuron* **17**: 115–124.

Suga, N. (1989). Principles of auditory information-processing derived from neuroethology. *J. Exp. Biol.* **146**: 277–286.

Sugiyama, J., Bowen, D. C., and Hall, Z. W. (1994). Dystroglycan binds nerve and muscle agrin. *Neuron* **13**: 103–115.

Sullivan, S. A., Moore, K. B., and Moody, S. A. (1999). Early events in frog blastomere fate determination. *In* "Cell Lineage and Determination" (S. A. Moody, Ed.), pp. 297–321. Academic Press, San Diego.

Sulston, J., and Horvitz, H. (1977). Postembryonic cell lineages of the nematode *Caenorhabditis elegans*. *Dev. Biol.* **56**: 110–156.

Sulston, J. E., Schierenberg, E., White, J. G., and Thompson, J. (1983). The embryonic cell lineage of the nematode *Caenorhabditis elegans*. *Dev. Biol.* **100**: 64–119.

Sulston, J., and White, J. (1980). Regulation and cell autonomy during postembryonic development of *Caenorhabditis elegans*. *Dev. Biol.* **78**: 542–576.

Sun, Y.-a., and Poo, M.-m. (1987). Evoked release of acetylcholine from the growing embryonic neuron. *Proc. Natl. Acad. Sci. USA* **84**: 2540–2544.

Super, H., and Soriano, E. (1994). The organization of the embryonic and early postnatal murine hippocampus. II. Development of entorhinal, commissural, and septal connections studied with the lipophilic tracer DiI. *J. Comp. Neurol.* **344**: 101–120.

Sur, M., Humphrey, A. L., and Sherman, S. M. (1982). Monocular deprivation affects X- and Y-cell retinogeniculate terminations in cats. *Nature* **300:** 183–185.

Sur, M., Weller, R. E., and Sherman, S. M. (1984). Development of X- and Y-cell retinogeniculate terminations in kittens. *Nature* **310:** 246–249.

Sutherland, M. L., Delaney, T. A., and Noebels, J. L. (1996). Glutamate transporter mRNA expression in proliferative zones of the developing and adult murine CNS. *J. Neurosci.* **16:** 2191–2207.

Sutter, A., Riopelle, R. J., Harris-Warrick, R. M., and Shooter, E. M. (1979). Nerve growth factor receptors: Characterization of two distinct classes of binding sites on chick embryo sensory ganglia cells. *J. Biol. Chem.* **254:** 5972–5982.

Suzue, T., Kaprielian, Z., and Patterson, P. H. (1990). A monoclonal antibody that defines rostrocaudal gradients in the mammalian nervous system. *Neuron* **5:** 421–431.

Swaab, D. F., and Hofman, M. A. (1988). Sexual differentiation of the human hypothalamus: Ontogeny of the sexually dimorphic nucleus of the preoptic area. *Dev. Brain Res.* **44:** 314–318.

Syková, E. (1992). Ion-sensitive electrodes. *In* "Monitoring Neuronal Activity: A Practical Approach" (J. A. Stamford, Ed.), pp. 261–282. IRL Press, New York.

Syková, E., Jendelová, P., Simonová, Z., and Chvátal, A. (1992). K+ and pH homeostasis in the developing rat spinal chord is impaired by early postnatal X-irradiation. *Brain Res.* **594:** 19–30.

Taghert, P. H., Doe, C. Q., and Goodman, C. S. (1984). Cell determination and regulation during development of neuroblasts and neurones in grasshopper embryo. *Nature* **307:** 163–165.

Takahashi, T., Momiyama, A., Hirai, K., Hishinuma, F., and Akagi, H. (1992). Functional correlation of fetal and adult forms of glycine receptors with developmental changes in inhibitory synaptic receptor channels. *Neuron* **9:** 1155–1161.

Tallal, P., Miller, S. L., Bedi, G., Byma, G., Wang, X., Nagarajan, S. S., Schreiner, C., Jenkins, W. M., and Merzenich, M. M. (1996). Language comprehension in language-learning impaired children improved with acoustically modified speech. *Science* **271:** 81–84.

Tallal, P., and Piercy, M. (1973). Defects of non-verbal auditory perception in children with developmental aphasia. *Nature* **241:** 468–469.

Tan, S. S., Kalloniatis, M., Sturm, K., Tam, P. P., Reese, B. E., and Faulkner-Jones, B. (1998). Separate progenitors for radial and tangential cell dispersion during development of the cerebral neocortex. *Neuron* **21:** 295–304.

Tanabe, Y., and Jessell, T. M. (1996). Diversity and pattern in the developing spinal cord. *Science* **274:** 1115–1123. Erratum (1997). *Science* **276:** 21.

Tanabe, Y., William, C., and Jessell, T. M. (1998). Specification of motor neuron identity by the MNR2 homeodomain protein. *Cell* **95:** 67–80.

Tang, J., Rutishauser, U., and Landmesser, L. (1994). Poly-

sialic acid regulates growth cone behavior during sorting of motor axons in the plexus region. *Neuron* **13:** 405–414.

Taniguchi, M., Yuasa, S., Fujisawa, H., Naruse, I., Saga, S., Mishina, M., and Yagi, T. (1997). Disruption of semaphorin III/D gene causes severe abnormality in peripheral nerve projection. *Neuron* **19:** 519–530.

Tata, J. R. (1966). Requirement for RNA and protein synthesis for induced regression of the tadpole tail in organ culture. *Dev. Biol.* **13:** 77–94.

Tear, G., Seeger, M., and Goodman, C. S. (1993). To cross or not to cross: A genetic analysis of guidance at the midline. *Perspect. Dev. Neurobiol.* **1:** 183–194.

Tepper, J. M., and Trent, F. (1993). *In vivo* studies of the postnatal development of rat neostriatum neurons. *Prog. Brain Res.* **99:** 35–50.

Thigpen, A. E., Davis, D. L., Gautier, T., Imperato-McGinley, J., and Russell, D. W. (1992). The molecular basis of steroid 5 α-reductase deficiency in a large Dominican kindred. *New England J. Med.* **327:** 1216–1219.

Thomas, K. R., and Capecchi, M. R. (1986). Targeting of genes to specific sites in the mammalian genome. *Cold Spring Harbor Symp. Quant. Biol.* **51:** 1101.

Thompson, W., Kuffler, D. P., and Jansen, J. K. S. (1979). The effect of prolonged, reversible block of nerve impulses on the elimination of polyneuronal innervation of newborn rat skeletal muscle fibers. *Neuroscience* **4:** 271–281.

Timney, B. (1981). Development of binocular depth perception in kittens. *Invest. Ophthalmol. Visual Sci.* **21:** 493–496.

Tinbergen, N. (1948). Social releasers and the experimental method required for their study. *Wilson Bull.* **60:** 6–51.

Tobias, M. L., Viswanathan, S. S., and Kelley, D. B. (1998). Rapping, a female receptive call, initiates male–female duets in the South African clawed frog. *Proc. Natl. Acad. Sci. USA* **95:** 1870–1875.

Tomaselli, K. J., Reichardt, L. F., and Bixby, J. L. (1986). Distinct molecular interactions mediate neuronal process outgrowth on non-neuronal cell surfaces and extracellular matrices. *J. Cell Biol.* **103:** 2659–2672.

Tomasiewicz, H., Ono, K., Yee, D., Thompson, C., Goridis, C., Rutishauser, U., and Magnuson, T. (1993). Genetic deletion of a neural cell adhesion molecule variant (N-CAM-180) produces distinct defects in the central nervous system. *Neuron* **11:** 1163–1174.

Toran-Allerand, C. D. (1980). Sex steroids and the development of the newborn mouse hypothalamus and preoptic area *in vitro*. II. Morphological correlates and hormonal specificity. *Brain Res.* **189:** 413–427.

Toran-Allerand, C. D., Hashimoto, K., Greenough, W. T., and Saltarelli, M. (1983). Sex steroids and the development of the newborn mouse hypothalamus and preoptic area *in vitro*: III. Effects of estrogen on dendritic differentiation. *Brain Res.* **283:** 97–101.

Tosney, K. W., and Landmesser, L. T. (1985). Growth cone morphology and trajectory in the lumbosacral region of the chick embryo. *J. Neurosci.* **5:** 2345–2358.

Trisler, D. (1990). Cell recognition and pattern formation in the developing nervous system. *J. Exp. Biol.* **153:** 11–27.

Trowe, T., Klostermann, S., Baier, H., Granato, M., Crawford, A. D., Grunewald, B., Hoffmann, H., Karlstrom, R. O., Meyer, S. U., Muller, B., Richter, S., Nusslein-Volhard, C., and Bonhoeffer, F. (1996). Mutations disrupting the ordering and topographic mapping of axons in the retinotectal projection of the zebrafish, *Danio rerio*. *Development* **123:** 439–450.

Troy, C. M., Stefanis, L., Greene, L. A., and Shelanski, M. L. (1997). Nedd2 is required for apoptosis after trophic factor withdrawal, but not superoxide dismutase (SOD1) downregulation, in sympathetic neurons and PC12 cells. *J. Neurosci.* **17:** 1911–1918.

Truman, J. W. (1992). Developmental neuroethology of insect metamorphosis. *J. Neurobiol.* **23:** 1404–1422.

Truman, J. W. (1983). Programmed cell death in the nervous system of an adult insect. *J. Comp. Neurol.* **16:** 445–452.

Truman, J. W., and Schwartz, L. M. (1984). Steroid regulation of neuronal death in the moth nervous system. *J. Neurosci.* **4:** 274–280.

Tsim, K. W., Ruegg, M. A., Escher, G., Kröger, S., and McMahan, U. J. (1992). cDNA that encodes active agrin. *Neuron* **8:** 677–689.

Tsuchida, T., Ensini, M., Morton, S. B., Baldassare, M., Edlund, T., Jessell, T. M., and Pfaff, S. L. (1994). Topographic organization of embryonic motor neurons defined by expression of LIM homeobox genes [see Comments]. *Cell* **79:** 957–970.

Turner, A. M., and Greenough, W. T. (1985). Differential rearing effects on rat visual cortex synapses. I. Synaptic and neuronal density and synapses per neuron. *Brain Res.* **329:** 195–203.

Turner, D. L., and Cepko, C. L. (1987). A common progenitor for neurons and glia persists in rat retina late in development. *Nature* **328:** 131–136.

Turner, D. L., and Weintraub, H. (1993). Expression of achaete–scute homolog 3 in *Xenopus* embryos converts ectodermal cells to a neural fate. *Genes Dev.* **8:** 1434–1447.

Turner, J. E., Barde, Y. A., Schwab, M. E., and Thoenen, H. (1982). Extract from brain stimulates neurite outgrowth from fetal rat retinal explants. *Brain Res.* **282:** 77–83.

Udin, S. B., and Keating, M. J. (1981). Plasticity in a central nervous pathway in *Xenopus*: Anatomical changes in the isthmotectal projection after larval eye rotation. *J. Comp. Neurol.* **203:** 575–594.

Uriel, J., Bouillon, D., Aussel, C., and Dupiers, M. (1976). α-Fetoprotein: The major high-affinity estrogen binder in rat uterine cytosols. *Proc. Natl. Acad. Sci. USA* **73:** 1452–1456.

Usdin, T. B., and Fischbach, G. D. (1986). Purification and characterization of a polypeptide from chick brain that promotes the accumulation of acetylcholine receptors in chick myotubes. *J. Cell Biol.* **103:** 493–507.

Valenzuela, D. M., Stitt, T. N., DiStefano, P. S., Rojas, E., Mattsson, K., Compton, D. L., Nuñez, L., Park, J. S., Stark, J. L., Gies, D. R., Thomas, S., Le Beau, M. M., Fernald, A. A., Copeland, N. G., Jenkins, N. A., Burden, S. J., Glass, D. J., and Yancopoulos, G. D. (1995). Receptor tyrosine kinase specific for the skeletal muscle lineage: Expression in embryonic muscle, at the neuromuscular junction, and after injury. *Neuron* **15:** 573–584.

Valverde, F. (1968). Structural changes in the area striata of the mouse after enucleation. *Exp. Brain Res.* **5:** 274–292.

Van der Loos, H., Dorfl, J., and Welker, E. (1984). Variation in pattern of mystacial vibrissae in mice. A quantitative study of ICR stock and several inbred strains. *J. Hered.* **75:** 326–336.

Van der Loos, H., and Woolsey, T. A. (1973). Somatosensory cortex: Alterations following early injury to sense organs. *Science* **179:** 395–398.

Van der Meer, A. L., Van der Weel, F. R., and Lee, D. N. (1995). The functional significance of arm movements in neonates. *Science* **267:** 693–695.

Van der Zee, C. E., Ross, G. M., Riopelle, R. J., and Hagg, T. (1996). Survival of cholinergic forebrain neurons in developing p75NGFR-deficient mice. *Science* **274:** 1729–1732.

Vassar, R., Chao, S. K., Sitcheran, R., Nunez, J. M., Vosshall, L. B., and Axel, R. (1994). Topographic organization of sensory projections to the olfactory bulb. *Cell* **79:** 981–991.

Vaughn, J. E. (1989). Review: Fine structure of synaptogenesis in the vertebrate central nervous system. *Synapse* **3:** 255–285.

Vaughn, J. E., Barber, R. P., and Sims, T. J. (1988). Dendritic development and preferential growth into synaptogenic fields: A quantitative study of golgi-impregnated spinal motor neurons. *Synapse* **2:** 69–78.

Vaughn, J. E., Henrikson, C. K., and Grieshaber, J. A. (1974). A quantitative study of synapses on motor neuron dendritic growth cones in developing mouse spinal cord. *J. Cell Biol.* **60:** 664–672.

Vervoort, M., Dambly-Chaudiere, C., and Ghysen, A. (1997). Cell fate determination in *Drosophila*. *Curr. Opin. Neurobiol.* **7:** 21–28.

Vicini, S., and Schuetze, S. M. (1985). Gating properties of acetylcholine channels at developing rat endplates. *J. Neurosci.* **5:** 2212–2224.

Vince, M. A. (1979). Effects of accelerating stimulation on different indices of development in Japanese quail embryos. *J. Exp. Zool.* **208:** 201–212.

Vince, M. A., and Salter, S. H. (1967). Respiration and clicking in quail embryos. *Nature* **216:** 582–583.

Vogel, M. W., and Prittie, J. (1995). Purkinje cell dendritic arbors in chick embryos following chronic treatment with an *N*-methyl-D-aspartate receptor antagonist. *J. Neurobiol.* **26:** 537–552.

Vogt, W. (1925). Gestaltungsanalyse am Amphibienkeim mit ortlicher Vitalfarbung I. Methodik und Wirkungsweise der ortlichen Vitalfarbung mit Agar als Farbtrager. *Arch Entw. Mech. organ* **106:** 542–610.

von Bartheld, C. S., Byers, M. R., Williams, R., and Bothwell, M. (1996). Anterograde transport of neurotrophins and axodendritic transfer in the developing visual system. *Nature* **379:** 830–833.

von Bernhardi, R., and Muller, K. J. (1995). Repair of the central nervous system: Lessons from lesions in leeches. *J. Neurobiol.* **27:** 353–366.

Voyvodic, J. T. (1989). Peripheral target regulation of dendritic geometry in the rat superior cervical ganglion. *J. Neurosci.* **9:** 1997–2010.

Wade, J., and Arnold, A. P. (1996). Functional testicular tissue does not masculinize development of the zebra finch song system. *Proc. Natl. Acad. Sci. USA* **93:** 5264–5268.

Waid, D. K., and McLoon, S. C. (1998). Ganglion cells influence the fate of dividing retinal cells in culture. *Development* **125:** 1059–1066.

Walk, R. D., and Gibson, E. J. (1961). A comparative and analytical study of visual depth perception. *Psychol. Monogr.* **75:** 1–44.

Wallace, B. G. (1994). Staurosporine inhibits agrin-induced acetylcholine receptor phosphorylation and aggregation. *J. Cell Biol.* **125:** 661–668.

Wallace, B. G. (1995). Regulation of the interaction of nicotinic acetylcholine receptors with the cytoskeleton by agrin-activated protein tyrosine kinase. *J. Cell Biol.* **128:** 1121–1129.

Wallace, B. G., Qu, Z., and Huganir, R. L. (1991). Agrin induces phosphorylation of the nicotinic acetylcholine receptor. *Neuron* **6:** 869–878.

Wallace, M. T., and Stein, B. E. (1997). Development of multisensory neurons and multisensory integration in cat superior colliculus. *J. Neurosci.* **17:** 2429–2444.

Walsh, F. S., and Doherty, P. (1997). Neural cell adhesion molecules of the immunoglobulin superfamily: Role in axon growth and guidance. *Annu. Rev. Cell Dev. Biol.* **13:** 425–456.

Walter, J., Henke-Fahle, S., and Bonhoeffer, F. (1987a). Avoidance of posterior tectal membranes by temporal retinal axons. *Development* **101:** 909–913.

Walter, J., Kern-Veits, B., Huf, J., Stolze, B., and Bonhoeffer, F. (1987b). Recognition of position-specific properties of tectal cell membranes by retinal axons *in vitro*. *Development* **101:** 685–696.

Walter, J., Muller, B., and Bonhoeffer, F. (1990). Axonal guidance by an avoidance mechanism. *J. Physiol.* **84:** 104–110.

Wang, F., Nemes, A., Mendelsohn, M., and Axel, R. (1998). Odorant receptors govern the formation of a precise topographic map. *Cell* **93:** 47–60.

Wang, H. U., and Anderson, D. J. (1997). Eph family transmembrane ligands can mediate repulsive guidance of trunk neural crest migration and motor axon outgrowth. *Neuron* **18:** 383–396.

Wang, J., Renger, J. J., Griffith, L. C., Greenspan, R. J., and Wu, C. F. (1994). Concomitant alterations of physiological and developmental plasticity in *Drosophila* CaM kinase II-inhibited synapses. *Neuron* **13:** 1373–1384.

Wang, T., Xie, K., and Lu, B. (1995). Neurotrophins promote maturation of developing neuromuscular synapses. *J. Neurosci.* **15:** 4796–4805.

Warren, R. A., and Jones, E. G. (1997). Maturation of neuronal form and function in a mouse thalamo-cortical circuit. *J. Neurosci.* **17:** 277–295.

Watanabe, T., and Raff, M. C. (1990). Rod photoreceptor development *in vitro*: Intrinsic properties of proliferating neuroepithelial cells change as development proceeds in the rat retina. *Neuron* **4:** 461–467.

Watkins, D. W., Wilson, J. R., and Sherman, S. M. (1978). Receptive-field properties of neurons in binocular and monocular segments of striate cortex in cats raised with binocular lid suture. *J. Neurophysiol.* **1:** 322–337.

Watson, J. B., and Raynor, R. (1920). Conditioned emotional reactions. *J. Exp. Psychol.* **3:** 1–14.

Watson, J. T., Robertson, J., Sachdev, U., and Kelley, D. B. (1993). Laryngeal muscle and motor neuron plasticity in *Xenopus laevis*: Testicular masculinization of a developing neuromuscular system. *J. Neurobiol.* **24:** 1615–1625.

Wechsler-Reya, R. J., and Scott, M. P. (1999). Control of neuronal precursor proliferation in the cerebellum by Sonic Hedgehog. *Neuron* **22:** 103–114.

Weinberg, C. B., and Hall, Z. W. (1979). Antibodies from patients with myasthenia gravis recognize determinants unique to extrajunctional acetylcholine receptors. *Proc. Natl. Acad. Sci. USA* **76:** 504–508.

Weintraub, H. (1993). The MyoD family and myogenesis: Redundancy, networks, and thresholds. *Cell* **75:** 1241–1244.

Werner, L. A., and Gray, L. (1998). Behavioral studies of hearing development. *In* "Development of the Auditory System" (E. W. Rubel, A. N. Popper, and R. R. Fay, Eds.), pp. 12–79. Springer–Verlag, New York.

Werner, L. A., and Marean, G. C. (1996). "Human Auditory Development." Westview, Boulder, CO.

Werner, L. A., Marean, G. C., Halpin, C. F., Spetner, N. B., and Gillenwater, J. M. (1992). Infant auditory temporal acuity: Gap detection. *Child Dev.* **63:** 260–272.

Wessells, N. K., and Nuttall, R. P. (1978). Normal branching, induced branching, and steering of cultured parasympathetic motor neurons. *Exp. Cell Res.* **115:** 111–122.

Westerfield, M., Liu, D. W., Kimmel, C. B., and Walker, C. (1990). Pathfinding and synapse formation in a zebrafish mutant lacking functional acetylcholine receptors. *Neuron* **4:** 867–874.

Westrum, L. E. (1975). Electron microscopy of synaptic structures in olfactory cortex of early postnatal rats. *J. Neurocytol.* **4:** 713–732.

White, F. A., Keller-Peck, C. R., Knudson, C. M., Korsmeyer, S. J., and Snider, W. D. (1998). Widespread elimination of naturally occurring neuronal death in Bax-deficient mice. *J. Neurosci.* **18:** 1428–1439.

White, K., Tahaoglu, E., and Steller, H. (1996). Cell killing by the *Drosophila* gene reaper. *Science* **271:** 805–807.

Wictorin, K., Brundin, P., Gustavii, B., Lindvall, O., and Bjorklund, A. (1990). Reformation of long axon pathways in adult rat central nervous system by human fore-brain neuroblasts. *Nature* **347:** 556–558.

Wiener-Vacher, S. R., Toupet, F., and Narcy, P. (1996). Canal and otolith vestibulo-ocular reflexes to vertical and off vertical axis rotations in children learning to walk. *Acta Oto-Laryngol.* **116:** 657–665.

Wiesel, T. N., and Hubel, D. H. (1962). Receptive fields, binocular interaction and functonal architecture in the cat's visual cortex. *J. Physiol.* **160:** 106–154.

Wiesel, T. N., and Hubel, D. H. (1963a). Single-cell responses in striate cortex of kittens deprived of vision in one eye. *J. Neurophysiol.* **26:** 1003–1017.

Wiesel, T. N., and Hubel, D. H. (1963b). Effects of visual deprivation on morphology and physiology of cells in the cat's lateral geniculate body. *J. Neurophysiol.* **26:** 978–993.

Wiesel, T. N., and Hubel, D. H. (1965). Comparison of the effects of unilateral and bilateral eye closure on cortical unit responses in kittens. *J. Neurophysiol.* **28:** 1029–1040.

Wigston, D. J., and Sanes, J. R. (1985). Selective reinnervation of intercostal muscles transplanted from different segmental levels to a common site. *J. Neurosci.* **5:** 1208–1221.

Williams, B. P., Park, J. K., Alberta, J. A., Muhlebach, S. G., Hwang, G. Y., Roberts, T. M., and Stiles, C. D. (1997). A PDGF-regulated immediate early gene response initiates neuronal differentiation in ventricular zone progenitor cells. *Neuron* **18:** 553–562.

Williams, J. R., Sharp, J. W., Kumari, V. G., Wilson, M., and Payne, J. A. (1999). The neuron-specific K-Cl cotransporter, KCC2—Antibody development and initial characterization of the protein. *J. Biol. Chem.* **274:** 12,656–12,664.

Williamson, T., Gordon-Weeks, P. R., Schachner, M., and Taylor, J. (1996). Microtubule reorganization is obligatory for growth cone turning. *Proc. Natl. Acad. Sci. USA* **93:** 15,221–15,226.

Wilson, D. M. (1968). The flight-control system of the locust. *Sci. Am.* **218:** 83–90.

Wilson, P. A., and Hemmati-Brivanlou, A. (1995). Induction of epidermis and inhibition of neural fate by Bmp-4. *Nature* **376:** 331–333.

Wilson, S. W., Brennan, C., Macdonald, R., Brand, M., and Holder, N. (1997). Analysis of axon tract formation in the zebrafish brain: The role of territories of gene expression and their boundaries. *Cell Tissue Res.* **290:** 189–196.

Wilson, S. W., Ross, L. S., Parrett, T., and Easter, S. S., Jr. (1990). The development of a simple scaffold of axon tracts in the brain of the embryonic zebrafish, *Brachydanio rerio. Development* **108:** 121–145.

Winberg, M. L., Mitchell, K. J., and Goodman, C. S. (1998). Genetic analysis of the mechanisms controlling target selection: Complementary and combinatorial functions of netrins, semaphorins, and IgCAMs. *Cell* **93:** 581–591.

Withington-Wray, D. J., Binns, K. E., and Keating, M. J. (1990). The developmental emergence of a map of auditory space in the superior colliculus of the guinea pig. *Dev. Brain Res.* **51:** 225–236.

Wolitzky, B. A., and Fambrough, D. M. (1986). Regulation of the $(Na^+ + K^+)$-ATPase in cultured chick skeletal muscle. Modulation of expression by the demand for ion transport. *J. Biol. Chem.* **261:** 9990–9999.

Woods, D. F., and Bryant, P. J. (1991). The discs-large tumor suppressor gene of *Drosophila* encodes a guanylate kinase homolog localized at septate junctions. *Cell* **66:** 451–464.

Woolsey, T. A., and Van der Loos, H. (1970). The structural organization of layer IV in the somatosensory region (SI) of mouse cerebral cortex. The description of a cortical field composed of discrete cytoarchitectonic units. *Brain Res.* **17:** 205–242.

Wright, L. L., and Smolen, A. J. (1987). The role of neuron death in the development of the gender difference in the number of neurons in the rat superior cervical ganglion. *Int. J. Dev. Neurosci.* **5:** 305–311.

Wu, G.-Y., and Cline, H. T. (1998). Stabilization of dendritic arbor structure *in vivo* by CaMKII. *Science* **279:** 222–226.

Wu, G.-Y., Malinow, R., and Cline, H. T. (1996). Maturation of central glutamatergic synapse. *Science* **274:** 972–976.

Wurst, W., Auerbach, A. B., *et al.* (1994). Multiple developmental defects in Engrailed-1 mutant mice: An early mid-hindbrain deletion and patterning defects in forelimbs and sternum. *Development* **120:** 2065–2075.

Xia, Z., Dickens, M., Raingeaud, J., Davis, R. J., and Greenberg, M. E. (1995). Opposing effects of ERK and JNK-p38 MAP kinases on apoptosis. *Science* **270:** 1326–1331.

Xie, Z.-p., and Poo, M.-m. (1986). Initial events in the formation of neuromuscular synapse: Rapid induction of acetylcholine release from embryonic neuron. *Proc. Natl. Acad. Sci. USA* **83:** 7069–7073.

Yaari, Y., Hamon, B., and Lux, H. D. (1987). Development of two types of calcium channels in cultured mammalian hippocampal neurons. *Science* **235:** 680–682.

Yang, X., Hyder, F., and Shulman, R. G. (1996). Activation of single whisker barrel in rat brain localized by functional magnetic resonance imaging. *Proc. Natl. Acad. Sci. USA* **93:** 475–478.

Yin, J. C., Del Vecchio, M., Zhou, H., and Tully, T. (1995). CREB as a memory modulator: Induced expression of a dCREB2 activator isoform enhances long-term memory in *Drosophila. Cell* **7:** 107–15.

Yin, J. C., Wallach, J. S., Del Vecchio, M., Wilder, E. L., Zhou, H., Quinn, W. G., and Tully, T. (1994). Induction of a dominant negative CREB transgene specifically blocks long-term memory in *Drosophila. Cell* **7:** 49–58.

Yool, A. J., Dionne, V. E., and Gruol, D. L. (1988). Developmental changes in K^+-selective channel activity during differentiation of the Purkinje neuron in culture. *J. Neurosci.* **8:** 1971–1980.

Yoon, M. G. (1975). Readjustment of retinotectal projection following reimplantation of a rotated or inverted tectal tissue in adult goldfish. *J. Physiol. (London)* **252:** 137–158.

Yoshihara, Y., and Mori, K. (1997). Basic principles and molecular mechanisms of olfactory axon pathfinding. *Cell Tissue Res.* **290:** 457–463.

Young, S. H., and Poo, M.-m. (1983). Spontaneous release of transmitter from growth cones of embryonic neurones. *Nature* **305:** 634–637.

Young, S. R., and Rubel, E. W. (1986). Embryogenesis of arborization pattern and topography of individual axons in n. laminaris of the chicken brain stem. *J. Comp. Neurol.* **254:** 425–459.

Yuan, J. Y., and Horvitz, H. R. (1990). The *Caenorhabditis elegans* genes ced-3 and ced-4 act cell autonomously to cause programmed cell death. *Dev. Biol.* **138:** 33–41.

Yuasa, J., Hirano, S., Yamagata, M., and Noda, M. (1996). Visual projection map specified by topographic expression of transcription factors in the retina. *Nature* **382:** 632–635.

Yuodelis, C., and Hendrickson, A. (1986). A qualitative and quantitative analysis of the human fovea during development. *Vision Res.* **26;** 847–855.

Zafra, F., Castrén, E., Thoenen, H., and Lindholm, D. (1991). Interplay between glutamate and γ-aminobutyric acid transmitter systems in the physiological regulation of brain-derived neurotrophic factor and nerve growth factor synthesis in hippocampal neurons. *Proc. Natl. Acad. Sci. USA* **88:** 10,037–10,041.

Zhang, L., Spigelman, I., and Carlen, P. L. (1991). Development of GABA-mediated, chloride-dependent inhibition in CA1 pyramidal neurones of immature rat hippocampal slices. *J. Physiol.* **444:** 25–49.

Zhang, L. I., Tao, H. W., Holt, C. E., Harris, W. A., and Poo, M.-m. (1998). A critical window for cooperation and competition among developing retinotectal synapses. *Nature* **395:** 37–44.

Zheng, C., Heintz, N., and Hatten, M. E. (1996). CNS gene encoding astrotactin which supports neuronal migration along glial fibers. *Science* **272:** 417–419.

Zheng, J. Q., Felder, M., Connor, J. A., and Poo, M.-m. (1994). Turning of nerve growth cones induced by neurotransmitters. *Nature* **368:** 140–144.

Zhong, Y., and Wu, C.-F. (1991). Altered synaptic plasticity in *Drosophila* memory mutants with a defective cyclic AMP cascade. *Science* **251:** 198–201.

Zippelius, H. (1972). Die Karawanenbildung bei Feld - und Hausspitzmaus. *Z. Tierpsychol.* **30:** 305–320.

Zipursky, S. L., and Rubin, G. M. (1994). Determination of neuronal cell fate: Lessons from the R7 neuron of *Drosophila. Annu. Rev. Neurosci.* **17:** 373–397.

Zirpel, L., and Rubel, E. W. (1996). Eighth nerve activity regulates intracellular calcium concentration of avian cochlear nucleus neurons via a metabotropic glutamate receptor. *J. Neurophysiol.* **76:** 4127–4139.

Ziskind-Conhaim, L., Geffen, I., and Hall, Z. W. (1984). Redistribution of acetylcholine receptors on developing rat myotybes. *J. Neurosci.* **4:** 2346–2349.

Zoran, M. J., Funte, L. R., Kater, S. B., and Haydon, P. G. (1993). Contact with a synaptic target causes an elevation in a presynaptic neurons's resting calcium set-point. *Dev. Biol.* **158:** 163–171.

Zou, D.-J., and Cline, H. T. (1996). Expression of constitutively active CaMKII in target tissue modifies presynaptic axon arbor growth. *Neuron* **16:** 529–539.

INDEX